Cardiac Imaging Update 2017

Cardiac Imaging Update 2017

Editors

GN Mahapatra
Senior Consultant and Head
Department of Nuclear Medicine
PET-CT, SPECT-CT
SevenHills Hospital
Mumbai, Maharashtra, India
Executive President, WCCICC–2017

PC Manoria
Director
Manoria Heart and Critical Care Hospital
Bhopal, Madhya Pradesh, India

Diwakar Jain
Professor of Medicine
Director of Nuclear Cardiology
New York Medical College
Westchester Medical Center
Valhalla, New York, USA

Forewords
Daniel S Berman, Jagat Narula

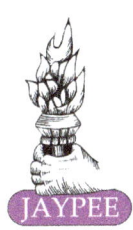

The Health Sciences Publisher
New Delhi | London | Panama

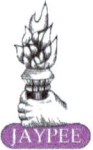 **Jaypee Brothers Medical Publishers (P) Ltd.**

Headquarters
Jaypee Brothers Medical Publishers (P) Ltd.
4838/24, Ansari Road, Daryaganj
New Delhi 110 002, India
Phone: +91-11-43574357
Fax: +91-11-43574314
E-mail: jaypee@jaypeebrothers.com

Overseas Offices

J.P. Medical Ltd.
83, Victoria Street, London
SW1H 0HW (UK)
Phone: +44-20 3170 8910
Fax: +44(0) 20 3008 6180
E-mail: info@jpmedpub.com

Jaypee-Highlights Medical Publishers Inc.
City of Knowledge, Bld 235, 2nd Floor
Clayton, Panama City, Panama
Phone: +1 507-301-0496
Fax: +1 507-301-0499
E-mail: cservice@jphmedical.com

Jaypee Brothers Medical Publishers (P) Ltd.
17/1-B, Babar Road, Block-B
Shaymali, Mohammadpur
Dhaka-1207, Bangladesh
Mobile: +08801912003485
E-mail: jaypeedhaka@gmail.com

Jaypee Brothers Medical Publishers (P) Ltd.
Bhotahity, Kathmandu, Nepal
Phone: +977-9741283608
E-mail: kathmandu@jaypeebrothers.com

Website: www.jaypeebrothers.com
Website: www.jaypeedigital.com

© 2017, Jaypee Brothers Medical Publishers

The views and opinions expressed in this book are solely those of the original contributor(s)/author(s) and do not necessarily represent those of editor(s) of the book.

All rights reserved. No part of this publication may be reproduced, stored or transmitted in any form or by any means, electronic, mechanical, photocopying, recording or otherwise, without the prior permission in writing of the publishers.

All brand names and product names used in this book are trade names, service marks, trademarks or registered trademarks of their respective owners. The publisher is not associated with any product or vendor mentioned in this book.

Medical knowledge and practice change constantly. This book is designed to provide accurate, authoritative information about the subject matter in question. However, readers are advised to check the most current information available on procedures included and check information from the manufacturer of each product to be administered, to verify the recommended dose, formula, method and duration of administration, adverse effects and contraindications. It is the responsibility of the practitioner to take all appropriate safety precautions. Neither the publisher nor the author(s)/editor(s) assume any liability for any injury and/or damage to persons or property arising from or related to use of material in this book.

This book is sold on the understanding that the publisher is not engaged in providing professional medical services. If such advice or services are required, the services of a competent medical professional should be sought.

Every effort has been made where necessary to contact holders of copyright to obtain permission to reproduce copyright material. If any have been inadvertently overlooked, the publisher will be pleased to make the necessary arrangements at the first opportunity.

Inquiries for bulk sales may be solicited at: jaypee@jaypeebrothers.com

Cardiac Imaging Update 2017

First Edition: 2017

ISBN: 978-93-86322-93-7

Contributors

Aamish Kazi
Junior Consultant
Picture This by Jankharia
Mumbai, Maharashtra, India

Abhiram GA
Department of Nuclear
Medicine
PGIMER, Chandigarh, India

AK Pancholia
Head
Department of Medicine,
Clinical and Preventive Cardiology
Arihant Hospital and Research Center
Indore, Madhya Pradesh, India

Anirban Mukherjee
Department of Nuclear Medicine
Eastern Diagnostics
Kolkata, West Bengal, India.

Anitha G
Arrhythmia—Heart Failure Academy
Department of Cardiac Electrophysiology
and Pacing
The Madras Medical Mission
Chennai, Tamil Nadu, India

Asha Moorthy
Lead Consultant
CG Heart Institute
Super-Speciality Hospitals
Chennai, Tamil Nadu, India

Ashwani Sood
Associate Professor
Department of Nuclear Medicine
PGIMER, Chandigarh, India

Bhavin Jankharia
Consultant Radiologist
Picture This by Jankharia
Mumbai, Maharashtra, India

BK Das
Director and Chief
Department of Nuclear Medicine
Utkal Institute of Medial Sciences
Bhubaneswar, Odisha, India

BR Mittal
Professor and Head
Department of Nuclear Medicine
PGIMER, Chandigarh, India

Chetan D Patel
Professor
Department of Nuclear Medicine
All India Institute of Medical Sciences
New Delhi, India

Debabrata Dash
Senior Interventional Cardiologist
Thumbay Hospital
Al Nuaimiyah, Ajman, UAE

Diwakar Jain
Professor of Medicine
Director of Nuclear Cardiology
New York Medical College
Westchester Medical Center
Valhalla, New York, USA

Eike Nagel
Head
Department of Interdisciplinary
Cardiovascular Imaging
DZHK Center for Cardiovascular Imaging
University Hospital Frankfurt
Frankfurt, Germany

Gawri Sankar
Senior Resident
Sanjay Gandhi Postgraduate Institute
of Medical Sciences
Lucknow, Uttar Pradesh, India

GN Mahapatra
Senior Consultant and Head
Department of Nuclear Medicine
PET-CT, SPECT-CT SevenHills Hospital
Mumbai, Maharashtra, India
Executive President, WCCICC–2017

HK Chopra
Chief Consultant Cardiologist
Moolchand Medcity
New Delhi, India

IB Vijayalakshmi
Professor
Department of Cardiology
PSSMY Super-Speciality Hospital
Victoria Hospital Complex
Bangalore Medical College and
Research Institute
Bengaluru, Karnataka, India

Jagat Narula
Professor
Department of Medicine and Radiology
Icahn School of Medicine at Mount Sinai
Mount Sinai, New York, USA

Jain T Kallarakkal
Interventional Cardiologist
St Mary's Hospital
Thodupuzha, Kerala, India

Jamshid Maddahi
Director
UCLA School of Medicine
Los Angeles, California, USA

Johann Christopher
Consultant Cardiologist
Director of Imaging
Care Hospital
Hyderabad, Telangana, India

Meera Venkatesh
IAEA, Vienna, Austria

MS Hiremath
Director
Cardiac Cath Lab
Ruby Hall Clinic
Pune, Maharashtra, India

Mudalsha Ravina
Senior Resident
Sanjay Gandhi Postgraduate Institute
of Medical Sciences
Lucknow, Uttar Pradesh, India

Mythri Shankar
Senior Consultant
Department of Nuclear Medicine
Cytecare Cancer Hospitals
Bengaluru, Karnataka, India

N Ramamoorthy
Former Head
Radiopharmaceutical Division
BARC-DAE
Mumbai, Maharashtra, India

Navin C Nanda
Professor
Department of Medicine
Director
Heart Station/Echocardiography
Laboratories
Birmingham, Alabama, USA

Neel Bhatia
Associate Consultant
Department of Noninvasive Cardiology
BLK Super-Speciality Hospital
Delhi, India

Nitin Yadav
Junior Resident
Sanjay Gandhi Postgraduate Institute
of Medical Sciences
Lucknow, Uttar Pradesh, India

Om Tavri
Consultant Radiologist
Asian Heart Institute
Mumbai, Maharashtra, India

Oma Shankar
Chief Technologist and RSO
Department of Nuclear Medicine
Utkal Institute of Medical Sciences
Bhubaneswar, Odisha, India

Padmakar V Kulkarni
Department of Radiology
The University of Texas Southwestern
Medical Center
Dallas, Texas, USA

Pankaj Manoria
Chief Interventional Cardiologist
Manoria Heart and Critical Care Hospital
Bhopal, Madhya Pradesh, India

Parang Sanghavi
Junior Consultant, Picture This by Jankharia
Mumbai, Maharashtra, India

PC Manoria
Director
Manoria Heart and Critical Care Hospital
Bhopal, Madhya Pradesh, India

Peeyush Jain
Head
Department of Preventive and
Rehabilitative Cardiology
Fortis Escorts Heart Institute
New Delhi, India

Piyush Manoria
Sr Resident
Department of Gastroenterology
Sri Aurobindo Institute of Medical Sciences
Indore, Madhya Pradesh, India

Prasanta Kumar Pradhan
Professor
Department of Nuclear Medicine
Sanjay Gandhi Postgraduate Institute
of Medical Sciences
Lucknow, Uttar Pradesh, India

Priya Chudgar
Consultant Radiologist
Asian Heart Institute
Mumbai, Maharashtra, India

René RS Packard
Department of Medicine (Cardiology) and
Department of Molecular and Medical
Pharmacology (Nuclear Medicine)
UCLA School of Medicine
Los Angeles, California, USA

Sameer Shrivastava
Director
Noninvasive Cardiology
Fortis Escorts Heart Institute
New Delhi, India

Sanjay Gambhir
Head
Department of Nuclear Medicine
Sanjay Gandhi Postgraduate Institute
of Medical Sciences
Lucknow, Uttar Pradesh, India

Satoshi Nakatani
Consultant Cardiologist
Division of Functional Diagnostics
Department of Health Sciences
Osaka University Graduate School
of Medicine
Yamadaoka Suita
Osaka, Japan

Shrikant Solav
Consultant
Department of Nuclear Medicine
SPECT Lab
Pune, Maharashtra, India

SK Parashar
Superintendent
SKS Medical College
Bhopal, Madhya Pradesh, India

Sudatta Ray
Consultant
Department of Nuclear Medicine
Utkal Institute of Medical Sciences
Bhubaneswar, Odisha, India

Tommaso D' Angelo
Section of Radiological Sciences
Department of Biomedical Sciences and
Morphological and Functional Imaging
University Hospital
Messina, Italy

Ulhas M Pandurangi
Head Arrhythmia-Heart Failure Academy
Department of Cardiac Electrophysiology
and Pacing
The Madras Medical Mission
Chennai, Tamil Nadu, India

Viney Jetley
Associate Director
Department of Cardiology
Senior Interventional Cardiologist
Fortis Escorts Heart Institute
New Delhi, India

Foreword

Over the past several decades, the field of cardiac imaging has developed at a remarkable rate. Powerful noninvasive tools for the diagnosis and management of patients with cardiovascular disease have come up. Noninvasive imaging of the heart has become a central component in the evaluation of nearly all cardiac patients. It is important for a practicing physician, using these methods, to be knowledgeable regarding the fundamentals, strengths and weaknesses of the methods, as well as of the evidences supporting their clinical use. In this book *Cardiac Imaging Update 2017*, GN Mahapatra has enlisted experts in all of the imaging fields as well as in specific clinical cardiology fields of the current interest, to write the chapters that cover the full range of clinical cardiac imaging and its applications, and the current topics in clinical cardiology, focusing on how the information derived can be used in clinical decision-making and patient management.

Section 1—Cardiac Imaging is devoted to noninvasive imaging. For echocardiography, it focuses on the major areas of strength with chapters on endocarditis, aortic stenosis, heart failure, and cardiomyopathy. From the technological standpoint, recent developments in speckle tracking are covered in a separate chapter. A chapter covers the applications of cardiovascular magnetic resonance (CMR), while another discusses the relative roles of CMR and cardiac CT. The book then delves deeply into recent developments on the use of nuclear scanning for assessment of the patients with known or suspected coronary artery disease and myocardial viability. Regarding SPECT and PET, a chapter covers how myocardial perfusion imaging (MPI) with these methods, is applied. Specifically, regarding PET, a chapter deals with rubidium-82 for MPI, which can be performed without the need for a cyclotron at a facility, which is dealing with the added value of quantitative myocardial perfusion reserve with PET MPI tracers. How myocardial viability imaging with PET combined with SPECT—an approach that could be widely available—can be performed even in sites that do not have access to a PET perfusion tracer, by combining the use of F-18 fluorodeoxyglucose (FDG) for metabolism, the standard PET tracer used for assessing cancer, with the standard SPECT agents that are used for MPI. This is followed by a chapter which that on the question as to how myocardial viability imaging applies to clinical practice, an area of controversy given the results of recent multicenter trials. Two chapters explore novel tracers and their evolution. The potential application of assessing cardiac dyssynchrony with nuclear medicine procedures and their possible applications in guiding cardiac resynchronization therapy, is also covered. The book then explores invasive approaches used for assessment of coronary plaque and flow physiology. In *Section 2—Clinical Cardiology*, consideration of several areas of current interest in cardiology outside of imaging, is explored. Overall, clinicians performing cardiac imaging as well as those who utilize these techniques in practice, will find the book very useful to provide a comprehensive update of the status of the clinical applications of the imaging approaches as well as an update of important issues of clinical cardiology.

Daniel S Berman MD FACC
Professor
Department of Medicine
UCLA School of Medicine
Los Angeles
Chief
Department of Cardiac Imaging
and Nuclear Cardiology
Cedars-Sinai Health Institute
Los Angeles, California, USA

Foreword

A compendium of chapters written by the stalwarts in the field of cardiovascular imaging is being released on the eve of the uniquely conceived, one of its kind in India, imaging conference—First World Congress on Cardiac Imaging and Clinical Cardiology-2017 (WCCICC-2017). It is a unique blend of cardiovascular diagnostic and prognostic imaging and the appropriateness of the clinical and procedural management. The content of the Congress and hence the collection of chapters included in this book, strive toward an ecumenical approach to imaging; promoting cooperation between the, now distinct, often competing, and parochially biased, imaging disciplines. This Congress and chapter collection, actively seek to change the thinking from imaging as a destination to imaging as a patient-care enhancer. It serves as a soapbox to encourage the development of an integrated cardiovascular imaging subspecialty.

These are exciting times for cardiovascular imaging. Rapid advances in technology have opened up a bewildering array of clinical applications. Although imaging is one of the major discoveries of the last millennium, and is growing at a rapid pace, there is intense scrutiny of its benefit and extensive controversy over who can best deliver it. The carefully selected chapters have exploited the uniqueness of each imaging modality and identified its strengths to best optimize the clinical care. Dr GN Mahapatra and colleagues are to be congratulated for bringing the best topics of the Congress together, and hope that the readers will be as thrilled as the authors are, and that whatever be your area of interest, this compendium has something for each one of you.

I wish the Congress as well as this collection every success!

Jagat Narula MD PhD MACC
Philip J and Harriet L Goodhart Chair in Cardiology
Professor, Medicine and Radiology, Icahn School of Medicine
Chief of Cardiology, Mount Sinai West and St Luke's Hospitals
Associate Dean, Arnhold Institute for Global Health
Director, Cardiovascular Imaging, Mount Sinai Health System
Mount Sinai, New York, USA
Editor-in-Chief, Journal of the American College of Cardiology—Imaging
Executive Editor, Journal of the American College of Cardiology

Preface

Cardiac Imaging Update 2017 is a unique attempt encompassing an amalgam of cardiac imaging and clinical cardiology. In the era of multiple super-specialties, it is an excellent step for maintaining unity among diversity in the field of medical sciences. This cohesiveness is, indeed, the need of the hour.

In this book, a talented group of experts, who have excelled in their fields, have provided the in-depth information on the topics covered.

The book begins with *Section—1: Cardiac Imaging*, and highlights current concepts of echocardiography, CT, CMR, PET-CT, SPECT, and multimodality imaging, in various cardiovascular diseases. Chapters have also been dedicated to the current interventional imaging techniques such as optical coherence tomography.

Section—2: Clinical Cardiology has chapters on emerging therapies such as PCSK9 inhibitors and DOACs in atrial fibrillation, STEMI, statin intolerance, and sudden cardiac death, etc.

We are sure the book will be of immense value to the postgraduates, physicians and specialists and will find a permanent place on their desk.

GN Mahapatra
PC Manoria
Diwakar Jain

Contents

SECTION 1: Cardiac Imaging

NONINVASIVE

1. **Echocardiographic Evaluation of Infective Endocarditis: The Current Status** — 3
   IB Vijayalakshmi
   - Evaluation of Infective Endocarditis *3*

2. **The Intricacies in Echocardiographic Evaluation of Aortic Stenosis** — 17
   Sameer Shrivastava, Neel Bhatia
   - Main Echocardiographic Indices Used to Assess AS Severity *17* • Aortic Valve Area *19*
   - Dimensionless Velocity Index *19* • Assessing Left Ventricle Contractile and/or Flow Reserve *20* • Distinguishing between True Severe and Pseudosevere Aortic Stenosis *21*

3. **Echocardiography of Heart Failure: How to Use It in Routine Clinical Practice?** — 24
   Satoshi Nakatani
   - How to Assess Systolic Function of the Heart? *24* • How to Assess Diastolic Function of the Heart? *25* • Left Ventricular Geometry and Abnormal Echoes *28*
   - Right Ventricular Function *28* • Intracardiac Pressure Estimation *29*

4. **Speckle Tracking Echocardiography: Basics and Clinical Applications** — 31
   Navin C Nanda
   - Cardiac Muscle Structure *31* • Methods of Speckle Tracking Echocardiography and Parameters Measured *32*

5. **A Gold Standard for Evaluation of Cardiomyopathies** — 43
   Johann Christopher
   - Idiopathic Dilated Cardiomyopathy *43* • Myocarditis *43*
   - Hypertrophic Cardiomyopathy *44* • Restrictive Cardiomyopathy *45*
   - Cardiac Amyloidosis *45* • Arrhythmogenic Right Ventricular Cardiomyopathy *46*
   - Left Ventricular Noncompaction *46* • Myocardial Sarcoidosis *46*
   - Iron Overload Cardiomyopathy *46*

6. **Real World Indications for Cardiac Magnetic Resonance Imaging: When is It Invaluable in Clinical Practice?** — 51
   Tommaso D'Angelo, Eike Nagel
   - Myocarditis *52* • Nonischemic Dilated Cardiomyopathies *53*
   - Hypertrophic Cardiomyopathy *53* • Coronary Artery Disease *54*
   - Viability/Hibernation *55* • Other Indications *55*
   - Contraindications and Limitations *55*

7. **Cardiac MRI and Cardiac CT: Indispensable Tools for the Diagnosis of Coronary Artery Disease** — 57
   Parang Sanghavi, Aamish Kazi, Bhavin Jankharia
   - Cardiac Computed Tomography *57* • Cardiac Magnetic Resonance Imaging *59*

8. **Cardiac Imaging: Current Scenario and Future Directions** — 61
   Om Tavri, Priya Chudgar
   - Computed Tomography Coronary Angiography *61* • Perfusion Imaging *62*
   - Virtual Computed Tomography—Fractional Flow Reserve *63* • Spectral Computed Tomography *63* • Plaque Characterization *63* • Hybrid Imaging *64*
   - Cardiac Magnetic Resonance Imaging *64* • T1 and T2 Mapping *65*

9. **Clinical Decision-making with Myocardial Perfusion Imaging in Patients with Known or Suspected Coronary Artery Disease** — 67
   Mythri Shankar
   - Diabetes Mellitus *68* • Women and Elderly *68* • Chronic Kidney Disease *69*

10. **Current Status of Rubidium-82 PET-CT Myocardial Perfusion Imaging** — 70
    Prasanta Kumar Pradhan, Gowri Sankar
    - Historical Perspective *70* • Characteristics of Sr-82/Rb-82 Generator and Physiology of Rb-82 *70* • Comparison with SPECT Agents *70* • Comparison between Rb-82 and N-13 Ammonia *71* • Dosimetry *71*

11. **Innovation of New Tracers in the Era of Multimodality Cardiac Imaging** — 74
    Padmakar V Kulkarni
    - Myocardial Function *75* • Myocardial Perfusion *75* • Fluorine-18-labeled Agents for Myocardial Perfusion Studies *75* • Energy Metabolism *76*
    - Imaging Atherosclerotic Plaques *76*

12. **Myocardial Imaging Products' Evolution: Change for the Better** — 80
    N Ramamoorthy, Meera Venkatesh
    - Thallium-201 as Myocardial Perfusion Marker *80* • Technetium-99m Compounds as Myocardial Perfusion Markers *81* • Labeled Fatty Acid as Marker for Metabolism: Iodine-123 Products *81* • PET Tracers as Myocardial Perfusion Markers *81*
    - PET Tracers as Marker of Myocardial Viability *82*

13. **Efficacy of Combining FDG-PET Metabolic and Tc-99m–MIBI Myocardial Perfusion Study in Assessment of Myocardial Viability** — 85
    BK Das, Sudatta Ray, Oma Shankar
    - What is Myocardial Viability? *85* • Methods of Assessment of Viability *85*
    - Combination of MPS with MIBI and FDG-PET *86*

14. **Myocardial Viability Assessment: Is it Alive?** — 88
    Shrikant Solav

15. **Hybrid Myocardial Imaging Techniques: Role in Functionally Relevant Coronary Disease** — 90
    Sanjay Gambhir, Mudalsha Ravina, Gawri Sankar, Nitin Yadav
    - Morphology Versus Anatomy *90* • Technical Developments *90*
    - Calcium Scoring and Myocardial Perfusion Imaging *91* • Hybrid PET-MR *96*

16. **Role of Coronary Flow Reserve in Coronary Artery Disease** — 100
    Ashwani Sood, Abhiram GA, BR Mittal
    - Diagnosis of Coronary Artery Disease *100*

17. **Nuclear Medicine in Assessment of Cardiac Dyssynchrony** — 106
   Anirban Mukherjee, Chetan D Patel
   - Introduction to Cardiac Dyssynchrony *106* • Nuclear Medicine Techniques in Assessment of Cardiac Dyssynchrony *106* • Clinical Utility of Assessment of Cardiac Mechanical Dyssynchrony *108*

INVASIVE

18. **Is Optical Coherence Tomography Ready to Replace Intravascular Ultrasound in Percutaneous Coronary Intervention?** — 112
   Debabrata Dash
   - Role of Optical Coherence Tomography before Percutaneous Coronary Intervention *112*
   - Optical Coherence Tomography in Assessment of Stenting *114* • Postintervention Assessment *114*
   - Artifacts *115* • Will Optical Coherence Tomography Replace Intravascular Ultrasound *115*

19. **Association of Coronary Stenosis and Plaque Morphology with Fractional Flow Reserve and Outcomes** — 117
   Jagat Narula
   - Severity of Luminal Stenosis and Fractional Flow Reserve *117* • Plaque Morphology and Fractional Flow Reserve *118* • Fractional Flow Reserve and Subsequent Clinical Events *119*
   - Plaque Morphology: A Link between Fractional Flow Reserve and Clinical Outcomes *119*
   - Article Information *122*

SECTION 2: Clinical Cardiology

EMERGING THERAPIES

20. **PCSK9 Inhibitors: Will they be the Next Wonder Drug after Statins?** — 127
   PC Manoria, Pankaj Manoria, Piyush Manoria, SK Parashar
   - Residual Atherogenic Risk Poststatin Therapy *127* • High Triglycerides as a Determinant of Residual Atherogenic Risk *128* • PCSK9 *128* • Clinical Approval in Europe and USA *130*

21. **Fighting the Devil of Stroke in Atrial Fibrillation: The New Weapons in the Armory** — 134
   PC Manoria, Pankaj Manoria, Piyush Manoria, SK Parashar
   - When to Use New Oral Anticoagulants? *135* • Limitations of New Oral Anticoagulants *136*
   - Comparison of TSOACs *140*

CORONARY ARTERY DISEASE

22. **Management of Prehospital Phase of Acute Myocardial Infarction** — 142
   AK Pancholia
   - Pathophysiology and Impact of Time *142* • Delays in Providing Treatment for Cardiac Emergencies *143* • Prehospital ECGs in Patients with STEMI: What are the Benefits? *143* • Current Guidelines for Prehospital ECGs among Patients with ST-segment Elevation Myocardial Infarction *144* • Treatment of Acute Coronary Syndromes in the Prehospital Phase *145* • Reperfusion Therapy: Prehospital Thrombolysis *146* • Prerequisites for Prehospital Thrombolysis *146*
   - Choice of Thrombolytic Agents for Prehospital Thrombolysis *146* • Prehospital versus In-hospital Thrombolysis *147* • Comparison of Thrombolysis with Percutaneous Coronary Intervention in Randomized Controlled Trials *147*

23. STEMI Care in India and the Real World: Pharmacoinvasive Approach — 153
HK Chopra

- Development of Thrombolytic Therapy *153* • Trends in Thrombolysis for STEMI *156* • STEMI Care in India: Problems and Solutions *159*
- Future Directions for STEMI Program in India *160*

24. Bioresorbable Vascular Scaffold — 163
MS Hiremath

- Polymer Based *164* • Metal Based *164* • Cohort A *164* • E-BVS Implantation: Tips and Traps *165* • Role of Intravascular Imaging in BVS Implantation and Follow-up *167*
- E-BVS from Clinical Trials to Clinical Practice *167* • Noninvasive Assessment of BVS *168*
- Restoration of Vasomotion *168*

25. Statin Intolerance — 174
Peeyush Jain, Col. Viney Jetley

- Statin Myopathy *174* • Common Concerns Associated with Long-term Use of Statins *174*

26. Sudden Cardiac Death: How to Predict and Prevent it? — 182
Pankaj Manoria, PC Manoria, Piyush Manoria

- Magnitude of the Problem *182* • Causes of Sudden Cardiac Death *182*
- Mechanism of Sudden Cardiac Death *182* • Risk Factors for Sudden Cardiac Death *183* • Treatment *183*

27. New Gadgets Knocking at the Door: Leadless Pacemakers, Subcutaneous Implantable Cardioverter Defibrillators, Wearable Defibrillators — 187
Anitha G, Ulhas M Pandurangi

- Leadless Pacemaker *187* • Wireless Cardiac Stimulation System *187*
- Subcutaneous Implantable Cardioverter Defibrillator *188*
- Wearable Cardioverter Defibrillator *189*

28. Echocardiographic Evaluation of Left Atrial Clot and Its Utility in Clinical Practice — 191
Asha Moorthy, Jain T Kallarakkal

29. Clinical Applications of Nuclear Cardiology Procedures and Its Future Directions — 193
GN Mahapatra

- Scope of Radionuclide Imaging Procedures *193* • Myocardial Perfusion *194*
- Stress-gated SPECT Tc-99m Myocardial Perfusion Imaging Agents *195*
- Clinical Applications of Myocardial Perfusion Imaging *197* • Pharmacological Stress Perfusion Imaging *199* • Dipyridamole Myocardial Perfusion Imaging *199*
- Mechanism of Action of Dipyridamole *200* • Adenosine Myocardial Perfusion Imaging *200* • Dobutamine Myocardial Perfusion Imaging *200* • Pharmacological Stress Perfusion Imaging with Low Level Treadmill/Bicycle Exercise *202* • New Options in Pharmacological Stress *202* • Regadenoson Myocardial Perfusion Scintigraphy *202*
- Dual Isotope Imaging Using Tl-201 and F-18 FDG Imaging *208* • Fluorodeoxyglucose Positron Emission Tomography versus Fluorodeoxyglucose Single Photon Emission Computed Tomography *210* • Emerging Concepts in Nuclear Cardiology *211*
- Computation of Myocardial Blood Flow with Rubidium-82 and Comparison to N13 Ammonia *212* • Dynamic Single Photon Emission Computed Tomography (SPECT) *215*
- F-18 Flurpiridaz Positron Emission Tomography Myocardial Perfusion Imaging Tracer *217*

- F-18 BMS Myocardial PET Tracer *218* • C-11 Hydroxyephedrine/C-11 Epinephrine/I-*123* MIBG and Tc99m tetrofosmin/Sestamibi SPECT MPI *218* • Tracers for Detecting Chronic Inflammatory Disorders such as Cardiac Sarcoidosis/Amyloidosis *218* • Tracers for Detecting Atheromatous Plaque Particularly Vulnerable Plaque Imaging *219* • Tracers for Stem Cells Tracking *219* • Tracers for Patients with Infectious Endocarditis and Aortic Graft Prosthetic Infection *219* • Useful Combined Nuclear Cardiology Techniques *221*

30. Cardiac Positron Emission Tomography Perfusion Tracers: Current Status and Future Directions   225
Jamshid Maddahi, René RS Packard

- Current Myocardial Perfusion Positron Emission Tomography Tracers *225*
- Future Directions *226* • Funding *228* • Disclosure *228*

Index   *231*

SECTION 1

Cardiac Imaging

Noninvasive

- Echocardiographic Evaluation of Infective Endocarditis: The Current Status
- The Intricacies in Echocardiographic Evaluation of Aortic Stenosis
- Echocardiography of Heart Failure: How to Use it in Routine Clinical Practice?
- Speckle Tracking Echocardiography: Basics and Clinical Applications
- A Gold Standard for Evaluation of Cardiomyopathies
- Real World Indications for Cardiac Magnetic Resonance Imaging: When is it Invaluable in Clinical Practice?
- Cardiac MRI and Cardiac CT: Indispensable Tools for the Diagnosis of Coronary Artery Disease
- Cardiac Imaging: Current Scenario and Future Directions
- Clinical Decision-making with Myocardial Perfusion Imaging in Patients with Known or Suspected Coronary Artery Disease
- Current Status of Rubidium-82 PET-CT Myocardial Perfusion Imaging
- Innovation of New Tracers in the Era of Multimodality Cardiac Imaging
- Myocardial Imaging Products' Evolution: Change for the Better
- Efficacy of Combining FDG-PET Metabolic and Tc-99m–MIBI Myocardial Perfusion Study in Assessment of Myocardial Viability
- Myocardial Viability Assessment: Is it Alive?
- Hybrid Myocardial Imaging Techniques: Role in Functionally Relevant Coronary Disease
- Role of Coronary Flow Reserve in Coronary Artery Disease
- Nuclear Medicine in Assessment of Cardiac Dyssynchrony

Invasive

- Is Optical Coherence Tomography Ready to Replace Intravascular Ultrasound in Percutaneous Coronary Intervention?
- Association of Coronary Stenosis and Plaque Morphology with Fractional Flow Reserve and Outcomes

NONINVASIVE

1 Echocardiographic Evaluation of Infective Endocarditis: The Current Status

IB Vijayalakshmi

INTRODUCTION

Infective endocarditis (IE) is a very serious infective disease of cardiac valves with high mortality, if not diagnosed and treated in time. It is defined as infection of a native or prosthetic heart valve/the endocardial surface, or an indwelling implanted cardiac device. The yearly incidence is about 3–10 per 1,00,000 people.[1] In spite of improvements in culture sensitivity tests and availability of higher antibiotics, IE remains associated with high morbidity and mortality. Echocardiography plays a key role not only in the diagnosis of IE but also in prognostication, follow-up during therapy and during surgery. Technological development of two-dimensional (2D) transthoracic echocardiography (TTE) and later transesophageal echocardiography (TEE) and recently three-dimensional (3D) or four-dimensional image (4D) echocardiography has led to its increased diagnostic capabilities and its broad use in routine everyday clinical practice.

EVALUATION OF INFECTIVE ENDOCARDITIS

In clinical practice, the diagnosis of IE usually relies on the association between an infective syndrome and underlying damaged (rarely normal) valves. The diagnosis of IE necessitates integration of clinical findings, microbiological analysis and imaging results. The modified Duke's clinical diagnostic criteria incorporates all these findings as either major or minor criteria. A definite diagnosis requires either two major or one major with three minor, or five minor criteria.[2] The Duke's criteria have reduced sensitivity in patients with suspected prosthetic valve endocarditis (PVE), right-sided IE and cardiac device infection and hence should be used as a diagnostic guide rather than a replacement for a good clinical judgment.[3] The echocardiography, positive blood cultures and clinical features remain the cornerstone of diagnosis for IE. Further microbiological studies are required when blood cultures are negative. The European Society of Cardiology (ESC) 2015 modified criteria for the diagnosis of IE **(Table 1)** have included newer imaging modalities (MRI, CT, PET/CT), which may improve the sensitivity of the modified Duke criteria in difficult cases.[4]

Indications for Echocardiography in IE

Echocardiography, either transthoracic echocardiography (TTE) or TEE has a key role in the diagnosis of IE and detection of complications. Echocardiography should be performed at the earliest in all the cases, in which IE is clinically suspected. The knowledge of clinical history is important as echocardiography does not provide substantial tissue characterization or pathologic information.[5] Echocardiography must be performed as soon as IE is suspected in cases with pyrexia of unknown origin (PUO). TTE must be performed first in all cases, because it is a noninvasive technique that provides useful information for both the diagnosis and the assessment of IE severity. TTE is better than TEE for the detection of anterior cardiac abscesses and for hemodynamic assessment of valvular dysfunction. TEE must also be performed in the patients with suspected IE, because of its better image quality and better sensitivity, particularly for the diagnosis of perivalvular involvement.[6] 3D TEE provides incremental value over 2D in TEE in its ability to accurately identify and localize vegetations and to identify complications such as abscesses, perforations and ruptured chordae.[7,8] Although in clinical practice 3D TTE is increasingly performed, it should still be regarded as a supplement to standard echocardiography in most cases.[4]

The indications of echocardiographic examination for diagnosis and follow-up of patients with suspected IE are described in **Table 2**, as per the ESC guidelines.[4]

Table 1 European Society of Cardiology 2015 modified criteria for the diagnosis of infective endocarditis[2,4]

Major criteria

• Blood cultures positive for IE
  – Typical microorganisms consistent with IE from 2 separate blood cultures:
    - *Viridans streptococci, Streptococcus gallolyticus (Streptococcus bovis)*, HACEK (*Haemophilus, Aggregatibacter, Cardiobacterium, Eikenella corrodens, Kingella*) group, *Staphylococcus aureus*; or
    - Community-acquired enterococci, in the absence of a primary focus; or
  – Microorganisms consistent with IE from persistently positive blood cultures:
    - ≥2 positive blood cultures of blood samples drawn >12 hours apart; or
    - All of 3 or a majority of ≥4 separate cultures of blood (with and last samples drawn ≥1 hour apart); or
    - Single positive blood culture for *Coxiella burnetii* or phase I IgG antibody titer >1:800
• *Imaging positive for IE*
  – Echocardiogram positive for IE:
    - Vegetation
    - Abscess, pseudoaneurysm, intracardiac fistula
    - Valvular perforation or aneurysm
    - New partial dehiscence of prosthetic valve
  – Abnormal activity around the site of prosthetic valve implantation detected by ^{18}F-FDG PET/CT (only if the prosthesis was implanted for >3 months) or radiolabelled leukocytes SPECT/CT
  – Definite paravalvular lesions by cardiac CT

Minor criteria
• Predisposition such as predisposing heart condition, or injection drug use • Fever, as temperature >38°C • Vascular phenomena (including those detected by imaging only): major arterial emboli, septic pulmonary infarcts, infectious (mycotic) aneurysm, intracranial hemorrhage, conjunctival haemorrhages, and Janeway's lesions • Immunological phenomena: glomerulonephritis, Osler's nodes, Roth's spots, and rheumatoid factor • Microbiological evidence: positive blood culture but does not meet a major criterion as noted above or serological evidence of active infection with organism consistent with IE

Abbreviation: IE, infective endocarditis

Table 2 Role of echocardiography in infective endocarditis[4]

Recommendations	Class[a]/Level[b]
Diagnosis	
TTE is recommended as the first-line imaging modality in suspected IE	I B
TOE is recommended in all patients with clinical suspicion of IE and a negative or nondiagnostic TTE	I B
TOE is recommended in patients with clinical suspicion of IE, when a prosthetic heart valve or an intracardiac device is present	I B
Repeat TTE and/or TOE within 5–7 days is recommended in case of initially negative examination when clinical suspicion of IE remains high	I C
Echocardiography should be considered in *Staphylococcus aureus* bacteremia	IIa B
TOE should be considered in patients with suspected IE, even in cases with positive TTE, except in isolated right-sided native valve IE with good quality TTE examination and unequivocal echocardiographic findings	IIa C
Follow-up under medical therapy	
Repeat TTE and/or TOE are recommended as soon as a new complication of IE is suspected (new murmur, embolism, persisting fever, HF, abscess, atrioventricular block)	I B
Repeat TTE and/or TOE should be considered during follow-up of uncomplicated IE, in order to detect new silent complications and monitor vegetation size. The timing and mode (TTE or TOE) of repeat examination depend on the initial findings, type of microorganism, and initial response to therapy	IIa B
Intraoperative echocardiography	
Intraoperative echocardiography is recommended in all cases of IE requiring surgery	I B
Following completion of therapy	
TTE is recommended at completion of antibiotic therapy for evaluation of cardiac and valve morphology and function	I C

Abbreviations: HF, heart failure; IE, infective endocarditis; TOE, transesophageal echocardiography; TTE, transthoracic echocardiography
[a]Class of recommendation
[b]Level of evidence

Anatomical and Echocardiographic Features in IE

Infective endocarditis is anatomically characterized by a combination of vegetations, destructive lesions of valves and walls of cardia and abscess formation. The major echocardiographic criteria for IE are vegetation, abscess and new dehiscence of a prosthetic valve. The anatomical and echocardiographic definitions are described in **Table 3**.[4]

Vegetation

The presence of vegetation is the hallmark of IE. The vegetation is a fuzzy echo structure/mass attached to a valve/endocardium, with oscillating chaotic motion independent of the valve **(Figs 1A and B)**. They are typically attached on the low-pressure side of the valve structure, but may be located anywhere on the components of the valvular and subvalvular apparatus, as well as on the mural endocardium **(Fig. 2)** of

Table 3 Anatomical and echocardiographic definitions[4]

	Surgery/necropsy	Echocardiography
Vegetation	Infected mass attached to an endocardial structure or on implanted intracardiac material	Oscillating or nonoscillating intracardiac mass on valve or other endocardial structures, or on implanted intracardiac material
Abscess	Perivalvular cavity with necrosis and purulent material not communicating with the cardiovascular lumen	Thickened, nonhomogeneous perivalvular area with echodense or echolucent appearance
Pseudoaneurysm	Perivalvular cavity communicating with the cardiovascular lumen	Pulsatile perivalvular echo-free space, with color Doppler flow detected
Perforation	Interruption of endocardial tissue continuity	Interruption of endocardial tissue continuity traversed by color Doppler flow
Fistula	Communication between two neighboring cavities through a perforation	Color Doppler communication between two neighboring cavities through a perforation
Valve aneurysm	Saccular outpouching of valvular tissue	Saccular bulging of valvular tissue
Dehiscence of a prosthetic valve	Dehiscence of the prosthesis	Paravalvular regurgitation identified by TTE/TEE, with or without rocking motion of the prosthesis

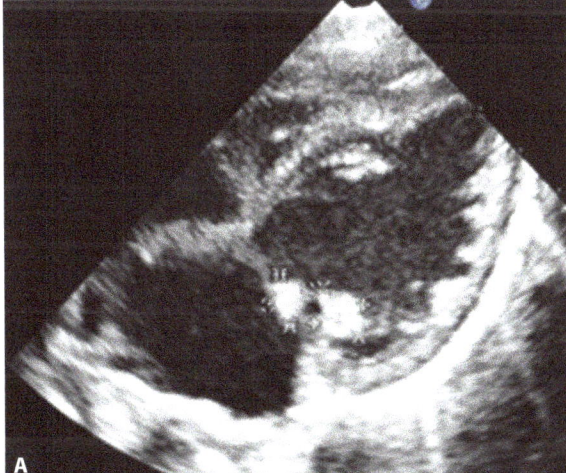 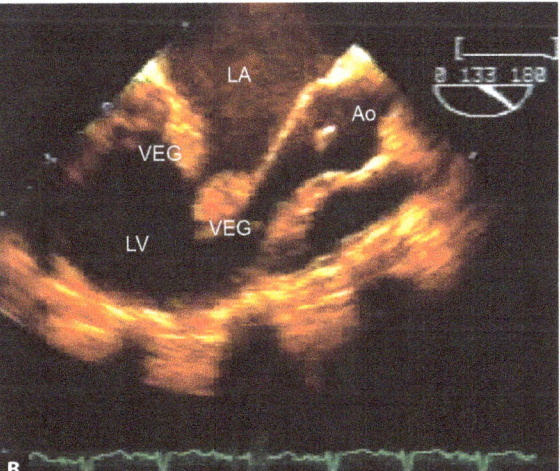

Figs 1A and B: (A) TTE modified 2-chamber view shows large vegetations on anterior and posterior mitral leaflets with mild pericardial effusion in a 12 years old girl of RHD; (B) TEE shows large mobile vegetation attached to both anterior and posterior mitral leaflets in a 30 years old lady of RHD with history of fever of one month
Abbreviations: VEG, vegetation; LA, left atrium, Ao, aorta; LV, left ventricle

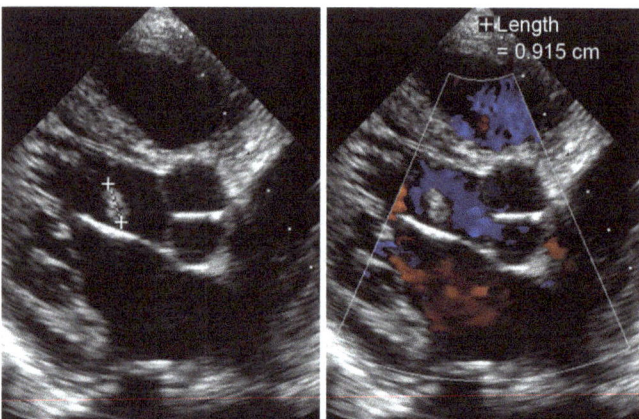

Fig. 2: TTE in parasternal long-axis shows large highly mobile vegetation in LVOT in a 7 years old boy operated for shoulder injury

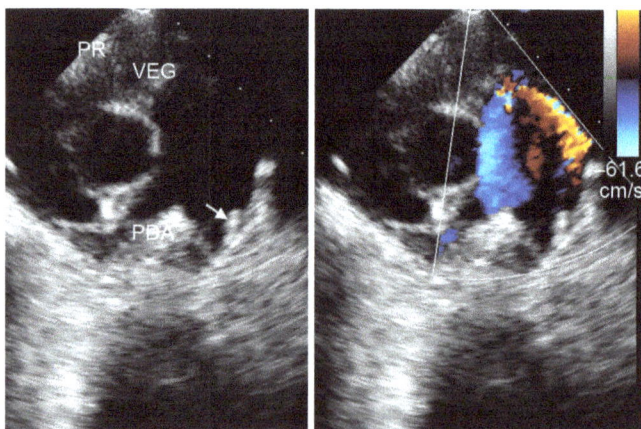

Fig. 3: TTE in short-axis view shows vegetation in the pulmonary artery in a case of small patent ductus arteriosus (PDA)
Abbreviation: VEG, vegetation

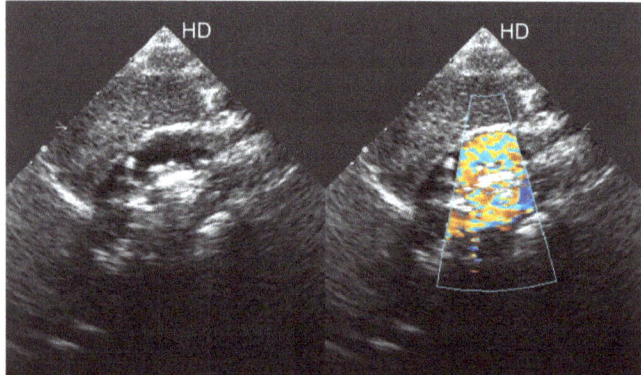

Fig. 4: TTE in suprasternal view showing multiple vegetations in arch of aorta with color Doppler showing turbulence in arch of aorta in a 3-year old boy with bicuspid aortic valve

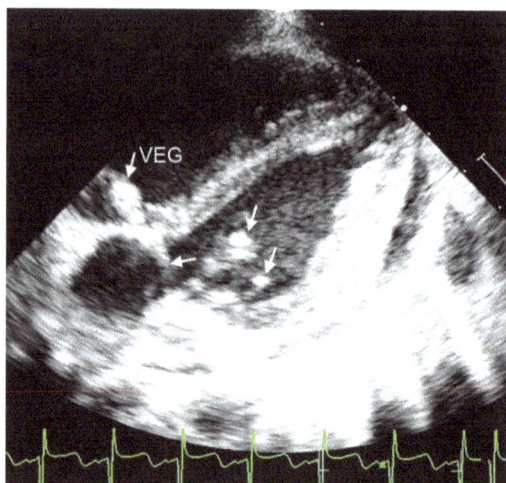

Fig. 5: TTE in modified 5-chamber view shows small vegetations on aortic and mitral valves but large vegetation on RV side almost closing VSD in a 5 years old boy with small VSD

the cardiac chambers or the ascending aorta **(Fig. 3)** and pulmonary artery **(Fig. 4)**. The vegetation can vary in size and number **(Fig. 5)**. The large and mobile vegetations are more prone for embolization **(Fig. 6)** and less frequently to valve or prosthetic obstruction.[6] The diagnostic yield of the technique in the detection of vegetations is influenced by several factors: image quality; echogenicity and vegetation size (<2–3 mm); vegetation location; presence of previous valvar disease (mitral valve prolapse, degenerative calcified lesions) or valvular prosthesis; recent embolization and in nonvegetant IE; experience and skill of the examiner; and pretest probability of endocarditis.[4,9] Diagnosis may be particularly challenging in IE affecting intracardiac devices, even with the use of TEE.[4] The detailed echocardiographic features of vegetation is given in **Table 4**.[5] Sanfilippo et al. characterized vegetation by echocardiography based on its mobility, size, extent and consistency **(Box 1)**.[10]

Vegetations can be detected in 42–86% of IE patients with echocardiography. In diagnosis of vegetations in native and prosthetic valves, TTE sensitivity is 70% and 50% respectively and TEE sensitivity is 96% and 92% respectively.[6,11] Specificity has been reported to be around 90% for both TTE and TEE.[9] The sensitivity of 3D and 4D TEE in diagnosis of IE is similar to 2D TEE, while its specificity is much higher (100%). However, sensitivity of TTE is much lower in detecting vegetations in patients with artificial valves, implanted pacemaker or implantable cardioverter-defibrillator. About 15% of patients with endocarditis have normal echocardiographic finding. Echocardiography may not detect vegetations in too early stage of disease or in case when vegetation caused an embolic event.[12] In patients with high clinical suspicion of IE and a negative initial echocardiographic examination, TTE and/or TEE should be repeated within 5–7 days later or even earlier

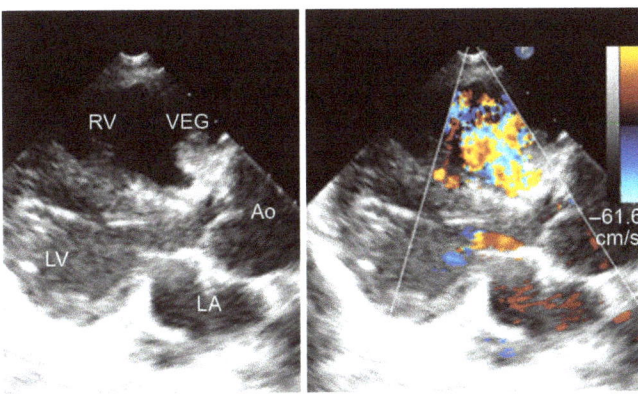

Fig. 6: TTE in parasternal long-axis shows large highly mobile vegetation in a RVOT in a 11 years old boy operated for tetralogy of Fallot

in the case of *Staphylococcus aureus* infection.[13] Follow-up echocardiography to monitor complications and response to treatment is mandatory.

Abscess and Perivalvular Involvement

The presence of a perivalvular abscess is a second major echocardiographic criterion for IE. The echo features of an abscess are given in **Table 4**.[5] Abscesses are more frequent in aortic native valve (10–40%) and PVE (56–100%) and may be complicated by pseudoaneurysm or fistulous track formation (**Figs 7 and 8**). In mitral valve IE, perivalvular abscesses are usually located posteriorly or laterally.[4] If a clear free space is present in the aortic root, the diagnosis is easy but it may be much more difficult at the early stage of the disease when only a thickening of the aortic root is observed.[6]

Table 4 Echocardiographic features of infectious vegetations and abscesses[5]

Vegetations
- *Echogenicity/echo texture*: Gray scale, myocardial texture, however, healed vegetations are more echogenic and often are calcified
- *Size*: Highly variable
- *Aspect/shape*: Usually amorphous, shaggy, lobulated, less commonly linear or round
- *Location*: Atrial side of atrioventricular valves, ventricular side of the aortic valve, but may affect any side
- *Motion*: High-frequency flutter, oscillating, chaotic, orbiting, independent of valve motion; if large, prolapses into ventricles in diastole
- *Associations*: Valvular regurgitation, valvular mycotic aneurysms, valvular destruction, perivalvular abscess, prosthetic dehiscence
- *Differential diagnosis*: Native valve noninfectious vegetations, papillary fibroelastoma, valvular strands and Lambl's excrescences, mitral annular calcification with mobile components, left ventricular outflow tract calcification with mobile components; prostheses: thrombosis, mitral subvalvular tissue remnants, platelet thrombi and microcavitations associated to mechanical prosthetic valves
- *"Healed vegetations"*: Similar to any inflammatory process, once resolved, infective vegetations may scar and may appear as echogenic calcific nodules

Abscesses
Echolucent or echogenic-heterogeneous space or tissue thickening, which may or not "fill" with Doppler color signal, adjacent to valvular structure, usually paravalvular but may affect any myocardial region
  Affects the aortic valve more commonly and may result in fistulous tract formation (i.e., aorta-ventricle, aorta-atrium) as well as pseudoaneurysm (typically of the aortic root)

BOX 1 Characterization of vegetation by Sanfilippo et al.[10]

Vegetation size
Measurements are made in two orthogonal dimensions of the identified vegetations, one perpendicular to the leaflet surface and a second parallel to the leaflet, at the point of maximal thickness. For both mitral and aortic valves, the vegetation was measured in the parasternal long-axis view during diastole.

Vegetation mobility grading
- *Grade l*: A fixed vegetation with no detectable independent motion
- *Crude 2*: A vegetation with fixed base but with a mobile free edge and larger in its parallel dimension than its perpendicular dimension
- *Crude 3*: A pedunculated vegetarian defined as a lesion that has a stalk and a perpendicular dimension greater than the parallel dimension but that remains within the same chamber throughout the cardiac cycle
- *Grade 4*: A prolapsing vegetation that is one that crosses the coaptation plane of the leaflets at some point during the cardiac cycle

Vegetation extent grading
The maximal extension of each vegetation assessed in multiple echocardiographic views and graded as:
- *Grade l*: A single vegetation
- *Grade 2*: Multiple vegetations limited to a single valve leaflet
- *Grade 3*: Involvement of multiple valve leaflets
- *Grade 4*: A vegetation that extended to extravalvular structures

Vegetation consistency
The consistency or texture of each vegetation is assessed by using the appearance of the myocardial echoes as a reference. Calcifications is assessed on the basis of characteristic bright reflections
- *Grade l*: A completely calcified vegetation
- *Grade 2*: A partially calcified vegetation
- *Grade 3*: Consistency denser than myocardial echoes but without calcification
- *Grade 4*: Consistency equal to that of myocardial echoes

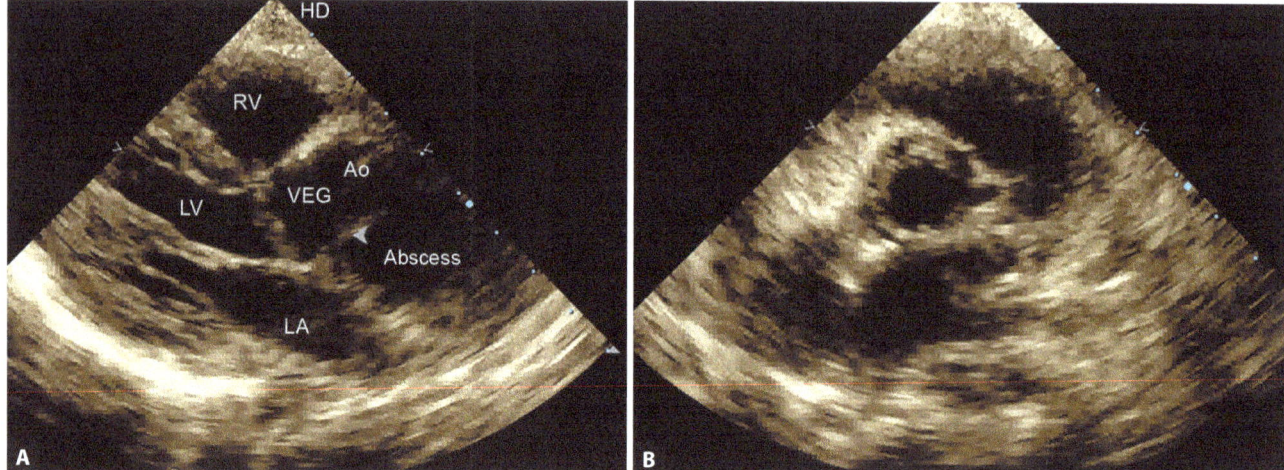

Figs 7A and B: (A) TTE parasternal long-axis shows large abscess (arrow) in the para-aortic region; (B) Short-axis shows multiple aortic para-annular abscesses in a 6 years old girl of bicuspid aortic valve with critical stenosis, who had undergone aortic balloon valvuloplasty, who presented with a history of fever for 15 days

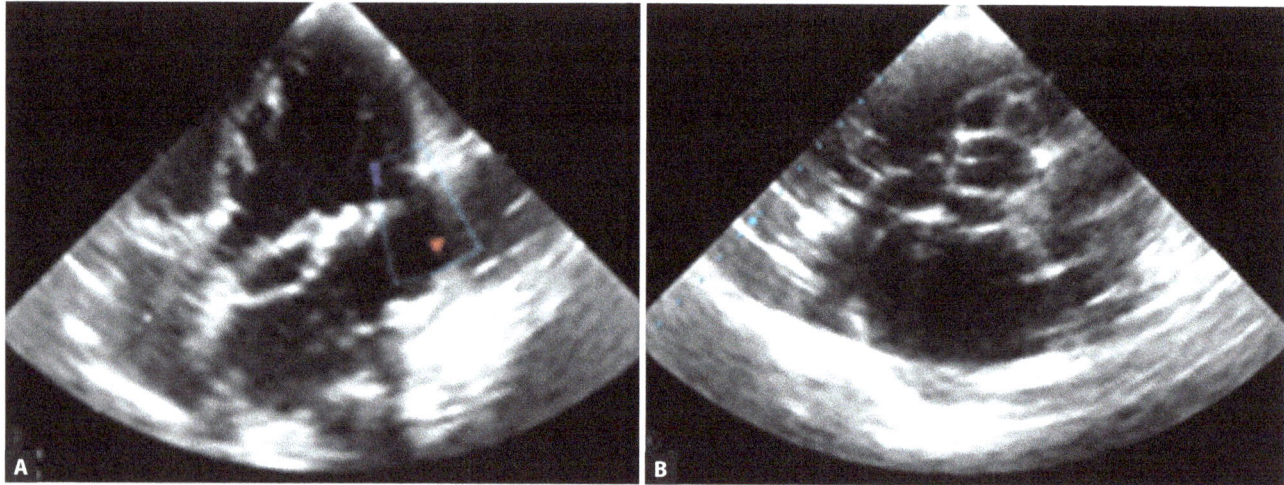

Figs 8A and B: (A) TTE apical four-chamber; and (B) Short-axis view shows multiple aortic abscess in a 28 years old pregnant lady, a known case of RHD, history of fever for 15 days with a fatal outcome

Similarly, small abscesses may be difficult to identify, especially in the early stage of the disease, in the postoperative period and in the presence of a prosthetic device (particularly in the mitral position).[14] Serial echocardiographic studies have shown that abscess formation is a dynamic process, starting with aortic root wall thickening and extending to the development of fistulae.[15]

The pseudoaneurysms and fistulae are severe complications of IE and are frequently associated with very severe valvular and perivalvular damage.[16-18] The anatomical and echocardiographic appearance of pseudoaneurysm and fistula is described in **Table 3**. Formation of a fistula may be a complication of both abscesses and pseudoaneurysm. The frequency of fistula formation in IE has been reported to be 1.6%, with *S. aureus* being the most commonly associated organism (46%).[18] The sensitivity of TTE for the diagnosis of abscesses is about 50%, compared with 90% for TEE **(Fig. 9)**. Specificity higher than 90% has been reported, for both TTE and for TEE.[6,11] TEE needs to be performed in all cases of aortic valve IE and as soon as an abscess is suspected. Both TTE and TEE are mandatory in suspected perivalvular involvement.[6]

New Dehiscence of a Prosthetic Valve

The third main diagnostic criterion for IE is dehiscence of a prosthetic valve.[19] IE must be suspected in the presence of new perivalvular regurgitation, even in the absence of a vegetation or abscess. TEE has a better sensitivity than TTE for this diagnosis, especially in mitral PVE. IE must always be suspected in patients with new periprosthetic regurgitation, even in the absence of other echocardiographic findings of IE.[6]

Other Echocardiographic Features in IE

The other features of IE are destructive valve lesions. They are not main criteria for IE, but may be suggestive of the diagnosis. They are very frequently associated with vegetations or may be observed alone. The usual final consequences of these lesions are severe valve regurgitation and heart failure. Valvular regurgitation in native IE may occur as a result of mitral chordal rupture, leaflet rupture (flail leaflet), leaflet perforation or interference of the vegetation mass with leaflet closure.[6,20] The most frequent is anterior mitral valve leaflet perforation **(Figs 10A and B)** which is usually a consequence of a regurgitant jet through an infected aortic valve and is best visualized by TEE.[21] Also both TTE and TEE are useful for assessing the underlying valve disease and for the evaluation of consequences of IE, including: left ventricular size/function, quantification of valve regurgitation/obstruction, right ventricular function, estimation of pulmonary pressures, presence and quantification of a pericardial effusion.[6]

Echocardiography for the Diagnosis of Complications of IE

The three most frequent and severe complications of IE are heart failure, perivalvular extension, embolic events. Echocardiography plays a key role in the diagnosis (vegetation, abscess, new regurgitation or new prosthetic valve dehiscence) and management of these complications. Echocardiography helps clinicians not only for taking the decision to operate or not, but also for choosing the optimal timing of surgery **(Figs 11A and B)**.[6]

The most frequent complication of IE is heart failure and is the main indication for urgent valve surgery in IE. It is observed in 42–60% of cases overall and is more often present when IE affects the aortic (29%) rather than the mitral (20%) valve. It can be caused by severe aortic or mitral insufficiency, intracardiac fistulae or more rarely, by valve obstruction, when a large vegetation partially obstructs the valve orifice.[4,20] TTE is of crucial importance for initial evaluation and follow-up. The complications can be assessed on 2D echocardiography (TTE/TEE) with pulsed, continuous, and color Doppler, which

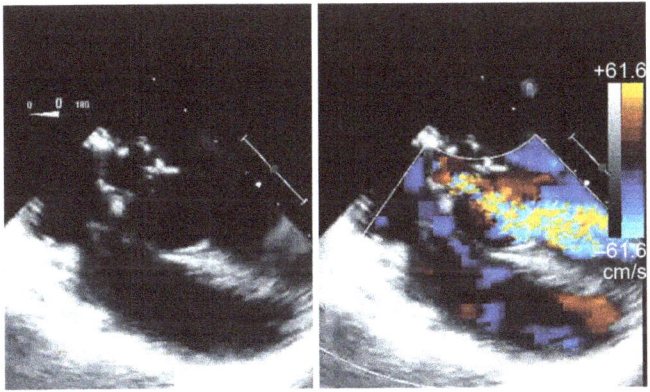

Fig. 9: TEE showing aortic valve abscess with perforation and color Doppler showing severe aortic regurgitation

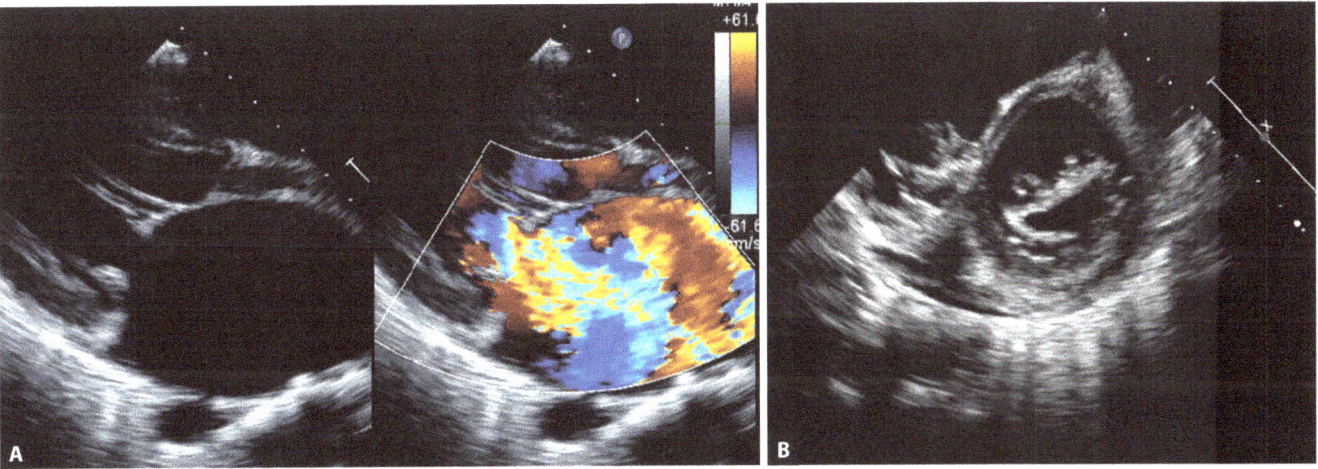

Figs 10A and B: (A) TTE parasternal long-axis view shows perforation of anterior mitral leaflet with severe mitral regurgitation on color Doppler; (B) Short-axis shows the perforation in anterior mitral leaflet (arrow) in an 11 years old boy with RHD

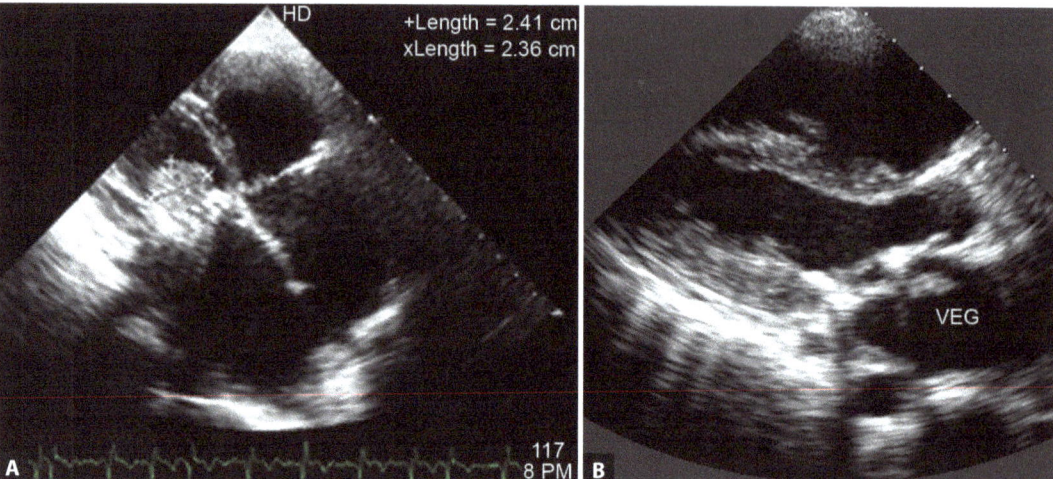

Figs 11A and B: (A) TTE in four-chamber view shows large thrombus over prosthetic valve in a 35 years old lady who had undergone mitral valve replacement; (B) PLAX view showing vegetation on left atrial side of mitral valve in a 16 years old post-mitral valve repair girl

allows identification of the mechanisms (valve perforation, cusp fenestration, torn leaflet, flail mitral leaflet due to ruptured infected chordae, or interference of the vegetation mass with leaflet closure) and quantification and evaluation of the hemodynamic tolerance of the regurgitation (cardiac output, left and right ventricular filling pressures, pulmonary arterial pressure, left and right ventricular function). Valve perforation, secondary mitral lesions and aneurysms are best assessed using TEE.[6,11,22] Careful echocardiographic examination of the mitral leaflets is required in all patients with aortic IE, because small aneurysms or perforations may be easily missed.

In patients with uncontrolled infection and at risk for perivalvular extension, prompt TTE and TEE are required. Perivalvular extensions are present in around 20% of cases and indicate valve surgery.[23] TEE is preferred for the diagnosis of perivalvular extension and its resulting complications but TTE seems better in case of anterior abscess of the aortic annulus.[24]

Embolic events are a frequent and life-threatening complication of IE-related to the migration of cardiac vegetations, which are symptomatic in around 20–25% of cases[25-28] and silent (only detected by cerebral imaging) in almost 50% of cases.[25,26] The risk of embolism is highest during the first 2 weeks of antibiotic therapy and is clearly related to the size, location, and mobility of the vegetation. The highest risk is observed for large (>10–15 mm) and very mobile vegetations **(Fig. 12)**. The echocardiographic grading of mobility of vegetation gives the idea of risk for embolization **(Box 1)**. Echocardiography, particularly TEE, is the key examination for the diagnosis and description of characteristics of vegetations. The occurrence of embolic events requires systematic TTE and TEE examination.[6] Echocardiographic predictors of systemic embolism and stroke are given in **Box 2**.[5]

Though purulent pericarditis is rare in IE, infection involving the mitral or tricuspid annulus may extend to

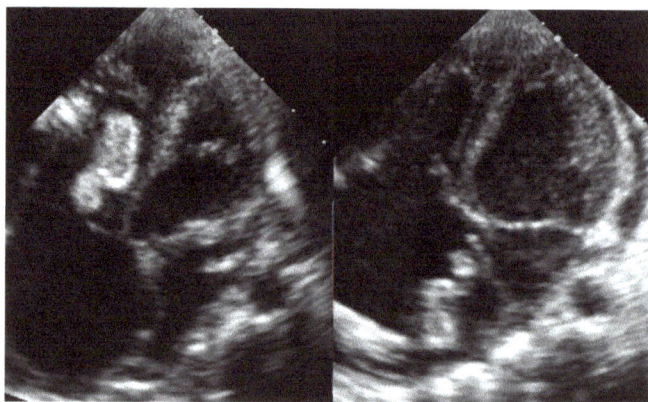

Fig. 12: TTE in four-chamber view shows highly mobile and pedunculated vegetation on a Gerbode ventricular septal defect

---

BOX 2 Echocardiographic and other predictors of systemic embolism and stroke[5]

- Echocardiographic predictors of systemic embolism and stroke
  - Visible vegetations by both TTE and TEE
  - Abscess formation
  - Highly mobile vegetation
  - Vegetation size >10–15 mm
  - MV endocarditis, particularly the anterior leaflet
- Bivalvular vegetation
- Other predictors
  - Fungal IE
  - *S. aureus* IE
  - *Streptococcus bovis* IE
  - Antibiotic therapy, as risk for stroke decreases after 1–2 weeks of antibiotic therapy

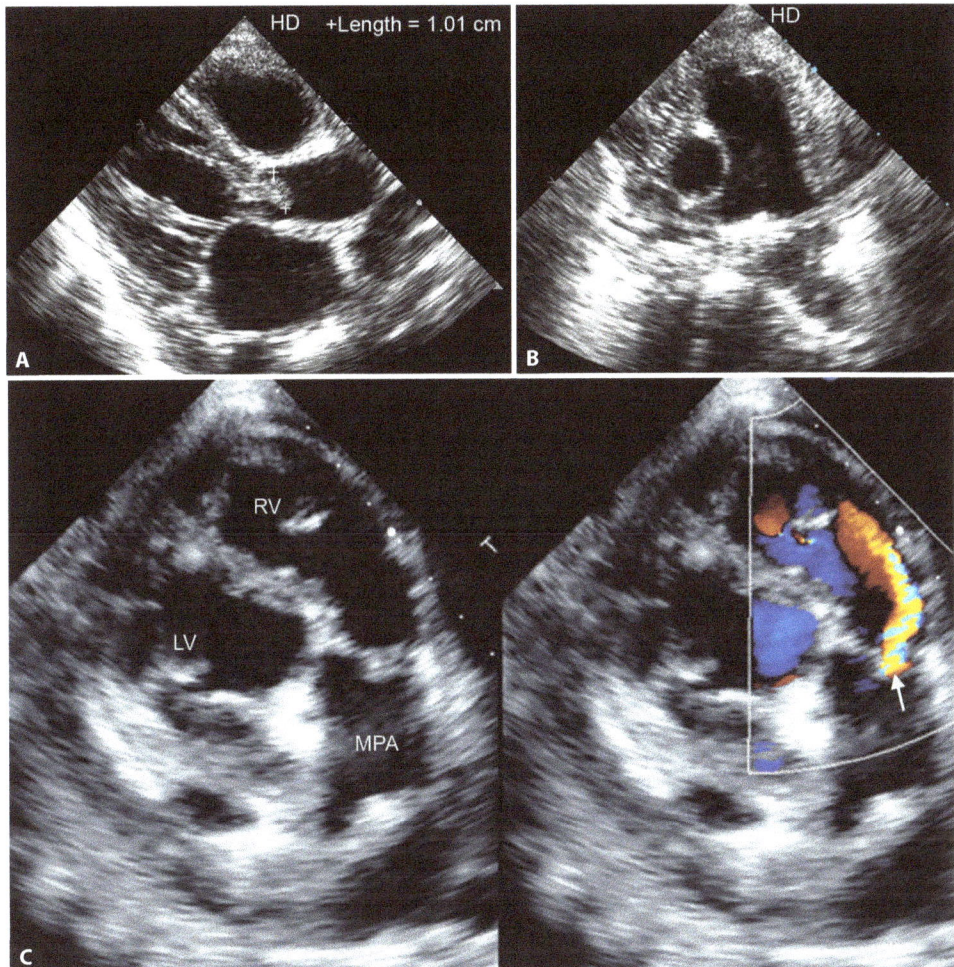

Figs 13A to C: (A) TTE in parasternal long-axis shows large vegetation on aortic valve; (B) Short-axis showed thick pus churning like contrast and small vegetation on pulmonary valve; (C) Color Doppler showed perforation of pulmonary valve and regurgitant jet coming out through the perforated valve
Abbreviations: RV, right ventricle; LV, left ventricle; MPA, main pulmonary artery

the pericardium. We have reported a case of purulent pericarditis with quadruple valve endocarditis.[29] In this case of a 7 years old boy with history of fall sustaining fracture of head of humerus with hemarthrosis of left shoulder; aspiration and open nailing was done just a week back. He developed high degree fever with chills and rigors and breathlessness. He was referred for cardiac evaluation despite the severe wound infection at the site of surgery. Emergency TTE done showed pericardial effusion which turned out to be frank pus on aspiration and large mobile vegetation attached to aortic valve **(Figs 13A and B)**. He also had vegetations on the mitral, tricuspid, and the pulmonary valves **(Fig. 13C)**.

Purulent pericarditis may also be secondary to a pseudoaneurysm of the proximal aorta, a myocardial abscess, a myocarditis, or a septic coronary embolus. Rarely, ruptured pseudoaneurysms or fistulae may communicate with the pericardium, with dramatic and often fatal consequences. Echocardiography is the best examination to diagnose and appreciate the hemodynamic tolerance of pericarditis and is guide to drainage. In the rare cases of coronary obstruction due to vegetation embolism, coronary compression, or ostial occlusion by large vegetation, echocardiography may visualize a new left ventricular segmental wall motion abnormality. Myocarditis is an uncommon complication of IE, generally associated with abscess formation. TTE plays a key role for the evaluation of global and regional left and right ventricular function in this situation.[6]

Echocardiography for the Follow-up of IE

Along with clinical follow-up, echocardiography must be used for follow-up of patients with IE under antibiotic therapy and after surgery **(Fig. 14)**. Depending on the clinical presentation, the type of microorganism and the initial echocardiographic findings, the number, type, and timing of repeat examinations is decided. In noncomplicated streptococcal native IE, weekly TTE may be sufficient, while more frequent TEE and TTE can be necessary in postoperative staphylococcal early PVE.

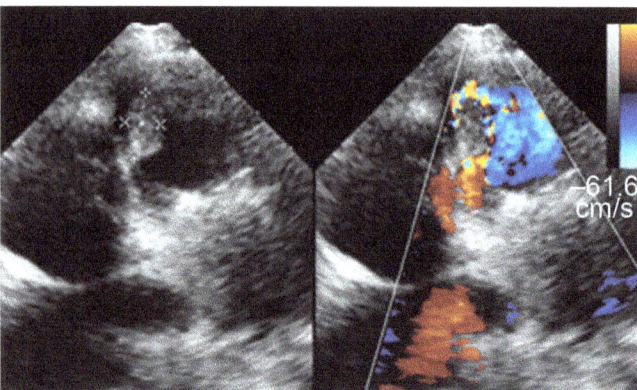

Fig. 14: TTE in short-axis with color Doppler shows large vegetation attached to VSD patch in a 10 years old boy who had undergone VSD closure

Serial echocardiographic studies during hospitalization, may show a gradual reduction in size, decrease in mobility, and increase in echogenicity of vegetations.[6] These lesions may either disappear or remain unchanged long after the acute phase of the disease, even after healing of the disease. Increasing vegetation size under therapy must be considered as a risk factor for new embolic event, while unchanged or reduced vegetation size under therapy may be more difficult to interpret. After hospital discharge, the main complications include recurrence of infection, heart failure, need for valve surgery and death. Thus, clinical and echocardiographic periodic close follow-up (at 1, 3, 6 and 12 months) is mandatory during the first year after the end of antibiotic treatment.[4]

Echocardiography during Surgery

Even though meticulous echocardiographic evaluation, including TEE, is performed to select patients referred for surgery, infective lesions may grow or embolize since the last preoperative examination. Hence, intraoperative TEE is mandatory in patients being operated on for IE.[4] It provides the surgeon with a final anatomical evaluation of valvular and perivalvular damage, and is particularly useful for assessing the immediate result of conservative surgery, as well as in cases of complex perivalvular repair. In a recent series, systematic pre-pump intraoperative TEE changed the initial operative plan in 11% of cases.[30]

Post-pump intraoperative TEE is fundamental in the evaluation of the immediate surgical result in patients with infected and friable tissues, especially to assess the result of valve repair (highly sensitive to detect a significant residual regurgitation), valve replacement (analysis of prosthesis function, detection, localization, and quantification of perivalvular leaks), and complex perivalvular repair.[30,31] The role of the surgeon to ascertain macroscopic eradication of all infected tissue remains fundamental because intraoperative TEE is not sensitive enough to identify all foci of residual infection. Post-pump intraoperative TEE also serves as a reference document of the surgical result for subsequent postoperative echocardiography.

Echocardiography in Specific Situations

Prosthetic Valve IE

Prosthetic valve endocarditis is the most severe form of IE and occurs in 1–6% of patients with valve prostheses, accounting for 10–30% of all cases of IE[32] with similar incidences observed in mechanical and bioprosthetic valves. There is a lower incidence of vegetations and higher incidence of abscesses and perivalvular complications.[33] The anatomical involvement differs between PVE affecting mechanical versus bioprosthetic valves.[34] In mechanical valves, the infection usually involves the junction between the sewing ring and the annulus, leading to perivalvular abscess, dehiscence, pseudoaneurysms, and fistula in mechanical valves, whereas it is more frequently located on the leaflets, leading to cusp rupture, perforation, and vegetations in bioprosthetic IE. The usual consequence of PVE is new prosthetic regurgitation causing heart failure and less frequently prosthetic valve obstruction due to large vegetations.[6]

Both TTE and TEE are mandatory in suspected or definite PVE. In the diagnosis and evaluation of PVE, TEE plays the key role though fluoroscopy is valuable. The sensitivity and specificity of both TTE and TEE are lower in PVE than in native valve endocarditis probably due to presence of intracardiac material. In both mechanical and bioprosthetic valves, the sewing ring and support structures are strongly echogenic and may prevent vegetation detection within the valve apparatus or its shadow. The vegetative growth appears as thickening and irregularity of the normally smooth contor of the sewing ring.[35] Both thrombus and pannus **(Table 5)** have a similar appearance and cannot be distinguished from vegetative material.[5] Similarly differentiation between bioprosthetic degeneration and infective lesions is difficult. The diagnosis of an abscess is frequently more difficult in PVE, particularly in the early postoperative period. Hence a negative echocardiogram

Table 5 Echocardiographic evaluation of prosthetic valve obstruction mechanism

Favors pannus
- Mechanical prosthesis in the aortic position
- No significant decrease in occluder motion
- Therapeutic anticoagulation
- Identified mass not significantly mobile

Favors thrombus
- Mechanical prosthesis in the tricuspid or mitral position
- Abnormal occluder motion with obstruction
- Attachment to the occluder itself
- Subtherapeutic anticoagulation
- Large and mobile identified mass

is frequently observed in PVE and does not rule out the diagnosis and repeat examination must be done if clinical suspicion is high. Identification of a new periprosthetic leak is a major criterion, even in the absence of a vegetation or abscess, in which case an additional imaging modality could be considered. Echocardiography is also recommended for the preoperative and postoperative assessment of operated patients and for the follow-up of patients treated by medical therapy alone, because of the risk of late prosthetic dysfunction.[4,6]

Cardiac Device-related IE

Infection of cardiac implantable electronic devices (CIEDs) is a severe disease associated with high mortality.[36] Cardiac device-related IE (CDRIE) is defined as an infection extending to the electrode leads, cardiac valve leaflets or endocardial surface.[4] Echocardiography and blood cultures are the cornerstones of diagnosis. In suspected or definite CDRIE, although TEE is superior to TTE, both are mandatory, but their sensitivity and specificity are lower than in native IE. Echocardiography is also useful for the measurement of vegetation size and should be repeated after device extraction. Vegetations may be attached to the electrode lead, the tricuspid leaflets, and to the endocardial wall. Echocardiography also can assess tricuspid regurgitation, right heart chamber dilatation, and quantitation of pulmonary artery pressure. The whole infectious lead course, from the superior vena cava to the right ventricle, should be evaluated for vegetations. The vegetations attached to the electrode lead present with a typical motion and morphology. In other cases, lead vegetations may have a sleeve-like appearance and are difficult to distinguish from thrombi.[37] Hence, the clinical scenario and a repeat echocardiogram may help the diagnosis.

Right Heart Infective Endocarditis

Right-sided IE accounts for 5–10% of IE cases.[38,39] It is most commonly observed in patients with intravenous drug abuser (IVDA) and the most frequently affected valve is the tricuspid valve (58–80%).[40-42] In the assessment of patients with right-sided IE, TTE is of major value, due to the anterior location of the tricuspid valve and usually large vegetations. TEE is not mandatory in isolated right-sided native valve IE with good-quality TTE examination and unequivocal echocardiographic findings. TEE may be useful in detecting perivalvular abscess and unusual localizations of right-sided IE such as infection on the Eustachian valve[43,44] or on the Chiari network. TEE is also indicated with poor image quality with TTE, in those who have negative TTE despite a moderate or high level of clinical suspicion of IE (especially in the setting of staphylococcal bacteremia),[45] and when an associated left heart involvement is suspected. The size of the tricuspid vegetation and the severity of the tricuspid regurgitation must be evaluated by echocardiography, because these measurements have the potential to influence the therapeutic strategy.[4,6] Extensive valve destruction and severe regurgitation are a common sequel of right-sided IE. Vegetations may rarely be sufficiently large to mimic an intracardiac tumor and large vegetations (>2 cm) have been identified as an independent predictor of mortality together with fungal etiology.[46,47] Embolized vegetations have been seen floating free in the right ventricle or pulmonary artery and pulmonary embolism in the setting of high-grade fever may be the first clinical sign of right-sided endocarditis.[48] Mural vegetations have been observed in patients with congenital heart diseases and left-to-right shunts. Iatrogenic right-sided IE in children with congenital heart diseases has also been reported.[49] In one of our 5 years old boy weighing 12 kg who presented with history of fever for 1½ months; treated as bronchopneumonia **(Fig. 15A)** with parenteral antibiotics and IV fluids. When his condition deteriorated, became very moribund, developed CCF, he was referred to tertiary center. Emergency echocardiography was done showed a small ventricular septal defect (VSD) in parasternal long axis view **(Fig. 15B)**, which could not explain CCF. The subcostal view showed dilated noncollapsing inferior vena cava (IVC) with mobile vegetations **(Fig. 15C)** and apical four-chamber view showed huge grape-like highly mobile vegetations attached to tricuspid valve causing tricuspid stenosis (TS) and tricuspid regurgitation (TR) **(Fig. 15D)**. But the repeated blood cultures were negative. Probably contaminated IV fluids had caused right-sided IE and vegetations causing pulmonary embolism and CCF.[49]

Incidence of negative blood cultures endocarditis varies from 5% to more than 10% in most series.[50] The use of both TTE and TEE should be recommended in this setting. Routine echocardiography allows an early diagnosis and evidence-based treatment approach and, therefore, overcomes partially the worse natural history of these patients.[51,52]

Limitations of Echocardiography in IE

The sensitivity and specificity of both TTE and TEE are not 100%. Also a negative echocardiogram may be observed in about 15% of cases of IE and does not rule out IE. The imaging diagnosis may be particularly challenging in some cases, such as with intracardiac devices, valvular prostheses, the presence of pre-existing severe lesions (mitral valve prolapse, degenerative lesions), very small vegetations (<2 mm) or no vegetation and abscesses. In addition, the diagnosis may be difficult at the early stage of the disease.[53] False diagnosis of IE by echocardiography may occur in several situations. Appearances resembling vegetations may be seen in (i) torn rolled up chordae tendineae, (ii) degenerative or myxomatous valve disease, (iii) systemic lupus (inflammatory Libman–Sacks lesions), (iv) rheumatoid disease, (v) primary antiphospholipid syndrome, (vi) valvular thrombus, advanced malignancy (marantic endocarditis), (vii) in association with small intracardiac tumors (typically fibroelastomata).[54] Hence, the results of the echocardiographic study must be interpreted with

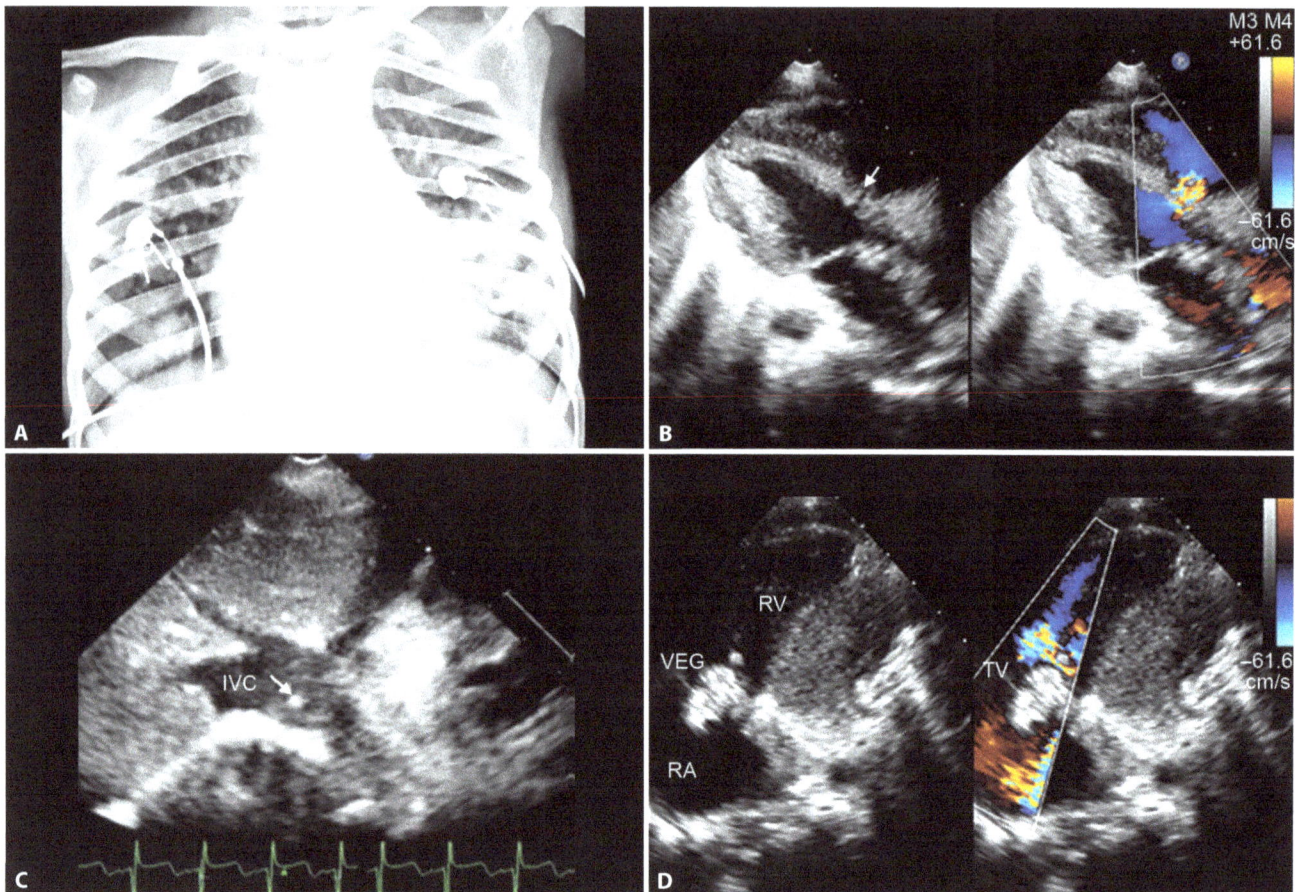

Figs 15A to D: (A) X-ray chest shows nonhomogeneous opacity; (B) TTE in parasternal long-axis view shows small VSD; (C) Subcostal view shows dilated noncollapsing inferior vena cava (IVC) with vegetation; (D) Apical four-chamber view with color Doppler shows TS, TR causing CCF

caution, taking into account the patient's clinical presentation and the likelihood of IE. Vegetation persisting after effective treatment must not be interpreted as a clinical recurrence of the disease unless supported by clinical features and bacteriologic evidence.[9]

Prosthetic findings that may be confused with vegetation include: (a) prosthetic strands, (b) thrombosis, (c) remnants of mitral subvalvular tissue, (d) microcavitations. Microcavitations are high-velocity, tiny, bright echoes that occur at, the inflow zone of mechanical valves (both aortic and mitral, more frequent mitral) at the time of valve closure, when flow velocity and pressure drop abruptly. They represent a normal phenomenon and, in fact, may disappear with valve obstruction or thrombosis, only to return after thrombolysis.[55] Vegetations on pacemaker leads,[56] indwelling catheters and right-sided prostheses are particularly difficult to diagnose with TTE because reverberations and artefacts produced by the intracardiac material may mask small vegetations attached to these structures.

In right-sided endocarditis, normal anatomical variants such as Chiari network or prominent Eustachian valve may cause diagnostic confusion, more particularly with TTE. Right atrial thrombus may be distinguished from vegetation in that it is less likely to lie in the path of the jet and tends to layer on the right atrial wall. Previous infection with damage to the tricuspid valve is commonly seen and hence presence of vegetation does not in itself signify the presence of active infection. Older or healed vegetations tend to be hyperechogenic and may even be calcified. But echocardiographic findings always need to be taken in their clinical context.

CONCLUSION

Echocardiography is a simple accurate method for detecting vegetations and endocardial damage in IE. It also helps in risk stratification and follow up. TEE has a major role both before surgery and during surgery. Recent advances in 3D imaging offers additional importance to the echocardiographic evaluation of patients with IE. But in all IE cases, echocardiographic findings must be interpreted based on clinical features of the patient. Imaging of IE remains a diagnostic challenge because echocardiography has several limitations, which can impact on patient prognosis. Newer imaging modalities are emerging and offer hope of better management of the disease and thus a reduction in mortality. The future in imaging of IE will be multimodal.

ACKNOWLEDGEMENT

Sincere thanks to Dr Chitra Narasimhan for kind assistance.

REFERENCES

1. Cahill TJ, Prendergast BD. Infective endocarditis. Lancet. 2016;387(10021):882-93.
2. Li JS, Sexton DJ, Mick N, et al. Proposed modifications to the Duke criteria for the diagnosis of infective endocarditis. Clin Infect Dis. 2000;30:633-8.
3. Prendergast BD. Diagnostic criteria and problems in infective endocarditis. Heart. 2004;90:611-3.
4. Habib G, Lancellotti P, Antunes MJ, et al. 2015 ESC Guidelines for the management of infective endocarditis: The Task Force for theManagement of Infective Endocarditis of the European Society of Cardiology (ESC). Endorsed by: European Association for Cardio-Thoracic Surgery (EACTS), the European Association of Nuclear Medicine (EANM). Eur Heart J. 2015;36(44):3075-128.
5. Saric M, Armour AC, Arnaout MS, et al. Guidelines for the Use of Echocardiography in the Evaluation of a Cardiac Source of Embolism. J Am Soc Echocardiogr. 2016;29(1):1-42.
6. Habib G, Badano L, Tribouilloy C, et al. Recommendations for the practice of echocardiography in infective endocarditis. Eur J Echocardiogr. 2010;11(2):202-19.
7. Hansalia S, Biswas M, Dutta R, et al. The value of live/real time three-dimensional transesophageal echocardiography in the assessment of valvular vegetations. Echocardiography. 2009;26:1264-73.
8. Liu YW, Tsai WC, Lin CC, et al. Usefulness of real-time three-dimensional echocardiography for diagnosis of infective endocarditis. Scand Cardiovasc J. 2009;43:318-23.
9. Evangelista A, Gonzalez-Alujas MT. Echocardiography in infective endocarditis. Heart. 2004;90(6):614-7.
10. Sanfilippo AJ, Picard MH, Newell JB, et al. Echocardiographic assessment of patients with infectious endocarditis: prediction of risk for complications. J Am Coll Cardiol. 1991;18:1191-9.
11. Mugge A, Daniel WG, Frank G, Lichtlen PR. Echocardiography in infective endocarditis: reassessment of prognostic implications of vegetation size determined by the transthoracic and the transesophageal approach. J Am Coll Cardiol. 1989;14:631-8.
12. Vincelj J. Echocardiography in Diagnosis and Management of Infective Endocarditis. J Cardiol Curr Res. 2016;5(2):00158.
13. Eudailey K, Lewey J, Hahn RT, George I. Aggressive infective endocarditis and the importance of early repeat echocardiographic imaging. J Thorac Cardiovasc Surg. 2014;147:e26-e28.
14. Hill EE, Herijgers P, Claus P, et al. Abscess in infective endocarditis: the value of transesophageal echocardiography and outcome: a 5-year study. Am Heart J. 2007;154:923-8.
15. Forteza A, Centeno J, Ospina V, et al. Outcomes in aortic and mitral valve replacement with intervalvular fibrous body reconstruction. Ann Thorac Surg. 2015;99:838-45.
16. Tingleff J, Egeblad H, Gotzsche CO, et al. Perivalvular cavities in endocarditis: abscesses versus pseudoaneurysms? A transesophageal Doppler echocardiographic study in 118 patients with endocarditis. Am Heart J. 1995;130:93-100.
17. Jenkins NP, Habib G, Prendergast BD. Aorto-cavitary fistulae in infective endocarditis: understanding a rare complication through collaboration. Eur Heart J. 2005;26:213-4.
18. Bashore TM, Cabell C, Fowler V Jr. Update on infective endocarditis. Curr Probl Cardiol. 2006;31:274-352.
19. Durack DT, Lukes AS, Bright DK. New criteria for diagnosis of infective endocarditis: utilization of specific echocardiographic finding: Duke Endocarditis Service. Am J Med. 1994;96:200-9.
20. Vilacosta I, San Roman JA, Sarria C, et al. Clinical, anatomic, and echocardiographic characteristics of aneurysms of the mitral valve. Am J Cardiol. 1999;84:110-3. A119.
21. Shiue AB, Stancoven AB, Purcell JB, et al. Relation of level of B-type natriuretic peptide with outcomes in patients with infective endocarditis. Am J Cardiol. 2010;106:1011-5.
22. Piper C, Hetzer R, Korfer R, et al. The importance of secondary mitral valve involvement in primary aortic valve endocarditis; the mitral kissing vegetation. Eur Heart J. 2002;23:79-86.
23. Selton-Suty C, Celard M, Le Moing V, et al. Preeminence of *Staphylococcus aureus* in infective endocarditis: a 1-year population-based survey. Clin Infect Dis. 2012;54:1230-9.
24. Graupner C, Vilacosta I, San Roman J, et al. Periannular extension of infective endocarditis. J Am Coll Cardiol. 2002;39:1204-11.
25. Cooper HA, Thompson EC, Laureno R, et al. Subclinical brain embolization in left-sided infective endocarditis: results from the evaluation by MRI of the brains of patients with left-sided intracardiac solid masses (EMBOLISM) pilot study. Circulation. 2009;120:585-91.
26. Duval X, Iung B, Klein I, et al. Effect of early cerebral magnetic resonance imaging on clinical decisions in infective endocarditis: a prospective study. Ann Intern Med. 2010;152:497-504.
27. Snygg-Martin U, Gustafsson L, RosengrenL, et al. Cerebrovascular complications in patients with left-sided infective endocarditis are common: a prospective study using magnetic resonance imaging and neurochemical brain damage markers. Clin Infect Dis. 2008;47:23-30.
28. Thuny F, Avierinos JF, Tribouilloy C, et al. Impact of cerebrovascular complications on mortality and neurologic outcome during infective endocarditis: a prospective multicentre study. Eur Heart J. 2007;28:1155-61.
29. Setty N. Vijayalaksmi IB, Chitra N, et al. Purulent pericarditis with quadruple valve endocarditis. Am J Case Rep. 2015;16:236-9.
30. Shapira Y, Weisenberg DE, Vaturi M, et al. The impact of intraoperative transesophageal echocardiography in infective endocarditis Isr. Med Assoc J. 2007;9:299-302.
31. Shapira Y, Vaturi M, Weisenberg DE, et al. Impact of intraoperative transoesophageal echocardiography in patients undergoing valve replacement. Ann Thorac Surg. 2004;78:579-83.
32. Vongpatanasin W, Hillis LD, Lange RA. Prosthetic heart valves. N Engl J Med. 1996;335:407-16.
33. Habib G, Thuny F, Avierinos JF. Prosthetic valve endocarditis: current approach and therapeutic options. Prog Cardiovasc Dis. 2008;50:274-81.
34. Piper C, Korfer R, Horstkotte D. Prosthetic valve endocarditis. Heart. 2001;85:590-93.
35. Lengyel M. The impact of transesophageal echocardiography on management of prosthetic valve endocarditis: experience of 31 cases and review of the literature. J Heart Valve Dis. 1997;6: 204-11.

36. Rundstrom H, Kennergren C, Andersson R, et al. Pacemaker endocarditis during 18 years in Goteborg. Scand J Infect Dis. 2004;36:674-9.
37. Klug D, Lacroix D, Savoye C, et al. Systemic infection related to endocarditis on pacemaker leads: clinical presentation and management. Circulation. 1997;95:2098-107.
38. Frontera JA, Gradon JD. Right-side endocarditis in injection drug users: review of proposed mechanisms of pathogenesis. Clin Infect Dis. 2000;30:374-9.
39. Wilson LE, Thomas DL, Astemborski J, et al. Prospective study of infective endocarditis among injection drug users. J Infect Dis. 2002;185:1761-6.
40. Mathew J, Addai T, Anand A, et al. Clinical features site of involvement bacteriological findings outcome of infective endocarditis in intravenous drug abusers. Arch Intern Med. 1995;155:1641-8.
41. Miro JM, Del Rio A, Mestres CA. Infective endocarditis in intravenous drug abusers and HIV-1 infected patients. Infect Dis Clin North Am. 2002;16:273.
42. Hubbell G, Cheitlin MD, Rapaport P. Presentation, management, follow-up evolution of infective endocarditis in drug addicts. Am Heart J. 1981;102:85-94.
43. Sawhney N, Palakodeti V, Raisinghani A, et al. Eustachian valve endocarditis: a case series and analysis of literature. J Am Soc Echocardiogr. 2001;14:1139-42.
44. San Roman JA, Vilacosta I, Sarria C, et al. Eustachian valve endocarditis: is it worth searching for? Am Heart J. 2001;142:1037-40.
45. Moss R, Munt B. Injection drug use and right sided endocarditis. Heart. 2003;89:577-81.
46. Scudeller L, Badano LP, Crapis M, et al. Population-based surveillance of infectious endocarditis in an Italian region. Arch Intern Med. 2009;169:1720-3.
47. Martin-Davila P, Navas E, Fortun J, et al. Analysis of mortality and risk factors associated with native valve endocarditis in drug users: the importance of vegetation size. Am Heart J. 2005;150:1099-106.
48. Nucifora G, Badano LP, Hysko F, et al. Pulmonary embolism and fever, when should right-sided infective endocarditis be considered? Circulation. 2007;115:e173-6.
49. Natraj S, Vijayalakshmi IB, Narasimhan C, et al. Iatrogenic Right-sided Infective Endocarditis In Children With CHD. Int J Cardiol Res. 2015;02(3):34-6.
50. Tunkel AR, Kaye D. Endocarditis with negative blood cultures. N Engl J Med. 1992;326:1215-7.
51. Zamorano J, de Isla LP, Moura L, et al. Impact of echocardiography in the short- and long-term prognosis of patients with infective endocarditis and negative blood cultures. J Heart Valve Dis. 2004;13:997-1004.
52. Zamorano J, Sanz J, Almeria C, et al. Differences between endocarditis with true negative blood cultures and those with previous antibiotic treatment. J Heart Valve Dis. 2003;12:256-60.
53. Thuny F, Gaubert JY, Jacquier A, et al. Imaging investigations in infective endocarditis: current approach and perspective. Arch Cardiovasc Dis. 2013;106(1):52-62.
54. Sanchez-Enrique C, Vilacosta I, Moreno HG, et al. Infected marantic endocarditis with leukemoid reaction. Circ J. 2014;78:2325-7.
55. Kaymaz C, Ozkan M, Ozdemir N, et al. Spontaneous echocardiographic microbubbles associated with prosthetic mitral valves: mechanistic insights from thrombolytic treatment results. J Am Soc Echocardiogr. 2002;15:323-7.
56. Vilacosta I, Sarriá C, San Román JA, et al. Usefulness of transesophageal echocardiography for diagnosis of infected transvenous permanent pacemakers. Circulation. 1994;89:2684-7.

2
The Intricacies in Echocardiographic Evaluation of Aortic Stenosis

Sameer Shrivastava, Neel Bhatia

In the developing world, aortic stenosis (AS) represents as one of the most prevalent valvular heart disease. Severe aortic stenosis is transformation of the aortic valve in a severely restricted, thickened, calcific valve; however, the initiating process is less likely to be a degenerative one, but rather similar to atherosclerotic plaque formation.

In the last few years more efforts have been put to predict aortic valve events more accurately. Today aortic stenosis patients are older and have been found to have higher incidence of hypertension, coronary disease, and diastolic dysfunction. Thus, the proportion of patients with low stroke volume due to left ventricular systolic function, small chamber size, increased vascular (in addition to valvular) afterload, and due to impaired longitudinal shortening may represent one-third of cases.[1]

Echocardiography has become the main diagnostic tool in assessing AS patients **(Table 1)**. Beyond gradient and area values, it provides a comprehensive assessment of the aortic valve and aortic root morphology, which is of interest when planning the surgery, and of coexistent cardiac pathologies **(Table 1)**. It is also instrumental in assessing special subgroups of patients with low gradients or decreased LV contractility, or those who may be considered for AVR even if asymptomatic. The central role of echocardiography in the management of AS patients is acknowledged by the use of echocardiographic indices to define AS severity and indications for surgery.[2]

MAIN ECHOCARDIOGRAPHIC INDICES USED TO ASSESS AS SEVERITY

Flow Velocities and Gradients

- Both peak flow velocity (V_{max}) and mean gradient are obtained by Doppler interrogation of aortic flow. As such, good alignment of the Doppler line and the flow direction (<20°) is required for accurate and reproducible results.

Table 1 Echocardiographic information in aortic stenosis patients

AV morphology:
• Tricuspid or bicuspid
• Severity of calcification
Aortic stenosis severity:
• Gradient
• Valve area
Aortic stenosis severity follow-up and progression of LV systolic function:
Global (LVEF)
LV contractile reserve
Severity of LV hypertrophy
Response to exercise
Aortic dimensions and pathology
Co-existent valvular disease

Abbreviations: LV, left ventricle; LVEF, left ventricular ejection fraction

- V_{max} is used rather than peak gradient to minimize the effect of small variations of velocity readings on the final result; this is less of a problem for the mean gradient that is obtained by integrating all the instantaneous gradients generated during ejection and is not a simple computation of mean velocity. For valvular jet velocities (V2) >3 m/s and subvalvular velocities (V1) <1.5 m/second, the latter can be ignored (simplified Bernoulli equation: $\Delta P = 4V2$), otherwise, both the proximal and the distal velocities have to be used (full Bernoulli equation). Furthermore, the cut-off values mentioned in **Table 2** are valid, if the LV ejection fraction (LVEF) is normal and there is no severe regurgitation across the valve.

Table 2 Stages of valvular aortic stenosis[33]

Stage	Definition	Valve anatomy	Valve hemodynamics	Hemodynamic consequences
A	At risk of AS	• Bicuspid aortic valve(or other congenital valve anomaly) • aortic valve sclerosis	Aortic V_{max} <2 m/s	None
B	Progressive AS	• Mild to moderate leaflet calcification of a bicuspid or trileaflet valve with some reduction in systolic motion or • Rheumatic valve changes with commissural fusion	• Mild AS: Aortic V_{max} 2.0–2.9 m/s or mean pressure <20 mm Hg • Moderate AS: Aortic V_{max} 3.0–3.9 m/s or mean pressure 20–39 mm Hg	• Early LV diastolic dysfunction may be present • Normal LVEF
C: Asymptomatic Severe AS				
C1	Asymptomatic Severe AS	Severe leaflet calcification or congenital stenosis with severely reduced leaflet opening	Aortic V_{max} ≥4 m/s or mean pressure ≥40 mm Hg • AVA typically is <1.0 cm² (or AVAi <0.6 cm²/m² Very severe AS is an aortic V_{max} >5 m/s or mean pressure >60 mm Hg	• LV diastolic dysfunction • Mild LV hypertrophy • Normal LVEF
C2	Asymptomatic Severe AS with LV dysfunction	Severe leaflet calcification or congenital stenosis with severely reduced leaflet opening	Aortic V_{max} >4 m/s or mean pressure >40 mm Hg AVA typically <1.0 cm² (or AVA <0.6 cm²/m²)	LVEF <50%
D: Symptomatic Severe AS				
D1	Symptomatic severe high gradient AS	Severe leaflet calcification or congenital stenosis with severely reduced leaflet opening	Aortic V_{max} >4 m/s or mean pressure >40 mm Hg AVA typically <1.0 cm² (or AVA <0.6 cm²/m²) but may be larger with mixed AS/AR	• LV diastolic dysfunction • LV hypertrophy pulmonary hypertension may be present
D2	Symptomatic severe low-flow/ low gradient AS with reduced LVEF	Severe leaflet calcification or congenital stenosis with severely reduced leaflet opening	AVA<1.0 cm² with resting aortic V_{max} 4 m/s or mean pressure <40 mm Hg Dobutamine stress echocardiography shows AVA <1.0 cm² with V_{max} >4 m/s at any flow rate	• LV diastolic dysfunction • LV hypertrophy • LVEF <50%

D3	Symptomatic Severe low gradient AS with normal LVEF or paradoxical low-flow severe AS	Severe leaflet calcification or congenital stenosis with severely reduced leaflet opening	AVA <1.0 cm² with aortic V_{max} <4 m/s or mean DP <40 mm Hg
			• Indexed AVA< 0.6 cm²/m² and
			• Stroke volume index <35 mL/m²
			• Measured when patient is normotensive (systolic BP <140 mm Hg)
				• Increased LV relative wall thickness
				  – Small LV chamber with low stroke volume
				  – Restrictive diastolic filling
				  – LVEF ≥50%

Sources of Error for Gradient Calculations

- Gradient underestimation is due to:
  - Malalignment of the Doppler line with the main flow direction; and
  - Missing the transducer position/window providing the optimal signal.
- Gradient overestimation is due to–
Confusion with a different, higher-velocity systolic flow (mitral regurgitation [MR], LV outflow tract [LVOT]

obstruction); and inclusion of a beat following a long diastole in measurements.

AORTIC VALVE AREA

Aortic valve area (AVA) is usually calculated using the continuity equation. All modern echocardiographic machines have incorporated analysis software to calculate AVA from the traced VTI and the measured LVOT diameter **(Fig. 1)**. An alternative method to obtain the AVA is by direct planimetry of the valve orifice in parasternal short-axis view, using either transthoracic or transesophageal echocardiography (TEE).

Sources of Error for Aortic Valve Area Calculations

The continuity equation method is subject to gradient error calculations and inaccurate LV outflow tract measurements, for which inter- and intra-observer variability may reach 8%.[2] This dimension, being squared in the continuity equation formula, can result in significant error and underestimation of valve area. The direct planimetry of the aortic valve orifice requires good-quality images, occasionally available only with TEE. Even with TEE, aortic valve direct planimetry may be inaccurate with a heavily calcified valve and is therefore considered to be an acceptable alternative when Doppler measurements are unreliable, but it is not a primary method to assess AVA.

DIMENSIONLESS VELOCITY INDEX

It is ratio between subvalvular (LVOT level) and valvular peak velocities, it is a version of the continuity equation that ignores LVOT diameter and thus is not subject to errors related to its measurements. A dimensionless velocity index (DVI) <0.25 is indicative of severe AS, with a valvular area of 25% of the expected normal valve area for the patient's body size. DVI does not provide a valve area but rather confirms or weakens the qualitative diagnosis of severe AS. The velocity index is also useful to differentiate between high valvular gradients due to truly severe AS and mild AS with increased velocities due to high-flow conditions such as sepsis or hyperthyroidism, when the DVI remains >0.3 as both the valvular and subvalvular velocities are high.

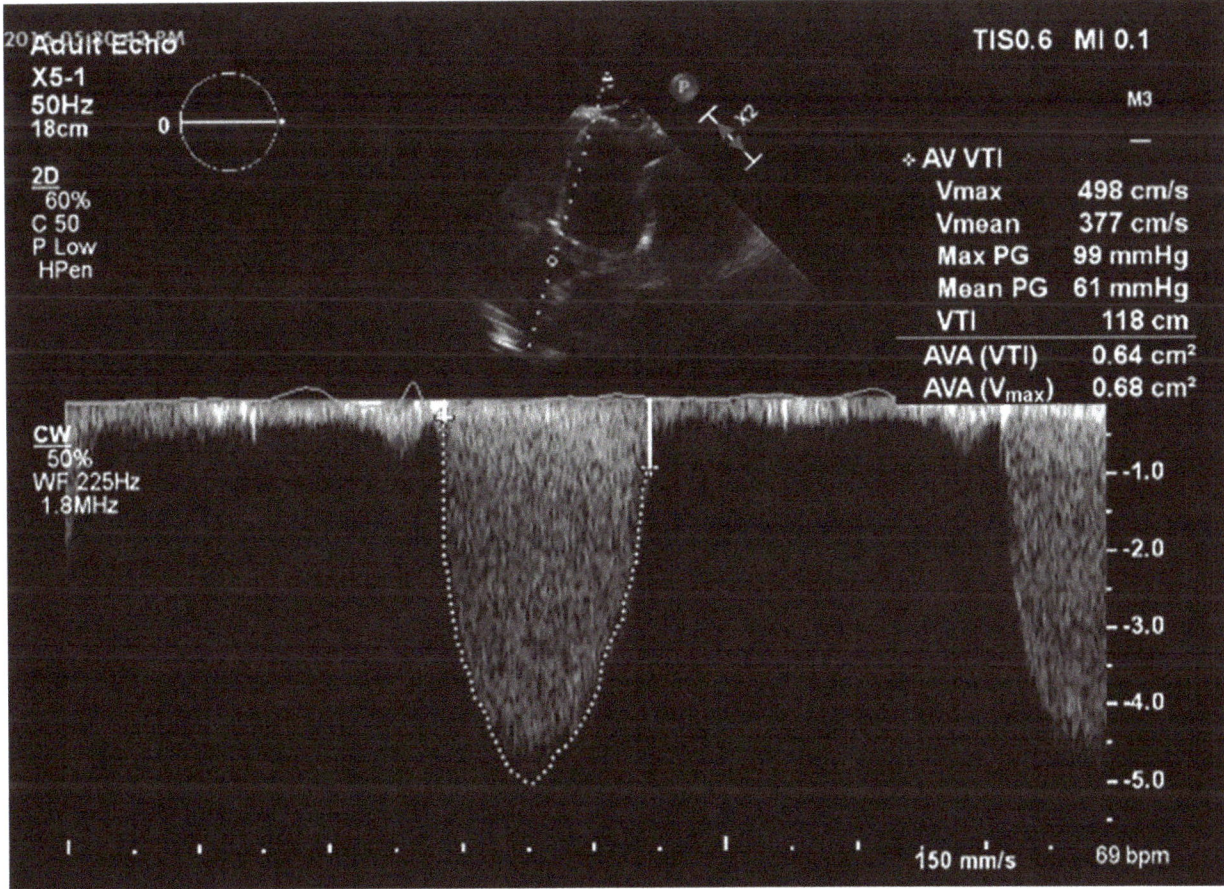

Fig. 1: Severe aortic stenosis by continuity equation

Real Dilemmas in the Diagnosis of Aortic Stenosis

The limitations and possible errors described above are generally well-known and, although occasionally confusing, their avoidance by appropriate technique and awareness is expected from a good echo study.

The echocardiographic uncertainties one may encounter in the diagnosis of AS relate mainly to contradictory results and lack of concordance between accepted echocardiographic indices of AS severity or between echocardiographic and catheterization results. The challenge of appropriate quantification of AS in patients with decreased LV function is well recognized. However, even patients with good LV contractility exhibit a mixture of hemodynamic patterns. In their review of 3,483 echocardiographic studies of patients with various degrees of AS and normal EF, Minners, et al. found in 30% of cases a lack of concordance between the different criteria of AS severity. Moreover, V_{max} and gradient were in the range of severe AS in 40–45% of patients, while by AVA 69–76% of them were diagnosed as having severe AS.[3]

Aortic stenosis severe by gradient but mild to moderate by aortic valve area. Occasionally, high (>4 m/s) peak velocities and elevated mean gradients (>30–40 mm Hg) are found in patients whose AVA by continuity equation is only in the mild to moderate range (>1 cm^2).
Frequently, the reasons for this discordance are related to execution errors of the echocardiographic study:
- Incorrect positioning of the pulsed-wave Doppler sample volume too close to the aortic valve, so that the LVOT signal is contaminated by the high-velocity valvular flow; and
- Erroneous measurement resulting in overestimation of the LVOT diameter. Real discrepancies, i.e. high velocities and gradients in the absence of significant AS, can occur in patients with a high cardiac output state, such as sepsis, hyperthyroidism, anemia or with AV fistulas. Awareness of the patient's clinical condition and a DVI >0.25 should clarify this condition. Aortic stenosis mild to moderate by gradient but severe by aortic valve area faced with this discrepancy, the first step is to establish the contractility of the left ventricle and dichotomise these low-gradient severe AS patients into those with reduced or normal EF.

Low-flow-Low-gradient Aortic Stenosis (LF/LGAS) with LV Systolic Dysfunction

It is defined as a combination of AVA <1 cm^2 (0.6 cm^2/m^2), mean gradient <40 mm Hg and LVEF <40%, and is described in 5–10% of patients with AS.[4,5] can be present in AS patients as a result of either concomitant pathology (coronary artery disease or cardiomyopathy) or of long-standing severe AS.

Other criteria which have been proposed in the literature to define the LF state in AS, include a cardiac index 3.0 L/min/m^2 and a stroke volume index 35 mL/m^2.[2,16,22]

Given that the gradient essentially depends on the flow per beat (i.e. the stroke volume) rather than on the flow per minute (i.e. the cardiac output), the former is the most frequently used parameter in this context.[22,25-27]

The main diagnostic challenge in LF-LGAS with low LVEF is to distinguish true severe from pseudosevere AS.

In the former, the primary culprit is deemed to be the valve disease, and the LV dysfunction is a secondary or concomitant phenomenon. Conversely, the predominant factor in pseudosevere AS is deemed to be myocardial disease, and AS severity is overestimated due to incomplete opening of the valve in relation to the LF state. Distinction between these two entities is essential because patients with true severe AS generally benefit from aortic valve replacement (AVR), whereas those with pseudosevere AS may not benefit.

ASSESSING LEFT VENTRICLE CONTRACTILE AND/OR FLOW RESERVE

The term "flow reserve" is utilized rather than "contractile reserve" because several mechanisms not necessarily related to intrinsic contractility may contribute to the lack of stroke volume increase during DSE, including: (1) afterload mismatch due to an imbalance between the severity of the stenosis and myocardial reserve;[29] (2) inadequate increase of myocardial blood flow due to associated CAD; and/or (3) irreversible myocardial damage due to previous myocardial infarction or extensive myocardial fibrosis.

deFilippi et al.[15] were the first to demonstrate that low-dose dobutamine stress echocardiography (DSE) may be used in these patients to assess the presence of LV flow reserve and to distinguish true versus pseudo severe aortic stenosis and to risk-stratify the patient in terms of perioperative risk and possible benefit of AVR. The use of DSE for this purpose has received a Class IIa (Level of Evidence: B) recommendation in the American College of Cardiology/American Heart Association-European Society of Cardiology (ACC/AHA-ESC/EACTS) guidelines.[22-24]

The accepted approach is to perform low-dose dobutamine stress echo study (DSE) and to quantify the inotropic response and the changes in AVA and transvalvular gradient.

Dobutamine Stress Echo Study in Low-gradient Aortic Stenosis

The accurate assessment of aortic valve area in patients with a reduced stroke volume is difficult because the calculated valve area is proportional to stroke volume and the constant of the Gorlin equation varies with transvalvular flow.[12,13] As a result, some patients with AS and a low transvalvular pressure gradient have a reduced valve area because of inadequate stroke volume in the presence of thickened valve leaflets rather than a fixed, anatomic stenosis. Cannon et al[14] described 8 such patients who were identified as having severe AS using

Table 3 Hemodynamic response patterns to dobutamine in patients with low-flow-low-gradient aortic stenosis

Increase in stroke volume	Gradient	Aortic valve area	Conclusion
>20%	⇔	Increased >1–1.2 cm²	Contractile reserve present, pseudo-severe AS
>20%	Increased	⇔	Contractile reserve present, true severe AS
<20%	⇔	⇔	No contractile reserve ? AS

⇔ = no significant change

the Gorlin equation but only mild AS during inspection of the valve at the time of surgery. These individuals were thought to have "pseudo-AS"; i.e., their aortic valve had thickened leaflets, which opened in direct relation to systolic blood flow. If the stroke volume was small, the leaflets opened poorly, resulting in a demonstrable transvalvular pressure gradient and a small calculated valve area. As the stroke volume increased, the leaflets opened more effectively, resulting in a larger valve area.

Dose of dobutamine required is in range of 5–20 µ/kg/minute, and although the dose-response to dobutamine is unpredictable and the inotropic response does not necessarily parallel the chronotropic and blood pressure response,[6] an increase in heart rate is generally taken as proof of dopaminergic stimulation sufficient to elicit an inotropic response. CR is considered to be present if the dobutamine infusion results in ≥20% increase in cardiac output.[4,7] In subjects, who show an increase in peak velocity (0.6 m/s), stroke volume (20%), or mean transvalvular pressure gradient (10 mm Hg) with DSE have LV contractile reserve. Patients with true severe AS and evidence of CR have a clear indication for AVR. The possible response patterns to dobutamine in patients with LF/LGAS are summarized in **Table 3**.

DeFilippi et al.[15] demonstrated that DSE could be used to distinguish individuals with fixed AS from those with pseudo-AS. In patients with fixed AS, dobutamine induced an increase in peak velocity, mean transvalvular pressure gradient, and valve resistance and no change in valve area. In contrast, in those with pseudo-AS, dobutamine caused a considerable increase in valve area (0.3 cm²) without a substantial change in peak velocity, mean transvalvular pressure gradient, or valve resistance.

DISTINGUISHING BETWEEN TRUE SEVERE AND PSEUDOSEVERE AORTIC STENOSIS

The evaluation of the changes in EOA and gradient during dobutamine infusion are also helpful in differentiating true severe from pseudosevere AS. Typically, pseudosevere AS shows an increase in EOA and relatively little increase in gradient in response to increasing flow, whereas true severe AS is characterized by little or no increase in EOA and an increase in gradient that is congruent with the relative increase in flow. Several parameters and criteria have been proposed in the literature to identify patients with pseudosevere AS during DSE, including a peak stress mean gradient 30 or 40 mm Hg depending on studies, a peak stress EOA 1.0 or 1.2 cm², and/or an absolute increase in EOA 0.3 cm²;[15,16,22,26,28,30] thus, the optimal cut-off values remain to be determined. The prevalence of pseudosevere AS is reported to be between 20% and 30%.[15,26,28,31]

Some patients may nonetheless have an ambiguous response to DSE due to variable increases in flow [15,26,27] and interpreting the changes in EOA and gradients without considering the relative changes in flow may often be problematic. Hence, to overcome this limitation, the investigators of the TOPAS (Truly or Pseudo-Severe Aortic Stenosis) study proposed to calculate the projected EOA that would have occurred at a standardized flow rate of 250 mL/s (EOAProj) [26,27] and this new parameter has been shown to be more closely related to actual AS severity, impairment of myocardial blood flow, LV flow reserve, and survival than the traditional DSE parameters.[5,26,27,32] Patients with no increase in stroke volume may nonetheless have an increase in mean flow rate sufficient to allow a reliable measurement of EOAProj; this is due to shortening of LV ejection time in relation to an increase in heart rate.[26,27] However, there are 10–20% of patients in whom the increase in flow rate is insufficient to allow calculation of EOAProj. In such cases or those with ambiguous results during DSE, quantification of valve calcification by multislice computed tomography may also be useful.

Therefore, DSE clearly can help to differentiate patients with fixed low-gradient AS from those with pseudo-AS.

In the study of Quere et al.[17] published in Circulation, the operative mortalities for those with and without LV contractile reserve were 6% and 33%, respectively.

From a previously reported French multicenter trial,[16] Quere et al.[17] identified 66 patients with symptomatic AS, a mean transvalvular pressure gradient 40 mm Hg, and an LVEF 40% who survived valve replacement surgery and underwent an evaluation of functional status and LVEF postoperatively. It was found that most patients with severe AS and a low transvalvular pressure gradient manifested a substantial improvement in symptomatic status and LVEF after valve replacement surgery, and these improvements occurred with similar frequency in subjects with and without LV contractile reserve.

Normal Left Ventricular Contractility and Low-gradient Severe Aortic Stenosis

The above term is reserved for patients with normal left ventricular ejection fraction but with reduced stroke volume and reduced systolic function seen secondary to left ventricular hypertrophy secondary to aortic stenosis known as increased concentric hypertrophy (ICR). This ICR in turn leads to decreased LV filling and reduced stroke volume (SV). Lower SV results in lower gradients across aortic valve.[18]

Inaccurate measurements and underestimation can occur due to LVOT shape which can alter the calculation of SV and AVA. This is in turn can lead to inconsistent measurement of Severity of AS.[19] It is here that role of TEE becomes important for planimetry of aortic valve.

Role of tissue Doppler imaging is important as it there would be impaired long axis shortening with reduced contractility. It was concluded in SEAS substudy[20] that LV myocardial systolic dysfunction is common in asymptomatic AS in particular in patients with low-flow AS and increased valvuloarterial afterload, whereas EF is generally preserved. A condition similar to LF-LGAS was seen in these patients with low SV and transaortic gradients. The major concern in these cases is that underestimation of AVA can lead to underutilization of valve replacement.[11]

Hachicha[11] et al described ventriculoarterial impedance (Zva), an index of global hemodynamic load and related this to the onset of symptoms and adverse events.

$$\text{Ventriculoarterial impedance (Zva)} = \frac{\text{Systolic arterial pressure + mean net transaortic gradient}}{\text{Stroke volume/m}^2}$$

Height can be substituted instead of BSA if SV is indexed to height in this formula. A value of Zva ≥4.5 mm Hg/mL m² may be useful to identify patients who are at risk of deterioration of myocardial function as per previously reported studies.[20,21]

Normal LVEF does not mean normal SV. Hachicha et al[11] showed that one-third of patients with severe AS had reduced SV Index (SV/BSA <35 mL/m²) despite preserved LVEF. This will lead to low flow situation and which in turn leads to low transvalvular gradients. In their study of 512 consecutive patients with echocardiographically determined low gradient severe AS (AVA ≤ 0.6 cm²/m²) and LVEF ≥50%, Hachicha et al[11] concluded that normal flow (NF) having SV index ≥35 mL was seen in 65% of cases and paradoxically low flow (PLF) having SV index ≤35 mL in 35% of cases. During 5 year follow-up, patients with PLF had a reduced survival compared to those with NF.

Guidelines[22] regarding diagnostic and therapeutic recommendations for LF-LGAS. Further prospective studies are needed to determine the prognosis and most appropriate timing of AVR in these asymptomatic paradoxically LF-LGAS patients with preserved LV function.

In clinical practice we are not infrequently challenged by the reality of patients with severe AS by both valve appearance and calculated valve area (AVA <1 cm²) and who present with a mean gradient in the mild-to-moderate range (<40 mm Hg) despite normal LV contractility. Obviously, technical errors have to be excluded, but this possible presentation of severe AS has recently been increasingly recognized[8-11] and has been described in up to 42% of patients with severe AS and normal LV contractility. Importantly, these patients do not seem to have a better prognosis than their 'high-gradient' counterparts.[9-11] Possible explanations for this hemodynamic pattern include:[9-11]

- Relatively low stroke volume, which is not suggested by an apparently normal EF—this could be related to small LV cavity (small-sized patients, severely hypertrophic ventricles) or occult L systolic dysfunction (elderly patients, LV hypertrophy); and
- Higher systemic vascular resistance and LV afterload. The importance of recognizing this not uncommon hemodynamic pattern cannot be overemphasised, since AVR, when appropriate, should not be denied to these patients due to a possibly misleading 'not severe enough' gradient.

CONCLUSION

Echocardiography is the first-line diagnostic tool in the assessment of patients with AS. Cut-off values define severity criteria used to decide appropriateness of intervention. A large number of patients do not fulfill all accepted criteria and may present with perplexing hemodynamic patterns and echocardiographic results. Awareness of the sources of possible errors and of less typical echocardiographic results is essential for the correct management of AS patients whose echocardiographic studies are, apparently, confounding.

REFERENCES

1. Briand M, Dumesnil JG, Kadem L. Reduced systemic arterial compliance impacts significantly on left ventricular afterload and function in aortic stenosis: implications for diagnosis and treatment. J Am Coll Cardiol. 2005;46:291-8.
2. Baumgartner H, Hung J, Bermejo J, et al. Echocardiographic assessment of valve stenosis: EAE/ASE recommendations for clinical practice. Eur J Echocardiogr. 2009;10:1-25.
3. Minners J, Allgeier M, Gohlke-Baerwolf C, et al. Inconsistencies of echocardiographic criteria for the grading of aortic valve stenosis. Eur Heart J. 2008;29(8):1043-8.
4. Tribouilloy C, Levy F, Rusinaru D, et al. Outcome after aortic valve replacement for low-flow/low-gradient aortic stenosis without contractile reserve on dobutamine stress echocardiography. J Am Coll Cardiol. 2009;53:1865-73.
5. Clavel MA, Fuchs C, Burwash IG, et al. Predictors of outcomes in low-flow, low-gradient aortic stenosis: results of the multicentre TOPAS Study. Circulation. 2008;118:S234-42.
6. Chenzbraun A, et al. Am J Cardiol. 2003;92(12):1451-4.
7. Bermejo J, Yotti R. Low-gradient aortic valve stenosis. Value and limitations of dobutamine stress testing. Heart. 2007;93:298-302.
8. Dumesnil JG, Pibarot P, Carabello B. Paradoxical low flow and/or low gradient severe aortic stenosis despite preserved left ventricular ejection fraction: implications for diagnosis and treatment. Eur Heart J. 2010;31(3):281-9.
9. Flachskampf FA. Severe aortic stenosis with low gradient and apparently preserved left ventricular systolic function—under-recognized or overdiagnosed? Eur Heart J. 2008;29(8):966-8.

10. Barasch E1, Fan D, Chukwu EO, et al. Severe isolated aortic stenosis with normal left ventricular systolic function and low transvalvular gradients: pathophysiologic and prognostic insights. J Heart Valve Dis. 2008;17(1):81-8.
11. Hachicha Z, Dumesnil JG, Bogaty P. Parodoxical low flow, low gradient severe aortic stenosis despite preserved ejection fraction is associated with higher after load and reduced survival. Circulation. 2007;115:2856-64.
12. Burwash IG, Thomas DD, Sadahiro M, Pearlman AS, Verrier ED, Thomas R, Kraft CD, Otto CM. Dependence of Gorlin formula and continuity equation valve areas on transvalvular volume flow rate in valvular aortic stenosis. Circulation. 1994;89:827-35.
13. Cannon SR, Richards KL, Crawford M. Hydraulic estimation of stenotic orifice area: a correction of the Gorlin formula. Circulation. 1985;71:1170-8.
14. Cannon JD, Zile MR, Crawford FA Jr, Carabello BA. Aortic valve resistance as an adjunct to the Gorlin formula in assessing the severity of aortic stenosis in symptomatic patients. J Am Coll Cardiol. 1992;20:1517-23.
15. deFilippi CR, Willett DL, Brickner ME, Appleton CP, Yancy CW, Eichhorn EJ, Grayburn PA. Usefulness of dobutamine echocardiography in distinguishing severe from non-severe valvular aortic stenosis in patients with depressed left ventricular function and low transvalvular gradients. Am J Cardiol. 1995;75:191-4.
16. Monin JL, Quere JP, Monchi M, Petit H, Baleynaud S, Chauvel C, Pop C, Ohlmann P, Lelguen C, Dehant P, Tribouilloy C, Gueret P. Low gradient aortic stenosis: operative risk stratification and predictors for long-term outcome: a multicenter study using dobutamine stress hemodynamics. Circulation. 2003;108: 319-24.
17. Quere JP, Monin JL, Levy F, Petit H, Baleynaud S, Chauvel C, Pop, C, Ohlmann P, Lelguen C, Dehant P, Gueret P, Tribouilloy C. Influence of preoperative left ventricular contractile reserve on postoperative ejection fraction in low-gradient aortic stenosis. Circulation. 2006;113:1738-44.
18. Jander Nikolaus. Low-gradient 'severe' aortic stenosis with preserved ejection fraction: new entity, or discrepant definitions? Eur Heart J. 2008;10(Suppl E):E11-E15.
19. Minners J, Allegeier M, Gohlke-Baerwolf C. Inconsistencies of echocardiographic criteria for the grading of aortic valve stenosis. Eur Heart J. 2008;29:1043-8.
20. Cramariue Dana, Cioffi Giovanni, Ashild E. Low-flow aortic stenosis in asymptomatic patients. JACC: Cardiovasc Imaging. 2009;2:390-99.
21. Briand M, Dumesnil JG, Kaedm L. Reduced systemic arterial compliance impacts significantly on left ventricular afterload and function in aortic stenosis: implications for diagnosis and treatment. J Am Coll Cardiol. 2005;46:291-8.
22. Vahanian A, Alfieri O, Andreotti F, et al. Guidelines on the management of valvular heart disease (version 2012): The Joint Task Force on the Management of Valvular Heart Disease of the European Society of Cardiology (ESC) and the European Association for Cardio-Thoracic Surgery (EACTS). Eur Heart J 2012;33:2451-96.
23. Bonow RO, Carabello BA, Chatterjee K, et al. 2008 focused update incorporated into the ACC/AHA 2006 guidelines for the management of patients with valvular heart disease: a report of the American College of Cardiology/American Heart Association Task Force on Practice Guidelines. J Am Coll Cardiol. 2008;52: e1-142.
24. Connolly HM, Oh JK, Schaff HV, et al. Severe aortic stenosis with low transvalvular gradient and severe left ventricular dysfunction. Result of aortic valve replacement in 52 patients. Circulation. 2000;101:1940-6.
25. Schwammenthal E, Vered Z, Moshkowitz Y, et al. Dobutamine echocardiography in patients with aortic stenosis and left ventricular dysfunction: predicting outcome as a function of management strategy. Chest. 2001;119:1766-77.
26. Blais C, Burwash IG, Mundigler G, et al. Projected valve area at normal flow rate improves the assessment of stenosis severity in patients with low flow, low-gradient aortic stenosis: the multicentre TOPAS (Truly or Pseudo Severe Aortic Stenosis) study. Circulation. 2006;113:711-21.
27. Clavel MA, Burwash IG, Mundigler G, et al. Validation of conventional and simplified methods to calculate projected valve area at normal flow rate in patients with low flow, low gradient aortic stenosis: the multicenter TOPAS (True or Pseudo Severe Aortic Stenosis) study. J Am Soc Echocardiogr. 2010;23:380-6.
28. Nishimura RA, Grantham JA, Connolly HM, Schaff HV, Higano ST, Holmes DR Jr. Low-output, low-gradient aortic stenosis in patients with depressed left ventricular systolic function: the clinical utility of the dobutamine challenge in the catheterization laboratory. Circulation. 2002;106:809-13.
29. Carabello BA, Green LH, Grossman W, Cohn LH, Koster JK, Collins JJ Jr. Hemodynamic determinants of prognosis of aortic valve replacement in critical aortic stenosis and advanced congestive heart failure. Circulation. 1980;62:42-8.
30. Zuppiroli A, Mori F, Olivotto I, Castelli G, Favilli S, Dolara A. Therapeutic implications of contractile reserve elicited by dobutamine echocardiography in symptomatic, low-gradient aortic stenosis. Ital Heart J. 2003;4:264-70.
31. Fougères É, Tribouilloy C, Monchi M, et al. Outcomes of pseudosevere aortic stenosis under conservative treatment. Eur Heart J. 2012;33(19):2426-33.
32. Burwash IG, Lortie M, Pibarot P, et al. Myocardial blood flow in patients with low flow, low gradient aortic stenosis: differences between true and pseudo-severe aortic stenosis. Results from the multicenter TOPAS (Truly or Pseudo-Severe Aortic Stenosis) Study. Heart. 2008;94:1627-33.
33. Rick A Nishimura, Catherine M Otto, Robert O Bonow, et al. 2014 AHA/ACC Guideline for the Management of Patients With Valvular Heart Disease: Executive Summary: A Report of the American College of Cardiology/American Heart Association Task Force on Practice Guidelines. J Am Coll Cardiol. 2014;63(22):2438-88.

3 Echocardiography of Heart Failure: How to Use it in Routine Clinical Practice?

Satoshi Nakatani

INTRODUCTION

American College of Cardiology Foundation/American Heart Association (ACCF/AHA) guideline for the management of heart failure (HF) classify it into four stages according to severity from stage A (patients at high risk of developing HF but with no functional abnormalities of the heart) to stage D (patients with refractory HF).[1] HF can progress from stage A to stage D over its course. Echocardiography is an essential tool in HF management in the clinical practice, which is not only useful for disease staging based on noninvasive repeated evaluations of cardiac function, hemodynamics, and other parameters, but is also capable of measuring indices that are effective in predicting disease outcomes. Echocardiography is also very useful to define etiology which causes HF such as myocardial infarction, valvular heart disease and congenital heart disease.

HOW TO ASSESS SYSTOLIC FUNCTION OF THE HEART?

Since the heart works as a pump to allow blood circulation throughout the body, quantitative analysis of the left ventricular (LV) pumping function is the basis of cardiac function assessments.

Ejection Fraction

Ejection fraction (EF), which is a common pumping function index, is calculated using the following formula:

$$EF = (LVEDV - LVESV)/LVEDV \times 100\ (\%)$$

where LVEDV is the LV end-diastolic volume and LVESV is the LV end-systolic volume. In echocardiographic evaluations, it is recommended to calculate EF by the modified Simpson's method using the apical 4- and 2-chamber views. In applying this method, the shape of LV is assumed to be a lump of ellipsoid disks. Another frequently used method is the visual estimation of EF, in which interobserver variability is considered sufficiently small as long as the observers are well experienced; however, caution is required as the results are highly dependent upon the observers' skills. Visually estimated EF is often expressed in 5% increments, e.g. 20–25%. EF can also be obtained by three-dimensional (3D) echocardiography. Since 3D echocardiography determined LV volumes and EF are not dependent on geometric assumptions, 3D echocardiography may become a standard method of measurements in the near future.

Fractional Shortening

Another popular index, fractional shortening (FS) is calculated by the following formula:

$$FS = (LVEDD - LVESD)/LVEDD \times 100\ (\%)$$

where LVEDD is the LV end-diastolic diameter and LVESD is the LV end-systolic diameter. This measure represents a change in the LV internal diameter along a single plane. Thus, it reflects the contraction of the measured site but does not necessarily reflect whole LV contraction. Nevertheless, as FS is a simple method, it can be used for cases in which LV performance is diffusely impaired. The site of measurement may vary depending on the observer; measurement must be performed at the same site as in the previous measurements to evaluate changes over time.

Stroke Volume

Stroke volume (SV) is the difference between LVEDV and LVESV. SV is also obtained by multiplying the velocity time integral (VTI) of the LV outflow tract velocity with the cross-sectional area of the LV outflow tract obtained by Doppler

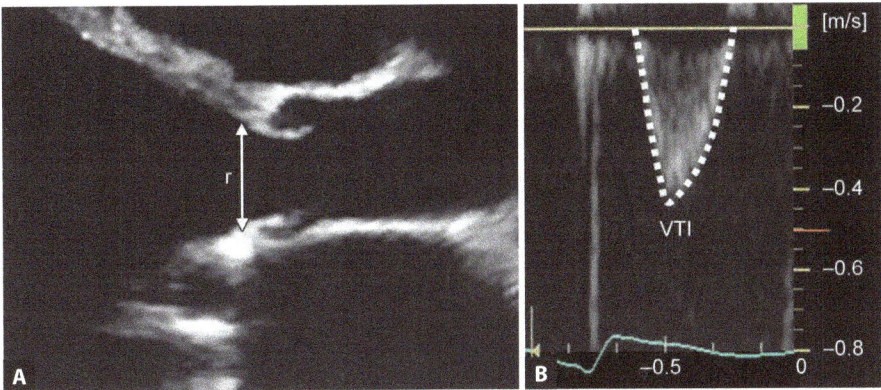

Figs 1A and B: Measurements of LV outflow diameter (r) at the zoomed view (A) and velocity time integral (VTI) of ejection flow (B)

echocardiography **(Figs 1A and B)**. In this calculation, it should be noted that outflow tract diameter measurement errors and inappropriate placement of a sample volume in the LV outflow tract will also cause errors in the results. VTI values <15 cm suggest reduced SV. Changes in VTI over time are a helpful index of change in the chronic HF (CHF) state. In patients with CHF, moderate or severe mitral regurgitation due to LV enlargement-related factors, such as tethering and annular dilation are often observed. In such cases, Doppler echocardiographic SV determination is recommended, since indices obtained based on volume changes do not necessarily reflect the forward flow. However, it should be noted that both SV measurement methods may result in overestimations of the forward flow in the presence of aortic regurgitations which has the backward flow.

Myocardial Strain

In echocardiography, regional contraction is evaluated based on visual observations of the systolic endocardial inward motion and degree of systolic wall thickening, which are subjective assessments. Establishment of an objective assessment method based on quantitative measures has been warranted. Myocardial strain is an index proposed for this purpose; this index reflects the level of regional myocardial shortening and lengthening in one direction and is calculated by the following formula:

Myocardial strain = (myocardial length after change − initial myocardial length)/initial myocardial length

The end-diastolic length is usually used to represent the initial myocardial length. Myocardial strain can be assessed as circumferential and radial strains from the short-axis windows or longitudinal strains from the apical windows. Additionally, area strains in 3D echocardiography can be quantified based on the percentage change in the regional area.[2]

Myocardial strain is an index for local cardiac motion; in contrast, global strain, e.g. the average strain of all segments, measures the entire LV myocardial motion, and it is gaining popularity as a new systolic index. The global longitudinal strain (GLS), which is the average of the segmental longitudinal strains obtained from the apical 4-, 3- and 2-chamber views, is commonly used **(Figs 2 and 3)**. Average GLS in healthy subjects is approximately −20%.[3,4] Although EF and GLS are correlated to a certain degree, they may differ in some cases. Further, GLS may be able to detect systolic abnormalities that are not evaluable by EF, and it could possibly be superior to EF in predicting the outcomes in patients with HF and other patient populations.[5-7]

HF with Reduced EF and HF with Preserved EF

Generally, HF with reduced EF, or HFrEF, is associated with a poor prognosis. LVEF and LV dimensions, such as LVEDD and volume, are significant outcome predictors. On the other hand, patients may exhibit an HF state despite preserved LVEF, which is called HF with preserved EF (HFpEF). HFpEF accounts for approximately 40% of the entire HF cases and is considered to be associated with a poor prognosis, as is HFrEF.[8] However, because of the lack of LV dilatation, marked LVEF decline, and visually recognizable diastolic dysfunction, HFpEF is often not recognized as HF. Therefore, it is important to evaluate both diastolic and systolic functions using comprehensive echocardiography.

HOW TO ASSESS DIASTOLIC FUNCTION OF THE HEART?

In HF evaluation, diastolic function is also important and can be an index for treatment strategy-related decision making and outcome prediction.

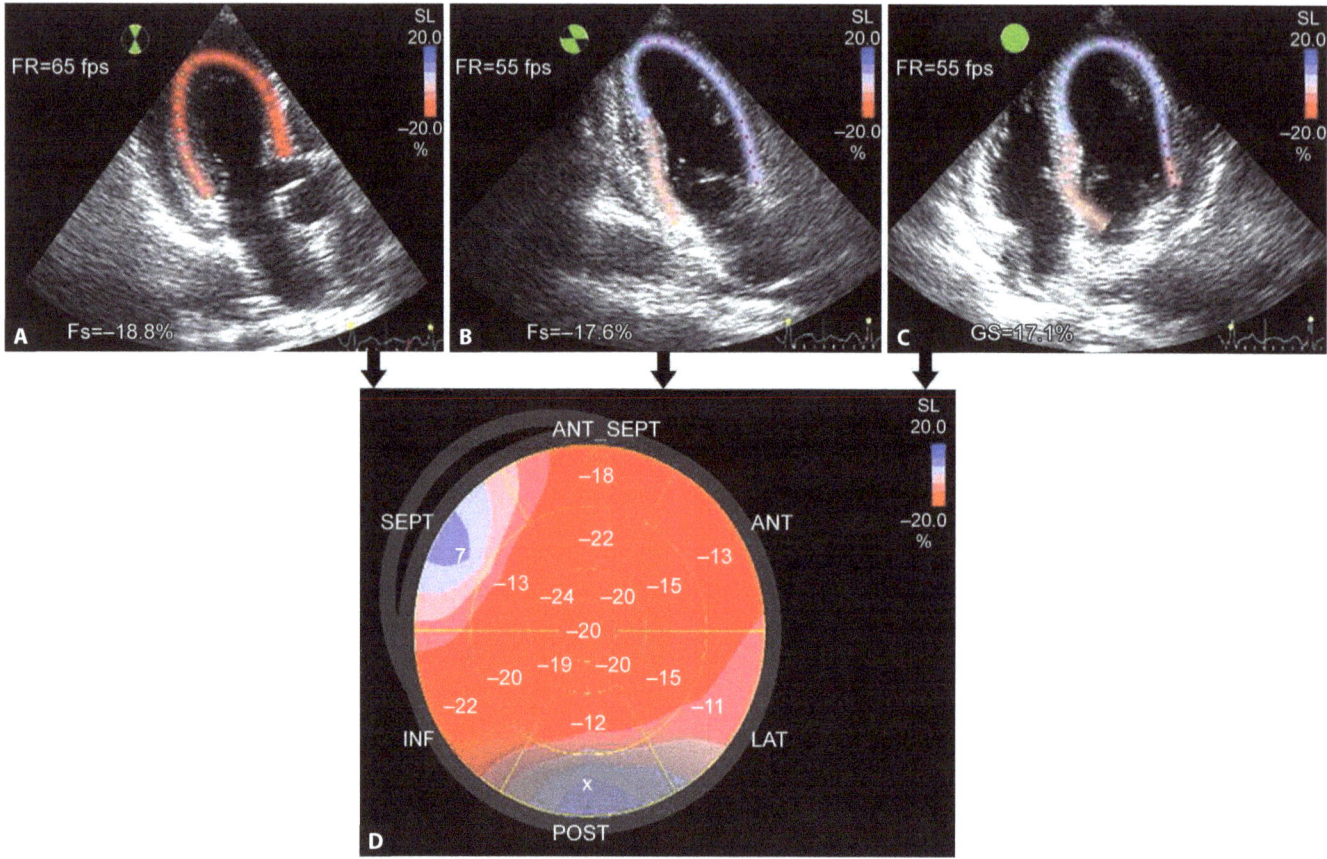

Figs 2A to D: Bull's eye view of longitudinal strain. Upper panels show measurements of longitudinal strains from apical 3-, 2- and 4-chamber views (A to C). By combining these 3 strains, Bull's eye view of strain is obtained (D)

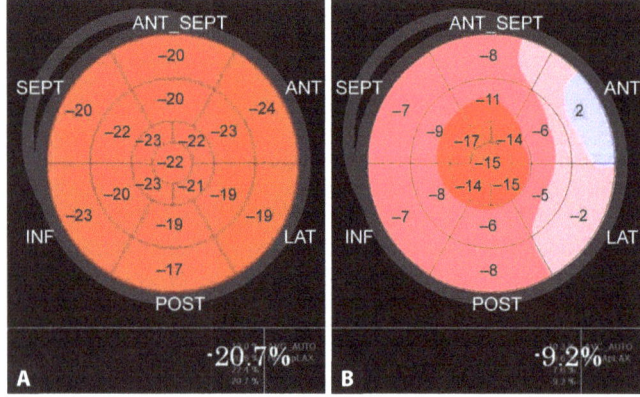

Figs 3A and B: Bull's eye views of longitudinal strain of a normal subject (A) and a patient with dilated cardiomyopathy (B). Global longitudinal strain is -20.7% for a normal subject and -9.2% for a patient with dilated cardiomyopathy

Transmitral Flow Velocity

Transmitral flow velocity is determined by the pressure gradient between the left ventricle and left atrium. The E-wave is generated in early diastole and the A-wave in late diastole. The main factors involved in LV diastolic performance are active LV relaxation during early to mid-diastole and LV stiffness during mid- to late diastole. These factors and left atrial (LA) pressure affect the E- and A-velocity ratio (E/A), generating normal or abnormal relaxation or pseudonormal or restrictive filling patterns **(Figs 4A to D)**. In the presence of abnormal relaxation, the E/A ratio diminishes to <1, and the E-wave deceleration time is prolonged. If disease progression increases LV stiffness and filling pressure, the E/A ratio will indicate a pseudonormalization pattern, and with further disease advancement, a restrictive filling pattern, i.e. E/A ratio ≥2. Cases with a persistent restrictive filling pattern after HF treatment initiation are reported to have a poor outcome.[9] Differentiating normal and abnormal relaxation patterns is important and can be achieved by reducing the preload via the Valsalva maneuver; this test will not result in marked E/A ratio changes in patients with normal LV filling pressures, as opposed to a significant change (by ≥50%) in those with increased pressures. However, since the Valsalva maneuver does not necessarily work successfully in all patients, other indices described further should also be utilized.[10]

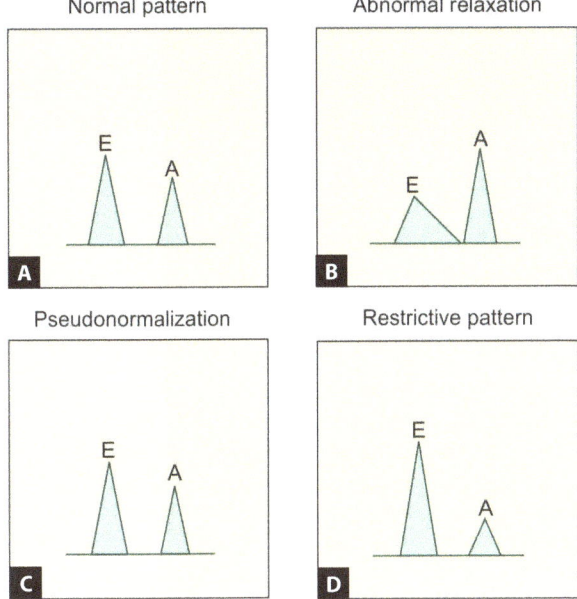

Figs 4A to D: Four types of transmitral flow patterns

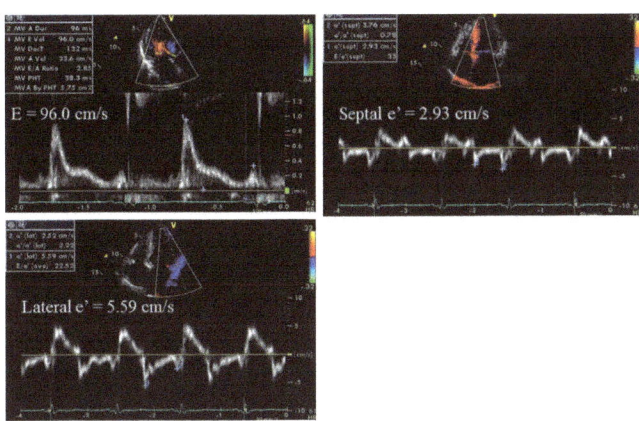

Fig. 5: A case with congestive heart failure. Transmitral flow shows a restrictive pattern with an E-velocity of 96 cm/s. Since averaged e' is 4.3 cm/s, E/e' is as high as 22.3 suggesting elevated LA pressure

Mitral Annular Velocity

Mitral annular early diastolic velocity (e') obtained from tissue Doppler echocardiography reflects LV relaxation and indicates relaxation abnormalities if septal e' is <8 cm/s and if lateral e' is <8.5 cm/s. A previous study reported an increased cardiovascular accident risk with an average e' <3 cm/s at four sites: septum, lateral wall, anterior wall, and inferior wall.[11] If diastolic dysfunction progresses and LA pressure increases, E-velocity is elevated while e' is reduced, further increasing the E/e' ratio. Even in cases with preserved diastolic function, the E/e' ratio has been shown to correlate well with LA pressure. Using septal e' measurements, an E/e' ratio <8 indicates normal LA pressure, whereas E/e' ratio >15 strongly suggests an increased LA pressure. Further, in cases of preserved systolic functions, an advanced diastolic dysfunction is suspected. The E/e' ratio 8–15 is considered to be a border zone. However, it has been reported that the E/e' ratio does not reflect LA pressure in cases of hypertrophic cardiomyopathy with HF symptoms nor the pulmonary wedge pressure in the presence of severely impaired cardiac functions, indicating a limitation of the E/e'-based LA pressure assessments.[10] **Figure 5** shows a case with congestive heart failure. Transmitral flow shows a restrictive pattern with an E-velocity of 96 cm/s. Septal e' is 2.93 cm/s, lateral e' is 5.59 cm/s and averaged e' is 4.3 cm/s. E/e' is 22.3 suggesting elevated LA pressure.

Pulmonary Venous Flow Velocity

Pulsed Doppler echocardiographic recording is performed on the apical 4-chamber view, with the sample volume positioned approximately 1 cm distal from the orifice of the right upper pulmonary vein where it joins the left atrium to obtain pulmonary venous (PV) flow velocity. A typical PV flow pattern consists of biphasic forward flow waves (S1 and S2) in systole, monophasic forward flow wave (D) in diastole, and backward flow wave (reversed A), i.e. a retrograde flow from the left atrium into the pulmonary veins at atrial contraction. Transthoracic approach often fails to clearly record the S1 and records only the S2 as a monophasic wave; if a monophasic wave is obtained, this should be recorded as the S-wave. In the presence of abnormal LV relaxation, poor D-wave progression occurs, reflecting poor transmitral E-wave progression, which increases the S/D ratio. In a compensatory response, LA contraction is enhanced, causing a slight increase in the reversed A-wave velocity in some instances. If LV diastolic dysfunction progresses with increased LV end-diastolic pressure and LA pressure, the E-wave velocity increases, resulting in a higher D-wave velocity and diminished S/D ratio. At atrial contraction, blood is ejected from the left atrium into the left ventricle and pulmonary veins. HF-associated LV filling pressure elevation raises resistance against blood flow from the left atrium into the left ventricle, resulting in a relatively elevated blood flow into the pulmonary veins. This increases the reversed A-wave velocity and prolongs the wave duration; consequently, the forward EF (A-wave duration, Ad) during atrial systole exceeds the retrograde flow duration (PV flow duration, Ard). Such duration difference (Ar –Ad) of >30 ms allows the identification of cases with increased LV end-diastolic pressures.[10]

Left Atrial Volume

Left atrial volume is an important predictor of cardiovascular events. Dilated LA reflects a chronically increased LA pressure. It is common to measure the anterior-posterior dimension of the left atrium in the parasternal long-axis view; however, this dimension is not the sole parameter that reflects LA

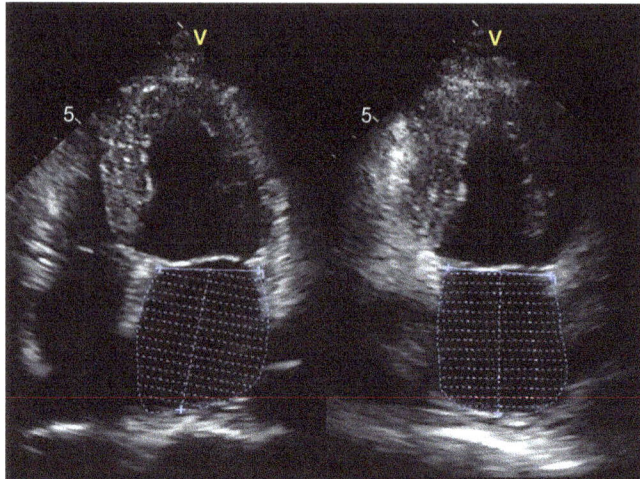

Fig. 6: Measurement of left atrial volume from apical 4- and 2-chamber views by the modified Simpson method

enlargement. Other methods are available: (a) the modified Simpson's method from the apical 4- and 2-chamber views **(Fig. 6)** and (b) the Ellipsoid method, which assumes the left atrium as a spheroid. LA volume obtained by the Ellipsoid method tends to be underestimated compared to that by the modified Simpson's method. Regarding cardiac events, larger LA volumes have been reported to be associated with higher incidences: 3.4 and 4.9 times higher in the groups with 34–53 mL/m^2 and >53 mL/m^2 LA volume indices (LA volume divided by the body surface area), respectively, compared with the incidence in the group with ≤34 mL/m^2 index.[12]

LEFT VENTRICULAR GEOMETRY AND ABNORMAL ECHOES

Some patients with HF may have LV morphological abnormalities; thus, echocardiographic assessments are required. Using a combination of echocardiographically obtained LV mass index and relative wall thickness, LV morphological characteristics can be classified into four groups: normal, concentric remodeling, concentric hypertrophy and eccentric hypertrophy. Eccentric hypertrophy is considered to be associated with a poor prognosis.[13]

Pericardial effusion is often found in a patient with CHF. Echocardiography should be used to assess the amount of pericardial effusion and if there is a possibility of cardiac tamponade. Diastolic collapse of RV or systolic collapse of the right atrium is a clue to diagnose cardiac tamponade. In a situation of blood stasis, a thrombus may be generated. Therefore, LV thrombi are sometimes found in a patient with a dilated ventricle using transthoracic echocardiography. LA thrombi may be found in a patient with atrial fibrillation which transesophageal echocardiography is helpful to detect.

RIGHT VENTRICULAR FUNCTION

In HF, the left ventricle receives more attention, but the right ventricle has its own functions that include delivering blood to the left ventricle via pulmonary vessels and influencing the pulmonary arterial (PA) pressure and right atrial (RA) pressure. Although echocardiographic right ventricular (RV) function assessments have limitations, they are useful for monitoring the course of the disease; RV function can be a decisive factor in disease outcomes.

Tricuspid Annular Plane Systolic Excursion

In an apical 4-chamber view focused on the right ventricle, the M-mode cursor is placed on the lateral tricuspid annulus, and the excursion of the tricuspid annulus (tricuspid annular plane systolic excursion, TAPSE) is measured. The TAPSE method only assesses the tricuspid annular motion, which does not reflect the entire RV function; however, it can be readily performed. TAPSE <16 mm is considered abnormal,[14] and TAPSE <14 mm is considered to suggest a poor prognosis.[15]

Right Ventricular Fractional Area Change

The EF of the right ventricle (RVEF) is difficult to determine because the right ventricle has a complex 3D structure. RV fractional area change (RVFAC) assessment is an alternative method; RV systolic function is estimated based on the RV end-diastolic and end-systolic areas measured in the apical 4-chamber view **(Fig. 7)**.

RVFAC = (RV end-diastolic area − RV end-systolic area)/RV end-diastolic area x 100 (%)

RVFAC values <35% are considered abnormal.

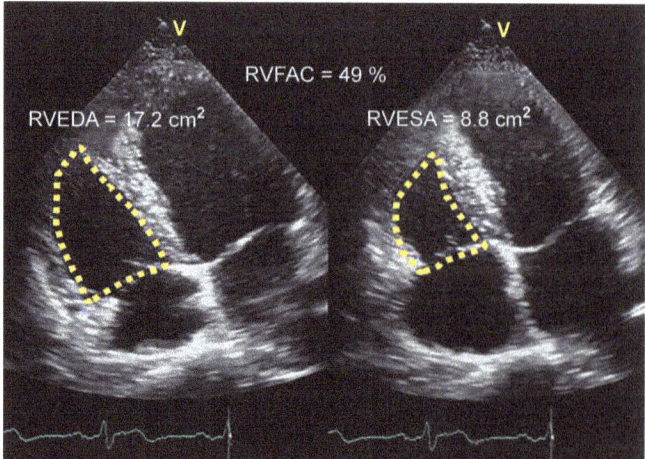

Fig. 7: Assessment of right ventricular fractional area change (FAC)

Systolic Tricuspid Annular Velocity by Tissue Doppler Echocardiography

An apical 4-chamber window is used. The sample volume is placed at the level of the tricuspid annulus of the RV free wall. Tricuspid annular motion is recorded by tissue Doppler echocardiography, and systolic tricuspid annular velocity (s') is obtained; s' values <10 cm/s are considered abnormal,[14] and s' values <9.5 cm/s have been reported as a predictor of a poor disease outcome.[16]

Others

Besides the abovementioned methods, RV global strain measured by speckle tracking echocardiography and RVEF obtained with 3D echocardiographic evaluation have been recently considered as promising RV function assessment methods.

INTRACARDIAC PRESSURE ESTIMATION

Echocardiography allows for noninvasive repeated estimations of the intracardiac pressure.

Assessment of Right Atrial Pressure

HF-associated body fluid retention and RA pressure elevation lead to dilatation of the inferior vena cava (IVC) and disappearance of inspiratory collapse. The American Society of Echocardiography Guidelines in 2010 report the following[14]: (a) IVC diameter ≤21 mm that collapses >50% with a sniff suggests an RA pressure of 3 mm Hg (0–5 mm Hg), (b) IVC diameter >21 mm that collapses <50% with a sniff suggests an RA pressure of 15 mm Hg (10–20 mm Hg), and (c) in other cases, an intermediate value of 8 mm Hg (5–10 mm Hg) may be used.

Estimation of Systolic Pulmonary Arterial Pressure (RV Systolic Pressure)

Peak tricuspid regurgitation flow velocity can be obtained by continuous-wave Doppler echocardiography, and RV-RA pressure difference can be calculated using the simplified Bernoulli equation. By adding an estimated RA pressure provided above to the calculated value, an estimate of the systolic PA pressure (systolic RV pressure) can be obtained.

Estimation of LV Diastolic Pressure and Mean Pulmonary Wedge Pressure

The PA-RV pressure difference can be calculated with the simplified Bernoulli equation using the pulmonary regurgitation end-diastolic flow velocity recorded by continuous-wave Doppler echocardiography. Addition of an estimated RA pressure provided above to the calculated difference can approximate the end-diastolic PA pressure. Mean PA pressure can be obtained from the systolic and diastolic PA pressures described earlier. As the first peak of pulmonary regurgitation velocity reflects a diastolic notch after the pulmonic valve closure, the PA-RV pressure difference during early diastole is considered to reflect mean PA pressure.

CONCLUSION

How to assess HF by using echocardiography has been described here. Recently, HF treatment options have broadened from conventional medical therapies to device-assisted therapies, such as cardiac resynchronization therapies, ventricular assist device therapies, and even heart transplantations. Because echocardiography is useful in each step, from determining the indication of a certain device-assisted therapy to evaluating the effects of the therapy provided, it is indispensable for HF management in the clinical practice.

REFERENCES

1. Yancy CY, Jessup M, Bozkurt B, et al. 2013 ACCF/AHA guideline for the management of heart failure. J Am Coll Cardiol. 2013;62:e147-239.
2. Seo Y, Ishizu T, Enomoto Y, Sugimori H, Aonuma K. Endocardial surface tracking for assessment of regional LV wall deformation with 3D speckle tracking imaging. JACC Cardiovasc Imaging. 2011;4:358-65.
3. Marwick TH, Leano RL, Brown J, et al. Myocardial strain measurement with 2-dimensional speckle-tracking echocardiography: definition of normal range. JACC Cardiovasc Imaging. 2009;2: 80-4.
4. Takigiku K, Takeuchi M, Izumi C, et al. Normal range of left ventricular 2-dimensional strain: Japanese ultrasound speckle tracking of the left ventricle (JUSTICE) study. Circ J. 2012;76: 2623-32.
5. Stanton T, Leano R, Marwick TH. Prediction of all-cause mortality from global longitudinal speckle strain: comparison with ejection fraction and wall motion scoring. Circ Cardiovasc Imaging. 2009;2:356-64.
6. Nahum J, Bensaid A, Dussault C, et al. Impact of longitudinal myocardial deformation on the prognosis of chronic heart failure patients. Circ Cardiovasc Imaging. 2010;3:249-56.
7. Mignot A, Donal E, Zaroui A, et al. Global longitudinal strain as a major predictor of cardiac events in patients with depressed left ventricular function: a multicenter study. J Am Soc Echocardiogr. 2010;23:1019-24.
8. Owan TE, Hodge DO, Herges RM, et al. Trends in prevalence and outcome of heart failure with preserved ejection fraction. N Engl J Med. 2006;355:251-9.
9. Pinamonti B, Zecchin M, Di Lenarda A, et al. Persistence of restrictive left ventricular filling pattern in dilated cardiomyopathy: an ominous prognostic sign. J Am Coll Cardiol. 1997;29:604-12.
10. Nagueh SF, Smiseth OA, Appleton CP, et al. Recommendations for the evaluation of left ventricular diastolic function by echocardiography. An update from the American Society of Echocardiography and the European Association of Cardiovascular Imaging. J Am Soc Echocardiogr. 2016;29:277-314.

11. Wang M, Yip G, Yu CM, et al. Independent and incremental prognostic value of early mitral annulus velocity in patients with impaired left ventricular systolic function. J Am Coll Cardiol. 2005;45:272-7.
12. Tamura H, Watanabe T, Nishiyama S, et al. Increased left atrial volume index predicts a poor prognosis in patients with heart failure. J Card Fail. 2011;17:210-6.
13. Dini FL, Capozza P, Donati F, et al. Patterns of left ventricular remodeling in chronic heart failure: prevalence and prognostic implications. Am Heart J. 2011;161:1088-95.
14. Rudski LG, Lai WW, Afilalo J, et al. Guidelines for the echocardiographic assessment of the right heart in adults: a report from the American Society of Echocardiography endorsed by the European Association of Echocardiography, a registered branch of the European Society of Cardiology, and the Canadian Society of Echocardiography. J Am Soc Echocardiogr. 2010;23:685-713.
15. Dini FL, Conti U, Fontanive P, et al. Right ventricular dysfunction is a major predictor of outcome in patients with moderate to severe mitral regurgitation and left ventricular dysfunction. Am Heart J. 2007;154:172-9.
16. Damy T, Viallet C, Lairez O, et al. Comparison of four right ventricular systolic echocardiographic parameters to predict adverse outcomes in chronic heart failure. Eur J Heart Fail. 2009;11:818-24.

4
Speckle Tracking Echocardiography: Basics and Clinical Applications

Navin C Nanda

Traditionally, left ventricular (LV) systolic function has been evaluated echocardiographically by assessing inward motion of the ventricular walls during systole and estimating the ejection fraction. With the advent of Doppler echocardiography, mitral inflow velocities were used to gain an understanding of LV diastolic function. Subsequently, with the realization that the LV also shortened longitudinally with the base moving towards the apex in systole, an attempt was made to study this motion using Doppler by filtering out high frequency signals from blood components and retaining only high amplitude waves from wall motion (tissue Doppler imaging). However, for accurate estimation of longitudinal motion by this technique, the ultrasonic beam needs to be kept parallel to wall motion with the Doppler intercept angle close to zero. This becomes a challenge with the LV walls moving in and out of the ultrasound beam throughout the cardiac cycle. Also, a hypokinetic segment may go undetected because the adjacent normally moving segment may pull it with it, the so-called tethering effect. Because of this, attention has focused on using two-dimensional echocardiography, which does not have the angle insonation problem of Doppler, to derive various markers of segmental and global muscle deformation, in particular thickening and shortening parameters. The two-dimensional technique called speckle tracking echocardiography (2D STE) is based on the premise that the equipment can follow small groups of myocardial pixels called speckles (produced by the interaction of the ultrasonic beam with the myocardium) because each group has a unique ultrasonic signature enabling it to be tracked throughout the cardiac cycle.

> *Speckle tracking echocardiography is a new addition to the echocardiographic techniques assessing ventricular function. It is used to assess segmental and global muscle deformation. 3D STE is superior to 2D STE because it enables to interrogate the same group of speckles throughout the cardiac cycle.*

A potential problem does exist with this modality. Because each two-dimensional image represents only a thin slice through the LV, it is easy for the group of speckles (called kernels) to move out of the examining plane and in some instances the equipment may be tracking a similar but not the same group of pixels during the cardiac cycle, this could introduce errors in measurements. A potential solution is using three-dimensional echocardiography (3DE) which provides a large pyramidal shaped section of the heart increasing the chances of interrogating the same group of speckles throughout the cardiac cycle **(Figs 1A and B)**.

Comparing 2D STE data to a variety of modalities has allowed for validation of the technique. This has included validation by comparison with tissue Doppler imaging, hemodynamics, tagged magnetic resonance imaging, and sonomicrometry studies.[1-3] The intra- and interobserver reproducibility of STE is superior to tissue Doppler but it is still not in the ideal range and there are highly significant inter-vendor differences. Despite these limitations, the technique has been found useful in assessing various parameters of LV segmental and global function in a variety of clinical scenarios. To understand these parameters, it is important to gain an insight into the structure and function of cardiac muscle.

CARDIAC MUSCLE STRUCTURE

> *The geometry and mechanics of cardiac contraction are highly complex and involves not only inward thickening but also rotation and translation motion due to different orientation and function of muscle fibers.*

Controversies exist regarding the orientation and function of muscle fibers in the heart.

In the helical model introduced by Torrent Guasp and popularized by Dr Buckberg, an eminent cardiac surgeon, a

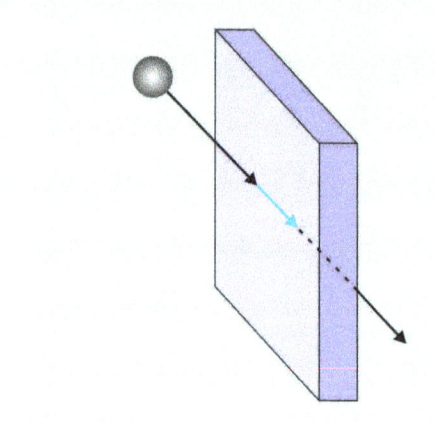
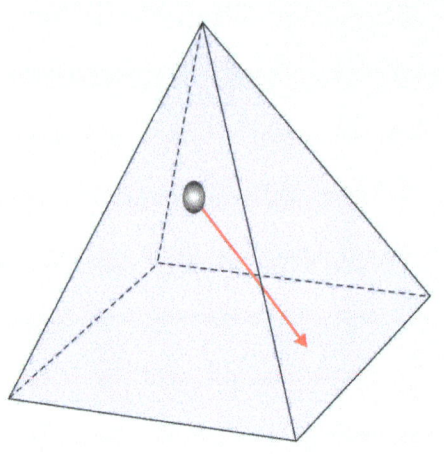

Figs 1A and B: Advantage of three-dimensional speckle tracking echocardiography over the two-dimensional (2D) technique. (A) As 2D echocardiography represents only a thin slice through the cardiac structures, it is easy for the speckle particle to move out of the scanning plane as the heart moves, making it difficult or impossible to track the same speckle during the cardiac cycle; (B) On the other hand, with the three-dimensional (3D) technique, a much larger pyramidal-shaped section is obtained, making it more difficult for the speckle particle to move out of the 3D data set (Figure courtesy of Toshiba Medical Systems Europe BV)
Reproduced from: Biswas M, Sudhakar S, Nanda NC, Buckberg G, Pradhan M, Roomi AU, et al. Two- and Three-dimensional Speckle Tracking Echocardiography: Clinical Applications and Future Directions. Echocardiography. 2013;30:88-105.

single myocardial muscle band consisting of helical fibers is folded upon itself. In this model, the cardiac muscle is formed of three layers.[4-6] The inner (descending segment) and outer oblique (ascending segment) layers each occupy a quarter of the total muscle mass whereas the middle layer which wraps around two-thirds of the ventricles transversely sparing the apex occupies approximately half of the total cardiac muscle mass[4,6-9] **(Fig. 2)**.

This complex arrangement of muscle fibers results in not only inward thickening of the LV walls and longitudinal shortening, but also rotation and translation motion. All these movements are important and contribute to normal functioning of the ventricles.

Contraction of the outer layer (ascending segment) leads to counterclockwise rotation of the apex in systole. During the same time, the base of the ventricle rotates in an opposite clockwise direction. Opposite movements occur in diastole with the apex rotating clockwise (presumably due to contraction of the inner/descending segment) and the base in a counterclockwise direction.[9]

METHODS OF SPECKLE TRACKING ECHOCARDIOGRAPHY AND PARAMETERS MEASURED

There are two methods for speckle tracking. The conventional method tracks groups of adjacent speckles, to judge the direction, speed, and distance of movement between areas in the myocardium. Velocity vector imaging is a similar concept

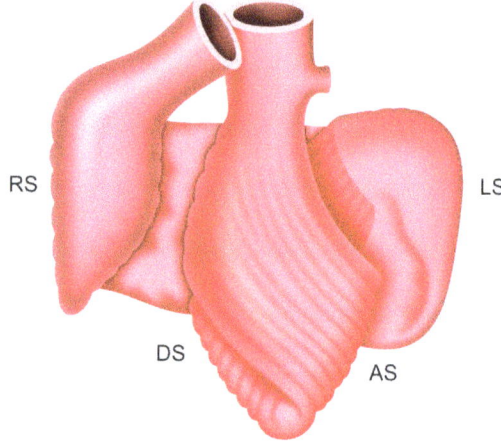

Fig. 2: Schematic model. It shows apical and basal loops. The apical loop consists of an outer ascending segment (AS) with oblique counterclockwise fiber orientation and an inner descending segment (DS) with fibers oriented in an oblique clockwise direction. The basal loop covers the upper two-thirds of the apical loop and its fibers are oriented in a circumferential or transverse direction. It can be considered to have 2 segments—right (RS) and left (LS)
Reproduced from: Buckberg G, Hoffman JI, Nanda NC, et al. Ventricular torsion and untwisting: further insights into mechanics and timing interdependence: a viewpoint. Echocardiography 2011;28:782-804, with permission from Wiley-Blackwell.

but builds on the conventional method by applying additional physiologic principles to track the speckles more closely[10] **(Fig. 3)**.

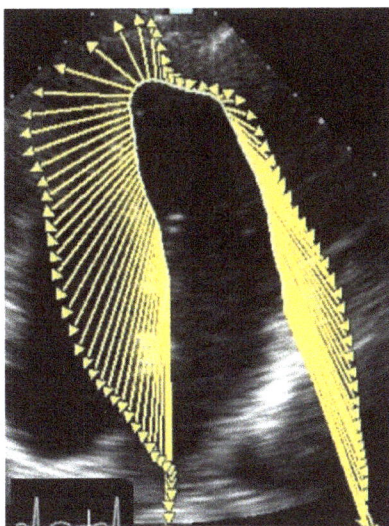

Fig. 3: Velocity vector imaging. Apical four-chamber view: The direction of the arrows indicates the direction of the movement of the left ventricular myocardium and the length of the arrows indicates the velocity of such movement
Reproduced from: Buckberg G, Hoffman J I, Nanda NC, et al. Ventricular torsion and untwisting: further insights into mechanics and timing interdependence: a viewpoint. Echocardiography. 2011;28:782-804, with permission from Wiley-Blackwell

The various measurements that can be measured by STE are as follows:

Global and segmental radial, transversal, circumferential and longitudinal strain, apical and basal rotation, twist and torsion, all by 2D STE. Strain rate can also be measured. In addition, area strain can be measured by 3D STE. These measurements are fully explained and illustrated in **Figures 4 to 7**.

> *Global longitudinal strain is considered to be the most reproducible and reliable parameter and is highest in the apex.*

Global longitudinal strain is considered to be the most reproducible and reliable parameter. The longitudinal strain is highest in the apex and there is an incremental gradient in longitudinal strain from the base to the apex. Additionally, strain values are lower in the subepicardium than they are in the subendocardium **(Fig. 8)**.

A distinct and clinically useful parameter measured only by 3DE is area strain. This represents a combination of longitudinal and circumferential strain. Approximate normal values of various parameters, some of which are not fully established yet are given in **Table 1**.

Image Acquisition

Acquisition protocols for STE are similar to routine echocardiography. Endocardial borders need to be identified for accurate circumferential, transverse, and radial tracking. Obtaining high quality images is necessary to identify the endocardial borders. This is an important consideration as poor quality 2D images will give inaccurate results. The ideal frame rate lies between 50 and 70 frames per second.[11] For 3D images, the suggested setting is between 20 and 30 volumes per second. Gated images are obtained with the patient's breath held in end-expiration and should be accompanied by a stable ECG trace. The images should be taken over three cardiac cycles. The software processing then averages the measurements to produce final values.

> *The images obtained must be of high quality with clear delineation of endocardial borders for optimizing the results of speckle tracking echocardiography.*

The quality of the images can be reduced by foreshortening the chamber of interest or by having an inappropriate frame rate. Foreshortening the chamber can limit visualization of the endocardial borders. Having a frame rate that is too high may lead to aberrations in calculations as the algorithms pick up minimal movements and magnify their effect. Conversely, a frame rate that is too low may underestimate and/or provide inaccurate tracking measurements by compromising temporal resolution.

In order to estimate left and right ventricular longitudinal and transverse strains and strain rates by 2D STE, two-chamber, three-chamber, and apical four-chamber views must be obtained. After obtaining these views, the operator can assess left and right ventricular strain. By obtaining parasternal short-axis views, the operator can obtain radial and circumferential strains and strain rates. The parasternal short-axis views are necessary for obtaining rotation, twist, and torsion analysis. Image acquisition should include a basal short-axis view from the tips of the papillary muscles and another view at apex at a location just proximal to the end of the left ventricular cavity. Myocardial segmentation varies widely between vendor software. Despite this the left ventricle is usually segmented into a 16- or 18-segment model.

Image Processing

The region of interest is first manually identified. Next, the appropriate view is used to evaluate each chamber. The short-axis or apical views are used to trace the endocardial border for the left ventricle. The apical four-chamber view is used to trace the endocardial border for the atria and right ventricle.

The wall thickness is manually adjusted but the epicardium is generally automatically traced by the system. The manual adjustment should be done particularly carefully when the relatively thin atrial and right ventricular walls are traced. The change of thickness is uniform between the inner and outer trace when the adjustments are made in 2D STE.

Segmental analysis is typically done, as mentioned earlier, in a 16- to 18-segment model. The atria are divided into three

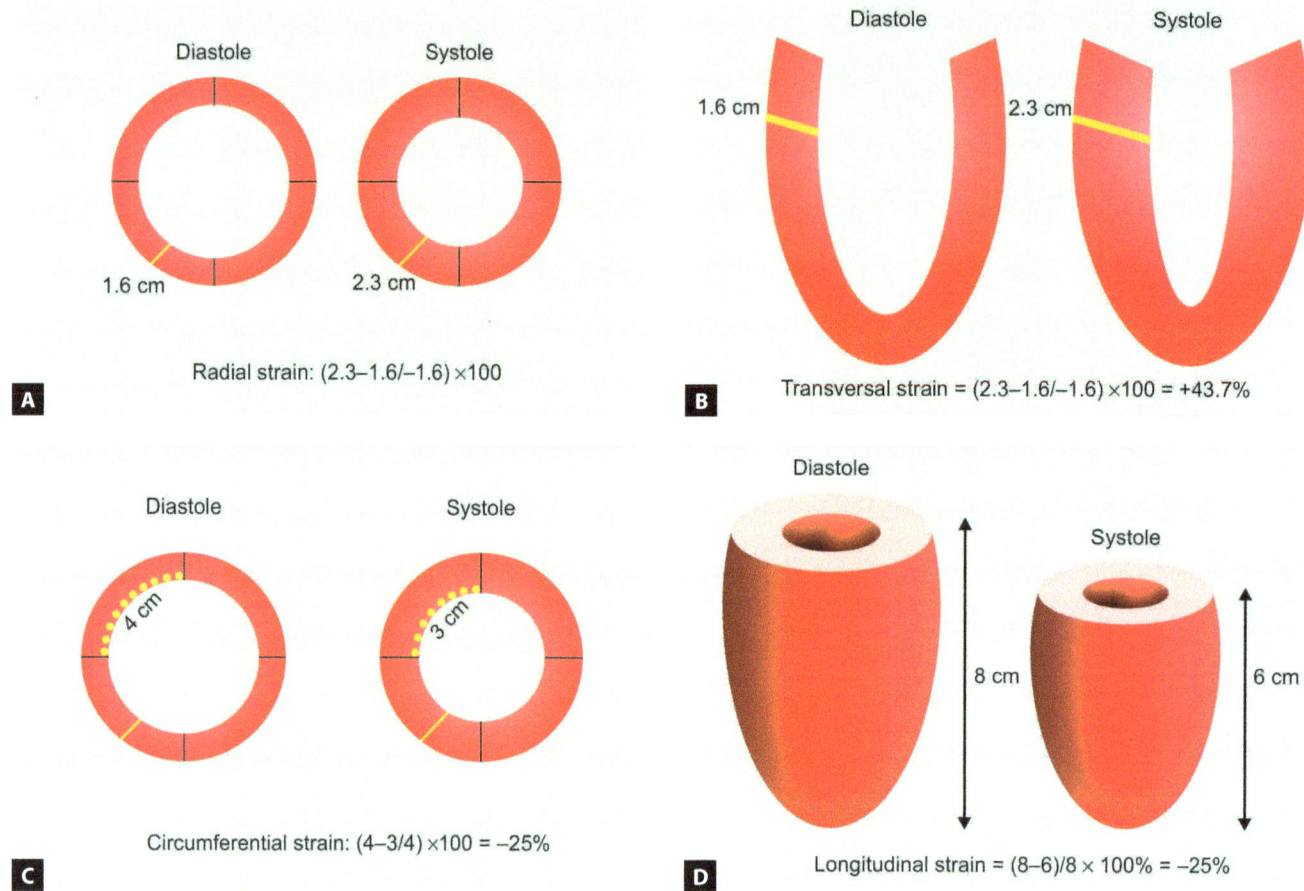

Figs 4A to D: (A) Radial strain shows radial thickening of the myocardium during systole. In the end-diastolic frame on the left the myocardial thickness is 1.6 cm and increases to 2.3 cm in end-systole as depicted on the right; hence, the radial strain will be +43.7%; (B) Transversal strain. The calculations are similar to radial strain except that the measurements are done using apical views; (C) Circumferential strain. This refers to the change in the circumference of each segment as denoted by the dotted yellow line. There is a 25% reduction in the circumferential length in end-systole from the baseline end-diastole; hence, the circumferential strain will be −25%; (D) Longitudinal strain shows shortening of ventricular length during systole. The figure on the left denotes end diastole and the one on the right depicts end systole. Note the downward descent of the mitral annulus toward the apex in systole. There is a reduction in length by 2 cm, which is a 25% decrease. As there is a decrease in the longitudinal length, it will be denoted by a negative (−) sign; hence the longitudinal strain will be −25%. Courtesy of Siemens Ultrasound. A and C are courtesy of Toshiba Medical system Europe BV.
Reproduced from: Biswas M, Sudhakar S, Nanda NC, Buckberg G, Pradhan M, Roomi AU, et al. Two- and Three-dimensional Speckle Tracking Echocardiography: Clinical Applications and Future Directions. Echocardiography. 2013;30:88-105

to six segments to correlate the roof, lateral wall, and interatrial septum. The right ventricle is divided into six segments, which correlate the following: apical left septum, mid-left septum, basal left septum, apical free wall, mid-RV free wall and basal RV free wall. When movements such as global twist are studied, mean measurements of the segments in the base are compared to mean values for segments in the apex. In order to ensure reliable tracking, vendors have developed a variety of tools. One such example is where the software identifies regions with suboptimal tracking. After identification, these segments are excluded from the final analysis and results. Other vendors also use scales to provide accuracy estimates of tracking. The clinical usefulness of both 2D and 3D STE are listed in **Tables 2 and 3**, respectively.

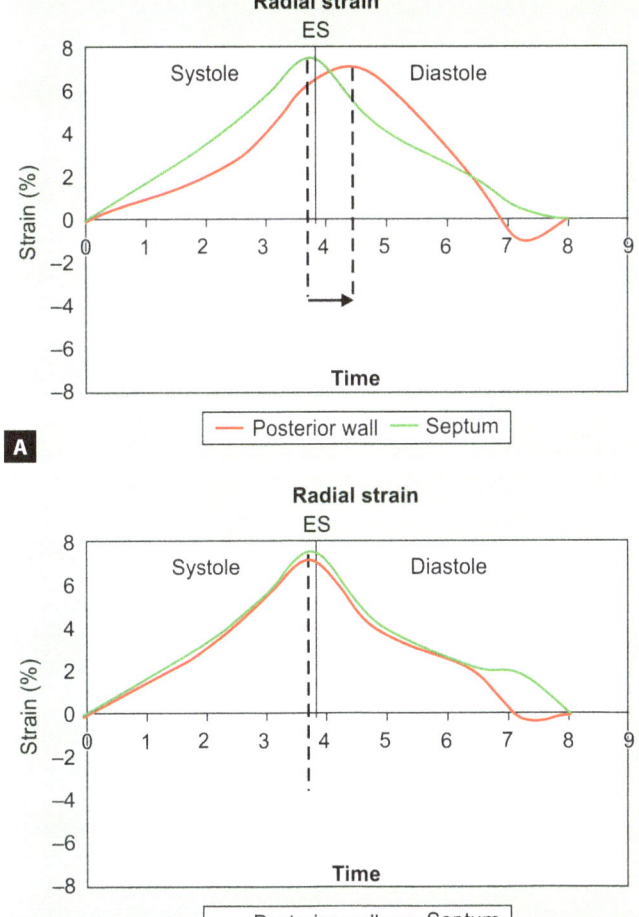

Figs 5A and B: Dysschronous left ventricular contraction depicted by radial strain. Note the time difference between peak strain of the posterior wall and ventricular septum denoted by the yellow arrow. The peak strain or contraction of the posterior wall is much delayed in comparison with the septum (A). The goal of resynchronization therapy is to get the peak strains (contractions) as close as possible to each other as depicted in (B).
Abbreviation: ES, end-systole.
Reproduced from: Biswas M, Sudhakar S, Nanda NC, Buckberg G, Pradhan M, Roomi AU, et al. Two- and Three-dimensional Speckle Tracking Echocardiography: Clinical Applications and Future Directions. Echocardiography. 2013;30:88-105

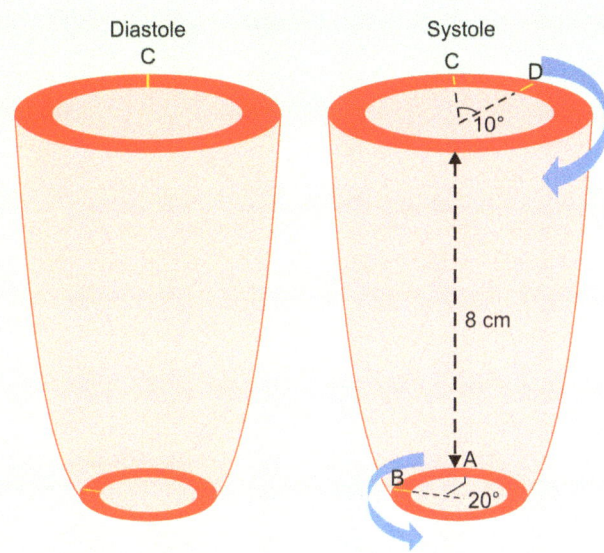

Fig. 6: Differential rotational movements of left ventricular apex and the base. In the normal individual, the apex rotates more than the base. By convention, counterclockwise motion is assigned a positive (+) sign and clockwise motion a negative (−) sign. In the above example, the apex rotates 20° in counterclockwise direction from end-diastole (point A) to end-systole (point B), hence the rotation of the apex will be +20°. As the base rotates at the same time 10° clockwise from point C to D, the rotation of the base will be −10°. 'Twist' is calculated as the algebraic difference in the rotation of the apex and base, in other words, how far apart a point in the apex and base move from each other. In the above example, the twist will be apex rotation (20°) minus base rotation (−10°), that is, 20-(-10) = +30° Twist can be calculated for any point in the myocardium compared to a reference basal point. 'Torsion' is a way of adjusting for the distance of a point of interest from the reference point in the base, as it is expected that the twist will be higher for the segments farther away from the base. Torsion = twist/the distance from the base or distance between any 2 points that are evaluated. In the above example, the torsion, calculated between apex and base, would be 30/8 = 3.75°/cm. As would be expected, the middle portion of the left ventricle would not show any rotation. Courtesy of Toshiba Medical Systems Europe BV.
Reproduced from: Biswas M, Sudhakar S, Nanda NC, Buckberg G, Pradhan M, Roomi AU, et al. Two- and Three-dimensional Speckle Tracking Echocardiography: Clinical Applications and Future Directions. Echocardiography. 2013;30:88-105

The STE is being increasingly utilized for early detection of chemotherapy induced cardiotoxicity by detecting diminished longitudinal strain. This change occurs before decrease in ejection fraction and withdrawing the culprit agent at this subclinical stage results in restoration of LV function

STE is also utilized for detection of subclinical myocardial disease in several diseases like diabetes, systemic hypertension, etc.

Tracking results can also be displayed as velocity vectors by some 2D STE applications. Each vector expresses the direction and magnitude of the velocity. Here the direction of the vector is used to denote the direction of the velocity. Similarly, the length of the arrow is used to depict the magnitude of the velocity. The velocity can then be qualitatively summarized with a series of arrows along the tracked contour of the chamber. The vectors can also be superimposed upon the echocardiographic images

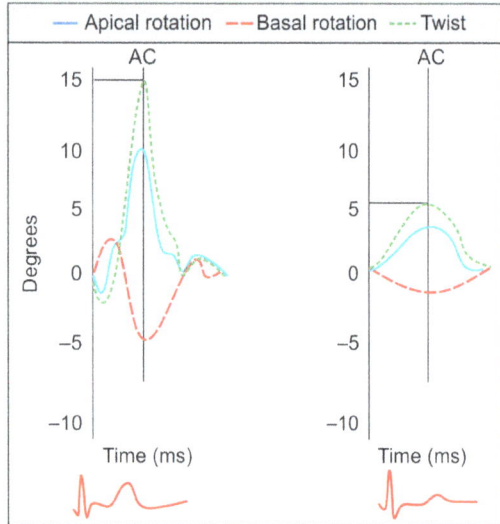

Fig. 7: Left ventricular (LV) rotation of the base and apex in a normal individual (A) compared with poor LV function (B). Note the decrease in basal and apical rotation as well as the twist in poor LV function

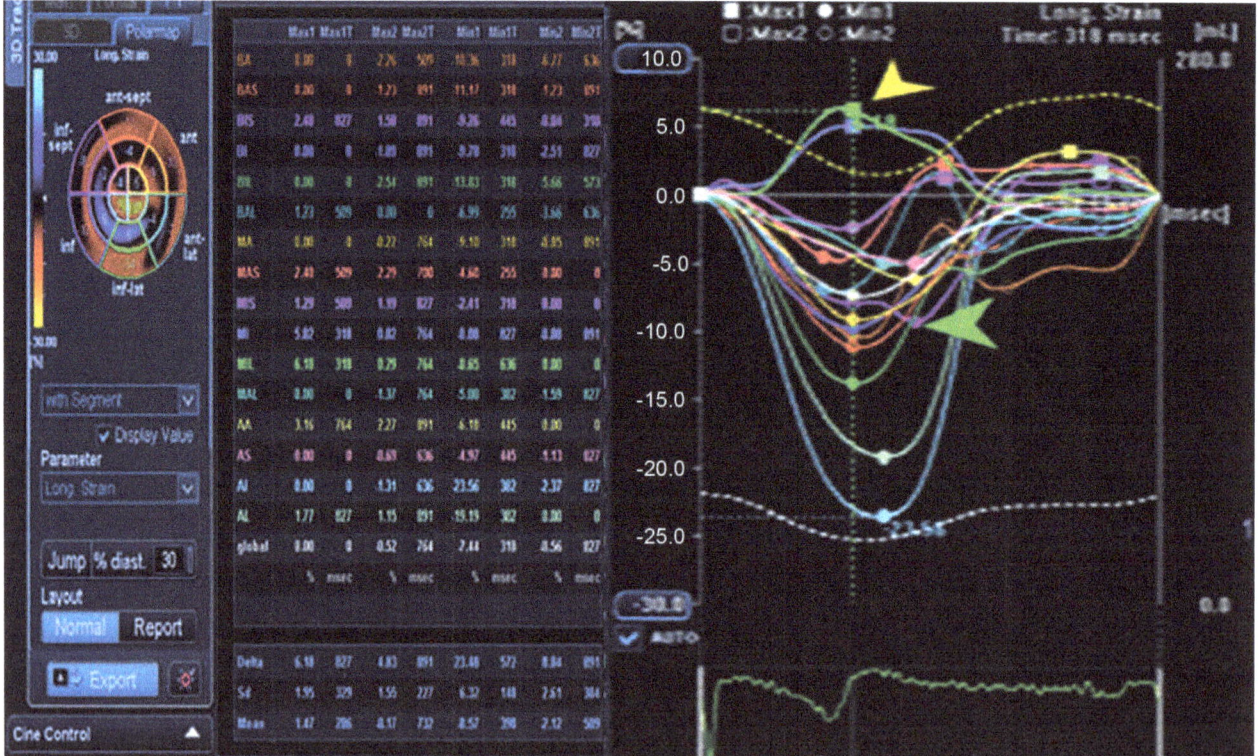

Fig. 8: An example of the display of information by a commercial software. The graph on the right side of the figure displays longitudinal strain values from a single cardiac cycle. Different myocardial segments are denoted by different colors of the curves. The dotted vertical green line indicates end-systole. As normal longitudinal strain is denoted by a negative sign, normal longitudinal strain curves would be plotted below the baseline with negative values and they would peak in end-systole. However, in this example, some curves are abnormal. For instance, the light green curve (yellow arrowhead) representing the mid-inferolateral segment (MIL) of the left ventricle is located above the baseline indicative of wall thinning during systole. The peak strain value can be read from the graph and in this case is abnormal at around +6%. Also, the purple curve (green arrowhead) representing the basal inferoseptal segment peaks way beyond end-systole and during diastole indicating postsystolic thickening. This finding is frequently associated with myocardial ischemia. All the values and curves shown in the illustration were obtained using 3D echocardiography.

Reproduced from: Biswas M, Sudhakar S, Nanda NC, Buckberg G, Pradhan M, Roomi AU, et al. Two- and Three-dimensional Speckle Tracking Echocardiography: Clinical Applications and Future Directions. Echocardiography. 2013;30:88-105

Table 1 Approximate normal left ventricular strain and rotation parameters by 2D STE from the literature[12-15]

Global longitudinal strain %	Mean = –20, (16–22)
Global circumferential strain %	Mean = –23, (21–28)
Global radial strain %	Mean = +47, (35–55)
Longitudinal strain rate (1/s)(rate of shortening)	Mean = –1.10
*Global area strain (longitudinal + circumferential)%	Mean = –39
Apical rotation	+10 degrees
Basal rotation	–5 degrees
Twist	+15 degrees
Torsion	1.87 degrees/cm

*Measured using three-dimensional (3D) STE. 2D STE: two-dimensional speckle tracking echocardiography.

Table 2 Clinical usefulness of two-dimensional speckle tracking echocardiography (2D STE)

1. Myocardial ischemia	• Reduction in strain by 2D STE more objective and accurate than the traditional method of assessing WMA[16] • Longitudinal, radial and circumferential strain reduced in ischemic areas in coronary artery disease[17,18] • Pansystolic thickening (deformation), detected by radial strain correlates with the severity of ischemia[19] • Postsystolic thickening/contraction occurring after aortic valve closure noted using radial strain by 2D STE has been found to be mainly associated with myocardial ischemia • 2D STE strain parameters may also help differentiate athlete's heart from hypertrophic cardiomyopathy **(Table 4)**
2. Myocardial infarction	• 2D STE successful in differentiating transmural from subendocardial infarction by showing lower circumferential strain in the former[20] • Reduced subendocardial LV twist noted in patients with ST-segment elevated myocardial infarction[21] • Decreased LV torsion and segmental longitudinal strain predicts progressive LV dilation after myocardial infarction[17-19,22-24]
3. Myocardial viability	Strain measurements by 2D STE more objective and accurate than visual WMA for assessment of myocardial viability during low-dose dobutamine stress echocardiography. 2D STE differentiates active contraction from passive motion due to tethering[25]
4. Heart failure with normal LVEF	Reduced and delayed LV untwisting at rest and exercise[26]
5. Cardiac resynchronization therapy (CRT)	• Combining longitudinal strain from TDI velocity with 2D STE radial strain may help in predicting response to CRT[27] • Longitudinal strain delay index (calculated from the difference between peak and end-systolic strain) of >25% predicts response to CRT (sensitivity 95%, specificity 83%)[28] • Speckle Tracking and Resynchronization (STAR) study showed radial and transversal strain superior to longitudinal and circumferential strain in predicting LVEF response and long-term survival after CRT[29] **(Fig. 5)** • Lack of dyssynchrony before CRT by 2D STE radial strain associated with death or hospitalization for heart failure after CRT[30]
6. Stress cardiomyopathy	Impaired longitudinal strain noted particularly in apical and mid-ventricular segments[31]

Contd...

Contd...

7. Restrictive cardiomyopathy	Impaired longitudinal deformation and twist mechanics are noted[32,33]
8. Constrictive pericarditis	Impaired LV circumferential deformation and torsion[33]
9. Detection of rejection and coronary stenosis in heart transplant patients	Sudden reduction of more ≥ 15% in global radial strain associated with acute rejection. Decrease in strain and strain rate at rest and with Dobutamine stress echo useful to detect significant coronary stenosis[6]
10. Early detection of chemotherapy induced cardiotoxicity	Reduction in radial strain may occur before changes in LVEF and associated with histological changes[34]
11. Detection of subclinical disease/early myocardial involvement	Reduction in strain may occur before changes in LVEF in systemic hypertension, diabetes mellitus, systemic sclerosis, amyloidosis, Duchenne's muscular dystrophy and Kawasaki syndrome[35-38]
12. Valvular heart disease	• Decreased radial, circumferential and longitudinal strain in patients with severe aortic stenosis and normal LVEF. Long-term follow-up after valve replacement show significant improvement with no change in EF[39] • Reduced preoperative 2D STE longitudinal strain in the ventricular septum (apical 4-chamber view) predicts a postoperative LVEF decrease of ≥10% in patients with chronic severe mitral regurgitation[40]
13. Congenital heart disease	• *Atrial septal defect*: Basal clockwise rotation during systole is reduced[41,42] • *Tetralogy of Fallot*: Right ventricular global longitudinal strain and strain rate are significantly decreased[43]
14. Chronic pulmonary hypertension (PH)	2D global free-wall longitudinal strain is reduced in patients with PH[44]
15. Advanced chronic renal disease	2D global longitudinal strain is superior to 2D LVEF in predicting cardiovascular mortality.[45]
16. Assessment of LV and RV function after mitral clip implantation	2D STE demonstrates significant increase in LV and RV longitudinal strains[46]

Abbreviations: CRT, cardiac resynchronization therapy; LV, left ventricle; LVEF, left ventricular ejection fraction; RV, right ventricle; TDI, tissue Doppler imaging; WMA, wall motion abnormality.
Reproduced from: Biswas M, Sudhakar S, Nanda NC, Buckberg G, Pradhan M, Roomi AU, et al. Two- and three-dimensional speckle tracking echocardiography: clinical applications and future directions. Echocardiography. 2013;30:88-105.

Table 3 Clinical usefulness of three-dimensional speckle tracking echocardiography (3D STE)

1. Ischemic LV dysfunction	3D STE longitudinal and area strains correlate with infarct size and scar extent evaluated by magnetic resonance imaging[47]
2. Acute myocardial infarction	Global 3D longitudinal strain superior to other echo findings in predicting LV function improvement following acute myocardial infarction[48]
3. LV wall-motion abnormalities (WMA)	• 3D STE superior to 2D STE for assessing LV WMA[49] • 3D area strain accurate and reproducible in deleting LV WMA as evaluated by experienced echocardiographers[50,51]
4. Early LV systolic dysfunction	3D global area strain identifies early LV systolic dysfunction in patients with risk factors for heart failure[52]
5. LV volume assessment	LV volume assessment more accurate and more reproducible by 3D STE as compared to 2D STE using cardiac magnetic resonance as a reference[53]
6. Left ventricular dyssynchrony	• Systolic dyssynchrony index of 9.8%, 93% sensitive and 75% specific in predicting response to CRT (meta-analysis of 73 studies)[54] • 3D STE assessment of strain is superior to 2D STE in LV lead positioning[55]
7. LV noncompaction	3D STE confirms 2D STE findings that LV twist is nearly absent with both apex and base moving in the same direction (clockwise) in systole[56]

Contd...

Contd...

8. Differentiation of hypertrophic cardiomyopathy from cardiac amyloidosis	3D LV basal radial strain more reduced in amyloidosis (7.5 ± 19.7%) than HCM (22.3 ± 22.7%, P < 0.0001); also, radial strain increased from base to apex in amyloidosis, but decreased in HCM (normal but reduced pattern)[57]
9. Takotsubo cardiomyopathy	3D STE provides rapid detection and follow-up of LV WMA[58]
10. Cardiac sarcoidosis	Global radial strain significantly lower in sarcoidosis (18.5 ± 8.4%) than dilated cardiomyopathy (28.5 ± 8.3%, P < 0.01). Global radial strain ≤ 21.1%, 70% sensitive and 88% specific in differentiating sarcoidosis from DCM[59]
11. Sickle cell disease	3D STE detects LV diastolic dysfunction[60]
12. Hypertension	3D STE global strain reduced in untreated early hypertensives compared with controls[61]
13. Transcatheter aortic valve replacement (TAVR)	3D STE similar to 2D STE in showing increased LV global longitudinal strain and twist following TAVR (especially when pre-TAVR LVEF was decreased), but faster image acquisition and data analysis[62]
14. Atrial septal defect	3D right ventricular ejection fraction and apical strain more sensitive predictors of unfavorable outcome than 2D Doppler indexes[63]
15. Chronic pulmonary hypertension (PH)	3D RV volume and 2D and 3D STE of RV found superior to conventional 2D parameters in detecting early RV failure in chronic PH and predicting mortality[44]
16. Post-cardiac surgery abnormal ventricular septal motion	Integrated cardioplegia found superior to antegrade cardioplegia by demonstrating improvement as opposed to deterioration of some ventricular septal segments using 3D strain parameters[64]
17. Assessment of LV and RV function after mitral clip implantation	3D LV and RV global free-wall longitudinal strain, 3D area strain and 3D RV EF improve significantly following Mitral Clip implantation[46]

Abbreviations: CRT, cardiac resynchronization therapy; EF, ejection fraction; LV, left ventricle; PH, pulmonary hypertension; RV, right ventricle; 2D, two-dimensional.
Reproduced from: Biswas M, Sudhakar S, Nanda NC, Buckberg G, Pradhan M, Roomi AU, et al. Two- and three-dimensional speckle tracking echocardiography: clinical applications and future directions. Echocardiography. 2013;30:88-105.

Table 4 Differentiation of athlete's heart from hypertrophic cardiomyopathy[16,61,65-70]

Athlete's heart	Hypertrophic cardiomyopathy
Normal longitudinal and other types of strain	Decreased longitudinal strain
Increased LVEDV Decreases after deconditioning for 3 months	Decreased LVEDV No change with deconditioning
Increased LV twist	Delayed LV untwisting
Increased early LA strain rate	Reduced LA strain and strain rate
No post systolic thickening	Postsystolic thickening present

Abbreviations: LA, left atrium; LV, left ventricle; EDV, end-diastolic volume.
Reproduced from: Biswas M, Sudhakar S, Nanda NC, Buckberg G, Pradhan M, Roomi AU, et al. Two- and three-dimensional speckle tracking echocardiography: Clinical applications and future directions. Echocardiography. 2013;30:88-105.

to facilitate understanding of the direction and velocity of movements in relation to the chamber.[10]

The assessment of LV volumes by 3-D STE is more accurate and reproducible and correlates with cardiac magnetic resonance

CONCLUSION

Despite some limitations which need to be overcome such as suboptimal reproducibility and inter-vendor differences, both 2D and 3D STE are finding increasingly useful applications in day to day clinical practice and show promise of becoming an important tool in the armamentarium of the echocardiographer and the cardiologist.

ACKNOWLEDGMENTS

This manuscript is reproduced with permission from the book "Emerging Concepts, Emerging Therapies and Emerging Technologies" published and printed by Dr PC

Manoria in Bhopal, Madhya Pradesh, India, in 2015, on behalf of the Integrated Society of Cardiology, Diabetology, Electrocardiography ECG and Critical Care.

REFERENCES

1. Nguyen JS, Lakkis NM, Bobek J, Goswami R, Dokainish H. Systolic and diastolic myocardial mechanics in patients with cardiac disease and preserved ejection fraction: impact of left ventricular filling pressure. J Am Soc Echocardiogr. 2010;23:1273-80.
2. Amundsen BH, Helle-Valle T, Edvardsen T, Torp H, Crosby J, Lyseggen E, et al. Noninvasive myocardial strain measurement by speckle tracking echocardiography: validation against sonomicrometry and tagged magnetic resonance imaging. J Am Coll Cardiol. 2006;47:789-93.
3. Cho G-Y, Chan J, Leano R, Strudwick M, Marwick TH. Comparison of two-dimensional speckle and tissue velocity based strain and validation with harmonic phase magnetic resonance imaging. The American Journal of Cardiology. 2006;97:1661-6.
4. Torrent-Guasp F, Buckberg GD, Clemente C, Cox JL, Coghlan HC, Gharib M. The structure and function of the helical heart and its buttress wrapping. I. The normal macroscopic structure of the heart. Seminars in Thoracic and Cardiovascular Surgery. 2001;13:301-19.
5. Torrent-Guasp F, Kocica MJ, Corno AF, Komeda M, Carreras-Costa F, Flotats A, et al. Towards new understanding of the heart structure and function. Eur J Cardiothorac Surg. 2005;27:191-201.
6. Buckberg G, Hoffman JIE, Nanda NC, Coghlan C, Saleh S, Athanasuleas C. Ventricular torsion and untwisting: Further insights into mechanics and timing interdependence: a viewpoint. Echocardiography. 2011;28:782-804.
7. Streeter DD, Spotnitz HM, Patel DP, Ross J, Sonnenblick EH. Fiber orientation in the canine left ventricle during diastole and systole. Circ Res. 1969;24:339-47.
8. Greenbaum RA, Ho SY, Gibson DG, Becker AE, Anderson RH. Left ventricular fibre architecture in man. Br Heart J. 1981;45:248-63.
9. Biswas M, Sudhakar S, Nanda NC, Buckberg G, Pradhan M, Roomi AU, et al. Two- and three-dimensional speckle tracking echocardiography: clinical applications and future directions. Echocardiography. 2013;30:88-105.
10. Vannan MA, Pedrizzetti G, Li P, Gurudevan S, Houle H, Main J, et al. Case reports: effect of cardiac resynchronization therapy on longitudinal and circumferential left ventricular mechanics by velocity vector imaging: description and initial clinical application of a novel method using high-frame rate B-mode echocardiographic images. Echocardiography. 2005;22:826-30.
11. Dandel M, Lehmkuhl H, Knosalla C, Suramelashvili N, Hetzer R. Strain and strain rate imaging by echocardiography - basic concepts and clinical applicability. Curr Cardiol Rev. 2009;5:133-48.
12. Yingchoncharoen T, Agarwal S, Popović ZB, Marwick TH. Normal ranges of left ventricular strain: a meta-analysis. Journal of the American Society of Echocardiography. 2013;26:185-91.
13. Marwick TH, Leano RL, Brown J, Sun J-P, Hoffmann R, Lysyansky P, et al. Myocardial strain measurement with 2-dimensional speckle-tracking echocardiography: definition of normal range. JACC: Cardiovascular Imaging. 2009;2:80-4.
14. Pérez de Isla L, Millán M, Lennie V, Quezada M, Guinea J, Macaya C, et al. Area strain: normal values for a new parameter in healthy people. Rev Esp Cardiol. 2011;64:1194-7.
15. Takahashi K, Al Naami G, Thompson R, Inage A, Mackie AS, Smallhorn JF. Normal rotational, torsion and untwisting data in children, adolescents and young adults. J Am Soc Echocardiogr. 2010;23:286-93.
16. Dandel M, Hetzer R. Echocardiographic strain and strain rate imaging—clinical applications. International Journal of Cardiology. 2009;132:11-24.
17. Shimoni S, Gendelman G, Ayzenberg O, Smirin N, Lysyansky P, Edri O, et al. Differential effects of coronary artery stenosis on myocardial function: the value of myocardial strain analysis for the detection of coronary artery disease. J Am Soc Echocardiogr. 2011;24:748-57.
18. Becker M, Hoffmann R, Kühl HP, Grawe H, Katoh M, Kramann R, et al. Analysis of myocardial deformation based on ultrasonic pixel tracking to determine transmurality in chronic myocardial infarction. Eur Heart J. 2006;27:2560-6.
19. Asanuma T, Uranishi A, Masuda K, Ishikura F, Beppu S, Nakatani S. Assessment of myocardial ischemic memory using persistence of post-systolic thickening after recovery from ischemia. J Am Coll Cardiol Img. 2009;2:1253-61.
20. Chan J, Hanekom L, Wong C, Leano R, Cho G-Y, Marwick TH. Differentiation of subendocardial and transmural infarction using two-dimensional strain rate imaging to assess short-axis and long-axis myocardial function. J Am Coll Cardiol. 2006;48:2026-33.
21. Bertini M, Delgado V, Nucifora G, Ajmone Marsan N, Ng ACT, Shanks M, et al. Left ventricular rotational mechanics in patients with coronary artery disease: differences in subendocardial and subepicardial layers. Heart. 2010;96:1737-43.
22. Jang JY, Woo JS, Kim W-S, Ha SJ, Sohn IS, Kim W, et al. Serial assessment of left ventricular remodeling by measurement of left ventricular torsion using speckle tracking echocardiography in patients with acute myocardial infarction. Am J Cardiol. 2010;106:917-23.
23. Park YH, Kang S-J, Song J-K, Lee EY, Song J-M, Kang D-H, et al. Prognostic value of longitudinal strain after primary reperfusion therapy in patients with anterior-wall acute myocardial infarction. J Am Soc Echocardiogr. 2008;21:262-7.
24. Nucifora G, Marsan NA, Bertini M, Delgado V, Siebelink H-MJ, van Werkhoven JM, et al. Reduced left ventricular torsion early after myocardial infarction is related to left ventricular remodeling. Circ Cardiovasc Imaging. 2010;3:433-42.
25. Ng ACT, Sitges M, Pham PN, Tran DT, Delgado V, Bertini M, et al. Incremental value of 2-dimensional speckle tracking strain imaging to wall motion analysis for detection of coronary artery disease in patients undergoing dobutamine stress echocardiography. Am Heart J. 2009;158:836-44.
26. Tan YT, Wenzelburger F, Lee E, Heatlie G, Leyva F, Patel K, et al. The pathophysiology of heart failure with normal ejection fraction: exercise echocardiography reveals complex abnormalities of both systolic and diastolic ventricular function involving torsion, untwist, and longitudinal motion. J Am Coll Cardiol. 2009;54:36-46.
27. Gorcsan J, Tanabe M, Bleeker GB, Suffoletto MS, Thomas NC, Saba S, et al. Combined longitudinal and radial dyssynchrony predicts ventricular response after resynchronization therapy. J Am Coll Cardiol. 2007;50:1476-83.
28. Lim P, Buakhamsri A, Popovic ZB, Greenberg NL, Patel D, Thomas JD, et al. Longitudinal strain delay index by speckle tracking imaging: a new marker of response to cardiac resynchronization therapy. Circulation. 2008;118:1130-7.

29. Tanaka H, Nesser H-J, Buck T, Oyenuga O, Jánosi RA, Winter S, et al. Dyssynchrony by speckle-tracking echocardiography and response to cardiac resynchronization therapy: results of the Speckle Tracking and Resynchronization (STAR) study. Eur Heart J. 2010;31:1690-1700.
30. Delgado V, van Bommel RJ, Bertini M, Borleffs CJW, Marsan NA, Arnold CT, et al. Relative merits of left ventricular dyssynchrony, left ventricular lead position, and myocardial scar to predict long-term survival of ischemic heart failure patients undergoing cardiac resynchronization therapy. Circulation. 2011;123:70-8.
31. Heggemann F, Weiss C, Hamm K, Kaden J, Süselbeck T, Papavassiliu T, et al. Global and regional myocardial function quantification by two-dimensional strain in Takotsubo cardiomyopathy. Eur J Echocardiogr. 2009;10:760-4.
32. Porciani MC, Cappelli F, Perfetto F, Ciaccheri M, Castelli G, Ricceri I, et al. Rotational mechanics of the left ventricle in AL amyloidosis. Echocardiography. 2010;27:1061-8.
33. Sengupta PP, Krishnamoorthy VK, Abhayaratna WP, Korinek J, Belohlavek M, Sundt TM, et al. Disparate patterns of left ventricular mechanics differentiate constrictive pericarditis from restrictive cardiomyopathy. JACC Cardiovasc Imaging. 2008;1:29-38.
34. Migrino RQ, Aggarwal D, Konorev E, Brahmbhatt T, Bright M, Kalyanaraman B. Early detection of doxorubicin cardiomyopathy using two-dimensional strain echocardiography. Ultrasound Med Biol. 2008;34:208-14.
35. D'Andrea A, Stisi S, Caso P, Uccio FS di, Bellissimo S, Salerno G, et al. Associations between left ventricular myocardial involvement and endothelial dysfunction in systemic sclerosis: noninvasive assessment in asymptomatic patients. Echocardiography. 2007;24:587-97.
36. Galderisi M, de Simone G, Innelli P, Turco A, Turco S, Capaldo B, et al. Impaired inotropic response in type 2 diabetes mellitus: a strain rate imaging study. Am J Hypertens. 2007;20:548-55.
37. Bellavia D, Abraham TP, Pellikka PA, Al-Zahrani GB, Dispenzieri A, Oh JK, et al. Detection of left ventricular systolic dysfunction in cardiac amyloidosis with strain rate echocardiography. J Am Soc Echocardiogr. 2007;20:1194-1202.
38. Mori K, Hayabuchi Y, Inoue M, Suzuki M, Sakata M, Nakagawa R, et al. Myocardial strain imaging for early detection of cardiac involvement in patients with Duchenne's progressive muscular dystrophy. Echocardiography. 2007;24:598-608.
39. Delgado V, Tops LF, van Bommel RJ, van der Kley F, Marsan NA, Klautz RJ, et al. Strain analysis in patients with severe aortic stenosis and preserved left ventricular ejection fraction undergoing surgical valve replacement. Eur Heart J. 2009;30:3037-47.
40. De Isla LP, de Agustin A, Rodrigo JL, Almeria C, del Carmen Manzano M, Rodríguez E, et al. Chronic mitral regurgitation: a pilot study to assess preoperative left ventricular contractile function using speckle-tracking echocardiography. J Am Soc Echocardiogr. 2009;22:831-8.
41. Dong L, Zhang F, Shu X, Guan L, Chen H. Left ventricular torsion in patients with secundum atrial septal defect. Circ J. 2009;73:1308-14.
42. Dong L, Zhang F, Shu X, Zhou D, Guan L, Pan C, et al. Left ventricular torsional deformation in patients undergoing transcatheter closure of secundum atrial septal defect. Int J Cardiovasc Imaging. 2009;25:479-86.
43. Li Y, Xie M, Wang X, Lv Q, Lu X, Yang Y, et al. Evaluation of right ventricular global longitudinal function in patients with tetralogy of fallot by two-dimensional ultrasound speckle tracking imaging. J Huazhong Univ Sci Technol Med Sci. 2010;30:126-31.
44. Vitarelli A, Mangieri E, Terzano C, Gaudio C, Salsano F, Rosato E, et al. Three-dimensional echocardiography and 2D-3D speckle-tracking imaging in chronic pulmonary hypertension: diagnostic accuracy in detecting hemodynamic signs of right ventricular (RV) failure. J Am Heart Assoc. 2015;4:e001584.
45. Krishnasamy R, Isbel NM, Hawley CM, Pascoe EM, Burrage M, Leano R, et al. Left ventricular global longitudinal strain (GLS) is a superior predictor of All-cause and cardiovascular mortality when compared to ejection fraction in advanced chronic kidney disease. PLoS ONE. 2015;10:e0127044.
46. Vitarelli A, Mangieri E, Capotosto L, Tanzilli G, D'Angeli I, Viceconte N, et al. Assessment of biventricular function by three-dimensional speckle-tracking echocardiography in secondary mitral regurgitation after repair with the MitraClip System. J Am Soc Echocardiogr; 2015.
47. Hayat D, Kloeckner M, Nahum J, Ecochard-Dugelay E, Dubois-Randé J-L, Jean-François D, et al. Comparison of real-time three-dimensional speckle tracking to magnetic resonance imaging in patients with coronary heart disease. Am J Cardiol. 2012;109:180-6.
48. Abate E, Hoogslag GE, Antoni ML, Nucifora G, Delgado V, Holman ER, et al. Value of three-dimensional speckle-tracking longitudinal strain for predicting improvement of left ventricular function after acute myocardial infarction. Am J Cardiol. 2012;110:961-7.
49. Maffessanti F, Nesser H-J, Weinert L, Steringer-Mascherbauer R, Niel J, Gorissen W, et al. Quantitative evaluation of regional left ventricular function using three-dimensional speckle tracking echocardiography in patients with and without heart disease. Am J Cardiol. 2009;104:1755-62.
50. Kleijn SA, Aly MFA, Terwee CB, van Rossum AC, Kamp O. Three-dimensional speckle tracking echocardiography for automatic assessment of global and regional left ventricular function based on area strain. J Am Soc Echocardiogr. 2011;24:314-21.
51. Saito K, Okura H, Watanabe N, Hayashida A, Obase K, Imai K, et al. Comprehensive evaluation of left ventricular strain using speckle tracking echocardiography in normal adults: comparison of three-dimensional and two-dimensional approaches. J Am Soc Echocardiogr. 2009;22:1025-30.
52. Wen H, Liang Z, Zhao Y, Yang K. Feasibility of detecting early left ventricular systolic dysfunction using global area strain: a novel index derived from three-dimensional speckle-tracking echocardiography. Eur J Echocardiogr. 2011;12:910-6.
53. Nesser H-J, Mor-Avi V, Gorissen W, Weinert L, Steringer-Mascherbauer R, Niel J, et al. Quantification of left ventricular volumes using three-dimensional echocardiographic speckle tracking: comparison with MRI. Eur Heart J. 2009;30:1565-73.
54. Kleijn SA, Aly MF, Knol DL, Terwee CB, Jansma EP, Abd El-Hady YA, et al. A meta-analysis of left ventricular dyssynchrony assessment and prediction of response to cardiac resynchronization therapy by three-dimensional echocardiography. Eur Heart J Cardiovasc Imaging. 2012;13:763-75.
55. Tanaka H, Hara H, Saba S, Gorcsan J. Usefulness of three-dimensional speckle tracking strain to quantify dyssynchrony and the site of latest mechanical activation. Am J Cardiol. 2010;105:235-42.

56. Nemes A, Kalapos A, Domsik P, Forster T. Identification of left ventricular "rigid body rotation" by three-dimensional speckle-tracking echocardiography in a patient with noncompaction of the left ventricle: a case from the MAGYAR-Path Study. Echocardiography. 2012;29:E237-40.
57. Baccouche H, Maunz M, Beck T, Gaa E, Banzhaf M, Knayer U, et al. Differentiating cardiac amyloidosis and hypertrophic cardiomyopathy by use of three-dimensional speckle tracking echocardiography. Echocardiography. 2012;29:668-77.
58. Baccouche H, Maunz M, Beck T, Fogarassy P, Beyer M. Echocardiographic assessment and monitoring of the clinical course in a patient with Takotsubo cardiomyopathy by a novel 3D-speckle-tracking-strain analysis. Eur J Echocardiogr. 2009;10:729-31.
59. Tsuji T, Tanaka H, Matsumoto K, Miyoshi T, Hiraishi M, Kaneko A, et al. Capability of three-dimensional speckle tracking radial strain for identification of patients with cardiac sarcoidosis. Int J Cardiovasc Imaging. 2013;29:317-24.
60. Ahmad H, Gayat E, Yodwut C, Abduch MC, Patel AR, Weinert L, et al. Evaluation of myocardial deformation in patients with sickle cell disease and preserved ejection fraction using three-dimensional speckle tracking echocardiography. Echocardiography. 2012;29:962-9.
61. Galderisi M, Esposito R, Schiano-Lomoriello V, Santoro A, Ippolito R, Schiattarella P, et al. Correlates of global area strain in native hypertensive patients: a three-dimensional speckle-tracking echocardiography study. Eur Heart J Cardiovasc Imaging. 2012;13:730-8.
62. Schueler R, Sinning J-M, Momcilovic D, Weber M, Ghanem A, Werner N, et al. Three-dimensional speckle-tracking analysis of left ventricular function after transcatheter aortic valve implantation. J Am Soc Echocardiogr. 2012;25:827-34.e1.
63. Vitarelli A, Sardella G, Roma AD, Capotosto L, De Curtis G, D'Orazio S, et al. Assessment of right ventricular function by three-dimensional echocardiography and myocardial strain imaging in adult atrial septal defect before and after percutaneous closure. Int J Cardiovasc Imaging. 2012;28:1905-16.
64. Bhaya M, Sudhakar S, Sadat K, Beniwal R, Joshi D, George JF, et al. Effects of antegrade versus integrated blood cardioplegia on left ventricular function evaluated by echocardiographic real-time 3-dimensional speckle tracking. The Journal of Thoracic and Cardiovascular Surgery. 2015;149:877-84.e5.
65. Butz T, Buuren F van, Mellwig KP, Langer C, Plehn G, Meissner A, et al. Two-dimensional strain analysis of the global and regional myocardial function for the differentiation of pathologic and physiologic left ventricular hypertrophy: a study in athletes and in patients with hypertrophic cardiomyopathy. Int J Cardiovasc Imaging. 2010;27:91-100.
66. Richand V, Lafitte S, Reant P, Serri K, Lafitte M, Brette S, et al. An ultrasound speckle tracking (two-dimensional strain) analysis of myocardial deformation in professional soccer players compared with healthy subjects and hypertrophic cardiomyopathy. Am J Cardiol. 2007;100:128-32.
67. Weiner RB, Hutter Jr. AM, Wang F, Kim J, Weyman AE, Wood MJ, et al. The Impact of Endurance Exercise Training on Left Ventricular Torsion. JACC: Cardiovascular Imaging. 2010;3:1001-9.
68. D'Ascenzi F, Cameli M, Zacà V, Lisi M, Santoro A, Causarano A, et al. Supernormal diastolic function and role of left atrial myocardial deformation analysis by 2D speckle tracking echocardiography in elite soccer players. Echocardiography. 2011;28:320-6.
69. Serri K, Reant P, Lafitte M, Berhouet M, Le Bouffos V, Roudaut R, et al. Global and regional myocardial function quantification by two-dimensional strain: application in hypertrophic cardiomyopathy. J Am Coll Cardiol. 2006;47:1175-81.
70. Sun JP, Stewart WJ, Yang XS, Donnell RO, Leon AR, Felner JM, et al. Differentiation of hypertrophic cardiomyopathy and cardiac amyloidosis from other causes of ventricular wall thickening by two-dimensional strain imaging echocardiography. Am J Cardiol. 2009;103:411-5.

5. A Gold Standard for Evaluation of Cardiomyopathies

Johann Christopher

INTRODUCTION

The term "cardiomyopathy" encompasses a broad and multietiologic spectrum of different entities, all of which are characterized by myocardial disease associated with cardiac dysfunction. The most commonly used classification system has been published in the 1995 World Health Organization/International Society and Federation of Cardiology task force report and classifies the cardiomyopathies according to the dominant functional impairment as follows:[1]
- Dilated cardiomyopathy
- Hypertrophic cardiomyopathy
- Restrictive cardiomyopathy
- Arrhythmogenic right ventricular (RV) cardiomyopathy
- Unclassified cardiomyopathies.

Cardiomyopathies may be idiopathic or associated with an underlying cardiac or systemic disorder, so-called "specific cardiomyopathies." The term "specific cardiomyopathy" includes ischemic, valvular, hypertensive, inflammatory and metabolic cardiomyopathies, and myocardial involvement by general systemic diseases, muscular dystrophies, neuromuscular disorders, sensitivity and toxic reactions, and peripartum cardiomyopathy.[1]

IDIOPATHIC-DILATED CARDIOMYOPATHY

Idiopathic-dilated cardiomyopathy (IDC) is characterized by dilation and impaired contractility of the left or both ventricles.[2] The atria is often dilated in addition to the ventricles. Atrial or ventricular thrombi are frequently observed.[3] Symptomatic patients present with left-sided or global heart failure, arrhythmias, thromboembolism, or sudden death.[4]

Echocardiographic criteria for the diagnosis of dilated cardiomyopathy include ejection fraction (EF) <45%,[5] fractional shortening <25%, and a left ventricular (LV) end-diastolic dimension >112% predicted value corrected for age and body surface area.[6]

Cine MR Imaging

Cine MR imaging accurately evaluates LV volume parameters and function with better reproducibility than 2D ECHO.[7] Features on cine MR images are as follows:
- Dilation of the left or both ventricles **(Figs 1A to D)**
- Diffuse hypokinesia of the left or both ventricles with decreased EF
- Increased myocardial mass secondary to chamber enlargement
- Normal myocardial thickness
- Preserved trabeculation (as opposed to infarct scar, where trabeculation is scarce).[8]

Delayed Enhanced MR Imaging

Delayed enhanced MR imaging is increasingly used to characterize various nonischemic cardiomyopathies.[9] In patients with IDC, delayed enhancement is thought to represent underlying fibrosis.[10] The three following patterns have been described in patients with IDC.[11]
1. No enhancement—59%.
2. Subendocardial or transmural enhancement—13%.
3. Patchy or longitudinal striae of midwall enhancement—28%.

The diagnosis of IDC should be considered when either no or midwall enhancement is seen in patients who have LV dysfunction. There are preliminary data demonstrating that the presence of delayed enhancement is associated with an unfavorable clinical outcome and may be a predictor of sudden death in patients with IDC.[12]

MYOCARDITIS

In acute and fulminant cases of heart failure, the diagnosis of acute myocarditis should be considered. The clinical diagnosis is often difficult. Endomyocardial biopsy is considered the gold standard for diagnosis and classification; however, it is

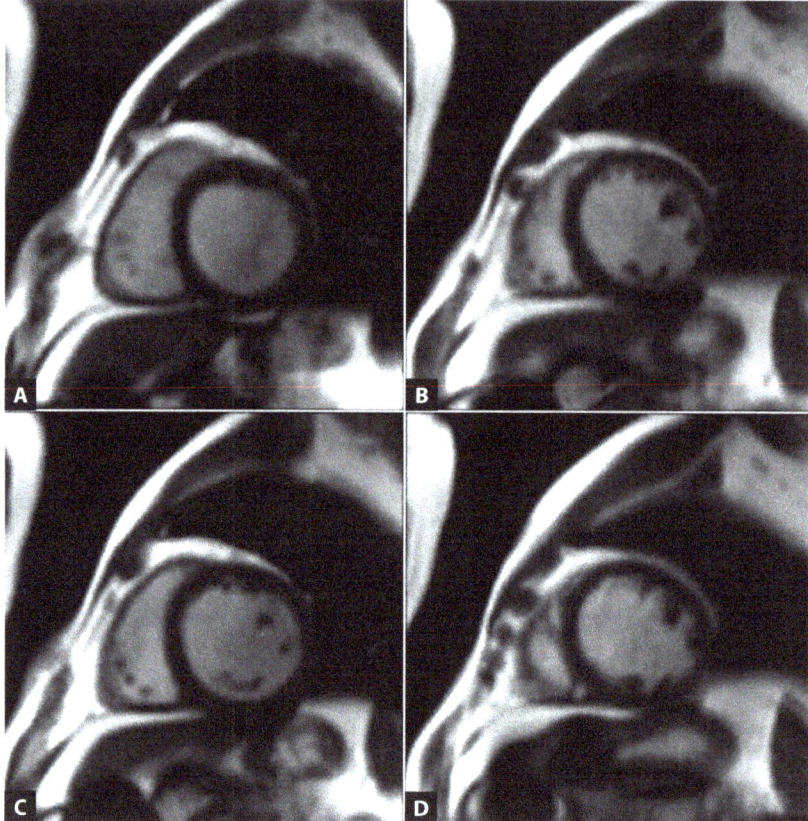

Figs 1A to D: Dilated cardiomyopathy

an invasive procedure and underestimates the true incidence of myocarditis.[13]

Delayed Enhanced MR Imaging

MR imaging aids in the diagnosis of acute, subacute, and chronic myocarditis.[14] A characteristic distribution of delayed enhancement in acute myocarditis involves the epicardial zone with varying degrees of progression toward the endocardium and sparing of the subendocardium.[15] The lateral and inferolateral walls are most frequently affected. The location of delayed enhancement may be used to guide endomyocardial biopsy.

Midwall hyperenhancement in a pattern identical to IDC has been shown to be present in 84% of patients with chronic active myocarditis by histological criteria.[16]

HYPERTROPHIC CARDIOMYOPATHY

Hypertrophic cardiomyopathy (HCM) is an autosomal-dominant inherited genetic disease characterized by LV hypertrophy in the absence of an underlying cause such as hypertension or aortic valve stenosis.[17] Rarely, the right ventricle may be involved.[18] HCM may be present in all age groups including the elderly with a prevalence of 1/500 in adults.[19] HCM is the most important cause of sudden death in young athletes.[20]

Cine and Phase Contrast MR Imaging

Cine MR imaging provides a comprehensive overview of the entire ventricular anatomy and is, therefore, very helpful for assessment of morphology and function in patients with established or suspected HCM.[21]

The typical features of HCM on cine MR images are as follows:
- Diffuse or focal increase of LV wall thickness (15 mm at end-diastole)
- Reduced systolic thickening of the hypertrophied myocardial segments
- Normal or decreased size of the LV cavity
- Normal or increased LV ejection fraction.

Asymmetric hypertrophy involving predominantly the basal septum is most common. Diffuse hypertrophy involving all myocardial segments is less frequently observed. Focal hypertrophy of the mid-myocardium or the apex have been described as distinct subtypes. The apical form is characterized by a spade-like configuration of the LV cavity.[22]

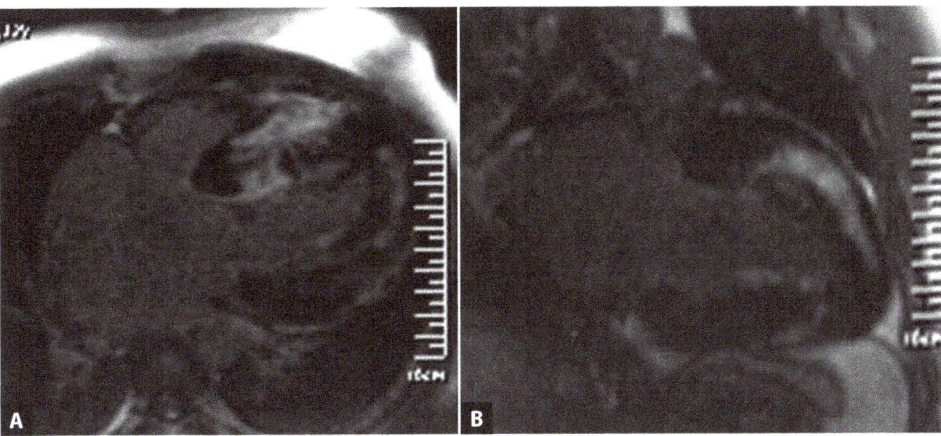

Figs 2A and B: Delayed enhancement in HCM

Patients with septal hypertrophy commonly demonstrate LV outflow tract obstruction, which is further accentuated by systolic anterior motion of the anterior mitral valve leaflet during systole. In these cases, cine MR imaging demonstrates turbulent flow as signal void in the LV outflow tract. Phase contrast imaging can be used to estimate the pressure gradient in the LV outflow tract.

Delayed Enhanced MR Imaging

Delayed enhancing lesions of the myocardium are frequently observed in patients with HCM, most commonly involve the thickened myocardial septum, and are thought to represent areas of fibrosis.[23] Most commonly, delayed enhancement is patchy. Delayed enhancement in HCM often involves the mid-myocardium at the junction of the interventricular septum and RV free wall.[24] There is preliminary data demonstrating a correlation of delayed enhancement with risk factors for sudden death **(Figs 2A and B)**.[25]

RESTRICTIVE CARDIOMYOPATHY

The characteristic feature of restrictive cardiomyopathy (RCM) is decreased diastolic ventricular compliance ("myocardial stiffness") with preserved systolic contraction. RCM may be idiopathic or occur with specific cardiomyopathies, particularly *amyloidosis*. Other disorders that can be associated with RCM are sarcoidosis, storage diseases, endomyocardial fibrosis, hypereosinophilic syndrome, neoplasm, radiation, or drug toxicity.[26]

CARDIAC AMYLOIDOSIS

The amyloidosis comprise a heterogeneous group of disorders that are characterized by deposition of fibrillar protein in the extracellular space. The different forms of amyloidosis are classified according to the type of abnormal protein fibril. Involvement of the heart is common in types AL, FAP, and ATTR. Secondary amyloidosis only rarely involves the heart.[27]

Amyloid infiltration of the heart is associated with a poor prognosis, with a median survival of 6 months.[27] Diagnosis in clinical practice is usually made by combined clinical and ECHO findings with a positive noncardiac biopsy.[28] Speckled appearance of the myocardium on ECHO and low voltage on electrocardiogram are classical features.[29]

Cine and Black-blood MR Imaging

The following findings may be observed in patients with cardiac amyloid deposition:[30]
- Concentric thickening of the wall of the left or both ventricles
- Increased thickness of the atrial walls and the interatrial septum
- Thickened valve leaflets
- Biatrial enlargement
- Small or normal-sized ventricles in early disease and increased ventricular size in late disease secondary to heart failure
- Impaired systolic function with decreased EF
- Atrial or ventricular thrombi
- Pleural and pericardial effusions.

Delayed Enhanced MR Imaging

Delayed enhancement is commonly found in patients with cardiac amyloidosis and is thought to be secondary to expansion of the extracellular space.[31] Different patterns of delayed enhancement have been described, including the following:[32]
- Diffuse subendocardial enhancement
- Limited focal enhancement
- Diffuse with transmural enhancement **(Fig. 3)**.

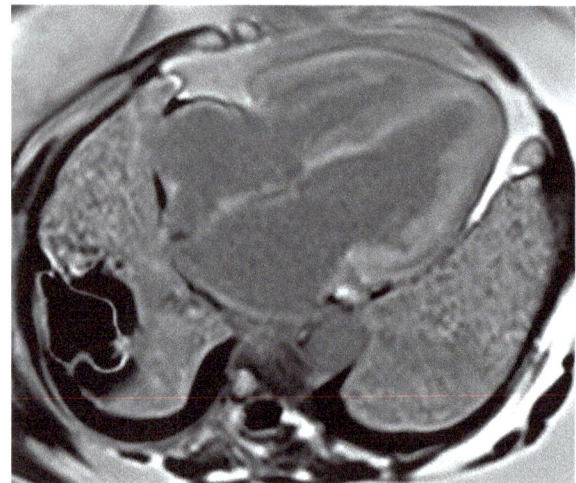

Fig. 3: Delayed enhancement in cardiac amyloidosis

ARRHYTHMOGENIC RIGHT VENTRICULAR CARDIOMYOPATHY

Arrhythmogenic right ventricular cardiomyopathy (ARVD/C) is characterized by progressive fatty or fibrofatty replacement of right ventricular myocardium, usually with sparing of the interventricular septum.[33]

Standardized criteria for the diagnosis have been developed by the Task Force of the Working Group on Cardiomyopathies. On the basis of these criteria, diagnosis of ARVD/C is made in the presence of the following:
- Two major criteria or
- One major plus two minor criteria or
- Four minor criteria from four different groups.

Cine and Black-blood MR Imaging

Cine MR imaging allows for accurate assessment of RV morphology and function and is currently the most reproducible component of the ARVD/C examination.[34] A detailed evaluation for global and segmental right ventricular dilation, regional wall motion abnormalities of the right ventricle can be made on cine MR based on the criteria for the diagnosis of ARVD/C **(Figs 4A to D)**.[35]

Delayed Enhanced MR Imaging

Delayed enhanced MR imaging is increasingly used to evaluate patients with suspected ARVD/C. There are preliminary data in a small number of patients demonstrating correlation of delayed enhancement with fibrofatty replacement on biopsy.[36]

LEFT VENTRICULAR NONCOMPACTION

Noncompaction has been categorized as an unclassified cardiomyopathy.[1] The apex and the midventricular lateral and inferior wall are most commonly affected.[37] Less frequently, the right ventricle may be involved as well.

MR Imaging

More recently, MR imaging has been used for the evaluation of noncompaction, with promising results. Particularly due to its consistent visualization of the apex, cine MR imaging has the potential to diagnose more subtle forms of noncompaction which may be overlooked by echo.[38] A study by Petersen and coworkers showed that an end-diastolic ratio of noncompacted to compacted myocardium of 2.3 on cine MR imaging had a sensitivity of 86% and a specificity of 99% for the diagnosis of noncompaction.[39]

Focal or global hypokinesia is common in noncompaction, and the LV ejection fraction is often reduced. Ventricular thrombi, which are common in patients with noncompaction, and may be visualized on cine and/or on delayed enhanced MR images. Patients with noncompaction may show delayed enhancement of the abnormal noncompacted myocardium and related papillary muscles likely representing fibrosis **(Figs 5A to H)**.[40]

MYOCARDIAL SARCOIDOSIS

Sarcoidosis is a multisystem granulomatous disorder of unknown etiology that occurs in all races but disproportionately affects blacks and females.[41] The diagnosis is based on clinical criteria in most patients and is suspected in all patients who present with arrhythmia, conduction block, or heart failure.

Cine MR Imaging

Cine MR imaging is not very sensitive for detection of myocardial sarcoidosis and may be completely normal, even in patients with strong clinical suspicion.[42]

The common findings on cine MR are:
- LV dilatation
- LV basal septal thinning
- Diffuse hypokinesis with decreased LV ejection fraction **(Figs 6A and B)**.[43]

Delayed Enhanced MR Imaging

Delayed enhanced MR imaging has shown promising results for detection of myocardial sarcoidosis.[44] Delayed enhancement in myocardial sarcoidosis is typically patchy or nodular.[45]

T2-weighted Imaging

Patients with myocardial sarcoidosis may show high signal intensity lesions within the myocardium on T2-weighted images, which correspond to myocardial inflammation.

IRON OVERLOAD CARDIOMYOPATHY

Heart failure due to iron overload is a leading cause of death in patients with transfusion-dependent anemias and hereditary

Chapter 5: A Gold Standard for Evaluation of Cardiomyopathies

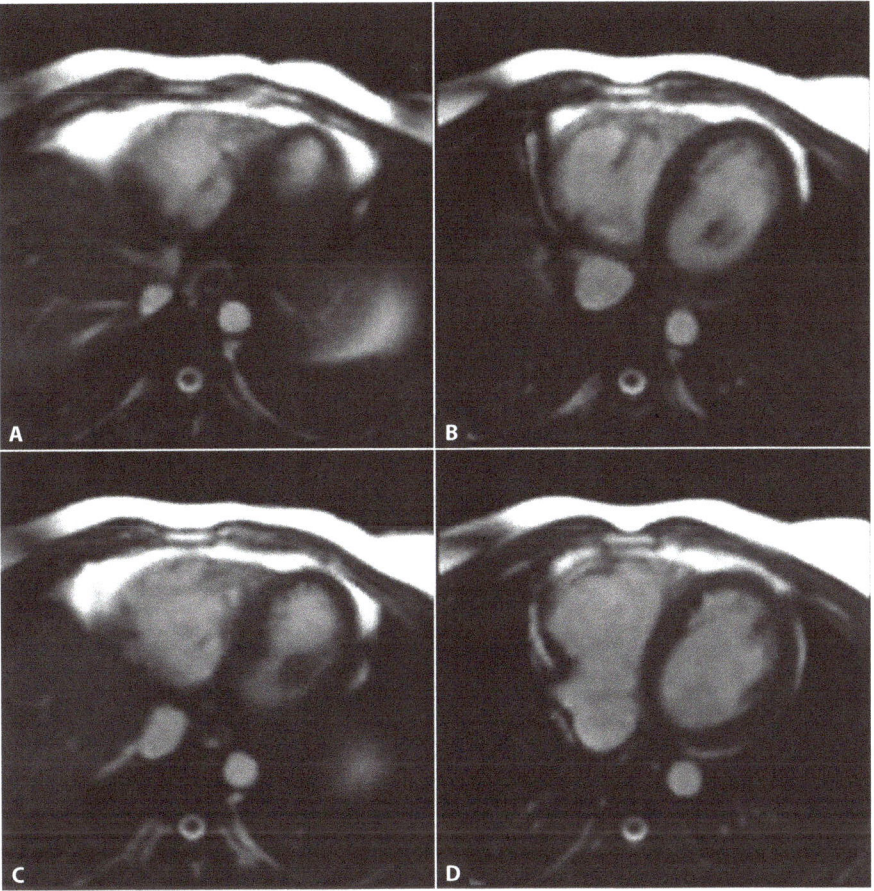

Figs 4A to D: RV dysfunction in ARVD/C

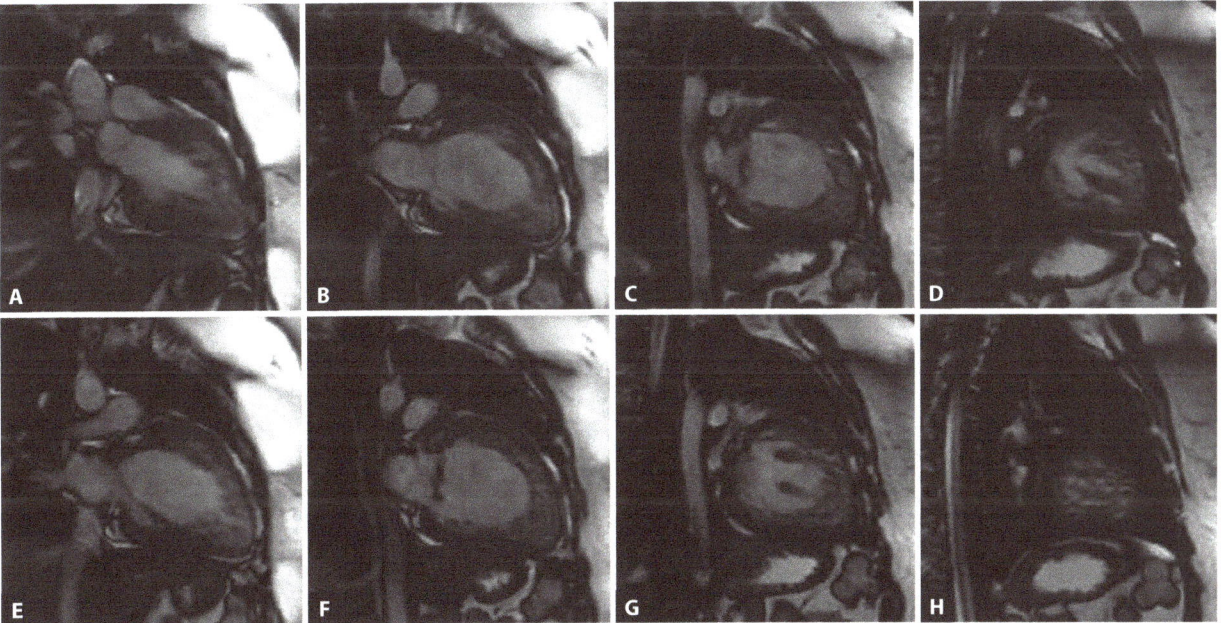

Figs 5A to H: Noncompaction of LV

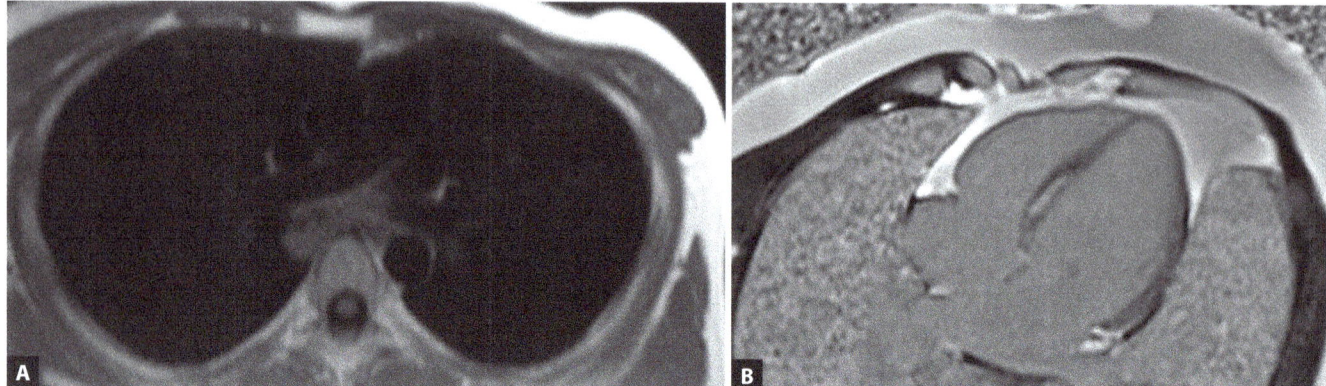

Figs 6A and B: Mediastinal nodes and scar in myocardial sarcoid

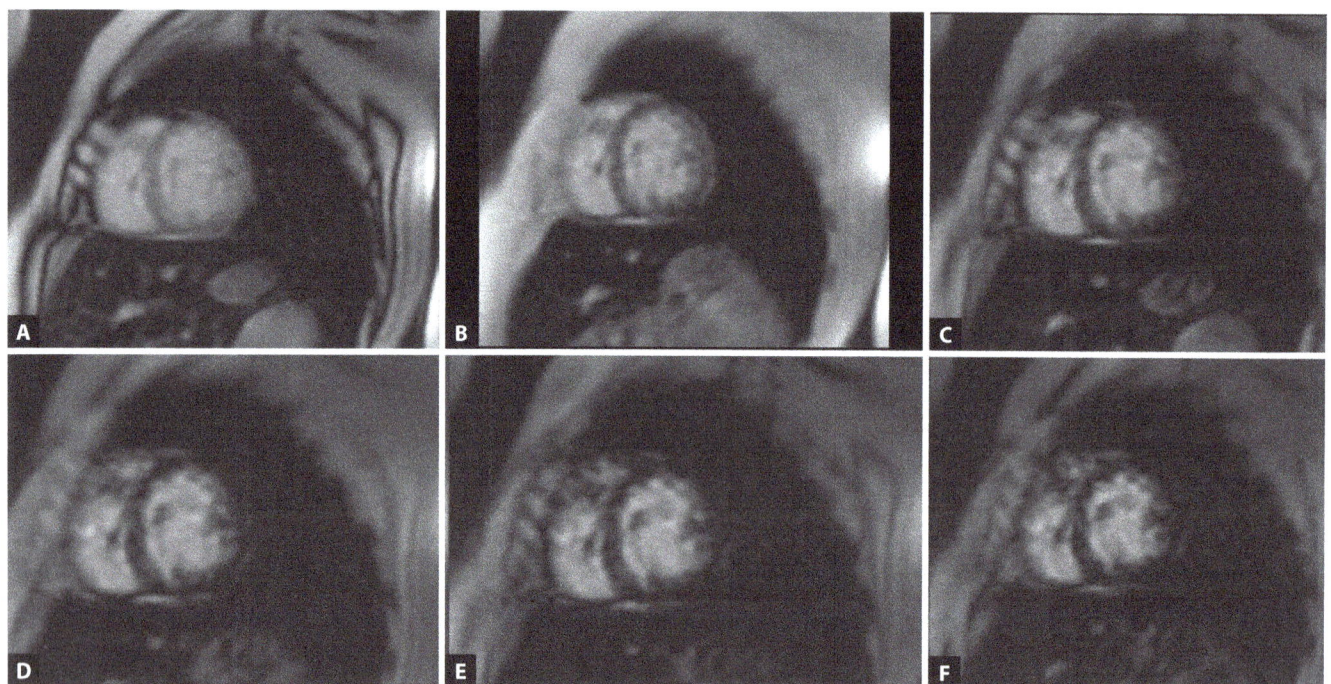

Figs 7A to F: Myocardial involvement in thalassemia

hemochromatosis. The ability to identify and monitor myocardial iron overload is of clinical importance as intensive chelation therapy may attenuate or reverse ventricular dysfunction in these patients **(Figs 7A to F)**.[46]

T2*-weighted Imaging

Quantification of myocardial iron content is performed with dedicated T2*-weighted sequences. Shortened myocardial T2* times correlate directly with increasing tissue iron levels, the occurrence of systolic and diastolic dysfunction, and the occurrence of clinical heart failure.[47] Vice versa, T2* values lengthen in patients receiving aggressive chelation therapy, heralding improvement in ventricular function.[48] Quantitative evaluation of myocardial iron content with dedicated T2*-weighted sequences is currently the only imaging modality capable of providing diagnostic and prognostic evaluation in patients with iron overload cardiomyopathy.

CONCLUSION

Cardiac MR imaging is an important diagnostic tool for evaluation of patients with various cardiomyopathies. Cardiac MR imaging provides an overview of the anatomy and physiology. Delayed enhanced MR imaging has been found to differentiate between pathology and normal variants, and also between different myocardial disease entities. Cardiac MR imaging of cardiomyopathies is no longer a sole research tool but is an invaluable part of routine clinical practice.

REFERENCES

1. Richardson P, McKenna W, Bristow M, et al. Report of the 1995 World Health Organization/International Society and Federation of Cardiology Task Force on the Definition and Classification of cardiomyopathies. Circulation. 1996;93(5):841-2.
2. Elliott P. Cardiomyopathy. Diagnosis and management of dilated cardiomyopathy. Heart. 2000;84(1):106-12.
3. Dec GW, Fuster V. Idiopathic dilated cardiomyopathy. N Engl J Med. 1994;331(23):1564-75.
4. Felker GM, Hu W, Hare JM, et al. The spectrum of dilated cardiomyopathy. The Johns Hopkins experience with 1,278 patients. Medicine (Baltimore). 1999;78(4):270-83.
5. Ichikawa Y, Sakuma H, Kitagawa K, et al. Evaluation of left ventricular volumes and ejection fraction using fast steady-state cine MR imaging: comparison with left ventricular angiography. J Cardiovasc Magn Reson. 2003;5(2):333-42.
6. Bellenger NG, Marcus NJ, Rajappan K, et al. Comparison of techniques for the measurement of left ventricular function following cardiac transplantation. J Cardiovasc Magn Reson. 2002;4(2):255-63.
7. Strohm O, Schulz-Menger J, Pilz B, et al. Measurement of left ventricular dimensions and function in patients with dilated cardiomyopathy. J Magn Reson Imaging. 2001;13(3):367-71.
8. Imai H, Kumai T, Sekiya M, et al. Left ventricular trabeculae evaluated with MRI in dilated cardiomyopathy and old myocardial infarction. J Cardiol. 1992;22(1):83-90.
9. Kim DH, Choi SI, Chang HJ, et al. Delayed hyperenhancement by contrast-enhanced magnetic resonance imaging: clinical application for various cardiac diseases. J Comput Assist Tomogr 2006;30(2):226-32.
10. Assomull RG, Prasad SK, Lyne J, et al. Cardiovascular magnetic resonance, fibrosis, and prognosis in dilated cardiomyopathy. J Am Coll Cardiol. 2006;48(10):1977-85.
11. McCrohon JA, Moon JC, Prasad SK, et al. Differentiation of heart failure related to dilated cardiomyopathy and coronary artery disease using gadolinium-enhanced cardiovascular magnetic resonance. Circulation. 2003;108(1):54-9.
12. Park S, Choi BW, Rim SJ, et al. Delayed hyperenhancement magnetic resonance imaging is useful in predicting functional recovery of non-ischemic left ventricular systolic dysfunction. J Card Fail. 2006;12(2):93-9.
13. Feldman AM, McNamara D. Myocarditis. N Engl J Med. 2000;343(19):1388-98.
14. Laissy JP, Hyafil F, Feldman LJ, et al. Differentiating acute myocardial infarction from myocarditis: diagnostic value of early- and delayed-perfusion cardiac MR imaging. Radiology. 2005;237(1):75-82.
15. Mahrholdt H, Goedecke C, Wagner A, et al. Cardiovascular magnetic resonance assessment of human myocarditis: a comparison to histology and molecular pathology. Circulation. 2004;109(10):1250-8.
16. De Cobelli F, Pieroni M, Esposito A, et al. Delayed gadolinium-enhanced cardiac magnetic resonance in patients with chronic myocarditis presenting with heart failure or recurrent arrhythmias. J Am Coll Cardiol. 2006;47(8):1649-54.
17. Maron BJ. Hypertrophic cardiomyopathy: a systematic review. JAMA. 2002;287(10):1308-20.
18. Severino S, Caso P, Cicala S, et al. Involvement of right ventricle in left ventricular hypertrophic cardiomyopathy: analysis by pulsed Doppler tissue imaging. Eur J Echocardiogr. 2000;1(4):281-8.
19. Maron BJ, Gardin JM, Flack JM, et al. Prevalence of hypertrophic cardiomyopathy in a general population of young adults. Echocardiographic analysis of 4111 subjects in the CARDIA Study. Coronary Artery Risk Development in (Young) Adults. Circulation. 1995;92(4):785-9.
20. Basavarajaiah S, Shah A, Sharma S. Sudden cardiac death in young athletes. Heart. 2007;93(3):287-9.
21. Rickers C, Wilke NM, Jerosch-Herold M, et al. Utility of cardiac magnetic resonance imaging in the diagnosis of hypertrophic cardiomyopathy. Circulation. 2005;112(6):855-61.
22. Eriksson MJ, Sonnenberg B, Woo A, et al. Long-term outcome in patients with apical hypertrophic cardiomyopathy. J Am Coll Cardiol. 2002;39(4):638-45.
23. Choudhury L, Mahrholdt H, Wagner A, et al. Myocardial scarring in asymptomatic or mildly symptomatic patients with hypertrophic cardiomyopathy. J Am Coll Cardiol. 2002;40(12):2156-64.
24. Bogaert J, Goldstein M, Tannouri F, et al. Original report. Late myocardial enhancement in hypertrophic cardiomyopathy with contrast-enhanced MR imaging. AJR Am J Roentgenol. 2003;180(4):981-5.
25. Moon JC, McKenna WJ, McCrohon JA, et al. Toward clinical risk assessment in hypertrophic cardiomyopathy with gadolinium cardiovascular Magnetic resonance. J Am Coll Cardiol. 2003;741(9):1561-7.
26. Kushwaha SS, Fallon JT, Fuster V. Restrictive cardiomyopathy. N Engl J Med. 1997;336(4):267-76.
27. Falk RH, Comenzo RL, Skinner M. The systemic amyloidoses. N Engl J Med. 1997;337(13):898-909.
28. Hamer JP, Janssen S, van Rijswijk MH, et al. Amyloid cardiomyopathy in systemic non-hereditary amyloidosis. Clinical, echocardiographic and electrocardiographic findings in 30 patients with AA and 24 patients with AL amyloidosis. Eur Heart J. 1992;13(5):623-7.
29. Leeson CP, Myerson SG, Walls GB, Maredia N, Ray SG. et al. Atrial pathology in cardiac amyloidosis: evidence from ECG cardiac amyloidosis. Clin Med. 2005;5(5):504-9.
30. Fattori R, Rocchi G, Celletti F, et al. Contribution of magnetic resonance imaging in the differential diagnosis of cardiac amyloidosis and symmetric hypertrophic cardiomyopathy. Am Heart J. 1998;136(5):824-30.
31. vanden Driesen RI, Slaughter RE, Strugnell WE. MR findings in cardiac amyloidosis. AJR Am J Roentgenol. 2006;186(6):1682-5.
32. Perugini E, Rapezzi C, Piva T, et al. Non-invasive evaluation of the myocardial substrate of cardiac amyloidosis by gadolinium cardiac magnetic resonance. Heart. 2006;92(3):343-9.
33. Fontaine G, Fontaliran F, Frank R. Arrhythmogenic right ventricular cardiomyopathies: clinical forms and main differential diagnoses. Circulation. 1998;97(16):1532-5.
34. Tandri H, Castillo E, Ferrari VA, et al. Magnetic resonance imaging of arrhythmogenic right ventricular dysplasia: sensitivity, specificity, and observer variability of fat detection versus functional analysis of the right ventricle. J Am Coll Cardiol. 2006;48(11):2277-84.

35. Corrado D, Fontaine G, Marcus FI, et al. Arrhythmogenic right ventricular dysplasia/cardiomyopathy: need for an international registry. Study Group on Arrhythmogenic Right Ventricular Dysplasia/Cardiomyopathy of the Working Groups on Myocardial and Pericardial Disease and Arrhythmias of the European Society of Cardiology and of the Scientific Council on Cardiomyopathies of the World Heart Federation. Circulation. 2000;101(11):E101-E106.
36. Tandri H, Saranathan M, Rodriguez ER, et al. Noninvasive detection of myocardial fibrosis in arrhythmogenic right ventricular cardiomyopathy using delayed-enhancement magnetic resonance imaging. J Am Coll Cardiol. 2005;45(1):98-103.
37. Jenni R, Oechslin E, Schneider J, et al. Echocardiographic and pathoanatomical characteristics of isolated left ventricular non-compaction: a step towards classification as a distinct cardiomyopathy. Heart. 2001;86(6):666-71.
38. Varghese A, Fisher NG, Pennell DJ. Late recognition of left ventricular non-compaction by cardiovascular magnetic resonance. Heart. 2005;91(3):282.
39. Petersen SE, Selvanayagam JB, Wiesmann F, et al. Left ventricular non-compaction: insights from cardiovascular magnetic resonance imaging. J Am Coll Cardiol. 2005;46(1):101-5.
40. McCrohon JA, Richmond DR, Pennell DJ, et al. Images in cardiovascular medicine. Isolated noncompaction of the myocardium: a rarity or missed diagnosis? Circulation. 2002;106(6):e22-e23.
41. Sartwell PE, Edwards LB. Epidemiology of sarcoidosis in the US Navy. Am J Epidemiol. 1974;99(4):250-7.
42. Tadamura E, Yamamuro M, Kubo S, et al. Effectiveness of delayed enhanced MRI for identification of cardiac sarcoidosis: comparison with radionuclide imaging. AJR Am J Roentgenol. 2005;185(1):110-5.
43. Smedema JP, Snoep G, van Kroonenburgh MP, et al. The additional value of gadolinium-enhanced MRI to standard assessment for cardiac involvement in patients with pulmonary sarcoidosis. Chest. 2005;128(3):1629-37.
44. Vignaux O. Cardiac sarcoidosis: spectrum of MRI features. AJR Am J Roentgenol. 2005;184(1):249-54.
45. Vignaux O, Dhote R, Duboc D, et al. Detection of myocardial involvement in patients with sarcoidosis applying T2-weighted, contrast-enhanced, and cine magnetic resonance imaging: initial results of a prospective study. J Comput Assist Tomogr. 2002;26(5):762-7.
46. Rahko PS, Salerni R, Uretsky BF. Successful reversal by chelation therapy of congestive cardiomyopathy due to iron overload. J Am Coll Cardiol. 1986;8(2):436-40.
47. Anderson LJ, Holden S, Davis B, et al. Cardiovascular T2-star (T2*) magnetic resonance for the early diagnosis of myocardial iron overload. Eur Heart J. 2001;22(23):2171-9.
48. Anderson LJ, Westwood MA, Holden S, et al. Myocardial iron clearance during reversal of siderotic cardiomyopathy with intravenous desferrioxamine: a prospective study using T2* cardiovascular magnetic resonance. Br J Haematol. 2004;127(3):348-55.

6

Real World Indications for Cardiac Magnetic Resonance Imaging: When is it invaluable in Clinical Practice?

Tommaso D' Angelo, Eike Nagel

INTRODUCTION

Cardiac magnetic resonance imaging (CMR) is a highly versatile noninvasive and nonionizing method for accurately evaluating function, structure, perfusion and tissue characteristics in a large variety of cardiac diseases. Due to its intrinsic flexibility, CMR represents an imaging modality that allows for the assessment of multiple different parameters within one examination. In particular, it can depict cardiovascular structure and anatomy, characterize tissue composition (including myocardial viability, inflammation and necrosis), measure cardiac function in terms of global and regional wall motion of the left and right ventricle or blood flow, assess metabolism with spectroscopic techniques, visualize and quantify myocardial perfusion and define the anatomy of epicardial coronary arteries.

The enthusiasm in which CMR was referred to be a "one stop shop" because of its capability to be a single solution to complex diagnostic problems, has matured towards a more balanced view about its effective clinical utility among the different diagnostic tools chosen by cardiologists with a stronger focus on the specific modules to answer a specific question as well as the economic need to shorten imaging times **(Fig. 1)**.

Commonly, CMR is not considered as the first diagnostic approach in patients presenting with heart related symptoms.

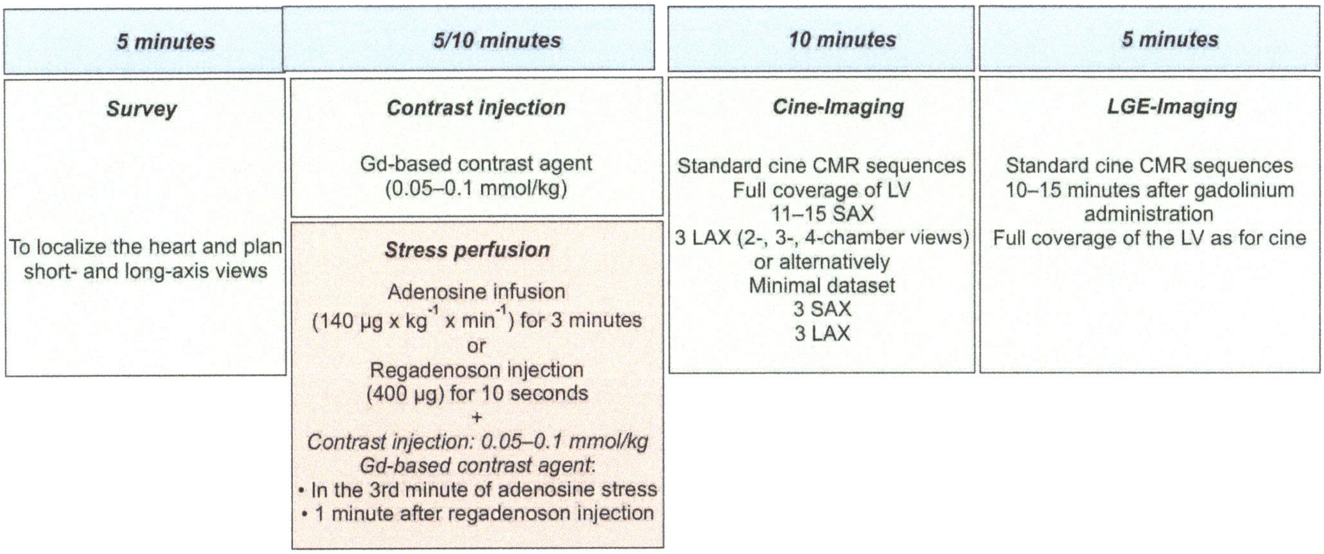

5 minutes	5/10 minutes	10 minutes	5 minutes
Survey	**Contrast injection**	**Cine-Imaging**	**LGE-Imaging**
To localize the heart and plan short- and long-axis views	Gd-based contrast agent (0.05–0.1 mmol/kg)	Standard cine CMR sequences Full coverage of LV 11–15 SAX 3 LAX (2-, 3-, 4-chamber views) or alternatively Minimal dataset 3 SAX 3 LAX	Standard cine CMR sequences 10–15 minutes after gadolinium administration Full coverage of the LV as for cine
	Stress perfusion Adenosine infusion (140 µg x kg^{-1} x min^{-1}) for 3 minutes or Regadenoson injection (400 µg) for 10 seconds + Contrast injection: 0.05–0.1 mmol/kg Gd-based contrast agent: • In the 3rd minute of adenosine stress • 1 minute after regadenoson injection		

Fig. 1: Typical CMR protocol. After individual patient planning using survey scans, intravenous adenosine (or regadenoson) is given prior to contrast injection, in case of stress perfusion imaging. Morphological assessment is therefore obtained by means of CINE-imaging and finally, a modified Look-Locker inversion time scout is performed prior to late-gadolinium enhancement imaging in short-axis (SAX) and long-axis (LAX) views

Table 1 Primary indications for CMR (from EuroCMR registry)[11]

Myocarditis/cardiomyopathies	32.2%	8950/27767
Suspected CAD/ischemia in known CAD	34.2%	9508
Myocardial viability	14.6%	4048
Valvular heart disease	5.4%	1495
Aortic disease	3.7%	1026
Congenital heart disease	2.2%	624
Ventricular thrombus	1.2%	330
Cardiac masses	1.0%	288
Pulmonary vessels	1.0%	282
Coronary vessels	0.2%	57
Other than above	10.7%	2963

In order to uncover the cause of such problems these patients should firstly be assessed by a careful review of clinical history, rest electrocardiography (ECG) and clinical examination. While an early CMR examination may actually shorten the pathway to diagnostic confidence and optimal therapy, most current guidelines and clinical routines tend to offer exercise ECG and transthoracic echocardiography as the first diagnostic tests. CMR should be considered in patients in whom these examinations do not provide adequate diagnostic information **(Table 1)**. In many patients, CMR is an invaluable method that might help understanding the presence and severity of morphological and functional abnormalities of the LV or RV myocardium, determining the underlying etiology (i.e. ischemic vs. nonischemic disease) of LV or RV dysfunction, identifying prognostic factors related to patient outcomes, and most importantly, guide towards individualized and optimized therapy **(Tables 2 and 3)**.[1-3]

In clinical routine CMR is mainly used in the work-up of *myocarditis and cardiomyopathies*, which may often present only mild and aspecific symptoms such as *chest pain* and *shortness of breath* or more severe *heart failure symptoms*, as well as in patients with known or suspected coronary artery disease or patients with unclear left ventricular (LV) hypertrophy. The strong case for CMR in congenital heart disease will not be discussed in this chapter.

MYOCARDITIS

Patients with myocarditis frequently present with unspecific symptoms, which include shortness of breath and chest pain. If symptoms are acute and combined with positive troponins they are often regarded as acute coronary syndromes and assessed with invasive angiography. CMR usually comes into play when invasive angiography shows normal coronary arteries. If symptoms are more protracted patients frequently present to CMR several weeks after the acute event.

In patients with suspected *myocarditis,* CMR allows for targeting several features such inflammatory hyperemia and edema, necrosis, contractile dysfunction, and pericardial effusion. In particular, regional necrosis is a frequent sign in severe myocarditis and its regional distribution allows for a typical distinction from ischemic lesions, which invariably include subendocardial layers, whereas myocarditis typically tends to exclude these areas. However, in less severe cases of myocarditis, necrosis may be absent and diagnosis harder. In

Table 2 Impact of CMR on patient management by indication[11]

	Myocarditis/CMP	Suspected CAD/Ischemia	Viability
All (from 27781 patients)	32.2%	34.2%	14.6%
Completely new diagnosis not suspected before	11.4%	8.1%	5.3%
Therapeutic consequences (change in medication)	25.3%	24.3%	33.2%
Therapeutic consequences (invasive procedure)	6.9%	23.1%	24.2%
Therapeutic consequences (hospital discharge)	10.4%	14.3%	6.9%
Therapeutic consequence (hospital admission)	1.1%	1.5%	1.9%
Impact on patient management (new diagnosis and/or therapeutic consequence	55.1%	71.4%	71.5%

Table 3 Additional diagnostic procedures avoided due to results of CMR in patients of EuroCMR registry[14]

	All (n = 10284)	No stress (n = 6933)	Stress (n = 3351)
Invasive angiography	21.5% (2,213)	10.2% (704)	45.0% (1,509)
Nuclear (SPECT/PET)	9.0% (928)	4.6% (319)	18.2% (609)
Coronary CT	2.0% (204)	1.9% (131)	2.2% (73)

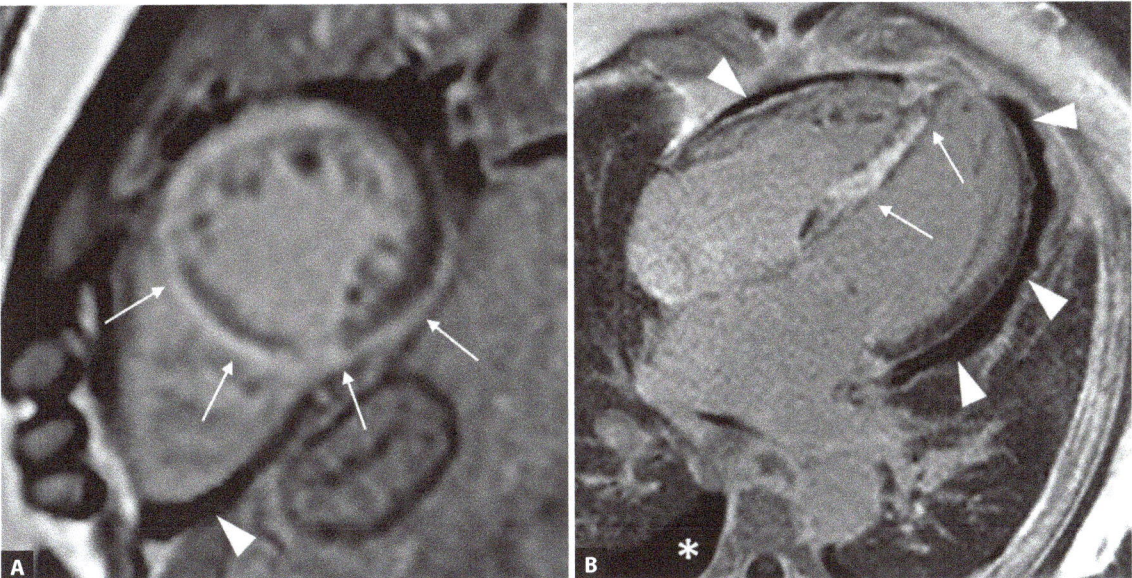

Figs 2A and B: Late gadolinium enhancement (LGE) images obtained along the apical short-axis view (A) and four-chambers view (B). CMR images clearly demonstrate the typically nonischemic, subepicardial LGE pattern (arrows). Pericardial effusion (arrowheads) and pleural effusion (asterisk) are also present

these cases, novel quantitative tissue characterization methods by native T1 and T2 mapping, have shown to provide important insight into inflammatory myocardial involvement, even with respect to disease recognition, allowing for monitoring of inflammatory activity and of response to anti-inflammatory treatment.[4,5]

NONISCHEMIC DILATED CARDIOMYOPATHIES

Many patients with cardiomyopathies are followed for years with various types and severities of symptoms. Echocardiographic imaging shows some grade of LV dilatation or dysfunction. CMR is frequently used, when the disease cannot be fully explained by echocardiography or before device placement to check for areas of irreversible necrosis. It is the strong belief of the authors, that CMR should be used earlier whenever possible to establish a diagnosis early and avoid deterioration into heart failure.

The CMR work-up of *nonischemic dilated cardiomyopathies* primarily consists on establishment of the correct diagnosis, i.e. ischemic versus nonischemic or the presence of a specific cardiomyopathy, which may be essential to guide therapy. The grade of LV dysfunction, the amount of irreversible necrosis, the presence of inflammation or ischemia or the observation of infiltrative disease are important measures of prognosis and support decision making for implantable cardioverter-defibrillators (ICDs), cardiac resynchronization therapy or revascularization.

Importantly, and in contrast to standard clinical assessment, LV volumes and function [ejection fraction (EF)] are important markers of outcome, however, they are outperformed significantly by the presence and extent of myocardial fibrosis (using late gadolinium enhancement (LGE) imaging) which is frequently found as a mid-myocardial stria in the interventricular septum **(Figs 2A and B)**. Ejection fraction further adds to the information obtained by fibrosis imaging alone.[6] More recently the use of mapping techniques (T1, ECV) have shown to provide even stronger prognostic information than the presence of regional scar.[7]

HYPERTROPHIC CARDIOMYOPATHY

Another problem of important clinical concern among cardiac diseases is represented by *hypertrophic cardiomyopathy (HCM)*. The average loss of individual lifetime caused by an HCM-induced lethal event is much higher than most of other heart diseases. This is due to the common early manifestation and to the fact that *sudden cardiac death* sometimes is the first symptom of the disease, especially in young patients. Most patients are sent to a CMR examination due to an unexplained left ventricular hypertrophy. This may be observed in healthy athletes, hypertensive or without obvious underlying cause.

The CMR is helpful to better assess the true regional wall thickness than echocardiography due to the better delineation of the epi- and endocardial border and independency of acoustic windows. In addition, it can detect and quantify the amount of myocardial scarring, which has been related to long-term clinical outcome and is—together with diffuse fibrosis—most likely the strongest predictor of outcome in these patients.[8] CMR findings may thus be much better predictor of lethal events than currently used individual or combined risk markers.

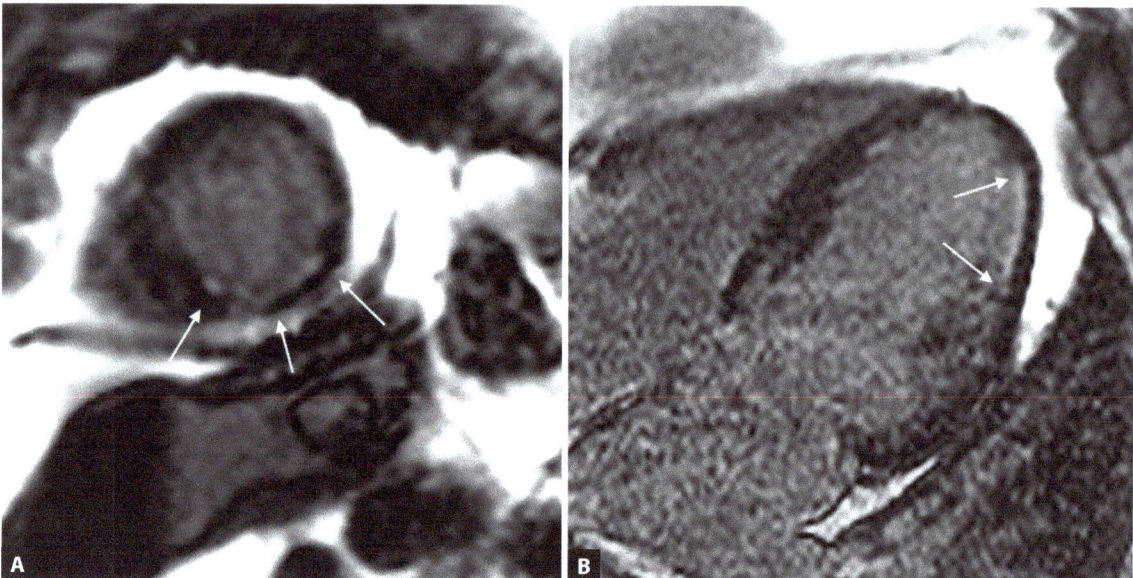

Figs 3A and B: Magnified late gadolinium enhancement (LGE) images obtained along the apical short-axis view (A) and four-chambers view (B). CMR images clearly demonstrate the typically ischemic, subendocardial LGE pattern (arrows)

When no evidence of myocardial scarring is seen at LGE imaging, the differential diagnosis of LV hypertrophy remains challenging, especially between HCM and increased myocardial wall thickness consequent to systemic hypertension or athletic lifestyle. In addition, it has been seen that a profibrotic state through genetically driven collagen metabolism usually precedes the overt phenotype with LV hypertrophy or fibrosis visible on LGE imaging. CMR can provide means of detecting these early myocardial tissue changes and thus distinguishing between these conditions by using the novel parametric techniques such as T1 mapping.[9]

CORONARY ARTERY DISEASE

Another outstanding indication for CMR is the detection and the risk assessment *in patients with known or suspected coronary artery disease (CAD)*. Recent guidelines provide Class I or IIa recommendation for the use of ischemia testing before invasive angiography in symptomatic patients (i.e. *chronic chest pain*) with an intermediate pre-test likelihood. The choice of imaging modality (SPECT, CMR or PET) is usually left to local conditions, physician or patient preference, and specific considerations. However, there is accumulating evidence, that the performance of CMR for the assessment of myocardial perfusion and ischemia is superior to SPECT imaging mainly due to its higher spatial resolution in combination with an excellent temporal resolution **(Figs 3 and 4)**. CMR is particularly indicated in symptomatic patients with medium to high pretest probability of CAD with or without inability to exercise or noninterpretable ECG as well as in patients with

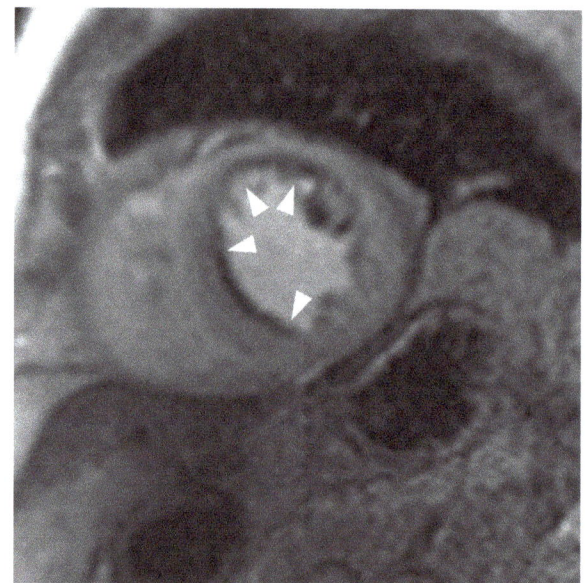

Fig. 4: CMR image obtained in short-axis view along the middle-slice during stress-perfusion sequence shows a septal subendocardial perfusion defect (arrowheads)

previous revascularization or myocardial infarction to assess the extent and severity of ischemia as well as the extent beyond areas of irreversible infarct damage.[10]

Symptomatic patients with low pretest probability of CAD might also appropriately undergo CMR, especially if they are unable to exercise or if they have an uninterpretative ECG.[10]

Table 4 Complications related to no-stress vs stress cardiovascular magnetic resonance according to EuroCMR registry[11]

Complications	All (n = 27396)	No stress (n = 17136)	Stress (n = 10228)
None	96.3% (26395)	98.6% (16893)	92.6% (9476)
Mild	3.6% (994)	1.4% (243)	7.3% (745)
Severe	0.0% (7)	0.0% (0)	0.1% (7)

In the work-up of asymptomatic individuals with high risk (regardless of ECG interpretability and ability to exercise) CMR stress test has also shown to be a valuable tool to assess risk stratification and thus, to reduce the number of patients who necessitate cardiac catheterization without a significant increase of procedural complications **(Table 4)**.[11]

In particular, a recent study has demonstrated the value of vasodilator stress perfusion CMR for risk stratification in patients with diabetes and found a yearly event rate of 0.5% for cardiac death or myocardial infarction in patients without scar or inducible ischemia, whereas those with inducible ischemia had an event rate of 8.2%.[10]

VIABILITY/HIBERNATION

The CMR is also used widely to assess *myocardial viability or hibernating myocardium* in patients with history of myocardial infarction.[12] LGE imaging with gadolinium is the most accurate and validated modality currently used as a mean to predict potential for functional recovery in hibernating or stunned myocardium, as well as overall risk and prognosis. A combination of LGE and ischemia imaging allows to assess whether there is any additional ischemia which may further weight in towards revascularization in patients with chronic infarction.

OTHER INDICATIONS

Finally, CMR is important in the diagnosis and follow-up of patients with *congenital heart disease, myocardial tumors, pericardial diseases* and in *valvular disease* usually as a complement to echocardiography, and it is increasingly used as an aid to determine the optimal timing for surgery. Several studies have also shown that CMR can also be used successfully in the screening, diagnosis, and follow-up of several aortic diseases, and especially in the diagnosis of *aortic dissection*.[11]

CONTRAINDICATIONS AND LIMITATIONS

The CMR possesses few contraindications such as incompatible devices. Some limitations, may need to be observed in patients with severe arrhythmia or severe or acute renal dysfunction.[13]

Arrhythmia was previously considered a problem for reduced quality of the images acquired. However, newer and faster imaging sequences, as well as improved arrhythmia rejection programming have reduced this problem. Occasionally a patient with reduced diagnostic accuracy may be encountered, especially for the quantification of end-systolic volumes.

Gadolinium-based contrast media are the main stone for "late gadolinium enhancement" imaging and first pass techniques that allow assessment of myocardial perfusion. In the last years, there have been reports about nephrogenic systemic fibrosis related to the use of gadolinium-based contrast agents in patients with *renal failure*. In order to avoid this extremely rare complications, current guidelines suggest that in patients with reduced renal function (eGFR <60 mL/min) only highly stable contrast media (cyclic structure) should be used. In patients with an estimated glomerular filtration, rate less than 30 mL/min contrast agents should only be given after a positive risk assessment and specific discussion with the patient.

Many patients with cardiac problems have implanted *pacemakers and cardiac devices*. The major concern with these devices in an MRI scanner is the possibility of heating and malfunctioning. However, there is an increasing focus on these problems among the manufacturers, and efforts are made to encounter these problems with the development of new MR-safe implants. In contrast to these devices, neither coronary stents, or mechanical valves should be considered as contraindications for performing CMR examinations.

REFERENCES

1. Dabir D, Child N, Kalra A, Rogers T, Gebker R, Jabbour A, Plein S, Yu CY, Otton J, Kidambi A, McDiarmid A, Broadbent D, Higgins DM, Schnackenburg B, Foote L, Cummins C, Nagel E, Puntmann VO. Reference values for healthy human myocardium using a T1 mapping methodology: results from the International T1 Multicenter cardiovascular magnetic resonance study. Journal of Cardiovascular Magnetic Resonance: Official Journal of the Society for Cardiovascular Magnetic Resonance. 2014;16:69. doi:10.1186/s12968-014-0069-x.
2. Kramer CM, Barkhausen J, Flamm SD, Kim RJ, Nagel E. Standardized cardiovascular magnetic resonance (CMR) protocols 2013 update. Journal of Cardiovascular Magnetic Resonance: Official Journal of the Society for Cardiovascular Magnetic Resonance. 2013;15:91. doi:10.1186/1532-429x-15-91.
3. Schulz-Menger J, Bluemke DA, Bremerich J, Flamm SD, Fogel MA, Friedrich MG, Kim RJ, von Knobelsdorff-Brenkenhoff F, Kramer CM, Pennell DJ, Plein S, Nagel E. Standardized image interpretation and post processing in cardiovascular magnetic resonance: Society for Cardiovascular Magnetic Resonance

(SCMR) board of trustees task force on standardized post processing. Journal of Cardiovascular Magnetic Resonance: Official Journal of the Society for Cardiovascular Magnetic Resonance. 2013;15:35. doi:10.1186/1532-429x-15-35.
4. Puntmann VO, Peker E, Chandrashekhar Y, Nagel E. T1 Mapping in Characterizing Myocardial Disease: A Comprehensive Review. Circulation research. 2016;119(2):277-99. doi:10.1161/circresaha.116.307974.
5. Puntmann VO, Nagel E. T1 and T2 mapping in nonischemic cardiomyopathies and agreement with endomyocardial biopsy. Journal of the American College of Cardiology. 2016;68(17):1923-24. doi:10.1016/j.jacc.2016.06.075.
6. Gulati A, Jabbour A, Ismail TF, Guha K, Khwaja J, Raza S, Morarji K, Brown TD, Ismail NA, Dweck MR, Di Pietro E, Roughton M, Wage R, Daryani Y, O'Hanlon R, Sheppard MN, Alpendurada F, Lyon AR, Cook SA, Cowie MR, Assomull RG, Pennell DJ, Prasad SK. Association of fibrosis with mortality and sudden cardiac death in patients with nonischemic dilated cardiomyopathy. JAMA. 2013;309(9):896-908. doi:10.1001/jama.2013.1363.
7. Hinojar R, Foote L, Sangle S, Marber M, Mayr M, Carr-White G, D'Cruz D, Nagel E, Puntmann VO. Native T1 and T2 mapping by CMR in lupus myocarditis: Disease recognition and response to treatment. International Journal of Cardiology. 2016;222:717-26. doi:10.1016/j.ijcard.2016.07.182.
8. Weng Z, Yao J, Chan RH, He J, Yang X, Zhou Y, He Y. Prognostic value of LGE-CMR in HCM: a meta-analysis. JACC Cardiovascular imaging. doi:10.1016/j.jcmg.2016.02.031.
9. Hinojar R, Varma N, Child N, Goodman B, Jabbour A, Yu CY, Gebker R, Doltra A, Kelle S, Khan S, Rogers T, Arroyo Ucar E, Cummins C, Carr-White G, Nagel E, Puntmann VO. T1 Mapping in discrimination of Hypertrophic Phenotypes: Hypertensive Heart Disease and Hypertrophic Cardiomyopathy: Findings From the International T1 Multicenter Cardiovascular Magnetic Resonance Study. Circulation Cardiovascular imaging. 2015;8(12). doi:10.1161/circimaging.115.003285.
10. Hendel RC, Friedrich MG, Schulz-Menger J, Zemmrich C, Bengel F, Berman DS, Camici PG, Flamm SD, Le Guludec D, Kim R, Lombardi M, Mahmarian J, Sechtem U, Nagel E. CMR first-pass perfusion for suspected inducible myocardial ischemia. JACC Cardiovascular Imaging. 2016;9(11):1338-48. doi:10.1016/j.jcmg.2016.09.010.
11. Bruder O, Wagner A, Lombardi M, Schwitter J, van Rossum A, Pilz G, Nothnagel D, Steen H, Petersen S, Nagel E, Prasad S, Schumm J, Greulich S, Cagnolo A, Monney P, Deluigi CC, Dill T, Frank H, Sabin G, Schneider S, Mahrholdt H. European Cardiovascular Magnetic Resonance (EuroCMR) registry--multi national results from 57 centers in 15 countries. Journal of Cardiovascular Magnetic Resonance : Official Journal of the Society for Cardiovascular Magnetic Resonance. 2013;15:9. doi:10.1186/1532-429x-15-9.
12. Schelbert EB, Cao JJ, Sigurdsson S, Aspelund T, Kellman P, Aletras AH, Dyke CK, Thorgeirsson G, Eiriksdottir G, Launer LJ, Gudnason V, Harris TB, Arai AE. Prevalence and prognosis of unrecognized myocardial infarction determined by cardiac magnetic resonance in older adults. JAMA. 2012;308(9):890-6. doi:10.1001/2012.jama.11089.
13. Hundley WG, Bluemke D, Bogaert JG, Friedrich MG, Higgins CB, Lawson MA, McConnell MV, Raman SV, van Rossum AC, Flamm S, Kramer CM, Nagel E, Neubauer S. Society for Cardiovascular Magnetic Resonance guidelines for reporting cardiovascular magnetic resonance examinations. Journal of Cardiovascular Magnetic Resonance : Official Journal of the Society for Cardiovascular Magnetic Resonance. 2009;11:5. doi:10.1186/1532-429x-11-5.
14. Bruder O, Schneider S, Nothnagel D, Dill T, Hombach V, Schulz-Menger J, Nagel E, Lombardi M, van Rossum AC, Wagner A, Schwitter J, Senges J, Sabin GV, Sechtem U, Mahrholdt H. EuroCMR (European Cardiovascular Magnetic Resonance) registry: results of the German pilot phase. Journal of the American College of Cardiology. 2009;54(15):1457-66. doi:10.1016/j.jacc.2009.07.003.

7

Cardiac MRI and Cardiac CT: Indispensable Tools for the Diagnosis of Coronary Artery Disease

Parang Sanghavi, Aamish Kazi, Bhavin Jankharia

INTRODUCTION

Coronary artery disease (CAD) affects 7–13% of urban and 2–7% of the rural populations in India and produces a significant disease burden.[1] Accurate evaluation of CAD helps to improve outcomes. Early diagnosis of CAD can help to institute aggressive measures to control disease and prevent progression to ischemic heart disease.[2]

Cardiac magnetic resonance imaging (MRI) and cardiac computed tomography (CT) in the last two decades have made great technological leaps that have allowed both of them to make a difference in the evaluation of CAD. Both of them have different indications and uses that we will discuss in the next few pages.

CARDIAC COMPUTED TOMOGRAPHY

For many years, this was the holy grail of imaging. While electron beam CT scanners (EBCT) had the temporal resolution to allow evaluation of the calcium content of the coronary arteries,[3] it was with the advent of four slice CT scanners,[4] with a slow heart rate of around 60, that it was possible to achieve a temporal resolution that could summate the coronary arteries over a few heart-beats and allow visualization of the coronary arteries. The current 256 and 320 slice scanners allow even faster acquisition of images, though good quality studies still need a low, steady heart rate and can be achieved with 64-slice CT scanners as well.

Calcium Scoring

This was the first modality to evaluate CAD risk. Outcome data over more than two decades has shown that a calcium (CA) score of 0 is associated with an extremely low coronary event risk.[5] As the calcium score increases, the event risk rises. It is an independent risk factor for coronary events and event-free survival. It is a modality ideally situated for mass screening.

- Plain scan
- Low radiation
- Easy to interpret.

Coronary Angiography

This requires intravenous contrast administration, a low heart rate as far as possible and a steady heart rate for the best images.

Conventional coronary angiography (CCA) is performed in the following situations:

To Rule Out Coronary Artery Disease

In patients with medium-to-high risk of CAD, who are otherwise asymptomatic or have equivocal symptoms or results of ECG or stress test, CCA is the modality of choice to evaluate the status of the coronary arteries. Outcome data is now available and shows that a normal coronary angiogram has a negligible coronary event risk with a negative predictive value approaching 100% **(Fig. 1)**.[6]

Conventional caronary angiography is also used in emergency rooms to triage chest pain. A "triple rule-out" study helps rule out coronary artery disease, pulmonary thromboembolism and aortic aneurysm with dissection.[7]

Stents

In-stent evaluation is still an issue. The larger the stent, the easier it is view the lumen **(Fig. 2)**. The faster scanners with iterative reconstructions have improved the ability to see the in-stent lumen **(Figs 3A to C)**, though with small stents, there are still issues.[8] While CCA is used in some instances to evaluate in-stent lumen, especially in patients with equivocal symptoms, often the reason to do CCA is to evaluate the rest of the vessels, with the same clinical indication as above.

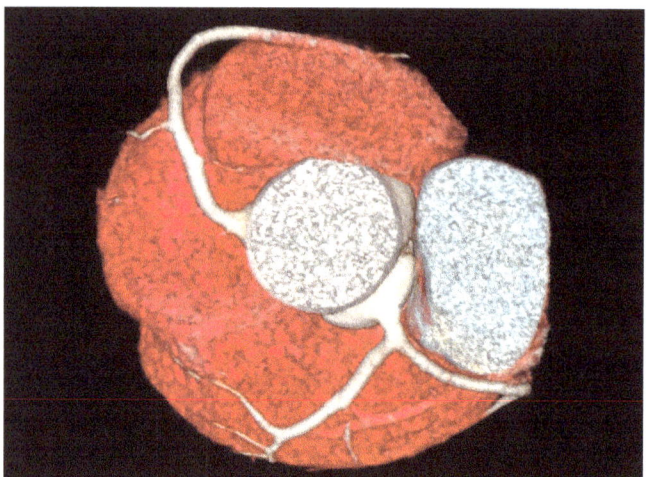

Fig. 1: Volume-rendered coronary CT angiogram (CTA) shows normal coronary arteries

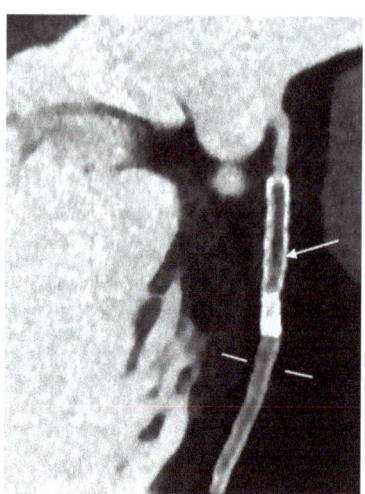

Fig. 2: Maximum intensity projection (MIP) CTA of the left anterior descending artery (LAD) using an iterative reconstruction algorithm shows in-stent occlusion (arrow)

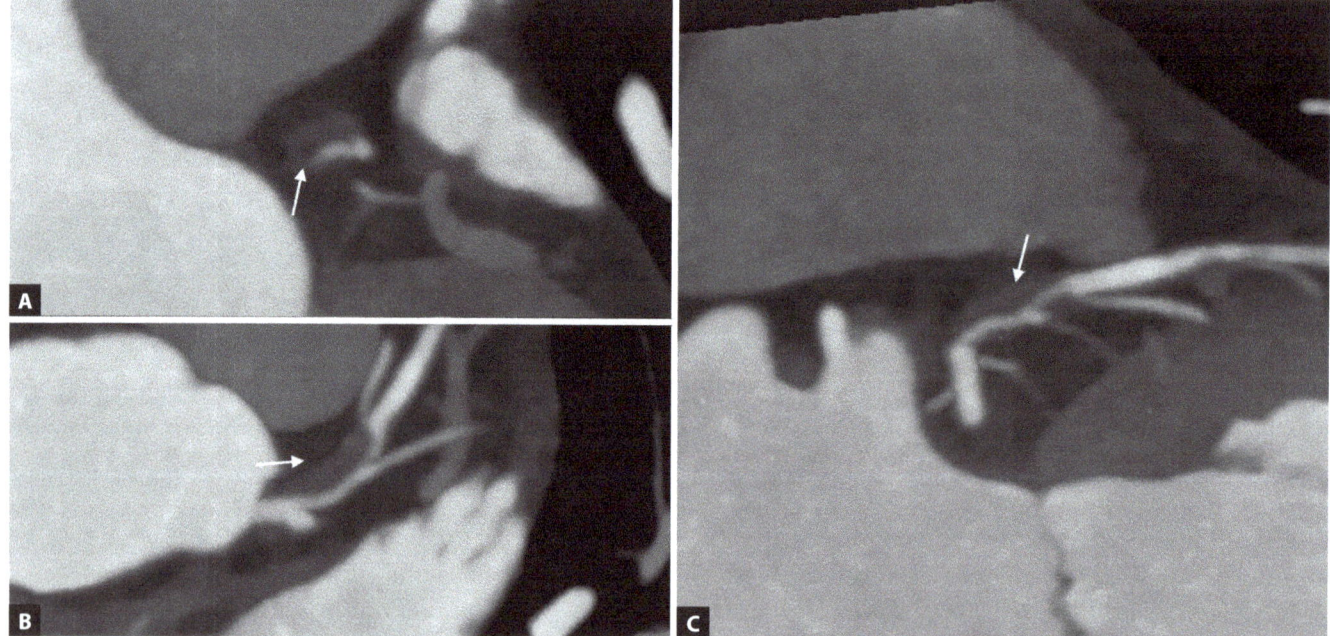

Figs 3A to C: MIP images in cross-section (A) and in two perpendicular longitudinal planes; (B, C) shows a complex plaque (arrows) with a lipid core (arrow in A) with significant stenosis

Plaque Evaluation

Cardiac CT is an excellent modality to evaluate plaque composition. The newer dual energy scanners with iterative reconstruction techniques have made plaque analysis **(Figs 3A to C)** more robust, though clinical utility is still suspect.[9] The analysis of plaque-at-risk using CCA is being evaluated in multiple clinical trials, but clinical utility may still be a few years away.[10]

Perfusion[11]

The newer scanners allow perfusion studies to be performed, but given the increased radiation and the availability of other equally good or better modalities with tested outcome data, it is unlikely that CT perfusion will assume an important role at least in the near future.

Following Bypass Surgery

Cardiac CT allows accurate evaluation of grafts, both venous and arterial and can serve as the first modality to evaluate graft patency, anastomotic site pathology and abnormalities of the post-graft vessel. A recent meta-analysis shows a sensitivity and specificity of 99% each for graft occlusion and 98% each for evaluation of >50% graft stenosis **(Fig. 4)**.[12]

CARDIAC MAGNETIC RESONANCE IMAGING

In the late 1990s, with the advent of faster gradients and balanced gradient sequences, it became easy to perform cardiac MRI studies in clinically acceptable times. This led to the use of cardiac MRI in myocardial, valvular and pericardial pathologies with an impact on management in many situations.

Coronary Arteries

While the first multicenter study on the use of CMR in the evaluation of coronary arteries showed good results, in practice, the visualization of coronary arteries by CMR is a time-consuming affair even with the use of whole heart techniques.[13]

Perfusion

Adenosine stress perfusion by CMR is a robust technique that is not inferior to nuclear medicine techniques.[14] The temporal and spatial resolution are now better and outcome data has shown results that are superior to nuclear medicine perfusion. Perfusion is usually combined with viability imaging, which improves the clinical utility of this test.

Viability Imaging

The discovery that 5–7 minutes after injection of gadolinium, it was possible to visualize infarcts **(Fig. 5)**, paved the way for the use of CMR in the assessment of viability after a coronary event. Today CMR is the gold standard for viability imaging and accurately predicts the presence of stunned, hibernating and nonviable segments, allowing correct clinical decision-making regarding revascularization, in patients with coronary artery stenoses and severe ischemia/infarction **(Fig. 6)**.[15]

CONCLUSION

Cardiac CT is anatomic tool that can be used in early diagnosis of CAD (calcium scoring) and in diagnosing coronary artery disease (cardiac CT angiography). Cardiac MRI is a functional tool that allows assessment of perfusion defects and is the gold standard for viability imaging.

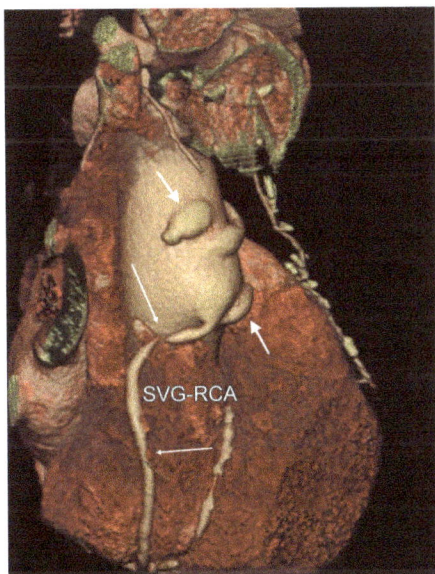

Fig. 4: VRT CT angiogram shows 2 occluded venous grafts (thick white arrows). The saphenous vein graft (SVG) to the posterior descending artery (PDA) shows focal severe stenosis (arrow) with another 50% stenosis more distally (arrow)

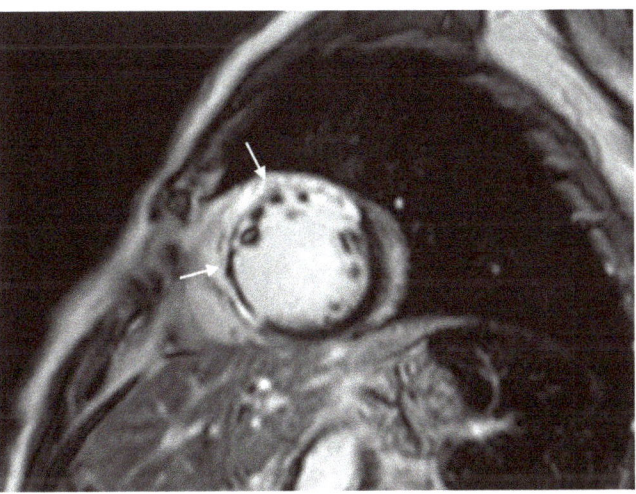

Fig. 5: Short axis (SA) mid-cavity, inversion recovery (IR) image obtained 7 minutes after intravenous (IV) gadolinium (Gd) injection shows a full-thickness LAD territory infarct involving the anterior wall and septum (arrows)

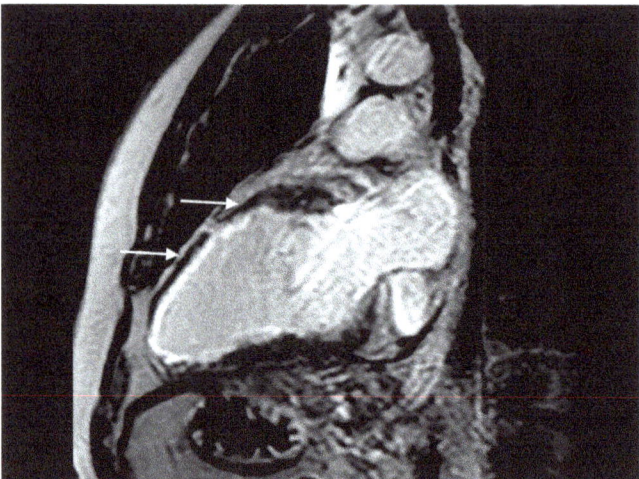

Fig. 6: 4-chamber (4C) IR image obtained 8 minutes after IV Gd injection shows an anterior wall infarct involving <50% of the thickness of the myocardium (arrows), suggesting hibernating, potentially viable myocardium, in this patient with LAD occlusion and akinesia of the septum

REFERENCES

1. Krishnan MN. Coronary heart disease and risk factors in India - on the brink of an epidemic? Indian Heart Jour. 2012;64:364.
2. Shah N, Soon K, Wong C, Kelly A-M. Screening for asymptomatic coronary heart disease in the young 'at risk' population: Who and how? IJC Heart Vascul. 2015;6:60.
3. Sechtem U. Electron beam computed tomography: on its way into mainstream cardiology? Eur Heart Jour. 2000;21:87.
4. Achenbach S, Giesler T, Ropers D, et al. Detection of coronary artery stenoses by contrast-enhanced, retrospectively electrocardiographically gated, multislice spiral computed tomography. Circulation. 2001;103:2535.
5. Greenland P, Bonow RO, Brundage BH, et al. ACCF/AHA 2007 clinical expert consensus document on coronary artery calcium scoring by computed tomography in global cardiovascular risk assessment and in evaluation of patients with chest pain: a report of the American College of Cardiology Foundation Clinical Expert Consensus Task Force (ACCF/AHA Writing committee to update the 2000 Expert Consensus Document on Electron Beam Computed Tomography) developed in collaboration with the Society of Atherosclerosis Imaging and Prevention and Society of Cardiovascular Computed Tomography. JACC. 2007;49:378.
6. Mowatt G, Cook JA, Hillis G, et al. 64-Slice computed tomography angiography in the diagnosis and assessment of coronary artery disease: systematic review and meta-analysis. Heart. 2008;94:1386.
7. Frauenfelder T, Appenzeller P, Karlo C, et al. Triple rule-out CT in the emergency department: protocols and spectrum of imaging findings. Eur Rad. 2009;19:789.
8. Taylor AJ, Cerqueira M, Hodgson JM, et al. ACCF/SCCT/ACR/AHA/ASE/ASNC/NASCI/SCAI/SCMR 2010 Appropriate Use Criteria for Cardiac Computed Tomography. A Report of the American College of Cardiology Foundation Appropriate Use Criteria Task Force, the Society of Cardiovascular Computed Tomography, the American College of Radiology, the American Heart Association, the American Society of Echocardiography, the American Society of Nuclear Cardiology, the North American Society for Cardiovascular Imaging, the Society for Cardiovascular Angiography and Interventions, and the Society for Cardiovascular Magnetic Resonance. Jour Cardiovasc Computed Tomogr. 2010;4:407e1-33.
9. Obaid DR, Calvert PA, Gopalan D, et al. Dual-energy computed tomography imaging to determine atherosclerotic plaque composition: a prospective study with tissue validation. Jour Cardiovasc Computed Tomogr. 2014;8:230.
10. Latif MA, Cury R, Akhlaq M, et al. A systematic review and meta-analysis: prevalence of coronary plaque high-risk features (low attenuation, enlarged diameter or positive remodeling, napkin ring, and spotty calcification (lens) in acute coronary syndrome as assessed by coronary computed tomographic angiography (CTA). JACC. 2016;67:1736.
11. Varga-Szemes A, Meinel FG, De Cecco CN, et al. CT myocardial perfusion imaging. Am J Roentgenol. 2015;204:487.
12. Barbero U, Innaccone M, d'Ascenzo F, et al. 64 slice-coronary computed tomography sensitivity and specificity in the evaluation of coronary artery bypass graft stenosis: a meta-analysis. Int J Cardiol. 2016;216:52.
13. Sakuma H. Coronary CT versus MR angiography: the role of MR angiography. Radiology. 2011;258:340.
14. Coelho-Filho OR, Rickers C, Kwong RY, Jerosch-Herold M. MR myocardial perfusion imaging. Radiology. 2013;266:701.
15. Rajiah P, Desai MY, Kwon D, Flamm SD. MR imaging of myocardial infarction. Radiographics. 2013;33:1383.

8. Cardiac Imaging: Current Scenario and Future Directions

Om Tavri, Priya Chudgar

INTRODUCTION

Over the past decade, technological improvements have led to the widespread use of imaging modalities in the prediction, diagnosis and follow-up of various cardiac diseases. From use of 4 slice multidetector computed tomography (MDCT) scanners, the CT scanners have evolved to 256 and beyond. It provides excellent anatomical details along with plaque morphology and luminal stenosis. CT coronary angiography today is considered well-established imaging tool for accurate interpretation of coronary artery disease.

Cardiac magnetic resonance imaging (MRI) with its multiplanar ability has added advantage of functional assessment. Cardiac magnetic resonance (CMR) has ability to quantify flow as well as ventricular volume. Though coronary vessels are better evaluated on CT scan, morphology of heart and its chambers is beautifully seen on MRI. Multiplanar imaging with excellent resolution makes MRI an ideal 'one stop shop 'for cardiac imaging. Newer machine allows rapid acquisition and also are more patient friendly. The amount of clinical information obtained is extremely important for planning of further management.

With the increasing incidence of heart disease, there is also need for early detection and accurate diagnosis. Recent advances in cardiac imaging have tremendously affected patient management. This article describes current scenario of cardiac imaging with insight into future direction.

COMPUTED TOMOGRAPHY CORONARY ANGIOGRAPHY

Cardiac CT will also provide more functional information in the future, and its use will continue to grow.

Advances in cardiac CT have brought its use in clinical routine to unprecedented levels. The main reason is that image acquisition optimization strategies allow radiologists to assess blood vessels with the same efficiency as coronary angiography, non-invasively and almost instantaneously.

CT is considered a wonderful technique for the evaluation of coronary arteries. It is really similar to coronary angiography, but without the risks **(Fig. 1)**. With newer machines, we have the ability to produce imaging very fast, reduce artefact, but especially reduce the dose of radiation in each patient.

Cardiac CT use in clinical routine will continue to rise in the near future. A paper published by the British Cardiovascular Society predicts that the number of cardiac CT examinations carried out will increase by up to 40 times by 2020. The use of cardiac CT is bound to increase and, by the next decade, it

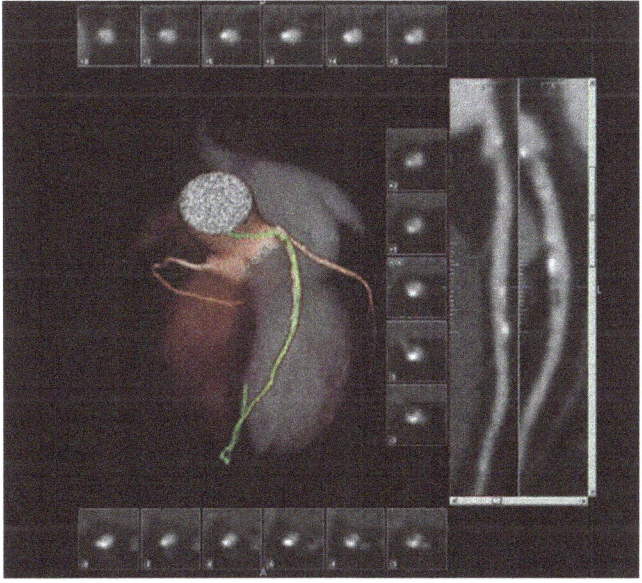

Fig. 1: Multiplanar reconstruction of CT coronary angiography to evaluate luminal narrowing with mixed density coronary plaque

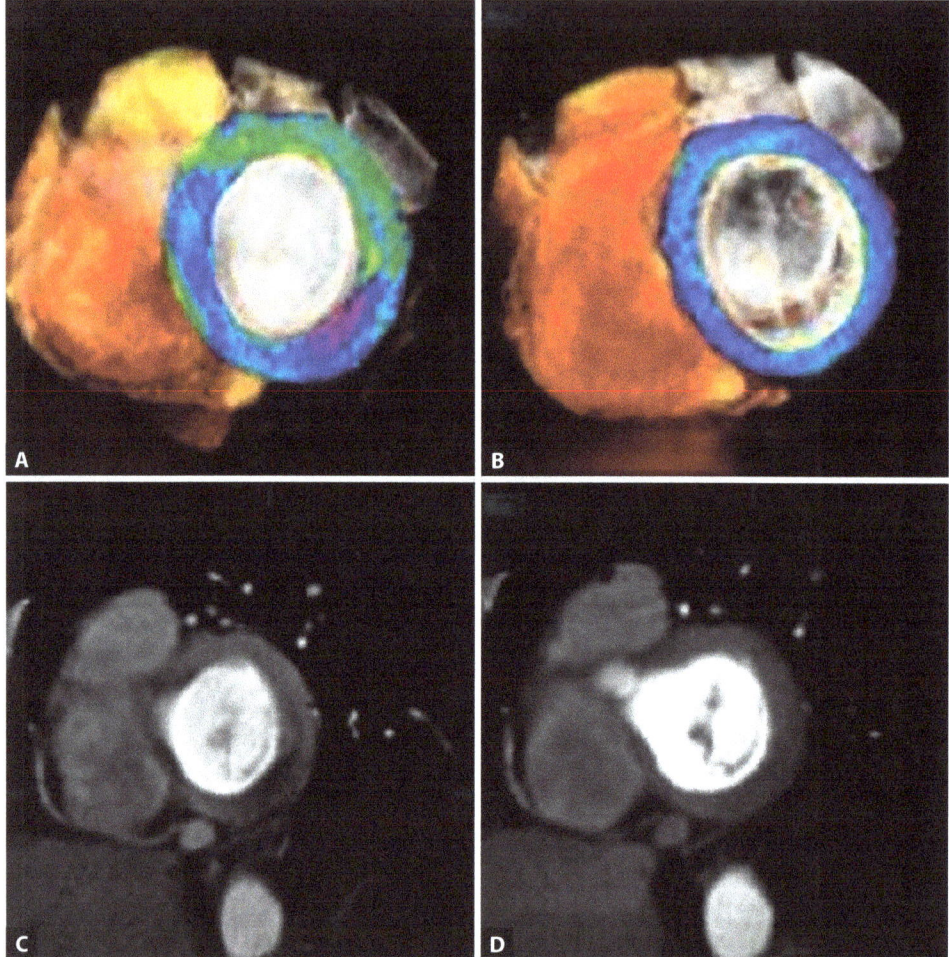

Figs 2A to D: CT myocardial perfusion image set showing perfusion defects in a color-coded iodine map and seen as darker areas of low contrast in the images

could penetrate everyday work, in both specialized and nonspecialized centers.

The Rule Out Myocardial Infarction/Ischemia Using Computer Assisted Tomography (ROMICAT II) trial aims to show that cardiac CT can be used in patients with acute chest pain, while the PROMISE trial looks at patients with stable chest pain. For the latter, 64-slice CT was tested against the conventional standard of care (ECG, lab tests, etc.), to show if a single CT examination can spare patients further tests.

By 2020, cardiac CT will have undergone further technical developments. Major advances have been made over the past five years to optimize image acquisition and reduce dose; specialized centers can now operate cardiac CT using one mSv. This dosage will become standard practice as demand for CT examinations grows.

Recent technical advances in multidetector row CT have resulted in lower radiation dose, improved temporal and spatial resolution, decreased scan time, and improved tissue differentiation. Lower radiation doses have resulted from the use of pre-patient z collimators, the availability of thin-slice axial data acquisition, the increased efficiency of ECG-based tube current modulation, and the implementation of iterative reconstruction algorithms. Faster gantry rotation and the simultaneous use of two X-ray sources have led to improvements in temporal resolution, and gains in spatial resolution have been achieved through application of the flying X-ray focal-spot technique in the z-direction. Shorter scan times have resulted from the design of detector arrays with increasing numbers of detector rows and through the simultaneous use of two X-ray sources to allow higher helical pitch. Some improvements in tissue differentiation have been achieved with dual energy CT.

PERFUSION IMAGING

CT perfusion software works by mapping iodine contrast distributions in the myocardium throughout the cardiac cycle **(Figs 2 and 3)**. These color-coded maps can be displayed as

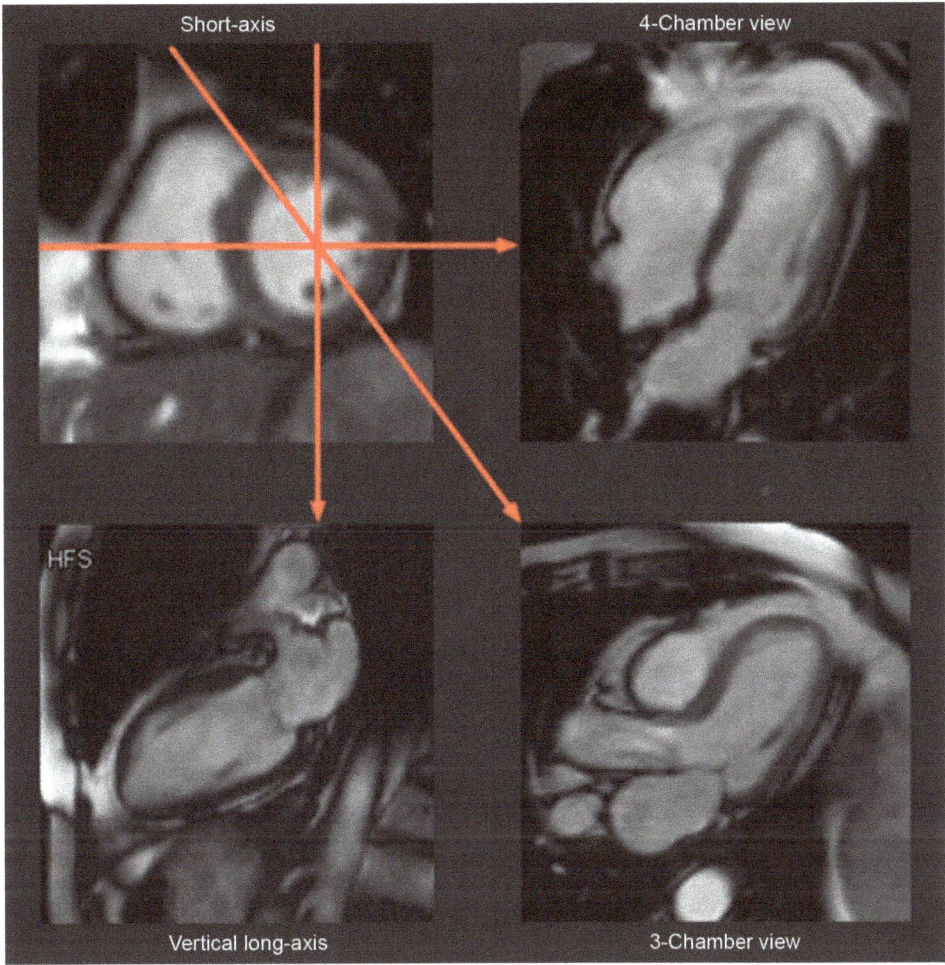

Fig. 3: Multiplanar capability of MRI evaluates cardiac chambers in different views

either bull's eye plots or overlaid on 3-D images of the heart, showing the wash in and wash out of contrast, which is used as a surrogate for blood. Areas of low contrast attenuation correlate with areas of low perfusion due to blocked arteries. Even without attenuation maps, many experienced cardiac CT readers can see shading defects in the myocardium caused by low areas of iodine contrast due to blockages.

VIRTUAL COMPUTED TOMOGRAPHY— FRACTIONAL FLOW RESERVE

A key component of this transformation is a new supercomputing technology called CT-fractional flow reserve (FFR), which may offer a noninvasive alternative to catheter-based FFR. Invasive FFR is the current gold standard for determining if a stent is required for a particular lesion. Cardiac CT advocates said this, combined with CT myocardial perfusion imaging, will make CT diagnostics much more accurate. Current cardiac CT relies only on a visual, anatomical assessment of the coronary vessels without any way to qualify the functional impact of atherosclerosis.

SPECTRAL COMPUTED TOMOGRAPHY

Spectral CT uses two different kV energies to image the same area of anatomy simultaneously. On a molecular level, some elements have different attenuations at different energies, such as iodine or calcium. This enables the mapping and dialing in or out of these elements from an image to reduce or eliminate calcium blooming and beam hardening artifacts. The technology also allows creation of virtual noncontrast images without the need for a second scan protocol. These methods may help improve image quality and reduce CT radiation dose.

PLAQUE CHARACTERIZATION

All advanced visualization and CT manufacturers offer software to characterize plaque composition based on its Hounsfield

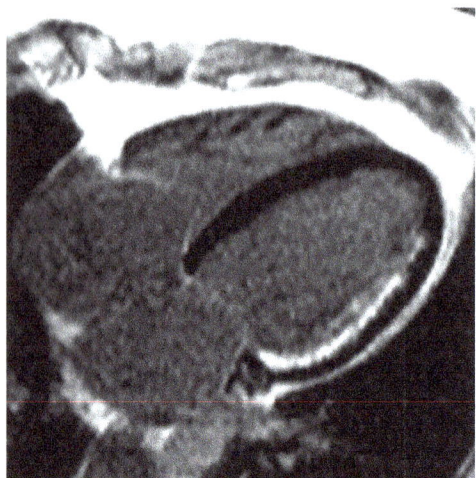

Fig. 4: Delayed hyperenhancement accurately depicts location and size of myocardial scar

unit measures. However, the software still requires additional clinical data for validation. Noninvasive CT plaque analysis could have a major impact on evaluating lesions without the need for catheterization, producing data and images similar to the invasive imaging methods of virtual histology intravascular ultrasound (IVUS) or near-infrared spectrography.

HYBRID IMAGING

Hybrid imaging, in particular positron-emission tomography (PET)-CT and the recently introduced MR-PET, should also offer information on both the myocardium and coronary arteries by 2020. Heart MRI, the golden standard for imaging the myocardium, will undergo several transformations, but this is further down the road, Researchers are currently testing the possibility of evaluating the myocardium with magnetic field strengths higher than 1.5T. So far they have not been very enthusiastic about the results, but things could change soon. Heart MRI is a very fast evolving modality. In the beginning we used low field, right now we are using medium field, and in the far future we could improve the evaluation with fields beyond 3T, helped by the development of new sequences, and provide new information about the heart structure.

CARDIAC MAGNETIC RESONANCE IMAGING

Cardiac MRI is a noninvasive, tomographic, nonionizing technique, thus it has been clinically used for assessing expansion of infarcted segments, late wall thinning of infarcted regions, left ventricular (LV) volumes, distortion of LV shape and compensatory hypertrophy of noninfarcted myocardium. MRI is mainly used for ischemic, nonischemic heart diseases, hypertrophic cardiomyopathy as well as heart failure and congenital heart disease.

Unlike echocardiography, PET and single-photon emission computed tomography (SPECT), MRI has the unique ability to provide quantitative information on cardiac function, perfusion and viability.

Due to excellent endocardial border delineation and no need for geometric assumptions of LV or RV shape, CMR is now regarded as the gold standard for the reproducible assessment of ventricular mass, volumes, and global ejection fraction. To detect a 10-gram change in LV mass (power 90%, error 0.05), a conventional echo study would need to enroll 505 patients, but the same CMR study would only need to recruit 14 patients. Similar, but less striking results are found with LV and RV functional assessment, creating a highly attractive research tool. Regional cardiac function can be assessed by myocardial deformation measured with cine MR tagging and myocardial strain and strain rate using harmonic phase analysis and velocity-encoded techniques, respectively.

Abnormal flow in the heart can be detected as a signal void on cine MRI (visually similar to color-flow Doppler). Unlike single-plane spectral Doppler techniques, multidirectional blood flow velocity can be calculated in any given plane with velocity-encoded MRI (phase velocity mapping). By combining the most accurate LV and RV volume assessment with this robust tool for arterial flow mapping, CMR should be considered the gold standard for the assessment of complex flow physiology as seen in complex congenital heart diseases and acquired multivalve lesions.

Delayed Enhancement MRI (DE-MRI)

It provides high contrast between viable and nonviable myocardium, thus it has been frequently used for detecting and measuring MI size. Furthermore, discrimination between viable and infarcted myocardium allows patients to avoid the risks associated with revascularization therapy when they are unlikely to benefit. MRI examination for evaluating suspected coronary artery disease consists of T2-weighted imaging for area at risk (AAR) demonstration and DE-MRI for infarct visualization **(Fig. 4)**.

Cardiac magnetic resonance (CMR) has a distinct advantage over echocardiography and nuclear scintigraphy in terms of fewer artifacts and unlimited acquisition windows. It is noninvasive, lacks ionizing radiation, and uses benign paramagnetic contrast agents without nephrotoxicity (unlike computed tomography). It has positioned itself to become a "one-stop diagnostic shop," offering extensive results during a single examination currently only available through a combination of multiple, separate, diagnostic procedures.

Computer software sophistication has developed to allow extremely rapid cardiac acquisitions. Even real-time imaging (acquisition of a single image within milliseconds) is now possible. Images can be scouted faster, resulting in less total time necessary for comprehensive cardiac examinations and provides a more robust environment for dobutamine stress MRI. Advancements in respiratory compensation techniques lessen the current need for patient cooperation and breath holding. This will further expand the utilization of CMR to include patients currently unable to cooperate because of age or underlying cardiopulmonary illness. Also, by eliminating breath holding, current time restraints can be removed and will allow even higher spatial resolution. Soon, the need for peripheral contrast administration will be removed entirely. Normal and pathologic tissue characteristics, as well as blood flow assessments, will be determined by their natural tissue variations in water content. This eliminates the need for IV administration and creates even faster examinations.

Dobutamine Stress MRI

It has proved to be highly accurate in detection of ischemia-induced minor reductions in wall thickening. Patients scheduled for echo stress testing with poor ultrasound windows are excellent candidates for dobutamine stress MRI examinations.

The spatial resolution of CMR (2–3 mm) is superior to positron emission tomography and single photon emission CT (4–8 mm), providing differentiating capabilities of partial myocardial thickness perfusion abnormalities. This has shown great promise in "syndrome X" patients where, for the first time, a diagnostic test could demonstrate an abnormal perfusion map (limited to the subendocardium), despite "normal" epicardial coronary arteries. Currently, myocardial stress perfusion is performed by measuring first-pass kinetics of gadolinium-based contrast agents. It is extremely likely that image acquisition will evolve to allow the measurement of myocardial perfusion without the need for additional contrast taking advantage of our "natural contrast." Furthermore, knowing that coronary disease alters the autonomic regulatory tone of coronary vessels, one could theoretically detect this in the resting state without the need for any additional stress agents.

Myocardial Viability

It is determined by CMR using dobutamine stress MRI (identical to low-dose dobutamine echo methods), metabolic imaging (magnetic resonance [MR] spectroscopy) or most commonly, quantifying delayed enhancement after contrast injection. Similarly, the prerequisite for injected contrast will likely surrender to natural contrast methods as MR progresses. This application of CMR may eventually become the diagnostic test of choice to detect heart transplant rejection, predict the likelihood of malignant cardiac dysrhythmias and potential benefit of implantable cardioverter-defibrillator implantation, and risk-stratify patients with hypertrophic and other cardiomyopathies.

T1 AND T2 MAPPING

T1 and T2 relaxation times with and without MR contrast media can be used for mapping myocardium LL, modified Look-Locker inversion-recovery (MOLLI) and shortened modified Look-Locker inversion-recovery (ShMOLLI) MRI sequences are the sequences of choice for T1 mapping. A quantitative T2 relaxation map (T2 mapping) has been introduced for quantifying myocardial edema and patients with MI. T2 mapping leverages the increased myocardial free water in the setting of AMI, taking advantage of the positive relationship between T2 signal intensity and tissue water content.

Coronary MR Angiography

It has already proven its value in the detection of anomalous coronary origins, the evaluation of coronary artery bypass graft obstruction, and the assessment of the most critical, proximal, and mid portions of native coronary arteries. Details of the arterial plaque, thick (stable) vs thin (vulnerable) fibrous caps, have been imaged in the larger aortic and carotid arteries. Although coronary artery plaques are much smaller, more tortuous, and highly mobile, these have also been imaged with success. As motion correction techniques advance, and designer contrast agents targeted to vulnerable plaques are developed, CMR will be able to accurately measure the plaque volume and composition, making this the tool of choice to serially follow the progression/regression of atherosclerosis ("noninvasive cellular imaging"). In time, these tools will combine to provide a robust and uncomplicated coronary angiographic technique, delivering information on coronary artery anatomy (obstruction and plaque vulnerability), as well as myocardial blood flow and microvascular integrity in a single examination.

CMR-guided Coronary Interventional Procedures

These eliminate the radiation exposure and contrast risks associated with conventional X-ray-guided angiographic techniques. As CMR-safe catheters are developed, the operator will combine complete three-dimensional data sets with coronary physiology and myocardial viability to immediately determine the success of the procedure. It has now become feasible to guide gene and stem cell transfer to the myocardium under MRI guidance.

The development of new tissue or lesion-specific contrast agents will make molecular imaging with MRI a reality and allow us to diagnose various pathologies noninvasively. Thrombus-specific agents based on small gadolinium-labeled peptides will soon become available, which will make CMR the gold standard for diagnosing thrombi.

MR Spectroscopy

MR spectroscopy for the assessment of myocardial metabolism in vivo is a powerful new development. It uses phosphate (31P), carbon (13C), and proton (1H). A detailed understanding of energy metabolism in normal and abnormal myocardium will help improve preventive, diagnostic, and therapeutic modalities for heart failure, ischemic heart disease, genetic cardiomyopathy, and even valvular heart disease.

Since cardiac MRI is rapidly becoming mainstream technology in the everyday clinical practice, the need for non-ferromagnetic devices is vital. New pacer leads with minor magnetic field interactions and relative lack of heating are on the horizon. As clinical research begins to utilize more CMR techniques to assess results of treatments and timing of interventions, patient management decisions will be based on the findings from CMR, rather than our current conventional noninvasive techniques.

Furthermore, as the amount of imaging data to review increases, it is imperative that a rapid, automated processing technique become uniform. Comparing this development to the early advances of nuclear scintigraphy is a relevant reminder of the common delay in processing capabilities compared to acquisition capabilities. It has only recently become possible to rapidly process the volume of imaging data routinely obtained with today's nuclear scanners. The "one-stop" cardiac patient examination demands an integrated, robust "one-stop" post-processing approach. Only then will CMR approach the clinical impact that nuclear and echo imaging enjoy.

CONCLUSION

Over the next 25 years, noninvasive cardiac imaging will experience an extraordinary transition! Patients will be imaged with a far greater spatial resolution. Coronary arteries in jeopardy will be identified. Currently utilized imaging modalities that have small but potential risks will be reduced, as will needless diagnostic interventional procedures and unnecessary surgeries. Our current clinical paradigms will be challenged by these data, and the evolution from disease management to disease prevention will be the physician's mantra.

BIBLIOGRAPHY

1. Advances Could Make Cardiac CT a One-Stop-Shop Imaging Modality. Dave Fornell, 2014.
2. Flohr T, Stierstorfer K, Bruder H, et al. New technical developments in multislice CT, part 1: Approaching isotropic resolution with sub-millimeter 16-slice scanning. 2002;174:839-45.
3. Gutberlet M, Fröhlich M, Mehl S, et al. Myocardial viability assessment in patients with highly impaired left ventricular function: Comparison of delayed enhancement, dobutamine stress MRI, end-diastolic wall thickness, and ti201-spect with functional recovery after revascularization. Eur Radiol. 2005;15:872-80.
4. Maythem Saeed, Tu Anh Van. Cardiac MR imaging: current status and future direction. Cardiovasc Diagn Ther. 2015;5(4):290-310.

9. Clinical Decision-making with Myocardial Perfusion Imaging in Patients with Known or Suspected Coronary Artery Disease

Mythri Shankar

INTRODUCTION

Myocardial ischemia often leading to infarction is caused by a critical coronary artery obstruction, which is also known as atherosclerotic coronary artery disease (CAD). It is the leading cause of death worldwide and witnessing a pattern of increasing expenditure each year for the diagnosis and management of CAD.

Diagnosing myocardial ischemia prior to a heart attack is important because of its fatality. CAD occurs in a significant number of patients and is often not diagnosed until after a heart attack. Recognizing CAD is very important, sometimes critical, since treatment options like medical therapies and revascularization surgeries help reduce the morbidity and mortality rates associated within to a great extent.

The diagnosis of CAD can be difficult to make since the symptoms of CAD vary. There is no screening method has been uniformly accepted for CAD and it is a disease which occurs across a varied patient population in all age groups and sex and patients with or without risk factors. Assessing the CAD risk level with given clinical information one can decide which type of workup is indicated, e.g. for low-risk population, exercise treadmill testing alone is frequently sufficient; however, in patients with a moderate-to-high risk for CAD, an imaging study is essential along with the stress test. Myocardial perfusion imaging (MPI) is the most effective initial imaging study for early detection of myocardial ischemia though may not widely and easily available. Quality control is also key in acquiring and processing good quality, artifact free images.[1]

Gated single-photon emission computed tomography (SPECT), stress thallium, cardiac SPECT are the different terminologies which have been in the Indian context all referring to MPI. MPI can accurately diagnose and risk stratify coronary artery disease (CAD) and has highest prognostic value in patients with intermediate pretest likelihood of disease. Lung uptake, transient ischemic dilatation (TID), summed stress scores (SSS), summed rest scores (SRS), ejection fraction (EF) have been used as prognostic parameters in assessing the perfusion status of the myocardium. With recent advances in technology, newer positron emission tomography (PET) perfusion tracers have added value by allowing us to estimate "Coronary Flow Reserve" (CFR) along with lesser attenuation artifacts. Overall sensitivity and specificity of perfusion imaging (SPECT or PET) has been comparable to cardiac magnetic resonance imaging (MRI). Myocardial perfusion imaging with SPECT depends on flow heterogeneity, and since chances of attenuation are higher sensitivity may be lesser than that seen in PET. PET myocardial perfusion imaging offers a high negative predictive value compared to SPECT and helps exclude obstructive CAD that further invasive testing is not needed, even in higher risk patients and abnormal CFR may help further classify extent of ischemia.[2,3]

Myocardial perfusion imaging can be abnormal in a small percentage of patients who had a normal treadmill, without symptoms of typical angina and have had a negative treadmill exam. Many patients with an abnormal treadmill test frequently directly undergo invasive coronary angiography (ICA), but the appropriate management of inconclusive tests is not well-defined. If such patients are subjected to myocardial perfusion imaging the probability of CAD changes from low to intermediate or high.[4]

Appropriate decision-making for diagnosis of CAD can be facilitated by myocardial perfusion imaging in patients with electrocardiogram (ECG) abnormalities, poor exercise capacity, or intermediate to high pretest likelihood of disease, patients with high-risk markers on exercise tolerance test (ETT) may benefit from noninvasive imaging. A negative exercise treadmill would signal low post-test likelihood of the disease, could be managed with lifestyle and risk factor modification and potential medical therapy. Patients with a positive ETT would benefit from invasive angiography. Patients with equivocal results and those with intermediate post-test likelihood should undergo noninvasive myocardial perfusion imaging with SPECT or PET. Patients who are not able to exercise or who have an abnormal resting ECG would also benefit from MPI with SPECT or PET. Many patients who are unable to exercise on the treadmill testing because of osteoarthritis, poor conditioning, and amputation (among other reasons) can be stressed pharmacologically.[5]

Myocardial perfusion imaging is performed for three indications in patients with or suspected CAD:
1. Diagnosis of CAD.
2. Risk stratification.
3. Assess treatment response.

Normal findings on a stress test can be followed by risk factor modification with lifestyle changes and medical therapy however, a positive test with inducible ischemia should prompt further investigations or management like invasive angiogram or aggressive medical therapy.

There is sufficient data to suggest that in patients with known or suspected CAD, SPECT myocardial perfusion imaging provides incremental prognostic value and enhanced risk stratification in patients with low, intermediate, and high risk patients. It has been over and again demonstrated that normal technetium 99m-sestamibi SPECT is associated with a low cardiac event rate of 0.6% per year and a normal- or low-risk stress. Myocardial perfusion imaging was associated with an annual cardiac event rate of only 0.6%. The presence, extent, and severity of perfusion abnormalities are strongly associated with increasing risk of a cardiovascular event. The highest strength of myocardial perfusion imaging lies in its negative predictive value. A normal stress myocardial perfusion imaging, even in the presence of angiographically documented CAD is associated with only a 1% annual risk of cardiac events for a period as long as 5 years.

Myocardial perfusion imaging SPECT has been demonstrated to effectively diagnose coronary disease and predict future cardiac risk in patients with diabetes and is highly effective at identifying at-risk diabetic and nondiabetic patients. It is also of significance in identifying CAD in women.

Myocardial perfusion imaging which will significantly influence the management of the patient, where the clinical decision is based on the results of MPI when used in the appropriate indications listed below.[6]

In detection of CAD in symptomatic patients in evaluation of CAD if:
- Pretest probability is low and intermediate with or ECG uninterpretable and patient is unable to exercise
- Pretest probability is intermediate and high regardless of ECG interpretability and ability to exercise
- There is a possibility of acute coronary syndrome, ECG shows no ischemic changes or with LBBB or electronically paced ventricular rhythm, low/high-risk TIMI score, troponin levels are peak or negative/borderline/equivocal/minimally elevated.

In detection of CAD in asymptomatic patients in evaluation of CAD if patient:
- Is high CHD risk (ATP 3 risk criteria)
- Has new onset heart failure with LV dysfunction without ischemic equivalent.
- Has ventricular tachycardia (low/moderate or high CHC risk)
- Has syncope, moderate or high CHD risk
- Has elevated troponin without additional evidence of acute coronary syndrome.

In risk assessment with prior test results and/or known chronic stable CAD if patient.[7]
- Has a prior noninvasive evaluation with equivocal, borderline or discordant stress testing where obstructive CAD remains a concern.
- Has new or worsening symptoms with abnormal coronary angiography or abnormal prior stress imaging study
- Has an angiogram shows abnormality of unclear significance
- Is asymptomatic prior coronary calcium Agatston score 100 and above and low-intermediate duke treadmill score.
- Is undergoing intermediate risk surgery or vascular, no active cardiac condition, more than clinical risk factor, poor or unknown functional capacity (less than 4 METS)

In risk assessment within 3 months of an acute coronary syndrome:
- To evaluate inducible ischemia, in STEMI/UA//NSTEMI, hemodynamically stable, no recurrent chest pain or no signs of HF and no prior coronary angiogram.

In risk assessment postvascularization (PCI or CABG) in:
- Symptomatic patients to evaluate ischemic component
- Asymptomatic patients if revascularization was incomplete, additional revascularization is feasible, more than 5 years of CABG.

There are 3 special patient populations where the role of MPI has a robust amount of prognostic value.

DIABETES MELLITUS

Patients with CAD and DM have a 2–8 times higher annual death rate, and cardiac event rates are not decreasing over time for patients with diabetes as they are in those without diabetes yearly cardiac death/nonfatal myocardial infarction rate is directly proportional to the degree of ischemia.[8]

WOMEN AND ELDERLY

Myocardial perfusion imaging is an especially important risk assessment tool in elderly patients, especially in those who have comorbidities or physical deconditioning that render them incapable of performing exercise stress, and in those patients who have age-related coronary artery calcification.

Women undergoing evaluation for ischemia tend to have higher false-positive rate on stress ECG alone and MPI would be beneficial.

CHRONIC KIDNEY DISEASE

Patients with chronic kidney disease (CKD) are at high risk of future cardiac events. Diabetic patients with CKD have a higher cardiac event rate than nondiabetic patients with CKD. Many patients with advanced CKD including those on dialysis may remain asymptomatic. There is evidence to suggest that larger the defect size was on vasodilator stress MPI, the worse the prognosis was for patients on long-term hemodialysis (in spite of presence of confounding variables including GFR and ejection fraction[9]).

The results of the MPI can add incremental prognostic value in determining the likelihood of cardiac death, with the greatest impact being in the patients with high likelihood of CAD. A mildly abnormal (<10% of myocardium involved) may be managed medically with lifestyle modifications/ moderately or severely abnormal MPI scan with aggressive medical treatment and revascularization. Patients with small amounts of inducible ischemia (5% to 10% myocardium ischemic) have a marginal survival advantage for medical therapy in women and no difference between therapies in men. Small survival advantages for revascularization over medical therapy in both men and women have been noted with moderate amounts of inducible ischemia (10% to 20% myocardium ischemic), more so in diabetic patients. With large amounts of inducible ischemia (>20% myocardium ischemic), the survival benefit for revascularization is increased more in women compared with men. Patients with >10% myocardium ischemic is associated with increased incidence of cardiac death. Early revascularization in such patients can result in a significant reduction of cardiac events. As stratifying by percent myocardium ischemic, mortality rates increases significantly in patients undergoing medical therapy, but not in patients referred for revascularization. An increasing survival benefit for revascularization over medical therapy is present with increasing amounts of inducible ischemia.[10]

REFERENCES

1. Semin Nucl Med. 2014;44(4):320-9. doi: 10.1053/j.semnuclmed.2014.04.006.
2. Cremer P, Hachamovitch R, Tamarappoo B. Clinical decision making with myocardial perfusion imaging in patients with known or suspected coronary artery disease. Semin Nucl Med. 2014;44(4):320-9.
3. ACCF/ACR/SCCT/SCMR/ASNC/NASCI/SCAI/SIR 2006. Appropriateness criteria for cardiac computed tomography and cardiac magnetic resonance imaging.
4. Roger D Des Prez, et al. Cost-effectiveness of myocardial perfusion imaging: A summary of the currently available literature. Jour of Nuc Cardio. 2005;12(6):750-9.
5. APPR/ACCF/ASNC/ACR/AHA/ASE/SCCT/SCMR/SNM 2009: Appropriate use criteria for cardiac radionuclide imaging. Jour of the Am Coll of Cardio. 2009;53(23):2201-29.
6. Berman, et al. Atlas of nuclear cardiology; 2003. p. 273.
7. Myocardial ischemia—Nuclear medicine and risk stratification: Thomas F Heston; 2015.
8. Wackers FJ, et al. Detection of silent myocardial ischemia in asymptomatic diabetic subjects: the DIAD study. Diabetes Care. 2004;27:1954-61.
9. Hachamovitch R, Hayes SW, Friedman JD, et al. Comparison of the short-term survival benefit associated with revascularization compared with medical therapy in patients with no prior coronary artery disease undergoing stress myocardial perfusion single photon emission computed tomography. Circulation. 2003;107(23):2900-7.
10. Jamieson M Bourque. Stress Myocardial Perfusion Imaging for Assessing Prognosis. JACC; 2011.

10
Current Status of Rubidium-82 PET-CT Myocardial Perfusion Imaging

Prasanta Kumar Pradhan, Gowri Sankar

HISTORICAL PERSPECTIVE

Rubidium has two naturally occurring and thirty artificially produced isotopes. Initial works in field of medicine were done with Rb-86 (a β-emitter with a half-life of 18.7 days), where its distribution was compared with that of potassium ions in various preclinical studies. It was established from these studies that the Rb uptake in myocardial tissue was higher than the plasma concentration and that it was dependent upon the coronary blood flow.[1] Initial clinical study with Rb-82 was done in 1982 [using Strontium-82 (Sr-82)/Rb-82 generator] when its uptake was studied in 5 healthy volunteers and in five patients with coronary artery disease. This study demonstrated reduced uptake of the tracer in ischemic patients. Further clinical studies done in the 1980s demonstrated the superiority of Rb-82 PET over Tc-99m-based single-photon emission computed tomography (SPECT) myocardial perfusion agents.[2,3] In 1989, the first Sr-82/Rb-82 generator was approved for clinical use in the USA (CardioGen-82; Bracco Diagnostics, Inc). Due to technological limitations in the PET-based cameras and in production of the parent molecule Sr-82, there was a delay in the widespread usage of Rb-82. However, in the past decade, with the advancements and widespread availability of the PET-CT systems, there is an increase in the utilization of the myocardial perfusion studies done with positron-emitting radionuclides.

CHARACTERISTICS OF SR-82/RB-82 GENERATOR AND PHYSIOLOGY OF RB-82

Rb-82 is a positron emitter with a half-life of approximately 75 seconds. Its parent molecule is strontium-82 (Sr-82) which has a half-life of 25 days. No carrier added Sr-82 is produced by proton spallation of molybdenum in an accelerator or by proton bombardment of Rb-85. Sr-82 thus produced is adsorbed on a stannic oxide column and is covered by a lead shield. Generator must be used with an infusion system specifically labeled for use with the generator and capable of accurate measurement and delivery of doses of rubidium chloride. Activity of Sr-82 at the calibration time is usually around 90–150 mCi. The generator should be stored at 20–25°C and needs to be replaced every 4–6 weeks.

As already mentioned, Rb-82 is a positron emitter. The maximum energy of the positron is 3.18 MeV. The mean positron range is 2.6 mm. The annihilation photons of 511 keV have an abundance of 192%. It also emits gamma rays of 777 keV, which have an abundance of 9%. Rb-82 decays to Kr-82 which is stable. Rb-82 rapidly crosses the capillary membrane after injection. The uptake of Rb-82 in viable myocardial cells is through an active process involving the Na/K adenosine triphosphate transporter (ATPase). However, this uptake is dependent on coronary flow. At low flow rates, the uptake bears a linear relationship to that of the blood flow but in higher flow rates, it becomes non-linear, i.e. the uptake decreases at higher flow rates.

COMPARISON WITH SPECT AGENTS

Tc-99m-based SPECT agents for myocardial perfusion imaging (MPI) performs poorly in obese patients, and in women with large breasts. There is reduced specificity in these patients owing to the attenuation artifacts. PET agents have superior specificity owing to the inherent camera properties like co-incidence imaging and better spatial resolution. Bateman et al. compared the image quality, accuracy and interpretive certainty between Rb-82-gated stress-rest MPI and Tc-99m sestamibi-gated stress-rest MPI in two patient populations which were matched for gender, and body mass index (BMI). There were a total of 112 patients in each group. Patients who were found to have significant defects in perfusion imaging were followed up with invasive coronary angiography within 60 days. Image quality was better in PET rather than

SPECT-MPI imaging (79% vs 62%, p < 0.05). Similarly, the accuracy was better in PET than SPECT-MPI at two levels of stenosis. In 70% stenosis, the accuracy was 89% vs 79%, for PET and SPECT-MPI respectively (p = 0.03); and in 50% stenosis, it was 87% vs 71% (p = 0.003). They finally concluded that gated stress-rest PET-MPI with Rb-82 performed significantly better than the SPECT-MPI in terms of image quality, accuracy and as well as in interpretive certainty. However, one should note that the SPECT-MPI done in this study did not use attenuation correction, which is much more commonly used now-a-days owing to better SPECT-CT imaging systems as well as improvement in the reconstruction algorithms. This might have led to poorer performance of SPECT-MPI.[4]

Another meta-analysis compared 15 Rb-82 PET-MPI studies (1344 patients) and 8 Tc-99m setamibi SPECT-MPI studies (1755 patients). The pooled sensitivity and specificity were 90% and 88% respectively for Rb-82 PET. The same for SPECT-MPI were 85% and 85% respectively. This analysis incorporated SPECT-MPI studies which used ECG gating as well as iterative reconstruction and/or attenuation correction. The drawback of this meta-analysis was that it was indirect and used pooling of studies. There were some referral and verification bias also. There was some heterogeneity in the study populations between Rb-82 and SPECT, and, sometimes, within them too.[5]

The recently concluded ARMI trial (Alternative Radiopharmaceutical for Myocardial Imaging), which is a multicenter, prospective study involving Rb-82 PET, showed excellent agreement between the various centers and the core center on the overall interpretation of the scans, with a κ = 0.94. In this study, they did a low dose (10 MBq/kg) rest and pharmacological stress (using dipyridamole) Rb-82 PET MPI. This was similar to that of SPECT-MPI studies.[6]

An ideal comparison between PET and SPECT-MPI should be made in the same population of patients. Studies like that are very few and were made in the initial phases of Rb-82 PET.

COMPARISON BETWEEN RB-82 AND N-13 AMMONIA

N-13 NH_3 (ammonia) is another PET tracer used for MPI which has a half-life of 10 minutes, but is cyclotron produced. There are no direct comparisons between Rb-82 and ammonia PET images. However, there are a few studies comparing the quantitative myocardial blood flow assessment between the two tracers. Quantitative myocardial flow reserve (MFR) is a good predictor of adverse cardiac events, which is independent of other imaging findings **(Figs 1A to E)**.

El Fakhri et al. studied the reproducibility and accuracy of quantitative myocardial blood flow assessment with Rb-82 PET. They also did a comparison with N-13 ammonia PET-MPI. They found that the reproducibility of Rb-82 studies were good. The correlation between myocardial flow at rest and those at peak stress between Rb-82 and N-13 NH_3 studies was very good ($R[2] = 0.857$). Bland-Altman plots comparing coronary flow reserve (CFR) between Rb-82 and N-13 NH_3 revealed an underestimation of CFR with Rb-82 in comparison with the later; the underestimation was within +/-1.96 SD.[8]

Renaud et al. tried to characterize the normal range of myocardial blood flow with Rb-82 and N-13 NH_3 PET imaging. Fourteen subjects with <5% risk of CAD underwent rest and stress Rb-82 and N-13 NH_3 dynamic PET imaging in a randomized order within 2 weeks. Myocardial blood flow was quantified using a one-compartment model for Rb-82, and a two-compartment model for N-13 NH_3. They concluded that the retention model may have higher sensitivity for detection and localization of abnormal flow and MFR using Rb-82 and N-13 NH_3, whereas the N-13 NH_3 two-compartment model has higher precision for absolute flow quantification.[9]

DOSIMETRY

A study in 2010 estimated dosimetry of Rb-82 in 10 healthy volunteers using the OLINDA/EXM 1.0 dosimetry software. The highest mean absorbed organ doses (μGy/MBq) were observed for the kidneys (5.81), heart wall (3.86) and lungs (2.96). Mean effective doses were 1.11 ± 0.22 and 1.26 ± 0.20 μSv/MBq using the tissue-weighting factors of the International Commission on Radiological Protection (ICRP) publications 60 and 103, respectively. On the basis of this study, a clinical Rb-82 injection of 2 × 1,480 MBq (80 mCi) would result in a mean effective dose of 3.7 mSv using the weighting factors of the ICRP 103, which is only slightly above the average annual natural background exposure.[10]

Dorbala et al. reported a way to reduce radiation dose with myocardial SPECT and PET imaging. They suggested that with the use of recent generation of 3D PET scanners and improvement in the software using a reduced dose of injected Rb-82 activity, i.e 2 MBq × 740 MBq or 2 mCi × 20 mCi), will lead to a preserved image quality while reducing the effective dose to 1.26 mSv for rest or stress. They also said that with the usage of stress-only 3D PET with MBF estimate, the radiation dose would come down to 1 mSv. This is half of the radiation dose with 99mTc-sestamibi or tetrofosmin.[11]

Another study compared the occupational exposure between Rb-82 and Tc-99m SPECT-MPI imaging. Electronic personal dosimeters were worn by staff involved in the administration and imaging of routine clinical Tc-99m SPECT and Rb-82 PET-MPI, and during tracer production and QC. Mean (SD) whole-body effective dose to staff during a single MPI procedure was 0.4 (0.4) μSv for Rb-82 PET (1110 MBq) and 3.3 (1.7) μSv for Tc-99m SPECT (350 MBq). Staff effective dose during tracer production and QC was low (<0.2 μSv/patient) and comparable between tracers. There was a significant reduction in effective dose during Rb-82 PET when compared with Tc-99m SPECT-MPI because of the short half-life of Rb-82 and reduced patient contact.[12]

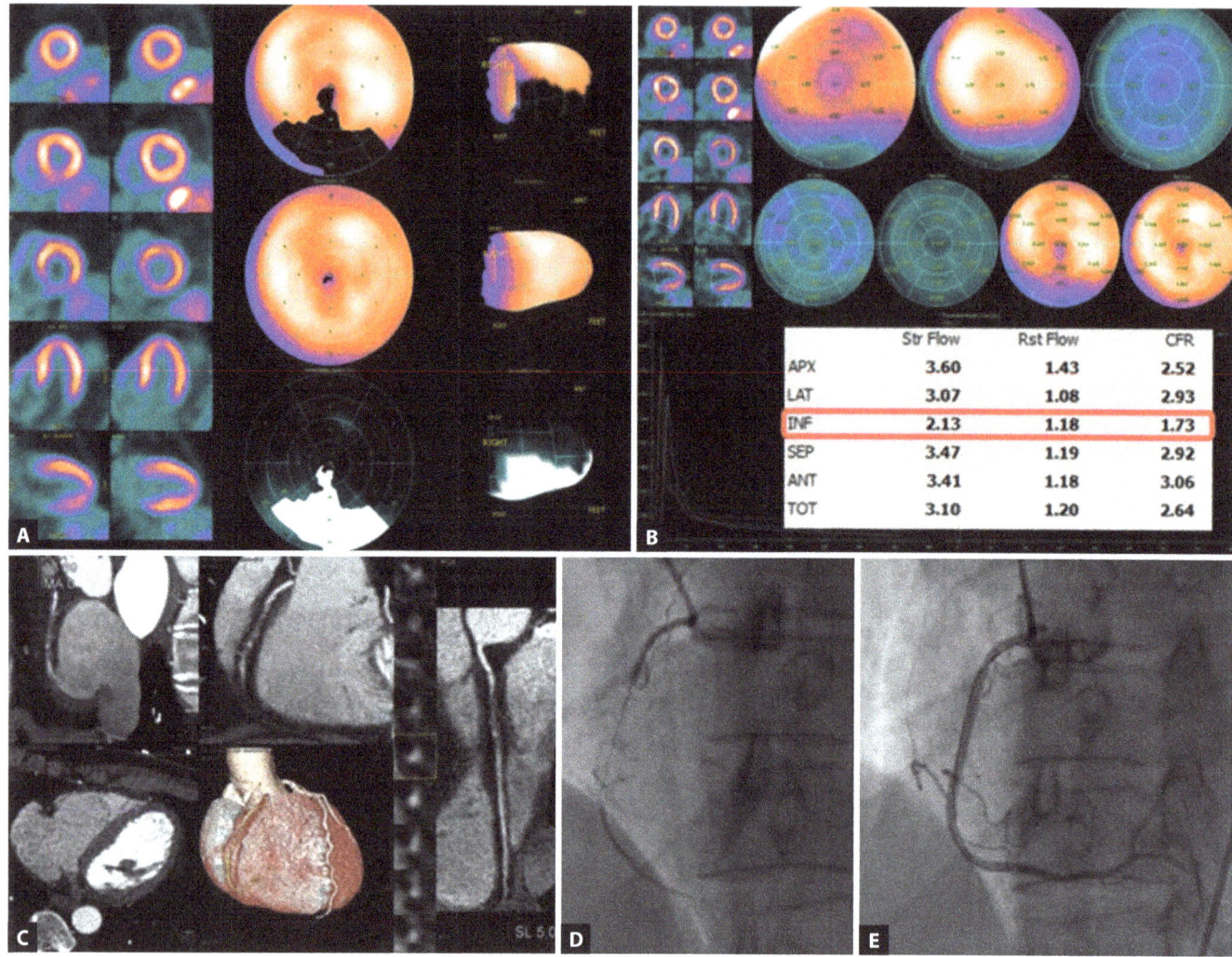

Figs 1A to E: Integrated ^{82}Rb PET/CTA study in a patient with chronic stable angina. Rest/stress ^{82}Rb PET scan demonstrates a large and severe stress-induced perfusion defect throughout inferior LV wall (A). Results of quantitative assessment of MBF from ^{82}Rb PET demonstrate impaired adenosine-stimulated flow in the inferior LV wall, resulting in a reduced MFR, compared to the other vascular territories in the LV (B). Cardiac CTA and coronary angiogram showing coronary stenosis in the right coronary artery (RCA) (C and D), and a normal postpercutaneous coronary intervention (PCI) angiogram (E). (*Source:* Adapted from Hagemann CE, et al. Am J Nuclear Med Mol Imaging; 2015)[7]

CONCLUSION

The advantages of Rb-82 PET is that it is generator produced, being a PET agent quantification of myocardial blood flow MBF) and myocardial flow reserve (MFR) can be done easily, it leads to reduced effective dose to the patients as well as reduced exposure to the medical personnel, has good interpretive confidence and good diagnostic accuracy. The disadvantages being that it has a very short half-life, cost of the procedure to the patient is high, availability of very few Sr-82 production sites in the world, higher positron range when compared with N-13 NH$_3$ and decrease in myocardial uptake at high flow rates. Its accuracy was significantly better than SPECT imaging particularly in obese or overweight patients and women with large breasts due to attenuation artifacts. Thus, more widespread use of Rb-82 PET in the future is expected owing to increase in the availability of dedicated cardiac PET cameras, may be beneficial to improve the accuracy of non-invasive detection of coronary artery disease.

REFERENCES

1. Love WD, Burch GE. Influence of the rate of coronary plasma flow on the extraction of Rb-86 from coronary blood. Circ Res. 1959;7:24-30.
2. Gould KL, Goldstein RA, Mullani NA, et al. Noninvasive assessment of coronary stenoses by myocardial perfusion imaging during pharmacologic coronary vasodilation. VIII.

Clinical feasibility of positron cardiac imaging without a cyclotron using generator-produced rubidium-82. J Am Coll Cardiol. 1986;7:775-89.
3. ACNP/SNM Task Force on Clinical PET. Positron emission tomography: clinical status in the United States in 1987. J Nucl Med. 1988;29:1136-43.
4. Bateman TM, Heller GV, McGhie AI, et al. Diagnostic accuracy of rest/stress ECG-gated Rb-82 myocardial perfusion PET: comparison with ECG-gated Tc-99m sestamibi SPECT. J Nucl Cardiol. 2006;13:24-33.
5. Mc Ardle BA, Dowsley TF, deKemp RA, et al. Does rubidium-82 PET have superior accuracy to SPECT perfusion imaging for the diagnosis of obstructive coronary disease? A systematic review and meta-analysis. J Am Coll Cardiol. 2012;60:1828-37.
6. Renaud JM, Mylonas I, McArdle B, et al. Clinical interpretation standards and quality assurance for the multicenter PET/CT trial rubidium-ARMI. J Nucl Med. 2014;55:58-64.
7. Hagemann CE, Ghotbi AA, Kjaer A, et al. Quantitative myocardial blood flow with Rubidium-82 PET: a clinical perspective. Am J Nuclear Med Mol Imaging. 2015;5(5):457-68.
8. El Fakhri G, Kardan A, Sitek A, et al. Reproducibility and accuracy of quantitative myocardial blood flow assessment with (82)Rb PET: comparison with (13) N-ammonia PET. J Nucl Med. 2009;50:1062-71.
9. Renaud JM, Dasilva JN, Beanlands RS, et al. Characterizing the normal range of myocardial blood flow with (82) rubidium and (13) N-ammonia PET imaging. J Nucl Cardiol. 2013;20:578-91.
10. Senthamizhchelvan S, Bravo PE, Esaias C, et al. Human biodistribution and radiation dosimetry of 82Rb. J Nucl Med. 2010;51:1592-9.
11. Dorbala S, Blankstein R, Skali H, et al. Approaches to reducing radiation dose from radionuclide myocardial perfusion imaging. J Nucl Med. 2015;56:592-9.
12. Tout D, Davidson G, Hurley C, et al. Comparison of occupational radiation exposure from myocardial perfusion imaging with Rb-82 PET and Tc-99m SPECT. Nucl Med Commun. 2014;35:1032-7.

11. Innovation of New Tracers in the Era of Multimodality Cardiac Imaging

Padmakar V Kulkarni

INTRODUCTION

Application of radiopharmaceutical agents to cardiology represents the study of function and physiologic condition rather than anatomy which is better accomplished with ultrasonography/echocardiology, computed tomography (CT) and magnetic resonance imaging (MRI). Nuclear cardiac imaging has evolved from being rather subjective to a more objective, digital-based quantitative technique providing insight into the physiological processes of cardiovascular disorders and predicting patient outcome. Radionuclide imaging of the cardiovascular system originated with the blood pool scan first described by Rejali and his colleagues in 1958.[1] Important changes came to blood pool imaging technology with the availability of the large-crystal scintillation camera and Tc-99m labeled tracers developed by Harper, et al.[2] The mainstays of the field have been the test of function by use of the blood pool agent Tc-99m labeled red blood cells and perfusion imaging of ischemia with tracers such as Tl-201 (thallous chloride). Agents for flow-perfusion have expanded to include a variety of Tc-99m chelates. Harper et al. demonstrated the clinical feasibility of myocardial imaging with N-13 (Ammonia) in 1972.[3] Routine clinical use of this agent had to wait the availability of positron emission tomography (PET), PET/CT scanners. Studies with radioisotopes of ionic potassium and rubidium in the 1950s, showed that uptake of these agents in the myocardium are related to blood flow as well as to structural and functional integrity of the myocardial cell membrane.[4] Noninvasive regional myocardial perfusion with radioactive potassium: study of patients with exercise and during angina pectoris. Potassium is the major intracellular cation in muscle, researchers focused on developing ionic myocardial perfusion tracers that have biological properties similar to those of potassium for myocardial imaging.[5-7] Positron emitting radioisotopes such as carbon, oxygen and nitrogen are ideally suited for labeling physiological substrates, but have very short half-lives (C-11: 20.4 min, O-15: 2.07 min, N-13: 9.96 min), an on-site cyclotron is required for production of these radioisotopes. Even though Rb-82 has been around for a while, recently US FDA approved the Rb-82 generator for routine clinical use. Limited availability and high cost associated with Rb-82 generator encouraged the development of F-18 labeled agents for myocardial perfusion with PET. F-18 has relatively longer half-life (110 min), it can be produced in a cyclotron and shipped to imaging sites nearby. Joint position statement from the American Society of Nuclear Cardiology, and the Society of Nuclear Medicine and Molecular Imaging highlights the attributes of myocardial perfusion PET both preferred and recommended in the era of high value initiative for appropriate patients.[8] Myocardial perfusion PET offers high image quality, high diagnostic accuracy, ability to accurately risk stratify patients with a wide array of clinical presentation, short acquisition times, low radiation exposure, and its unique ability to quantify myocardial blood flow. The presence of coronary artery calcium can also be identified when patients are imaged using a PET/CT scanner.[8] The purpose of the chapter is not to describe the many clinical applications of the wide variety of radiopharmaceutical agents available for cardiac imaging but to provide a brief overview of the currently available imaging agents as well as those under development. Many excellent reviews are available for additional background extended references.[9-16] Within the last decade there have been tremendous technical advancements in the field of cardiovascular imaging and has rapidly expanded to a variety of modalities to image morphology and function with cardiac PET/MRI, CT, PET/CT, and single photon emission tomography (SPECT)/CT. Recently, there have been efforts to develop combined imaging modalities with both functional and anatomical imaging for more accurate radiological diagnosis. PET and SPECT have high sensitivity quantitative measurement of imaging probes *in vivo*, while CT and MRI provide anatomical images with high spatial resolution.

The combined dual imaging modalities include PET/CT, SPECT/CT, PET/MRI and SPECT/MRI.[17] These technologies provide complementary functional information as regards myocardial blood flow and perfusion, viability, and, vulnerable arterial plaque burden. However, still they do need suitable radiopharmaceuticals to explore their full potential. Impact of these modalities on clinical practice with special attention to imaging parameters and protocols for use in practice and research have been described. The utility of multimodality imaging techniques for diagnosis and evaluation is discussed in the context of various clinical scenarios.[17]

MYOCARDIAL FUNCTION

Ventricular function may best be evaluated by echocardiography.[18,19] Imaging with Tc-99m labeled red blood cells[20] continues to be used for evaluating ventricular volume and ejection fraction.[21] Any agent that remains in the vascular space may be used for this purpose. Myocardial perfusion agents such as Tc-99m labeled sestamibi and tetrafosmin have permitted measurement of ventricular function by rapid images obtained during the first pass of the radiotracer through the left ventricle after intravenous injection.[22-25] Efforts are continuing to develop other SPECT and PET agents for determining left ventricular function.

MYOCARDIAL PERFUSION

The purpose of myocardial imaging is to determine the presence and extent of pathological condition. A number of radioisotope monovalent cations have shown to provide images of viable myocardium. Earlier, Tl-201 and Rb-82 were the most frequently used single-photon and PET isotopes, respectively. Rb-82 is available from a convenient generator and does not require an on-site cyclotron. This monovalent cation is taken up by viable myocardium and appears to be as predictive of tissue viability as 2-(F-18) fluoro-2-deoxyglucose.[26] Rb-82 chloride was found to identify a significant number of patients (18%) who had false negative results on Tl-201 scans two thirds of whom subsequently underwent revascularization.[23] Despite the early clinical practice with Tl-201, it is cyclotron produced, thus considerably more expensive than, for example Tc-99m based agents and has low photon energy (71 kev) emission which increases dose to the patient. This prompted the development of Tc-99m based agents for myocardial perfusion studies. Amongst the number of agents evaluated, the most useful were, technetium (I) isonitiles, notably hexakis-2-methoxyisobutyl isonitrile (Sestamibi, MIBI, and Cardiolite), tetraboroxime, (SQ30217, CardioTec), diphosphine complex tetrofosmin (Myoview), furifosmin (Q12 and TechneScan).[22-25] One characteristic of these technetium chelates is that they do not exhibit redistribution phenomenon of thallium-201: redistribution is advantageous in assessing ischemic, non-infarcted tissue which can be salvaged.

Breaks in the supply of technetium 99m(^{99m}Tc)—the main radiotracer for cardiac stress testing with single-photon emission CT myocardial perfusion imaging (SPECT-MPI) - can be linked to excess cardiac catheterizations, a study suggests. Venkatesh L Murthy, MD PhD, of University of Michigan, Ann Arbor, and colleagues followed what happened after a 6-month shortage of ^{99m}Tc, which is derived from highly-enriched uranium, due to shutdowns of two major nuclear reactors at the Petten High Flux and the Chalk River Laboratories facilities, located in the Netherlands and Canada, respectively.[27] A shortage of ^{99m}Tc necessitates a switch to thallium 201 and other radiotracers. But "thallium Tl 201 is associated with higher radiation exposure and lower specificity relative to ^{99m}Tc, the investigators noted.[27] This has encouraged development of alternative imaging agents and testing approaches.

Mitochondrial complex-1 (MC-1) inhibitors show great promise as molecular targets for novel cardiac radiotracers. Structurally the MC-1 derivatives are analogues of known inhibitors such as rotenone, deguelin, piericidin A, and pyridaben.[28-30] Development of iodine-123 labeled derivative of rotenone, denoted 123I-CMICE-013 has been reported with promising results for future clinical application.[28,29]

There are number of interesting chelates of PET radiotracers are available. These include the chelates of Gallium-68, available from a generator system, copper-64.[31-34] Other PET tracers include N-13 ammonia, O-15 H_2O, and carbon-11 acetate. However, they need an on-site cyclotron because of their very short half-lives.[35-37]

FLUORINE-18 LABELED AGENTS FOR MYOCARDIAL PERFUSION STUDIES

Myocardial perfusion imaging (MPI) with positron emission tomography (PET) has been shown to be superior to single photon emission computed tomography (SPECT). Nevertheless, widespread clinical use of PET MPI has been limited by the currently available PET myocardial perfusion tracers. PET tracers such as N-13 labeled ammonia ($^{13}NH_3$) and O-15 labeled water ($H_2^{15}O$) can be used for myocardial perfusion imaging (MPI), however they require an on-site cyclotron, and thus are impractical for widespread utilization. Rubidium-82 may be prepared on site using a generator, but it is not an ideal PET tracer due to high cost of the generator, high positron range that lowers image resolution and a very short (75 seconds) half-life that makes it incompatible with exercise stress imaging.

The positron range of F-18 is approximately seven times shorter than that of Rb-82, so it would be expected to produce images with higher resolution. **Table 1** shows physical characteristics and myocardial extraction properties. With a longer half-life (110 min), F-18 labeled agents may be produced at regional cyclotrons and delivered to imaging centers in much the same way as F-18 labeled fluorodeoxyglucose (FDG), thus obviating the need for an on-site cyclotron. The longer half-life

Table 1 Characteristics of PET tracers for cardiac imaging

Agent	Physical half-life	Positron energy (MeV)	Extraction
O-15 H$_2$O	2.05 min	1.73	100%
N-13 NH$_3$	9.96 min	1.19	80%
Rb-82	76 sec	3.15	50–60%
F-18 FDG	110 min	0.63	1–3%
F-18 pyridaben derivative (Flurpiridaz) F-18 fluorophenyl-triphenylphosphonium ion (BFPET) F-18 fluoro-3, 4-methyleneheptadecanoic acid (CardioPet)			>90%

of F-18 also ensures that the radiotracer is present long enough to allow a patient injected at peak treadmill exercise to move to the camera and still be effectively imaged. With this in mind recent efforts have focused on developing F-18 labeled MPI. Several ^{18}F-labeled perfusion PET tracers have been introduced for the evaluation of myocardial perfusion. Yu et al.[38] found that another mitochondrial complex I inhibitor, ^{18}F-RP1004, has a higher initial liver uptake compared to flurpiridaz F-18 (^{18}F-BMS-747158-02), possibly due to the higher lipophilicity of ^{18}F-RP1004. Mou et al.[39] synthesized [^{18}F] FP2OP, and biodistribution studies in mice have shown that [^{18}F] FP2OP has a significant high heart uptake, as well as good heart/liver, heart/lung, and heart/blood ratios and has therefore been proposed as a potential new MPI agent for PET. ^{18}F-FTPP is an analog of tetraphenylphosphonium (TPP$^+$) cation that concentrates in mitochondria, also demonstrated promising characteristics as a PET MPI tracer. Biodistribution and imaging studies with ^{18}F-FTPP in rats have shown rapid accumulation of activity in the heart (1–2 min) with stable retention for at least 1 h. Heart uptake of ^{18}F-FTPP in occluded heart ROIs was comparable to that of [^{13}N] NH$_3$ in rabbits[39,40] [^{18}F] Fluorophenyl-triphenylphosphonium ion is under investigation in animals and in human studies with encouraging results.[40,41] F-18 labeled rhodamine B has shown promise in myocardial PET studies in rats. A unique aspect of this agent is that it is inherently a dual modality imaging agent incorporating both F-18 label for PET and the intrinsic fluorescence of the rhodamine dye for fluorescence microscopy.[42]

Flurpiridaz F-18 is a new PET MPI radiopharmaceutical in clinical development. It is a structural analog of pyridaben and binds to mitochondrial complex I with high affinity.[43] Preclinical studies showed that the extraction fraction of F-18-Flurpiridaz was greater than 90 percent.[44-46] Phase I and phase II studies have been completed with F-18-flurpiridaz and Phase III studies are ongoing. These studies indicated the superiority of F-18-flurpiridaz to Tc-99m SPECT MPI in image quality, interpretative certainty, defect magnitude and detection of coronary artery disease.[47-51]

ENERGY METABOLISM

The uniqueness of nuclear imaging is the ability to measure biochemistry in a living system. Magnetic resonance imaging and echocardiographic methods frequently provide information as useful as that obtained with perfusion agents. Metabolism can be determined only with radiotracer method. Fatty acids are the primary source of energy for the normal myocardium. In ischemic myocardium, glucose becomes the primary source of energy. Therefore, energy metabolism can be traced with analogs of glucose and fatty acids. Earlier studies demonstrated feasibility of imaging fatty acid metabolism with C-11 labeled palmitic acid.[52,53] However, back diffusion and rapid oxidation of palmitic acid makes quantification difficult. A number fatty acid derivatives labeled with C-11, F-18 for PET studies and a variety of fatty acids labeled with I-123 for SPECT studies have been investigated.[54-60] Zemiva®, iodofiltic acid I-123, a fatty acid analog that detects cardiac ischemia by revealing abnormalities in fatty acid metabolism in the heart.[61] Phase II trials of 510 emergency department chest pain patients showed Zemiva® significantly increased sensitivity from 52.2 to 85% and negative predictive value from 72 to 89.6%. Phase III clinical trials are continuing.

IMAGING ATHEROSCLEROTIC PLAQUES

Atherosclerosis is largely an asymptomatic disease where plaque develops over decades and symptoms do not appear until greater than 70% of a vessel is occluded. This presents a significant risk of severe cardiovascular risk such as stroke or myocardial infarct. It would be highly desirable to have an early noninvasive diagnostic tool. A large number of imaging agents have been developed to detect specific aspects of vessel wall biology in atherosclerosis using various imaging modalities (**Tables 2 and 3**). Several new imaging modalities have emerged for noninvasive detection of vulnerable plaques likely to rupture. PET/CT has been explored as a technique to detect and quantify the presence of inflammation within carotid plaques.[62-74] Majority of PET studies utilized F-18

Table 2 Potential targets in imaging plaques

Target	Target name
Endothelial cell (EC)	VCAM-1 (vascular cell adhesion molecule)
EC, macrophage, SMC	IL-4 receptor
Monocyte	CCR2
	CCR5
Macrophage	Lyp-1
	Apo A-1 mimetic (Apolipoprotein)
	Apo E
Platelet	Integrin GPII, b-IIIa
Collagen	Type I
Fibrin	Type II

Table 3 PET agents for imaging plaques

Nonspecific agents
1. F-18 FDG
2. F-18 NaF
3. F-18 Fluorocholine
Specific agents
1. Cu-64 labeled D-Ala1-peptide T-amide (DAPTA) peptide (methacrylate)-core/polyethylene glycol-shell nanoparticles)
2. Cu-64 labeled A viral macrophage inflammatory protein II (vMIP-II)
3. Cu-64 labeled natriuretic peptide
4. Ga-68-Fucoidan (polysaccharidic ligand of P-selectin)
5. Cu-64 DOTA antiselectin monoclonal antibody

labeled fluorodeoxyglucose (FDG), as this agent accumulates in cells with high metabolic activity, such as inflammatory cells. However, implementation of the agent is limited due to high myocardial background level and nonspecific mechanism of action.

There have efforts towards developing more specifically targeted agents such as derivatives of RGD (Arg-Gly-Asp) peptide tracers labeled with F-18 and Ga-68. The RGD peptide binds to the cell surface glycoprotein receptor $\alpha_v\beta_3$ integrin, found on endothelial cells and macrophages. Macrophages within a developing plaque secrete proteases that function as regulators the atherosclerosis disease pathology. One class of proteases that are highly upregulated in activated macrophages is the cysteine cathepsins. A number of cysteine cathepsins probes have been developed for both optical and PET imaging. Researchers from Stanford, recently reported development of a dual modality optical and PET/CT probe to image activated macrophages in an experimental murine model of carotid inflammation. These probes provide accurate detection of lesions undergoing high levels of inflammatory activity and extracellular matrix modeling. The authors noted that these probes not only enable early detection, they can also provide real-time monitoring therapeutic response and clinical drug efficacy.[74] They demonstrated the use of both quenched fluorescent cathepsins ABP (BMV109) and a dual –modality optical, PET/CT probe (BMV101) labeled with Cu-64 for non-invasive diagnostic imaging of cardiovascular disease.

SUMMARY

Field of nuclear cardiac imaging has evolved from being rather subjective to a more objective, digital based quantitative technique providing insight into the physiological processes of cardiovascular disorders and predicting patient outcomes. Imaging techniques have moved from planar to SPECT, to SPECT-CT, PET, PET-CT, PET-MRI. Advances in chemistry have provided SPECT and PET agents in identifying specific molecular targets. It is anticipated that next quantum leap may come from PET radiotracers particularly F-18 labeled specific biomarkers fueled by availability of cyclotrons and multimodality imaging techniques.

REFERENCES

1. Rejali AM, MacIntyre WJ, Friedel HL. Radioisotope method of visualization of blood pools. Am J Roentgenol. 1958;79:129.
2. Harper PV, Lathrop KA, Jiminez F, Fink R, Gottschalk A. Technetium-99m as a Scanning agent. Radiology. 1965;85:101.
3. Harper PV, Lathrop KA, Krizek H, et al. Clinical feasibility of myocardial imaging with $^{13}NH_3$. J Nucl Med. 1972;13:278.
4. Love WD, Romney RB, Burch GE. A comparison of the distribution of potassium and exchangeable rubidium in the organs of the dog, using rubidium-86. Circ Res. 1954;2:112-22.
5. Zaret BL, Strauss HW, Martin ND, Wells HP, Flamm MD. Noninvasive regional myocardial perfusion with radioactive potassium: study of patients with exercise and during angina pectoris. N Engl J Med. 1973;288:809-12.
6. Lebowitz E, Green MW, Fairchild R. Thallium-201 for medical use: J Nucl Med. 1975;16:151-5.
7. Yano Y, Anger HO. Visualization of heart and kidneys in animals with ultra-short-lived Rb-82 and the positron scintillation camera: J Nucl Med. 1968;9:412.
8. Bateman MT, Dilsizian V, Beanlands RS, DePuey EG, Heller GV, and Wolinsky DA. American Society of Nuclear Cardiology and Society of Nuclear Medicine and Molecular Imaging Joint Position statement on the Clinical Indications for Myocardial Perfusion PET. JNM. 2016;57:1654-5.
9. Antar MA. radiopharmaceuticals for studying cardiac metabolism. Nucl Med Biol. 1990;17:103-28.
10. Kulkarni PV. Recent development in 99mTc and 123I - radiopharmaceuticals for SPECT imaging. Nucl Med Biol. 1981;18:647-54.
11. Stoklin G. Tracers for metabolic imaging of brain and heart. Eur J Nucl Med. 1992;19:527-51.
12. Syota A. In vivo investigations of myocardial perfusion, metabolism and receptors by positron emission tomography. Int J Microcirc Clin Exp. 1989;8:411-22.
13. Schindler TH, Quercioli A, Schelbert HR, Dilsizian VA. Cardiac PET imaging for detection and monitoring of coronary artery disease and microvascular health. J Am Coll Cardilo Img. 2010;3: 623-40.
14. Maddahi JA. Properties of an ideal PET perfusion tracer: New PET tracer cases and data. J Nucl Cardiol. 2012;19:S30-S37.
15. Dilsizian V, Taillefer R. Journey in evolution of Nuclear Cardiology: Will there be another quantum leap with the F-18 labeled myocardial perfusion tracers. JACC. 2012;5:1269-84.
16. Sogbein OO, Pelletier-Galarneau M, Schindler TH, Wei L, G, and Ruddy TD. New SPECT and PET Radiopharmaceuticals for Imaging Cardiovascular Disease. Article ID 942960, 25 pages http://dx.doi.org/10.1155/2014/942960.
17. Schindler TH, George RT, Lima JAC (Eds). Molecular and Multimodality Imaging in Cardiovascular Disease. Cham: Springer, 2015, NY, DOI 10.1007/978-3-319-19611-4.
18. Mele D, Teoli R, Cittanti C, et al. Assessment of left ventricular volume and function by integration of simplified 3D

echocardiography, tissue harmonic imaging and automated extraction of endocardial borders. Int J Cardiovasc Imaging. 2004; 20:191-202.
19. Ward RP, Mor-Avi V, Lang RM. Assessment of left ventricular function with contrast echocardiography. Cardiol Clin. 2004;22:211-9.
20. Atkins HL, Eckelman WC, Klopper JF. Vascular imaging with Tc-99m-red blood cells. Radiology. 1973;106:357-60.
21. Abidov A, Hachmovitch R, Rozanski A, et al. Prognostic implications of arterial fibrillation in patients undergoing myocardial perfusion single-photon emission computed tomography. J Am Coll Cardiol. 2004;44:1062-70.
22. Jones AG, Abrams MJ, Davison A, et al. Biological studies of a new class of technetium complexes: the hexakis-(alkylisonitrile)-technetium (I) cations. Int J Nucl Med Biol. 1984;11:225-34.
23. Seldin DW, Johnson LL, Blood DK, et al. Myocardial perfusion imaging with technetium-99m SQ30217: comparison with thallium-201 and coronary anatomy, J Nucl Med. 1989;30:312-9.
24. Cuocolo A, Maurea S, Pace L, et al. Structural characterization of the new myocardial imaging agent technetium-99m tetrofosmin (99mTc-P53). J Nucl Med. 1992;33:850-1.
25. Hendel RC, Verani MS, Miller DD, et al. Diagnostic utility of tomographic myocardial perfusion imaging with technetium-99m furifosmin (Q12) compared with thallium-201 : results with of a phase III multicenter trial. J Nucl Cardiol.1996;3:291-300.
26. Anagnostopoulos C, Georgakopoulos A, Pianou N, Nekolla SG. Assessment of myocardial perfusion and viability by positron emission tomography. Int. J Cardiol. 2013;167:1737-49.
27. Murthy VL, Lehrich J, Nallamothu BK. Cardiac stress testing and the radiotracer supply chain: nuclear freeze. JAMA Cardiol ; DOI: 10.1001/jamacardio. 2016.
28. Broisat A, Ruiz M, Goodman NC, et al. Myocardial uptake of 7'-(Z)-[^{123}I] iodorotenone during vasodilator stress in dogs with critical coronary stenosis. Circulation: Cardiovascular Imaging. 2011;4(6):685-92.
29. Wei L, Bensimon C, Lockwood J, et al. Synthesis and characterization of 123I-CMICE-013: a potential SPECT myocardial perfusion imaging agent. Bioorganic and Medicinal Chemistry; 2013;21(11): 2903-11.
30. Wei L, Bensimon C, Yan X, et al. Characterization of the four isomers of ^{123}I-CMICE-013: a potential SPECT myocardial perfusion imaging agent. Bioorganic & Medicinal Chemistry. 2014;22(7):2033-44.
31. Schoeder H, Friedrich M, Yopp H. Myocardial viability: what do we need? Eur J Nucl Med. 1993;20:792-803.
32. MacIntyre WJ, Go RT, King JL, et al. Clinical outcome of cardiac patients with negative thallium-201 SPECT and positive rubidium-82 PET myocardial perfusion imaging. J Nucl Med. 1993;34:400-04.
33. Green MA, Mathias CJ, Newmann WL, et al. Potential gallium-68 tracers for imaging the heart with PET. J Nucl Med. 1993;34:228-33.
34. Green MA, Mathias CJ, Newmann WL, et al. Copper-62 labeled pyruvaldehyde bis (N4-methylthiosemicarbazonato) copper(II):synthesis and evaluation as a positron emission tomography tracer for cerebral and myocardial perfusion. J Nucl Med. 1990;31:1989-96.
35. Schelbert HR, Phelphs ME, Huang SC, et al. N-13-ammonia as an indicator of myocardial blood flow. Circulation. 1981;63:1259-72.
36. Bergmann SR, Fox KA, Rand AL, et al. Quantification of regional myocardial blood flow in vivo with $H_2^{18}O$. Circulation. 1984;70:724-33.
37. Brown MA, Myears DR, Bergmann SR. Validity of estimates of myocardial oxidative metabolism with carbon-11-acetate and positron emission tomography despite altered patterns of substrate utilization. J Nucl Med. 1989;30:187-93.
38. Yu M, Guaraldi M, Kagan M, et al. Assessment of ^{18}F-labeled mitochondrial complex I inhibitors as PET myocardial perfusion imaging agents in rats, rabbits, and primates. European Journal of Nuclear Medicine and Molecular Imaging. 2009;36:63-72.
39. Mou T, Jing H, Yang W, et al. Preparation and biodistribution of [^{18}F]FP2OP as myocardial perfusion imaging agent for positron emission tomography. Bioorganic and Medicinal Chemistry. 2010;18:1312-20.
40. Madar I, Ravert HT, Du Y, et al. Characterization of uptake of the new PET imaging compound ^{18}F-fluorobenzyl triphenyl phosphonium in dog myocardium. J Nucl Med. 2006;47:1359-66.
41. Shoup TM, Elmaleh DR, Brownell A, Zhu A, Guerrero JL, Fischman AJ. Evaluation of (4-[^{18}F]Fluorophenyl) triphenylphosphonium ion. A potential myocardial blood flow agent for PET. Molecular Imaging and Biology. 2011;13: 511-7.
42. Bartholoma M, He H, Pacak C, et al. Biological characterization of F-18 labeled rhodamine B, a potential positron emission tomography perfusion tracer. Nucl Med Biol. 2013;40:1043-8.
43. Yalamanchili P, Wexler E, Hayes M, Yu M, Bozek J, Kagan M, et al. Mechanism of uptake and retention of F-18 BMS-747 158-02 in cardiomyocytes: a novel PET myocardial imaging agent. J Nucl Cardiol. 2007;14:782-8.
44. Huisman MC, Higuchi T, Reder S, Nekolla SG, Poethko T, Wester H-J, et al. Initial characterization of an 18F-labeled myocardial perfusion tracer. J Nucl Med. 2008;49:630-6.
45. Nekolla SG, Reder S, Saraste A, Higuchi T, Dzewas G, Preissel A, et al. Evaluation of the novel myocardial perfusion PET tracer 18F-BMS747158-02: Comparison to 13N-ammonia and validation with microspheres in a pig model. Circulation. 2009;119:2333-42.
46. Maddahi J. Properties of an ideal PET perfusion tracer: new PET tracer cases and data. J Nucl Cardiol. 2007;19(Suppl 1):S30-7.
47. Maddahi J, Czernin J, Lazewatsky J, Huang SC, Dahlbom M, Schelbert H, et al. Phase I, first-in-human study of BMS747158, a novel 18F-labeled tracer for myocardial perfusion PET: Dosimetry, biodistribution, safety, and imaging characteristics after a single injection at rest. J Nucl Med. 2011;52:1490-8.
48. Maddahi J, Bengel F, Huang SC, Czernin J, Schelbert H, Zhu Q, et al. Phase 1 rest-stress study of F-18 labeled BMS747158 myocardial perfusion PET tracer: Human safety, dosimetry, biodistribution, and myocardial imaging characteristics [abstract]. J Nucl Med. 2009;50:184.
49. Berman DS, Maddahi J, Tamarappoo BK, Czernin J, Taillefer R, Udelson JE, Gibson CM, Devine M, Lazewatsky J, Bhat G, Washburn D. Phase II safety and clinical comparison with single-photon emission computed tomography myocardial perfusion imaging for detection of coronary artery disease: flurpiridaz F-18 positron emission tomography. J Am Coll Cardiol. 2013;61(4):469-77.
50. Schelbert HR. Quantification of myocardial blood flow: What is the clinical role? Cardiol Clin. 2009;27:277-89.
51. Maddahi J, Huang S, Truong D, Lazewatsky JL, Ehlgen A, Schelbert H, et al. Preliminary results of absolute quantification of rest and stress myocardial blood flow with flurpiridaz F-18 PET in normal

and coronary artery disease patients in a single-center study [abstract]. J Nucl Cardiol. 2010;17:743.
52. Schon HR, Schelbert HR, Najafi A, et al. C-11 labeled palmitic acid for the noninvasive evaluation of regional myocardial fatty acid metabolism with positron computed tomography. I, Kinetics of C-11 palmitic acid in normal myocardium. Am Heart J. 1982;103:532-47.
53. Schon HR, Schelbert HR, Najafi A, et al. C-11 labeled palmitic acid for the noninvasive evaluation of regional myocardial fatty acid metabolism with positron computed tomography. II, Kinetics of C-11 palmitic acid in acutely ischemic myocardium. Am Heart J. 1982;103:538-61.
54. Elmaleh DR, Livni E, Alpert NM, et al. Myocardial extraction of 1-[11C] betamethyl heptadecanoic acid. J Nucl Med. 1994;35:496-503.
55. Ebert A, Herzog H, Stoklin GL, et al. Kinetics of 14(R-S)-fluorine-18-fluoro-6-thiaheptadecanoic acid in normal human hearts at rest, during exercise and after dipyridamole injection. J Nucl Med. 1994;35:51-6.
56. Rabinovitch MA, Kalif V, Allen R, et al. ω-^{123}I-Hexadecanoic acid metabolic probe of cardiomyopathy. Eur J Nucl Med. 1985;10:222-7.
57. Knapp FF, Ambrose KR, Goodman MM. New radio iodinated methyl branched fatty acids for cardiac studies. Eur J Nucl Med. 1986;12:S39-S44.
58. Wolfe CL, Kennedy PL, Kulkarni P, et al. Iodine-123 phenylpentadecanoic acid myocardial scintigraphy in patients with left ventricular hypertrophy: alterations in left ventricular distribution and utilization. Am Heart J. 1991;119:1338-7.
59. Kennedy PL, Corbet JR, Kulkarni PV, et al. I-123 phenylpentadecanoic acid myocardial scintigraphy: usefulness in the identification of myocardial ischemia. Circulation. 1986;74:1007-15.
60. Ugolini V, Hansen CL, Kulkarni PV, et al. Abnormal fatty acid metabolism in dilated cardiomyopathy detected by Iodine-123 phenylpentadecanoic acid and tomographic imaging. Am J Cardiol. 1988;62:923-8.
61. Zhao C, Shuk N, Okizaki A, et al. Comparison of myocardial fatty acid metabolism with left ventricular function and perfusion in cardiomyopathies: by 123I-BMIPP SPECT and 99mTC-tetrafosmin electrocardiographically gated SPECT. Ann Nucl Med. 2003;17:541-8.
62. Quilard T, Libby P. Molecular imaging of atherosclerosis for improving diagnosis and therapeutic development. Cir Res. 2012;111:231-44.
63. Tavakoli S, Vashist A, Sadeghi MM. Molecular imaging of plaque vulnerability. J Nucl Cardiol. 2014;21:1112-1128-1129, DOI: 10.1007/s1235-0-014-9959-4.
64. Liu Y, Pierce R, Luehmann HP, Sharp TL, Welch MJ. PET imaging of chemokine receptors in vascular injury-accelerated atherosclerosis. J Nucl Med. 2013;54:1135-41.
65. Li X, Bauer W, Israel I, Kreissl MC, Weirather J, Richter D, Bauer E, Herold V, Jakob P, Buck A, Frantz S, Samnick S. Targeting P-selectin by gallium-68-labeled fucoidan positron emission tomography for noninvasive characterization of vulnerable plaques: correlation with in vivo 17.6T MRI. Arterioscler Thromb Vasc Biol. 2014;34(8):1661-166, 2014 7. doi: 10.1161/ATVBAHA.114.303485.
66. Nakamura I, Hasegawa K, Wada Y, Hirase T, Node K, Watanabe Y. Detection of early stage atherosclerotic plaques using PET and CT fusion imaging targeting P-selectin in low density lipoprotein receptor-deficient mice. Biochem Biophys Res Commun 433: 47-51, 2013 doi: 10.1016/j.bbrc.2013.02.069. Epub 2013 Feb 26.
67. Irkle A, Vesey AT, Lewis DY, Skepper JN. Identifying active vascular microcalcification by (18)F-sodium fluoride positron emission tomography. Nat Commun. 2015;6: 7495,doi: 10.1038/ncomms8495.
68. Pressly ED, Detering L, Wang C, Pierce R, Woodard PK, Gropler RJ, Hawker CJ, Liu Y. PET/CT imaging of chemokine receptor CCR5 in vascular injury model using targeted nanoparticle. Luehmann HP. J Nucl Med. 2014;55(4):629-34.
69. Rudd JH, Hyfil F, Fayad ZA. Inflammation imaging in atherosclerosis. Arterioscler Thromb Vasc Biol. 2009;29:1009-16.
70. Alie N, Eldib M, Fayad ZA, Mani V. Inflammation, Atherosclerosis, and coronary Artery Disease: PET/CT for the evaluation of Atherosclerosis and Inflammation. Clin Med Insights Cardiol. 2014;8:13-21.
71. Dweck MR, Chow MW, Joshi NV, et al. Coronary arterial 18F-sodium fluoride uptake: a novel marker of plaque biology. J Am Coll Cariol. 2012;59:1539-48.
72. Menezes LJ, Kayani I, Ben-Haim S, Hutton B, Ell PJ, Groves AM. What is the natural history of 18F-FDG uptake in arterial atheroma on PET/CT? Implications for imaging the vulnerable plaque. Atherosclerosis. 2010;211:136-140.
73. Jezovnik MK, Zidar N, Lezaic L, Gersak B, Poredos P. Identification of inflamed atherosclerosis lesions in vivo using PET-CT. Inflammation. 2014;37:426-34.
74. Withana N, Saito T, Ma X, et al. Dual modality activity based probes molecular imaging agents for vascular inflammation. Journal of Nuclear Medicine, published online on May, 2016 doi:10.2967/jnumed.115.171553.

12 Myocardial Imaging Products' Evolution: Change for the Better

N Ramamoorthy, Meera Venkatesh

INTRODUCTION

Management of patients of coronary artery diseases (CAD) is an extremely large volume need in medical practice. Naturally role of nuclear medicine (NM) imaging for mapping the blood flow to the myocardium (myocardial perfusion) would be of considerable value, and hence, one of the very early aims of diagnostic nuclear medicine imaging was to visualize the myocardium. It is the functional evidence based demonstration by imaging the sites of low or nil perfusion, as well as of the viability of the corresponding zone(s) of myocardium, that would make NM add unique value for management of patients with ischemic heart disease (IHD). Those were the days of planar gamma camera dominance, while use of rectilinear scanner has not been altogether given up. This requirement literally drove hordes of researchers to undertake development of suitable products for myocardial imaging. The development was hindered due to nonavailability of a suitable gamma emitting short-lived potassium radionuclide, and the fact that the then emerging ^{99m}Tc products were mostly based on empirical approach to develop a suitable cationic complex species, to mimic K^+ or its analog Tl^+.

THALLIUM-201 AS MYOCARDIAL PERFUSION MARKER

The realization of the need for an analog to mimic intracellular K^+ (in light of nonavailability of a suitable potassium radionuclide [RN]) for myocardial imaging with the then prevalent planar gamma camera was the starting point in the evolution of myocardial perfusion imaging (MPI) agents. It is the advent in mid-1970s of $^{201}Tl^+$ tracer (74 hours half-life; Eγ 135 & 167 keV; 69–80 keV Hg X-rays)—mimic of intra-cellular K^+, due to similarity of ionic size and charge - that heralded a major milestone in the history of radiopharmaceutical and nuclear medicine practice. The very high myocardial extraction of Tl^+ ensured that 3–4% of injected dose of ^{201}Tl would be taken up by the myocardium. The added advantage of $^{201}Tl^+$ was the feature of its relatively slower uptake and slower wash-out from 'compromised but viable' myocardial tissue (ischemic areas), as compared to normal myocardial cells, and this helped obtain stress and rest images of myocardial perfusion, with a single injection of $^{201}TlCl$ and imaging twice, early (injection of tracer at peak exercise and imaging soon after) and a delayed image at 3–4 hours post-injection). This led to achieving an important place for ^{201}Tl imaging in NM, with as low as 50–75 MBq (about 1.5–2 mCi) administered dose, despite the relatively low resolution images obtained with the planar gamma camera. The term 'redistribution' was invariably cited while obtaining the delayed image, though it was a misnomer, as the difference was due to differential wash out of the tracer between high and low blood flow regions.

With the advent of SPECT, there was an important change for the better, as dose of ^{201}Tl was increased (up to 130 MBq [3.5 mCi]), and superior resolution image slices of myocardial perfusion were routinely registered and reported. ^{201}Tl has remained a good physiological tracer for MPI, while it is unfavorable from the point of view of image quality and higher absorbed radiation dose to the patients. Medical cyclotrons (MC) of 30 MeV protons (of a Belgium company) became highly popular for deployment for production of ^{201}Tl **(Table 1)**. ^{201}Tl has to be produced by (p, 3n) reaction (with its σ max being at 28 MeV) on enriched ^{203}Tl target, followed by a 2-stage processing, the first to quickly recover the ^{201}Pb produced from the thallium target, and then after about 30–32 hours, to separate and purify no-carrier-added ^{201}Tl as thallous chloride. Automated radiochemical processing module and high power 30 MeV cyclotron became popular in rendering reliable availability of ^{201}TlCl for medical use, and, in turn, made nuclear cardiology a regular facet of clinical NM.

TECHNETIUM-99M COMPOUNDS AS MYOCARDIAL PERFUSION MARKERS

The well-established merits of ^{99m}Tc (6 hours half-life; Eγ 140.5 keV [89%]) for high quality imaging **(Table 1)**, taken along with the vital need for a myocardial imaging agent, triggered in late 1970s and early 1980s much R&D efforts world over. This culminated in the development and launch of Tc(I) hexakis isonitirle mono-cationic complex, called ^{99m}Tc-sestamibi, by a US-based company. The concept in this development was to optimize a moderately lipophilic, cationic complex of ^{99m}Tc to mimic the thallous ion and facilitate uptake by the myocardium and fast clearance from the blood pool. This was subsequently supplemented by another similar monocationic complex product, called ^{99m}Tc-tetrofosmin, launched by a company in UK. The ^{99m}Tc based products understandably did not have the same features as ^{201}Tl$^+$, and thus two separate injections were necessary to elicit stress and rest perfusion patterns in patients. Further, their myocardial extraction efficiency was only 50–60% of that of ^{201}Tl (which was compensated partly by the larger injected dose of ^{99m}Tc activity. The phasing out of ^{201}Tl did not hence take place even after the next 10–15 years despite the edge ^{99m}Tc had in production logistics, patient dose and cost; and it is only since 2000, perceptible reduction in the use of ^{201}Tl has occurred.

The arrival of ^{99m}Tc based products for MPI and the entry of SPECT in NM however took place within the same span of time. This quickly led to MPI being done with SPECT and ^{99m}Tc products, both aspects making the image quality to be much superior to that obtainable with ^{201}Tl$^+$. The inevitable liver shadow with ^{99m}Tc products (being highly lipophilic) in planar imaging could also be avoided to a large extent by the SPECT images. The rest is history, with nearly 40–50% of all the large volume imaging done with ^{99m}Tc being that of myocardium—again, a change for the better. It is estimated that one ^{99m}Tc based imaging study is being done every second somewhere in the world, and thus, one myocardial imaging study using ^{99m}Tc is being done once every 2–2.5 seconds using one of the two products mentioned earlier. The quest for better agents led to R&D on promising ^{99m}Tc labeled molecules with novel ^{99m}Tc nitride core, but these however did not reach the clinics due to the lack of sustained efforts and funds necessary to complete development up to the stage of conducting clinical trials. The larger amount of injected dose possible in the case of ^{99m}Tc products (up to 740 MBq [20 mCi]), taken along with the ability to acquire ECG-gated images (when required), render it possible for also acquisition of data and deriving cardiac pumping parameter (left ventricular ejection fraction, LVEF), in addition to MP imaging. Echocardiography provides EF data and the role of NM is not unique.

LABELED FATTY ACID AS MARKER FOR METABOLISM: IODINE-123 PRODUCTS

Another early development involved iodine-123 fatty acid analogs, as tracer of myocardial metabolism imaging, a much welcome change for the better, but this could not however live up to its promise, unlike the above success story of ^{99m}Tc products. Since fatty acid is a primary source of energy for myocardium, radiolabeled (e.g. radioiodinated) analogs of fatty acid derivatives (ortho/para Iodo phenyl pentadecanoic acid [IPPA]) were attractive carrier molecules for myocardial imaging, e.g. ^{123}I-IPPA. ^{123}I (13.3 hours half-life; Eγ 159 keV [84%]) is an ideal agent for imaging with gamma camera and SPECT. The rather demanding production logistics (very highly enriched ^{124}Xe target use) as well as cost **(Table 1)**, and the then mindset that 13.3 hours half-life of ^{123}I is too short for facile transportation, severely impacted the exploitation of the actual utility of ^{123}I based myocardial agent. It is ironical that despite growth in the deployment of MC, and the paradigm-shift with respect to half-life of radionuclides in use nowadays—that is, the case of widespread distribution and use of 110 minutes half-life ^{18}F-interest in production and use of ^{123}I has remained rather low. ^{18}F labeled fatty acid analogs have been reported in quest of a PET tracer for myocardial metabolism imaging with limited success. It would be appropriate to revisit ^{123}I and product like IPPA for possible use. In light of emerging enhanced availability of PET and PET-CT systems, one can also consider use of ^{124}I-IPPA **(Table 1)**.

PET TRACERS AS MYOCARDIAL PERFUSION MARKERS

The fastest growing imaging modality since 2001, namely PET-CT, has also turned the focus on PET tracers for MPI, including by revisiting certain 'old' PET tracers **(Table 1)**. In this context, such a leaning to PET tracers could also be seen as arising from the inherent shortcoming of SPECT tracers owing to non-uniform attenuation and scatter photons from extra cardiac sources, while PET modality has the advantage of attenuation correction leading to superior resolution images of the 'defective' regions. ^{82}Sr-^{82}Rb generator, and the use of ^{82}Rb$^+$ (K$^+$ analogue) for PET imaging of myocardial perfusion, has been increasingly attracting global attention, more particularly after the 2008–2010 supply crisis of ^{99}Mo-^{99}Tc. ^{82}Sr with a half-life of 25 days renders generators of shelf-life of about a month or two. Half-life of ^{82}Rb (75 seconds) is favorable for repeat cardiac studies, wherever warranted, as for example, for certain need-based physiological and/or pharmacological intervention procedures. One can also cite the other PET tracer, ^{13}NH$_3$ (10 minutes half-life) here (as ^{13}NH$_4^+$) for MPI, though it is unlikely to be of large use (due to the requirement of on-site MC).

Advantage of Quantitation while Using PET Tracers

The NM procedures have been vital to the cardiologists in the management of patients with CAD/IHD. Over time, the role of NM imaging has also moved beyond perfusion imaging, responding to the importance and role of absolute quantitation of myocardial flow, expressed in terms of Coronary Flow Ratio (CFR—ratio of the myocardial blood flow at peak hyperemia to resting), in management of cardiac patients with coronary stenosis. To derive the CFR values, tracers whose uptake is directly proportional to the blood flow are required and the PET tracer, ^{15}O-water ($t_{1/2}$ 2.06 minutes) which diffuses freely across myocyte membranes, with 100% extraction fraction, would be the ideal tracer for the purpose. However, its use is limited due to practical disadvantages including the very short half-life of 2.06 minutes. Amongst the other myocardial perfusion PET tracers, ^{82}Rb$^+$ and ^{13}N-ammonia $^+$ are the ones used despite their non-ideal myocardial extraction fractions. Of these, ^{82}Rb which can be derived from a generator has an edge over ^{13}N-ammonia, and hence the preferred tracer currently for CFR estimation. But, ^{18}F - flurpiridaz, a compound in third phase clinical trial seems set to emerge as the winner, ticking all the required boxes—namely: uptake proportional to the flow; adequately long half-life; low positron energy enabling high resolution images; and cost relatively lower than that of ^{82}Rb$^+$ and ^{13}NH$_4^+$.

The growth in hybrid imaging using PET-CT (aimed at combining the functional imaging with anatomical imaging use of two modalities) has been rapid with nearly all PET centers currently equipped with PET-CT machines. The availability of CT along with PET proves to be an added advantage for estimation of another important parameter Fractional Flow Reserve (FFR), for management of patients with coronary stenosis. Recent advances in computational fluid dynamics and image-based modeling have made it possible to calculate FFR noninvasively without the need for additional imaging, modification of acquisition protocols, or administration of medications. This added possibility to the PET-CT imaging studies is yet another boost to the value-addition available with the use of nuclear (PET) cardiology.

PET TRACERS AS MARKER OF MYOCARDIAL VIABILITY

The role of nuclear medicine to directly show the extent of viability of the suspect segments or damaged or injured myocardium has been a well-recognized feature since early days, especially when ^{18}F-2-fluoro-2-deoxy glucose (^{18}FDG) entered the clinical NM scene. Now that medical cyclotrons (MC) and PET tracer like ^{18}FDG have become common place items (about 16 MC and 120 PET-CT now in India), NM's value addition to managing cardiac patients by demonstrating myocardial viability in an unequivocal manner can be increasingly put to clinical use. The blood flow starved lesion(s) shown on the MP images with ^{99m}Tc + SPECT, lighting up with ^{18}FDG on PET image, helps plan, or confirm the plan, for the subsequent interventions required (or otherwise). ^{18}FDG, well-known for its high value contributions to cancer patients, can be harnessed for the benefit of cardiac patients too. But, beyond FDG, several other ^{18}F labeled molecules are under investigation, and a few of these are in clinical trials. For example, ^{18}F-flurpiridaz is reported to have a very high first-pass extraction fraction by the heart, indicating its promising potential for myocardial perfusion imaging. While many PET radionuclides seem to be poised to enter fair to good use in nuclear cardiology, it is pertinent to note that among the PET nuclides, ^{18}F with the lowest positron energy (0.635 MeV) would be the best suited to provide high resolution images, and hence has an edge over other positron emitter nuclides. It is estimated that one PET study takes place every ten seconds, and that almost 90% is in oncology setting. Assuming 50% of the remaining PET study is in cardiology, one can cite that three PET cardiac studies are performed every ten minutes, though the need and scope for PET cardiac study are much larger.

Scope for Additional PET Tracers for Myocardial Imaging

The generator produced PET tracer ^{68}Ga (68 minutes half-life) is being already increasingly used in NM, mostly for its valuable role in tumor imaging. The availability of ^{68}Ga from reasonably long-lived ^{68}Ge-^{68}Ga generator is an important advantage, as it obviates the need for an on-site cyclotron or dependence on daily shipments. This aspect together with the amenability of trivalent gallium ion for complexation by a variety of chelating moieties have accelerated the R&D using ^{68}Ga. Thus a welcome development, another change for the better, will be development of a ^{68}Ga product for MP PET imaging in near future. This will enhance further the valuable role of ^{68}Ga, and in turn, demand for ^{68}Ge-^{68}Ga generator. Although several synthetic cationic complexes of Ga(III) have been explored as ^{68}Ga PET tracers (for example, gallium(III)-(bis(3-isopropoxy-2-phenolate -benzylidene) -N,N'-bis(2,2-dimethyl-3-amino-propyl) ethylenediamine) for MPI, a ^{68}Ga-complex with biochemical and pharmacokinetic properties ideally suited for PET MPI with high contrast perfusion images of the heart combined with rapid clearance from the liver has still not been achieved.

There is also potential to produce directly ^{68}Ga, using MC and highly enriched ^{68}Zn targets **(Table 1)**. This approach is deemed worthy of active pursuit, as it will reduce dependence on ^{68}Ge, which is being produced only in a few centers and is not freely commercially available.

Another positron emitting RN of high potential for further exploitation is Copper-64, which is already being much investigated for tumor imaging. The 12.4 hours half-life of

Chapter 12: Myocardial Imaging Products' Evolution: Change for the Better

Table 1 Radionuclides for myocardial imaging agents

RN & key features	Production route(s)	Logistics aspects	Chemical form(s)	Basis of imaging	Volume of use	General remarks
^{201}Tl, 74 hours 69–80 Hg X-rays	^{203}Tl(p,3n) ^{201}Pb→	Need 30 MeV MC	TlCl	K mimic	Very large in the past	Limitation of image quality
^{99m}Tc, 6 hours; 140.5 keV	^{99}Mo-^{99m}Tc generator	Widely available	Cationic complex; e.g. [Tc(RNC)$_6$]$^+$	Binding to mitochondria	Large to very large	^{99m}Tc being revisited with dithiocarbamate and bisphosphine chelates
^{123}I, 13.3 hours; 159 keV	^{124}Xe(p,2n) ^{123}Cs→^{123}Xe → ^{124}Te(p,2n) Te(p,xn)	Availability limited, can be increased	IPPA Rotenone-I-123	Fatty acid metabolism; Mitochondrial complex inhibitor	Very limited	Affected by earlier mind-set of distribution problems; But, recognized and being revived along with R&D on new compounds
^{82}Rb, 75 sec; β$^+$	^{82}Sr (25d) -^{82}Rb generator	Generator availability limited	RbCl	K mimic	Limited, but growing	Limited sources of ^{82}Sr & generator production Very high cost; need for large throughput
^{13}N, 10 minutes, β$^+$	^{16}O(p,α)	On site MC	NH$_4^+$	Conversion through glutamine synthase	Limited, but can grow further	Short T$_{1/2}$ problems
^{15}O, 2.06 minutes, β$^+$	^{14}N(d,n)	On site MC	^{15}O water	Passive diffusion	R & D	Very short T$_{1/2}$; no treadmill scope; pharmacological stress ^{15}O water is suboptimal due to a low myocardial-to-background count ratio
^{68}Ga, 68 minutes; β$^+$	^{68}Ge (271d) -^{68}Ga generator; ^{68}Zn(p,n)	Generator in wide use; direct production in MC feasible	[Ga(3-MeOsal)2BAPDMEN]$^+$ ^{68}Ga-RGD analogs	Mono-cationic species to mimic K$^+$ αVβ3 integrin molecular probes	R&D	Limited sources of ^{68}Ge production; ^{68}Ga to be explored more; compatible for various carrier moiety
^{64}Cu, 12.4 hours; β$^+$	^{64}Ni (p,n) 12- 9 MeV p	Availability growing	Cu-DOTA-VEGF121-	Imaging VEGF receptors in myocardial angiogenesis	R&D level; potential to grow	Compatible for various carrier moiety; can be better explored
^{11}C, 20 minutes; β$^+$	^{14}N (p, α)	On site MC	Glucose; Acetate; Palmitate	Metabolic/ Fatty acid pathway	Limited use	Mostly will serve as reference; other 11C-molecules being explored for metabolic studies
^{18}F, 110 minutes; β$^+$	^{18}O (p,n)	Widely produced and distributed	FDG	Shift to glycolytic pathway due to poor perfusion	Fair volume; growing further	Many new tracers being explored; e.g. F-18-flurpiridaz, etc.
^{124}I, 4.2 days; β$^+$	^{124}Te (p,n); ^{125}Te (p,2n)	Availability limited	IPPA	Fatty acid pathway	R&D level	I-123 and I-124 are often coproduced due to multiple concomitant reactions
^{62}Cu, 9.7 minutes; β$^+$	^{62}Zn-^{62}Cu gen ^{62}Ni(p,n)^{62}Cu 5-14 MeV p	Daily replacement of generator	Pyruval-dehyde-bis (N4 methyl-thiosemi-carbazone) PTSM		R&D	2.9 MeV β$^+$; Image resolution not the best; but being explored

^{64}Cu makes it more attractive for production and distribution logistics compared to ^{68}Ga. Both Ga and Cu have been used in NM with effective linker molecules to biologically (or biochemically) interesting carrier molecule (structures can be found in the paper of Yui-May Hsiao et al. cited in bibliography), thanks to their favorable complexation characteristics. This advantage can be further harnessed for development in future of a myocardial perfusion PET tracer. The superior resolution PET images and greater quantitation capability of PET are the key drivers for the suggested approach. That would help herald a distinct change for the better in the evolution of myocardial imaging agents. While ^{64}Cu has been explored for labeling with a VEGF analog to image VEGF receptor in angiogenesis, Copper-62, another positron-emitting radionuclide of copper (nearly 100% decaying by positron emission) is also being studied for use in cardiac imaging. ^{62}Cu ($T_{1/2}$ 9.7 minutes) is to be obtained essentially from its precursor ^{62}Zn ($T_{1/2}$ 9.2 hours), and requires virtually daily replacement of generator **(Table 1)**.

CONCLUSION

The recent emergence of (multi-slice) angio-CT has already added a powerful noninvasive imaging tool to the cardiologist in the investigation of patients of CAD; and so, what can NM and radiopharmaceuticals can do to advance nuclear cardiology further? If only there would be a suitable tracer that will lit up the interiors of the coronary arteries, almost in the same manner as the conventional angiography shows it all, that would be truly a phenomenal achievement, however tough the odds may be in the development of such a product and in achieving the resolution of the imaging instrumentation required. Some progress in terms of potential tracers for targeting arterial plaques has been covered in conferences and publications (e.g. by Orbay et al. cited in bibliography). PET imaging of atherosclerosis could be of great help to identify the at-risk individuals earlier in the disease process, as well as to monitor responses to therapy. Of the several PET tracers studied for imaging atherosclerosis, the most commonly cited is ^{18}F-FDG, while ^{11}C-choline, ^{18}F-galacto-RGD, ^{11}C-acetate, and ^{11}C-PK11195 have been tested clinically. But, the small size of the atherosclerotic lesions in coronary arteries in the vicinity of circulating tracer in blood, taken along with the respiratory and cardiac movements during the image acquisition, would lead to high degree of uncertainties. This could be better addressed by the use of PET/MR system, where MRI can provide high spatial resolution and exquisite soft tissue contrast, to complement PET. If a simple intravenous injection of a radiopharmaceutical, and after physiological stress too, would elicit what you can otherwise observe only in the cath lab., most groups of vulnerable people, and suspect or likely patients, could be investigated without branding them as 'cardiac patients' and avoiding the psychological consequences to the patient and his/her family. It would be worthwhile to aim for larger, concerted development efforts in this direction. Researchers in the field need to come together to see what may be achievable for such a larger role of NM in cardiac care and patient management in future.

BIBLIOGRAPHY

1. Green MA, Mathias CJ, Neumann WL, Fanwick PE, Janik M, Deutsch EA. Potential Gallium-68 tracers for imaging the heart with PET: Evaluation of four gallium complexes with functionalized tripodal tris (Salicylaldimine) Ligands. J NucI Med. 1993;34:228-33.
2. Maddahi J, Packard René RS. Cardiac PET perfusion tracers: current status and future directions. Semin Nucl Med. 2014;44:333-43 (*http://www.ncbi.nlm.nih.gov/pmc/articles/PMC4333146/pdf/nihms657665.pdf*).
3. Orbay H, Hong H, Zhang Y, et al. Positron emission tomography imaging of atherosclerosis. Theranostics. 2013;3: 894-902 (*http://www.thno.org/v03p0894.htm*).
4. Schelbert HR. Current status and prospects of new radionuclides and radiopharmaceuticals for cardiovascular nuclear medicine. Semin Nucl Med. 1987;17:145-81 (*http://www.seminarsinnuclearmedicine.com/article/S0001-2998(87)80019-3/pdf*).
5. Shoup TM, Elmaleh DR, Brownell AL, Zhu A, Guerrero JL, Fischman AJ. Evaluation of (4-[^{18}F] Fluorophenyl) triphenylphosphonium Ion. A potential myocardial blood flow agent for PET. Mol Imaging Biol. 2011;13:511-7.
6. Sogbein OO, Pelletier-Galarneau M, Schindler TH, Lihui Wei, Wells RG, Ruddy TD. New SPECT and PET radiopharmaceuticals for imaging cardiovascular disease. Hindawi publishing corporation; BioMed research international; Volume 2014, Article ID 942960.
7. Veeranna V, Dorbala S. Myocardial perfusion imaging with PET, PET/CT, PET/MRI: Technical advances and future applications. 'Perfusion imaging in clinical practice', Chapter 22, pp.398-411.
8. Yesen Li, Zhang W, HuaWu, Liu G. Advanced tracers in PET imaging of cardiovascular disease. Hindawi publishing corporation; BioMed research international; Volume 2014, Article ID 504532.
9. Yui-May Hsiao, Carla J Mathias, Shiaw-Pyng Wey, Phillip E Fanwick1, Mark A. Synthesis and Biodistribution of Lipophilic Monocationic Gallium Radiopharmaceuticals Derived from N, N'-bis (3-aminopropyl)-N, N'-dimethylethylenediamine: Potential Agents for PET Myocardial Imaging with 68Ga, Green, Nucl Med Biol. 2009;36:39-45.

13 Efficacy of Combining FDG-PET Metabolic and Tc-99m–MIBI Myocardial Perfusion Study in Assessment of Myocardial Viability

BK Das, Sudatta Ray, Oma Shankar

WHAT IS MYOCARDIAL VIABILITY?

Contractile function is the hallmark of myocardium. Myocardial contractile dysfunction represents hibernating or stunned myocardium. Hibernating myocardium has depressed myocardial contractility at rest due to persistently impaired coronary blood flow. The function can be partially or completely restored by improving coronary blood flow, by providing inotropic stimulation or by reducing oxygen demand. Several studies have shown that hibernating myocardium results from reduced myocardial blood flow. It is metabolically characterized by a switch from fat to glucose metabolism and accompanied by a reactivation of the fetal gene program. Myocardial territories that have normal blood flow at rest can also demonstrate depressed cardiac function if they undergo recurrent ischemic episodes with stress in a process known as repetitive myocardial stunning. These territories also improve with revascularization.

Viable myocardium thus can be defined as dysfunctional myocardium that resumes full contractile function if adequate blood supply is restored.

METHODS OF ASSESSMENT OF VIABILITY

Multiple imaging modalities exist for differentiating viable myocardium from scar in territories with contractile dysfunction. With the multiple modalities available, choosing the best modality for a specific patient can be at times difficult. The methods vary from echocardiography, cardiac magnetic resonance imaging, nuclear imaging with single photon emission computed tomography (SPECT) and positron emission tomography (PET) imaging and cardiac computed tomography. Dobutamine echocardiography and MRI rely on identifying the property of contractile reserve in hibernating myocardium in response to low-dose inotropic agents. Cardiac magnetic resonance (CMR) imaging and cardiac CT can assess the transmural extent of scar. This technology depends on an intact cellular membrane to prevent the extracellular contrast agent, gadolinium/iodinated contrast, from entering cells and thus allowing the gadolinium/iodinated contrast to concentrate in areas of increased interstitial space [scar, late gadolinium enhancement (LGE)]. It is not possible to describe the techniques in detail in this small write up. The ideal test for viability assessment would be easy availability, simple to perform, reasonably inexpensive, and safe with limited side effects. It would be reproducible and free from artifacts and also successfully differentiate patients who would benefit from revascularization from those who would not.

Nuclear studies, including SPECT and PET, rely on intact cellular membranes for active uptake of radiotracers like Thallium-20, intact sarcolemmal function to maintain electrochemical gradients across the cell membrane for radiotracer retention of Technetium-99m-labeled compounds and intact glucose uptake [Fluorine-18-labeled deoxyglucose (FDG)]. Modalities that depend on cell membrane function, a process that occurs early in the under-perfused state, show a low likelihood of recovery following revascularization if viability is not present (high sensitivity), while modalities that use contractile function, a change that occurs later in the under-perfused state, show a high likelihood of functional recovery if viability is present (high specificity).

Thallium-based myocardial perfusion and viability studies have declined due to poor physical imaging qualities of the radioisotope and prolonged study periods. Myocardial SPECT studies using Te99m agents have been widely used for years for assessment of perfusion as well as potential improvement possibility after revascularization. The biggest advantage of SPECT is that there is extensive clinical experience as well as a wealth of studies demonstrating the ability of SPECT to predict viability. SPECT imaging is widely available, easy to perform, and highly reproducible. Rest and stress perfusion scans can be performed on the same day using the appropriate protocol to evaluate the magnitude of stress-induced ischemia, global LV systolic function, and LV volumes. These factors influence postrevascularization recovery of function and determine patient management.

PET imaging can be used to assess viability by the measurement of myocardial perfusion and/or metabolism. Myocardial perfusion is assessed using Rubidium-82 or N-13 ammonia at rest and with pharmacologic stress to assess for stress-induced ischemia. Myocardial metabolism can be assessed by 18F-Fluoro-deoxy-glucose (FDG) (glucose metabolism), C-11 acetate (oxidative metabolism) or C-11 palmitate (fatty acid metabolism). Most commonly, however, myocardial metabolism is assessed by FDG, a glucose analog that is taken up by the glucose transporters on the myocytes and metabolized by hexokinase to F-18 FDG 6-phosphate, which is no longer metabolized and becomes trapped within the myocytes. FDG imaging is usually performed following a glucose load and intravenous insulin administration to improve image quality. In viable but jeopardized cells, FDG uptake increases due to a shift to anaerobic metabolism and a preference for glucose rather fatty acid metabolism.

The comparison between segmental myocardial perfusion, and metabolism provides information regarding the amount of normal, hibernating, and necrotic myocardium.

COMBINATION OF MPS WITH MIBI AND FDG-PET

PET-CT facilities are now available in many Nuclear Medicine departments. It has been possible to conduct combination of myocardial SPECT studies using Tc-99m agents and PET-CT for better assessment of myocardial viability. Reliable information about viability is vital for appropriate and evidence-based management of CAD. Moreover, many cardiologists are specifically asking for this information as assessment of myocardial perfusion is also available through other nonradio isotopic methods.

We have used this combination technique for a number of patients in whom SPECT studies alone could not provide sufficiently acceptable results. Evaluation of 23 such patients in whom SPECT and PET-CT studies were performed consecutively revealed following results:

Two patients in whom myocardial perfusion study (MPS-SPECT) had revealed strong suspicion of nonviable myocardium (scar tissue) in 4 segments showed adequate FDG uptake leading to medical management instead of invasive procedures. **Figures 1A and B** show one of the cases.

Three patients of sarcoidosis with strong indication of non-viable myocardium in 4 segments in MPS-SPECT who were subjected to FDG Study showed infiltration to myocardium revealing the cause of MPS findings. **Figures 2A and B** show one such case of myocardial infiltration of sarcoidosis along with findings of MPS with MIBI.

In this on-going study more cases will be recruited to reveal pattern of MPS-SPECT findings in myocardial sarcoidosis.

SUMMARY

Correct assessment of viability of myocardial tissue is extremely important for optimal management of CAD.

Several combination of studies with various protocols using different radiopharmaceuticals are in use with varying

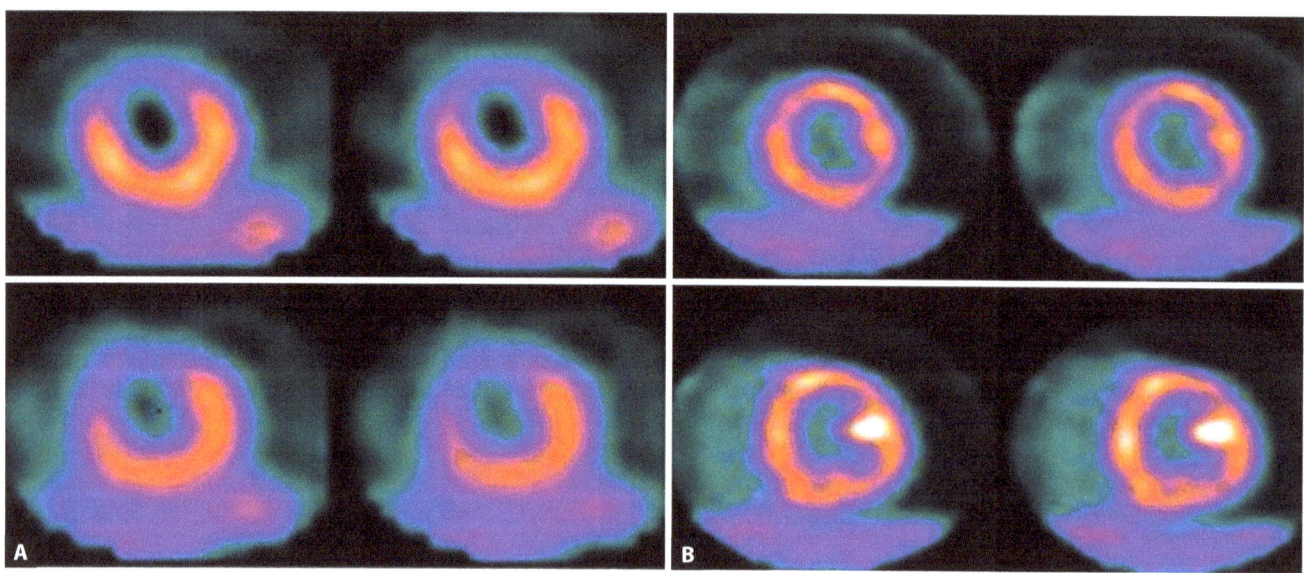

Figs 1A and B: (A) MIBI perfusion at rest (upper) and stress (lower); (B) PET-CT images. Mid to distal anterior wall and anteroseptum show non-transmural infarct with preserved glucose metabolism, suggestive of viable hibernating myocardium

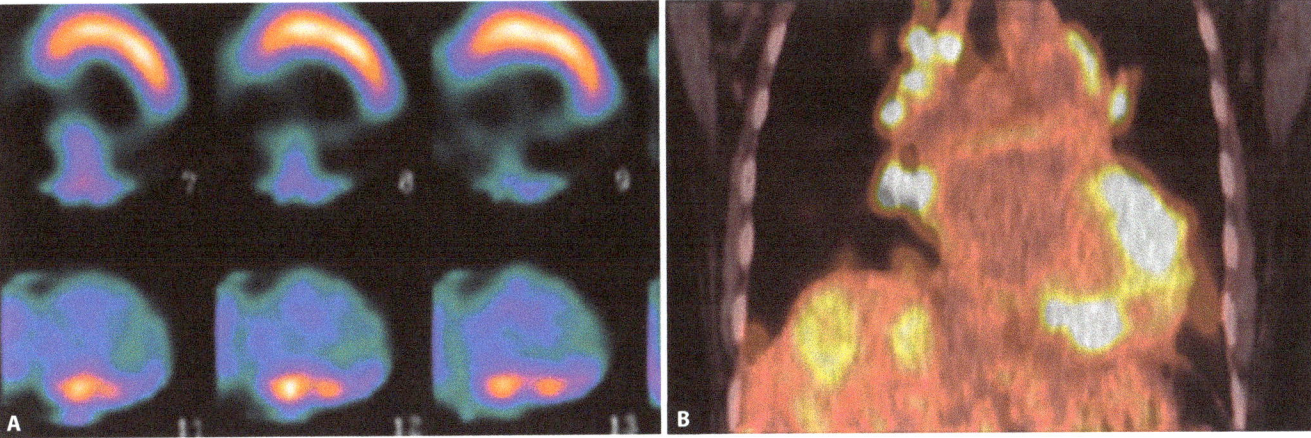

Figs 2A and B: (A) MIBI perfusion (upper) and FDG study (lower); (B) Sarcoidosis involving myocardium, mediastinum and liver. The patient had been meticulously prepared before FDG study to prevent glucose metabolism in normal myocardium. The focal patchy FDG uptake seen in this section in the mid to basal inferior and inferolateral wall is due to sarcoidosis infiltration to the myocardium

results. Now that PET-CT is available in many centers even in developing countries like India a combination of MIBI- MPS and metabolic assessment with FDG-PET may improve efficacy and prove to be more useful in management of CAD.

BIBLIOGRAPHY

1. Ahmadian A, Brogan A, Berman J, et al. Quantitative interpretation of FDG PET/CT with myocardial perfusion imaging increases diagnostic information in the evaluation of cardiac sarcoidosis. J Nucl Cardiol. 2014;21:925-39.
2. Bax JJ, Poldermans D, Elhendy A, Boersma E, Rahimtoola SH. Sensitivity, specificity and predictive accuracies of various noninvasive techniques for detecting hibernating myocardium. Curr Probl Cardiol. 2001;26:147-86.
3. Bonow RO. Identification of viable myocardium. Circulation. 1996;94:2674-80. [PubMed]
4. Di Carli MF, Prcevski P, Singh TP, Janisse J, Ager J, Muzik O, Vander Heide R. Myocardial blood flow, function, and metabolism in repetitive stunning. J Nucl Med. 2000;41:1227-34. [PubMed]
5. Dilsizian V, Rocco TP, Freedman NM, Leon MB, Bonow RO. Enhanced detection of ischemic but viable myocardium by the reinjection of thallium after stress-redistribution imaging. N Engl J Med. 1990;323:141-6.[PubMed]
6. Duncan BH, Ahlberg AW, Levine MG, McGill CC, Mann A, White MP, Mather JF, Waters DD, Heller GV. Comparison of electrocardiographic-gated technetium-99m sestamibi single-photon emission computed tomographic imaging and rest-redistribution thallium-201 in the prediction of myocardial viability. Am J Cardiol. 2000;85:680-4.
7. Eguchi M, Tsuchihashi K, Hotta D et al. Technetium-99 m sestamibi/tetrofosmin myocardial perfusion scanning in cardiac and noncardiac sarcoidosis. Cardiology. 2000;94:193-9.
8. Klein C, Nekolla SG, Bengel FM, Momose M, Sammer A, Haas F, Schnackenburg B, Delius W, Mudra H, Wolfram D, Schwaiger M. Assessment of myocardial viability with contrast-enhanced magnetic resonance imaging: comparison with positron emission tomography. Circulation. 2002;105:162-7. [PubMed]
9. Kuhl HP, Lipke CS, Krombach GA, Katoh M, Battenberg TF, Nowak B, Heussen N, Buecker A, Schaefer WM. Assessment of reversible myocardial dysfunction in chronic ischaemic heart disease: comparison of contrast-enhanced cardiovascular magnetic resonance and a combined positron emission tomography-single photon emission computed tomography imaging protocol. Eur Heart J. 2006;27:846-53. [PubMed]
10. Schinkel AF, Bax JJ, Poldermans D, Elhendy A, Ferrari R, Rahimtoola SH. Hibernating myocardium: diagnosis and patient outcomes. Curr Probl Cardiol. 2007;32:375-410. [PubMed]
11. Sciagra R, Pellegri M, Pupi A, Bolognese L, Bisi G, Carnovale V, Santoro GM. Prognostic implications of Tc-99m sestamibi viability imaging and subsequent therapeutic strategy in patients with chronic coronary artery disease and left ventricular dysfunction. J Am Coll Cardiol. 2000;36:739-45.

14. Myocardial Viability Assessment: Is it Alive?

Shrikant Solav

Hibernating myocardium is defined as chronic ischemic left ventricular dysfunction which is potentially capable of improving in function upon successful revascularization. Thus the gold standard for hibernating myocardium is "documentation of improvement in left ventricular function postrevascularization".[1]

This entity needs to be differentiated from scar related left ventricular dysfunction (which will not improve in function postrevascularization and also carries high perioperative mortality).[2]

It also needs to be differentiated from dilated cardiomyopathy, a condition in which the myocardium itself becomes weak in absence of coronary stenosis.

Chronic ischemic left ventricular dysfunction is a challenging entity in cardiology. It carries high long-term mortality rate if not revascularized.

There are three important parameters on the basis of which one can identify hibernating myocardium.
1. Perfusion status (thallium scan)
2. Functional reserve (low dose dobutamine-gated SPECT/echo study)
3. Metabolic reserve (FDG-PET scan)

If a segment of myocardium is dysfunctional as identified on echocardiogram, a simple way to look for viability is to check for perfusion status of the respective segment. An akinetic segment is considered to be viable if the perfusion of such a region is preserved.[3]

The perfusion in such abnormally functioning segments is not expected to be normal, but if the quantity of tracer uptake remains more than 35% of the noninfarcted territory, it is considered to be a reasonably good indicator of myocardial viability (85% of such segments will improve following revascularization).

Identification of functional reserve of the myocardium is used as a parameter of viability when the perfusion is preserved in the face of left ventricular dysfunction to distinguish between ischemic cardiomyopathy and dilated cardiomyopathy.

Using dobutamine challenge-gated SPECT study *a dual mode response* is a highly specific marker of hibernating myocardium (low left ventricular ejection fraction at rest which

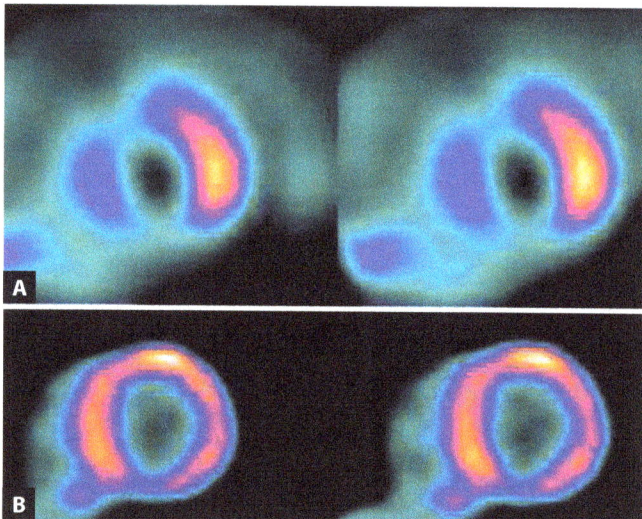

Figs 1A and B: (A) Myocardial perfusion study shows severe degree of perfusion defects in LAD and RCA territories; (B) FDG-PET scan images show preserved glucose metabolism in LAD and RCA territories thus showing perfusion- metabolism "mismatch" typical of Hibernating myocardium

Abbreviations: FDG-PET, fluorodeoxyglucose-positron-emission tomography; LAD, left anterior descending; RCA, right coronary artery

improves in response to low dose infusion of dobutamine and which shows deterioration in function as the rate of infusion is increased to higher level).[4]

The third important parameter is that of metabolic reserve. A dysfunctional segment which is devoid of perfusion (on Thallium scan) shows preserved metabolism on FDG-PET scan. This is called as perfusion metabolism mismatch.

Normal myocardium under fasting state preferentially uses fatty acids for its metabolism. In postprandial state there is a shift of metabolism to glucose.

A dysfunctional myocardial segment that is devoid of perfusion will continue to show glucose uptake in postprandial state as shown in **Figures 1A and B** (This is called as perfusion-metabolism mismatch).[5]

It is also important to understand that there is a prerequisite in all above conditions: that the revascularization is technically adequate.

REFERENCES

1. Heusch G, Schulz R, Rahimtoola SH. Myocardial hibernation: a delicate balance. Am J Physiol Heart Circ Physiol. 2005;288:H984-99.
2. Di Carli MF, Asgarzadie F, Schelbert HR, et al. Quantitative relation between myocardial viability and improvement in heart failure symptoms after revascularization in patients with ischemic cardiomyopathy. Circulation. 1995;92:3436-44.
3. Kiat H, Berman DS, Maddahi J, et al. Late reversibility of tomographic myocardial thallium defects: an accurate marker of myocardial viability. J Am Coll Cardiol. 1988;12:1456-63.
4. Picano E, Marzullo P, Gigli G, et al.Identification of viable myocardium by dipyridamole-induced improvement in regional left ventricular function assessed by echocardiography in myocardial infarction and comparison with thallium scintigraphy at rest. Am J Cardiol. 1992;70:703-10.
5. Bonow RO, Dilsizian V, Cuocolo A, et al. Identification of viable myocardium in patients with chronic coronary artery disease and left ventricular dysfunction: comparison of thallium scintigraphy with reinjection and PET imaging with F-18-fluorodeoxyglucose. Circulation.1991;83:26-37.

15
Hybrid Myocardial Imaging Techniques: Role in Functionally Relevant Coronary Disease

Sanjay Gambhir, Mudalsha Ravina, Gawri Sankar, Nitin Yadav

MORPHOLOGY VERSUS ANATOMY

Coronary artery disease (CAD) represents a major healthcare burden in developed and developing nations. Significant breakthrough treatments have been developed in the last two decades for the prevention and management of CAD.[1,2] Earlier for cardiac applications, the computed tomography (CT) data was useful only for attenuation correction, as the motion of the heart caused significant artifacts in the thoracic images of the mediastinum from the single slice CTs in these early scanners. Multidetector CT scanners for high-resolution cardiac imaging were integrated into hybrid systems starting in about 2002. For the first-time, it appeared that high-resolution cardiac anatomy would be easily correlated to myocardial perfusion imaging (MPI) using the same imager to acquire both images in a single scanning session.

In view of this, much has been done in the investigative armamentarium of CAD. Hybrid imaging permits the fused data from multiple different imaging modalities to provide valuable and complementary diagnostic data on physiology, and morphology in a single setting. This technology obviates the need for mental integration of functional and morphologic data. Dedicated hybrid scanners are now installed in specialized cardiac imaging centers to simplify image coregistration and improve patient care in a less time consuming process.[3] This approach helps to assess coronary artery calcium scores and coronary angiography with myocardial perfusion data and fusion in the same setting, thus revealing both the burden and its functional relevance noninvasively.

TECHNICAL DEVELOPMENTS

Early 4–16 slices, CT scanners did not allow good temporal and spatial resolution required for consistent and good delineation of the coronary tree. Clinical availability of hybrid imaging has been possible with attempts of new 64–256 slice CT scanners, dedicated cardiac fusion softwares, high powered postprocessing work stations.

Myocardial territories and their respective tributaries are best seen in 3D view unlike oncology images. The most important aspect of hybrid imaging is coregistration. Any kind of misalignment would imply wrong interpretation of perfusion data with coronary artery territory. Alignment can be done either by hardware or software-based approaches. In hardware-based approaches as in single-photon emission computed tomography-computed tomography (SPECT-CT) and positron emission tomography-computed tomography (PET-CT) both anatomic and nuclear medicine data sets are taken almost simultaneously with the patient lying still on the camera in the same position during both the scans. Software-based approaches allow to acquire images on different scanners and fusion is done by using landmark-based coregistration techniques.[4-6]

Protocols of Hybrid Cardiac Imaging Software

Thorough quality control has to be done during the imaging. Postimaging coregistration is the first and foremost step, followed by volume rendering, coronary tree segmentation and fusion images. These have been illustrated in the demonstrative cases.

SPECT-CT and PET-CT Hybrid Imaging—Added Advantages

SPECT-CT and PET-CT are well-established noninvasive tools for the diagnosis of ischemic CAD. It allows assessment of the physiological relevance of coronary lesions and offers a high prognostic predictive value. Although PET may achieve a higher accuracy than SPECT, its use has so far often been limited to large centers, especially with requirement of on-site cyclotron. However, rubidium-strontium generator is obviating the need for an onsite cyclotron.[7] Recent advances in image processing software and the advent of hybrid scanners have paved the way for fusion of images from different modalities.

SPECT-CT fusion software allows for identification of coronary artery calcium (CAC), flow limiting coronary stenosis and correlation of anatomic and physiologic data. PET-CT in addition to this allows for calculation of myocardial blood flow (MBF) and coronary flow reserve (CFR) and has superior accuracy compared to SPECT perfusion imaging.[8] Apart from that PET provides for a lesser radiation dose. Peak stress left ventricular ejection fraction (LVEF) is calculated easily from PET as opposed to poststress LVEF in SPECT-CT patients for revascularization.

The average sensitivity for detecting 50% angiographic stenosis is 87% (range, 71–97%), whereas the average specificity is 73% (range, 36–100%)[9] for SPECT-CT, whereas for PET-CT, the sensitivity is 91% (range, 83–100%), whereas the average specificity is 89% (range, 73–100%).[10]

CALCIUM SCORING AND MYOCARDIAL PERFUSION IMAGING

Hybrid PET/CT and SPECT-CT scanners were initially developed for accurate attenuation map. However, in these hybrid scanners calcium scoring may also be done in the same setting. Before discussing in detail about hybrid imaging lets first elucidate the role of coronary calcium scoring and its relevance alone and the incremental benefit with fusion imaging on risk profiling and coronary event rate.

Coronary artery calcification is pathognomonic of atherosclerosis, and a high calcium score is associated with greater burden of coronary atherosclerosis and ischemia, reflecting obstructive CAD.[11,12] Coronary artery calcium scoring has historically been used in asymptomatic, intermediate risk patients for assessment of cardiovascular risk. It has been shown to be a powerful marker of cardiovascular risk in intermediate risk populations and provides incremental value beyond traditional Framingham risk factors.

Usually, absence of coronary calcification (CAC 0), is associated with an excellent prognosis (0.4% annual rate of nonfatal MI or CD).[13] Also, patients with a low burden of calcified atherosclerosis and a normal myocardial perfusion imaging (MPI) are at low risk. Conversely, patients with high coronary calcification (CAC Z400) have higher event rates 2%, and higher frequency of ischemic burden on MPI (ischemic scan frequency: CAC 0, 1.6%, 1–399, 7.6%, and CAC Z 4, 28.8%, respectively).[13]

Rule Out Myocardial Infarction using Computer-assisted Tomography (ROMICAT) trial, only one patient of 368 low-intermediate risk patients presented with an acute coronary syndrome with zero calcium score.[14] Prognosticating CAD might significantly improve if CAC scoring with MPI might be done in a single dual modality study **(Flow chart 1)**.

Long-term risk of cardiac events in asymptomatic patients with high calcium score and normal MPI is high, while their short-term risk may be low. Likewise, symptomatic patients with a high burden of calcified coronary atherosclerosis (CAC score of Z1000 vs CAC o 1000) appear to be at a higher risk despite normal PET-MPI.[15]

After adjustment for clinical risk factors, obstructive plaque visualized by coronary computed tomography angiography (CCTA) and abnormal MPI were independent predictors of late events. An annual event rate of 1% was found in those with concordantly normal CCTA and MPI, and conversely those with concordantly abnormal CCTA and MPI had an event rate of 9%.[16] With significant incremental improved prediction of risk by the combination of the two modalities.

Because of its prognostic value and ability to potentially alter management, CAC is routinely being incorporated into perfusion protocols or estimated from an attenuation correction CT scan.[17-19]

Coronary CT Angiography and Myocardial Perfusion Imaging

Computed tomography coronary angiography (CTCA) has undergone rapid development in the last decade and has evolved as the most promising noninvasive tool for the visualization of the coronary anatomy. Its diagnostic performance has been studied by many. Pooled data demonstrates a consistent and unequalled high sensitivity (96%) and negative predictive value (NPV) of 94%, rendering it as an excellent tool to rule out obstructive coronary stenosis.[20-22] The high sensitivity and NPV are, however, subdued by a moderate specificity of 76% and positive predictive value (PPV) of 84%, although variability in between the studies is noted.

There is a frequent mismatch between anatomical and functional stenosis severity, and approximately half of the obstructive deemed lesions on CCTA are flow limiting.[23-25] Therefore, the stress perfusion information provides valuable clinical information regarding the physiological significance of anatomic stenoses for identification of patients in need of potential revascularization. This appears to hold true over a wide spectrum of CAD prevalence, in low-risk populations as well as in those with multivessel disease.[3]

In these patient cohorts, the value of dual-modality imaging lies far beyond the simple addition of a further diagnostic test as it allows accurate topographic anatomic association of perfusion defects and culprit lesion. By contrast, CTA improves the detection of multivessel CAD, which as discussed above, it is one of the main pitfalls of stress perfusion scintigraphy. We discuss a 60-year-old male patient (case 1), known diabetic, hypertensive with history of smoking, presented with complaints of angina on exertion (AOE) III for 2 months. Echocardiography revealed dilated LV cavity with global hypokinesia. The body mass index (BMI) was 23.4 and his total coronary artery calcium score (CACS) was 41. The patient underwent myocardial perfusion imaging initially which lead to suspicion of triple vessel disease **(Fig. 1)**.

The patient then underwent CTCA, which revealed significant stenosis in proximal part of left anterior descending artery (LAD) due to hard plaque, distal LAD, proximal part of first diagonal artery (D1), proximal and distal part of left circumflex artery (LCx), origin and proximal part of first obtuse marginal artery (OM1). It ruled out any significant stenosis in right coronary artery (RCA) which was also the dominant vessel **(Figs 2A and B)**. But there was still a doubt whether the reversible defect in the anterior wall was due to stenosis noted in the proximal LAD or D1.

Fusion imaging confirmed that the reversible defect in the anterior wall is due to disease in D1 **(Figs 3A and B)**.

Another case (case 2) is a 55-year-old male patient who is a known diabetic, not a known hypertensive and nonsmoker. Presented with complaints of DOE II, AOE II for past 6 months. His echocardiography showed ejection fraction (EF) of 20%; LAD and LCx territory were hypokinetic. The MPI findings were suggestive of severe dual vessel disease, involving LAD and RCA territories **(Fig. 4)**. CTCA showed heavy calcification in prox LAD and otherwise normal coronaries. Total CACS: 209 (Prox LAD: 205; Prox LCx: 4) **(Figs 5A and B)**. Fusion imaging was normal **(Figs 6A and B)**. Patient was kept on medical management. No cardiac events for 1 year postfusion imaging.

Fusion MPI with CTCA imaging also increased diagnostic confidence for categorizing intermediate lesions and equivocal perfusion defects, and in almost one-third of patients the fused analysis provided added diagnostic information not obtained on side-by-side analysis. As discussed above, the incremental value seems most pronounced for coronary stenoses in distal segments and diagonal branches and in vessels with extensive coronary lesions or heavy calcifications on CTA.

Santana and colleagues showed an improved diagnostic accuracy of hybrid SPECT-CT imaging compared to SPECT alone (P<0.001) and to the separate analysis of SPECT and CT (P=0.007) for diagnosis of obstructive CAD on conventional coronary angiography.[26] Similarly, Risper et al. compared the diagnostic accuracy of hybrid SPECT-CT in flow limiting coronary stenosis with CT angiography alone in 56 patients with angina pectoris. Hybrid SPECT-CT lead to remarkable improvement in specificity (from 63 to 95%) and PPV (from 31 to 77%) compared to CT alone, with no change in sensitivity and NPV.[27] These data validate the role of hybrid imaging in

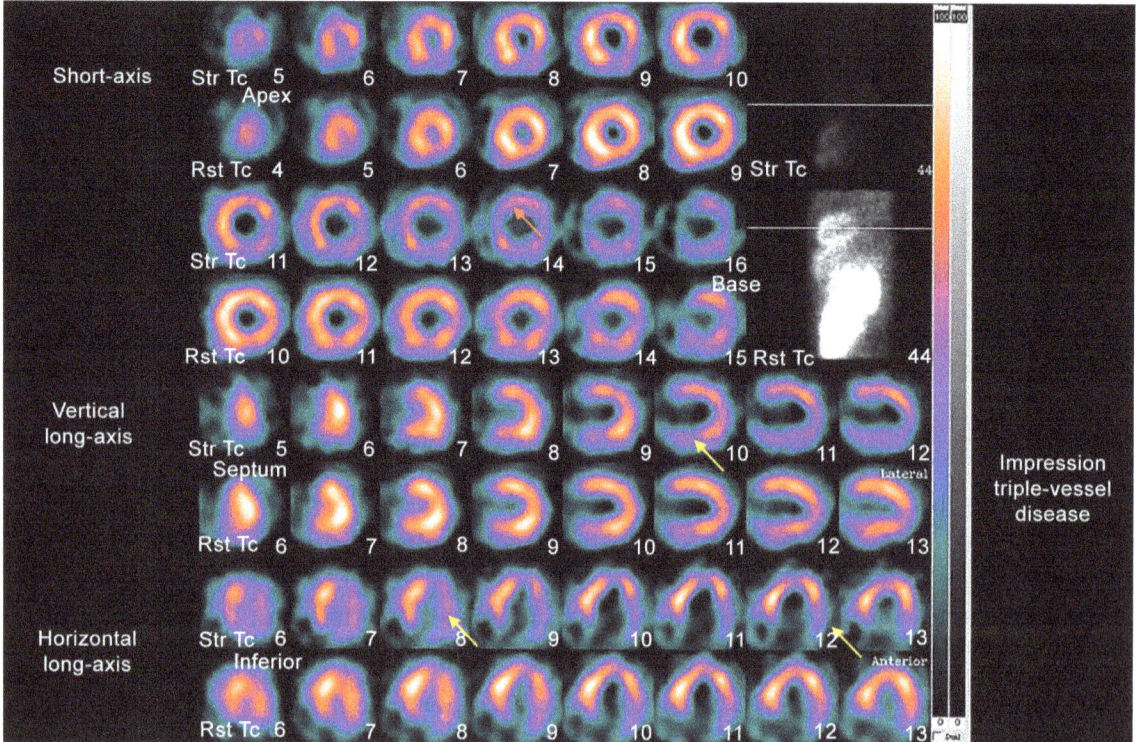

Fig. 1: Myocardial perfusion imaging (MPI) nonattenuated corrected slices of Case 1. There is severely reduced tracer uptake noted in the apex, mid and basal anterolateral, inferolateral, mid and basal inferior wall segments of the LV myocardium in the stress images (yellow arrows) which shows improvement in the rest images. Mild reversible ischemia is also noted in the entire anterior wall (orange arrow). Hence, MPI was suggestive of triple vessel involvement

Chapter 15: Hybrid Myocardial Imaging Techniques: Role in Functionally Relevant Coronary Disease

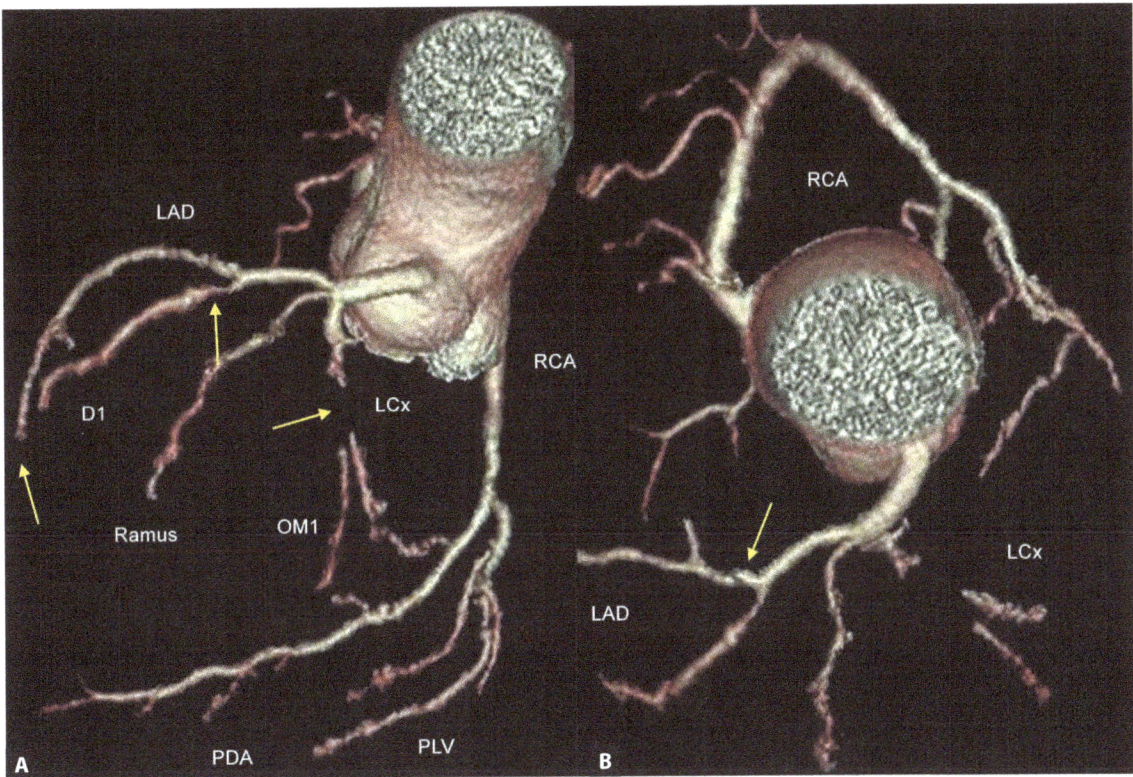

Figs 2A and B: 3-D reconstructed, volume rendered no cut images of the coronary vascular tree of Case 1. (A) Significant disease (yellow arrows) in distal LAD, proximal part of D1, proximal and distal part of LCx and origin and proximal part of OM1; (B) (Overhead view) shows hard plaque in the proximal part of the LAD (yellow arrow)
Abbreviations: LAD, left anterior descending artery; LCx, left circumflex artery; RCA, right coronary artery; D1, first diagonal artery; OM1, first obtuse marginal artery; PDA, posterior descending artery; PLV, posterior left ventricular branch

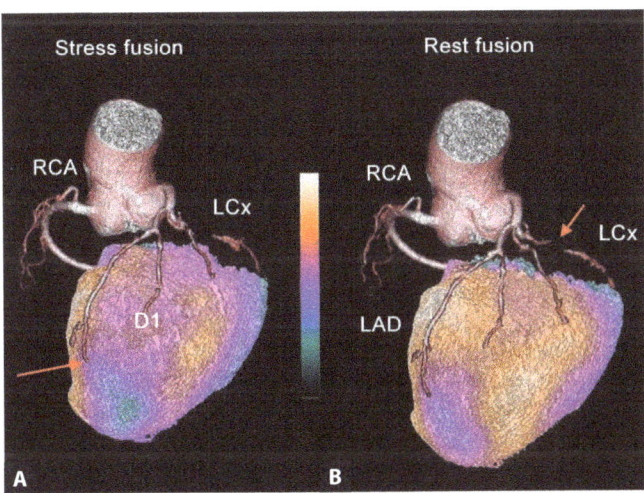

Figs 3A and B: SPECT/CTCA fusion images of Case 1. (A) Stress fusion image shows significant disease in distal part of LAD (red arrow) associated with significantly reduced perfusion in the LV myocardium distal to the disease (denoted by bluish green color in the perfusion image). Mildly reduced perfusion is noted in the anterior wall supplied by the diseased D1; (B) Rest fusion image shows improvement in perfusion in the region supplied by distal LAD in comparison to stress fusion image. Improvement is also noted in the entire anterior wall supplied by D1. A and B images also reveals significant disease in proximal LCx and OM1 (denoted by red arrow in image A) with significantly reduced perfusion in the area supplied by these vessels in the stress fusion image, which shows improvement, though not near normal, in the rest fusion image
Abbreviations: RCA, right coronary artery; LCx, left circumflex artery; D1, first diagonal artery; LAD, left anterior descending artery

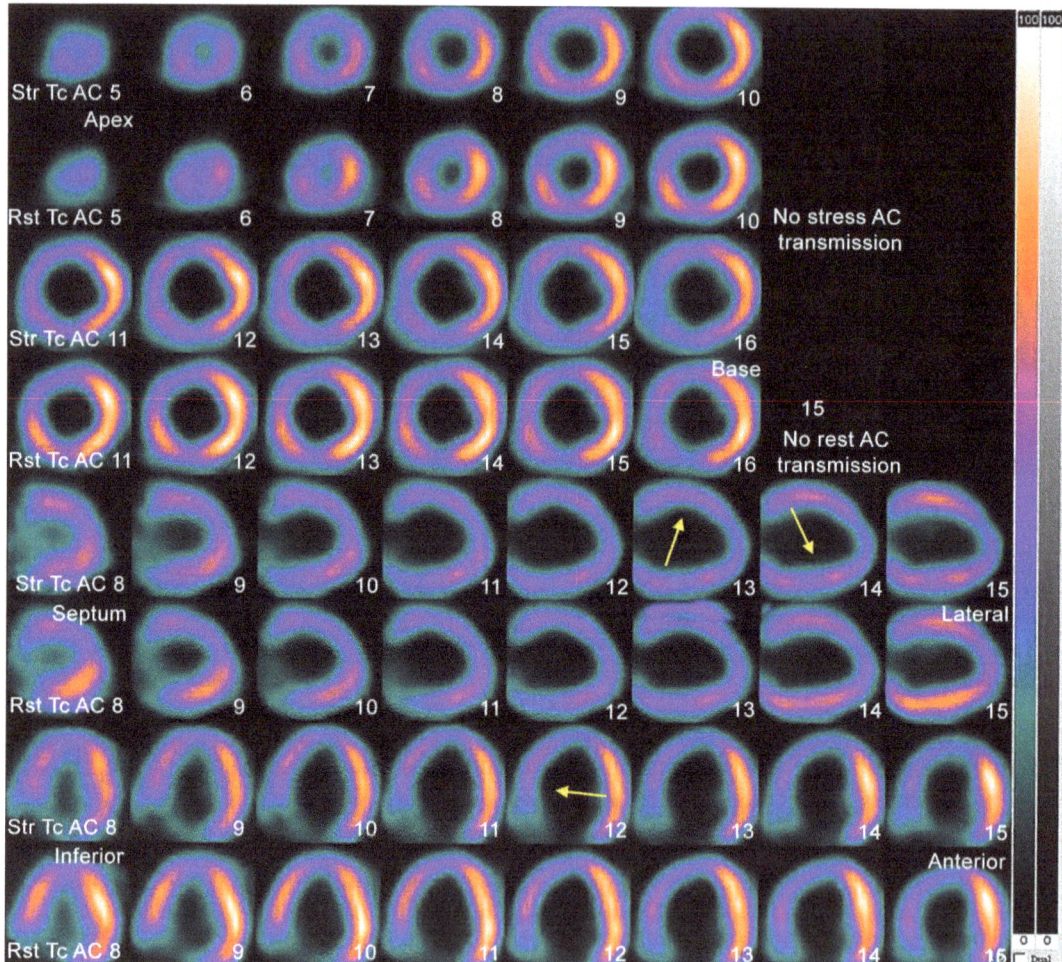

Fig. 4: Myocardial perfusion imaging (MPI) attenuated corrected slices of Case 2. There is severely reduced tracer uptake noted in all the myocardial segments except the lateral wall, in both stress and rest perfusion images (yellow arrows). Grossly dilated LV cavity was noted. Hence, MPI was suggestive of double vessel involvement (LAD and RCA territories)

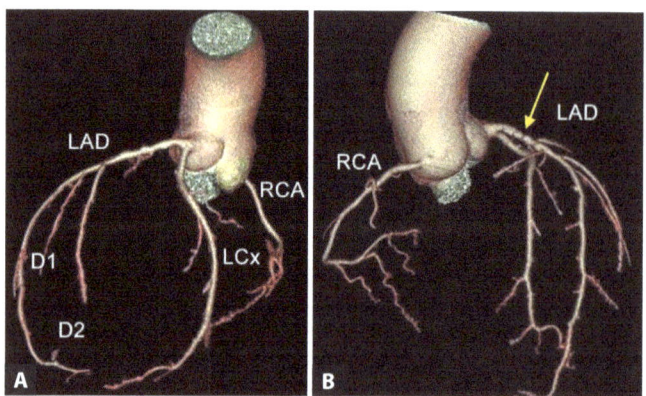

Figs 5A and B: 3-D reconstructed, volume rendered no cut images of the coronary vascular tree of Case 2. Images show normal coronaries with dominant RCA. Eccentric calcification is noted in proximal part of the LAD (yellow arrow)

Abbreviations: LAD, left anterior descending artery; LCx, left circumflex artery; RCA, right coronary artery; D1, first diagonal artery; D2, second diagonal artery

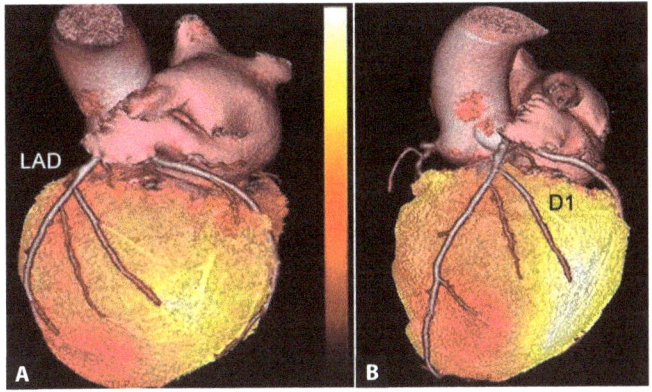

Figs 6A and B: SPECT/CTCA fusion images of Case 2. Stress fusion image (A) and rest fusion image (B) shows severely reduced perfusion in LAD territory, but there was no significant disease in the LAD in CTCA images, thus fusion imaging result was normal. The patient was diagnosed to have idiopathic dilated cardiomyopathy and patient was put on medical management
Abbreviations: LAD, left anterior descending artery; D1, first diagonal artery

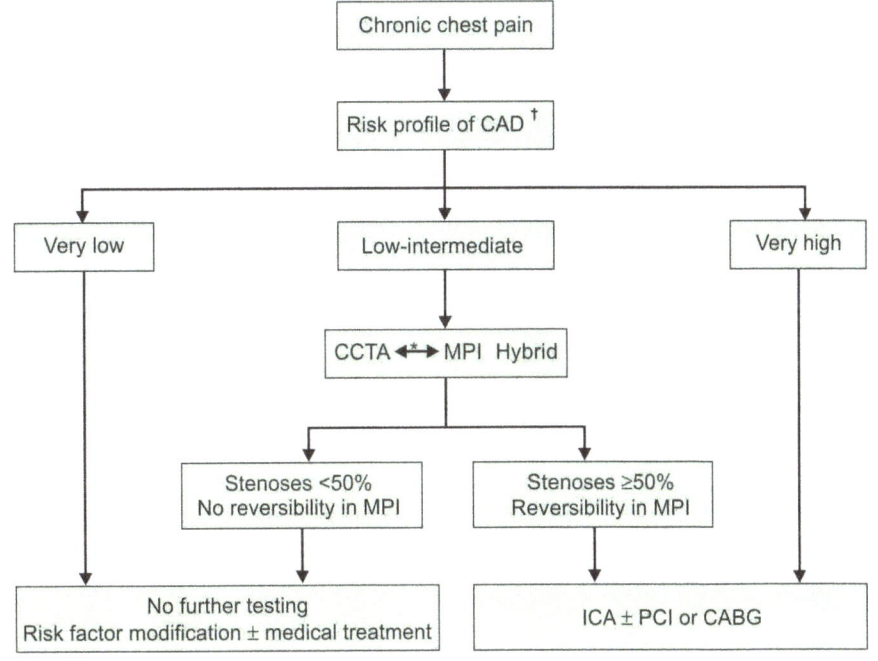

Flow chart 1: Proposed clinical algorithm for use in patients with chronic angina as stated in joint statement proposed by EANM, ESCR and ECNC. J Nucl Med Mol Imaging, 2010

†Type of chest pain, cardiovascular risk factors, stress testing, CAC score
*Inconclusive or equivocal test

Abbreviations: CAD, coronary artery disease; CAC, coronary artery calcium; CCTA, coronary computed tomography angiography; MPI, myocardial perfusion imaging; ICA, internal carotid artery; PCI, percutaneous coronary intervention; CABG, coronary artery bypass grafting

the noninvasive diagnosis of CAD as a decision-making tool for assessing the need for revascularization in obstructive CAD. Comprehensive noninvasive CAD assessment prior to revascularization is necessary in view of increasing debates over PCI with stable CAD **(Table 1)**.[28,29]

However, the specific impact of hybrid imaging on treatment strategy and subsequently on outcome remains to be determined in prospective and long-term studies.

In patients with multivessel CAD, there is so potential for underestimation of ischemia using qualitative MPI assessment, as qualitative analysis of myocardial perfusion images relies on identification of relative differences in blood flow from rest to stress perfusion. Therefore, only the areas of most significant relative coronary flow impairment are visually apparent.

Measurement of absolute MBF or CFR limits the risk of underestimating disease severity, as areas with low MBF or CFR

Table 1 Comparison between various international studies (fusion imaging)

Parameters	Jiang et al. China, 2013		Kadokami et al. Japan, 2011		Gaemperli et al. Switzerland, 2007		Risper et al. Israel, 2007	
	CTCA	Fusion	CTCA	Fusion	CTCA	Fusion	CTCA	Fusion
Total patients	54		49		25		44	
Segments analysed	216		145		339		170	
Patient population	Suspected or known CAD		Suspected or known CAD		Showing at least one defect in MPI		Angina pectoris	
Imaging	64 slice CTCA and SPECT with MIBI		64 slice CTCA and SPECT with MIBI and TI		64 slice CTCA and SPECT with tetrofosmin		16 slice CTCA and SPECT hybrid device	
Sensitivity (%)	90	90	77	80	85	Na	96	96
Specificity (%)	88	99	77	94	88	Na	63	95
PPV (%)	55	93	46	77	60	Na	31	77
NPV (%)	98	98	93	95	97	Na	99	99

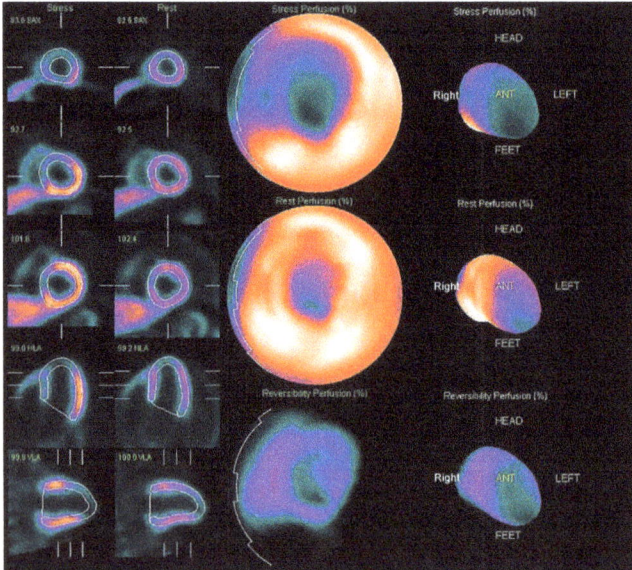

Fig. 7: A 60-year-old female patient with CAD, old history of AWMI. On CART-single vessel disease, LAD-100% block with LVEF of 35%. Both stress and rest perfusion images were acquired after injection of 20 mCi of ^{13}N-NH$_3$ using a dedicated LSO PET-CT scanner. Attenuation correction was performed using the CT image acquired during the study. Severely reduced tracer uptake is noted at the apex, apico and mid-anterior wall segments and the anteroseptal wall segments of LV myocardium in stress perfusion images which later shows improvement in rest images

will be identified as being abnormal regardless of the flow in other myocardial regions. The measurement of CFR provides additional opportunities for the assessment of coronary disease. For example, patients with no significant epicardial coronary disease may still have decreased CFR, consistent with impaired endothelial function or "small-vessel" disease.

Thus, in present hybrid PET-CTCA scanning can also is an independent predictor of cardiac events in this population.

The detection of reduced CFR in either of these scenarios could result in a change in clinical management (**Figs 7 and 8**). In the patient with probable multivessel CAD, there is a lower threshold for consideration of invasive catheterization for confirmation of diagnosis and subsequent revascularization. In the latter case, aggressive factor modification and/or medical therapy should contemplated.

HYBRID PET-MR

PET/MRI is a rapidly evolving imaging modality with enormous potential for cardiovascular applications. CMR provides high spatial resolution anatomic and functional detail as well as excellent tissue characterization, while PET provides the extremely high sensitivity needed to probe metabolic and molecular pathways and to detect myocardial inflammation. The combination is poised to provide novel insights into cardiac pathophysiology in a variety of cardiovascular diseases.

Functions

The CMR is widely recognized as the gold standard for assessment of myocardial function. Its versatility allows accurate quantification of ventricular volumes and mass and ejection fraction.[30,31] Likewise, PET provides accurate quantitative perfusion assessment with full ventricular coverage making it the gold standard for quantitative assessment of myocardial perfusion.

Challenges and Pitfalls including Radiation Dosimetry

Hybrid scanners offer advantages justifying the higher costs compared to software fusion of data sets obtained from

Chapter 15: Hybrid Myocardial Imaging Techniques: Role in Functionally Relevant Coronary Disease

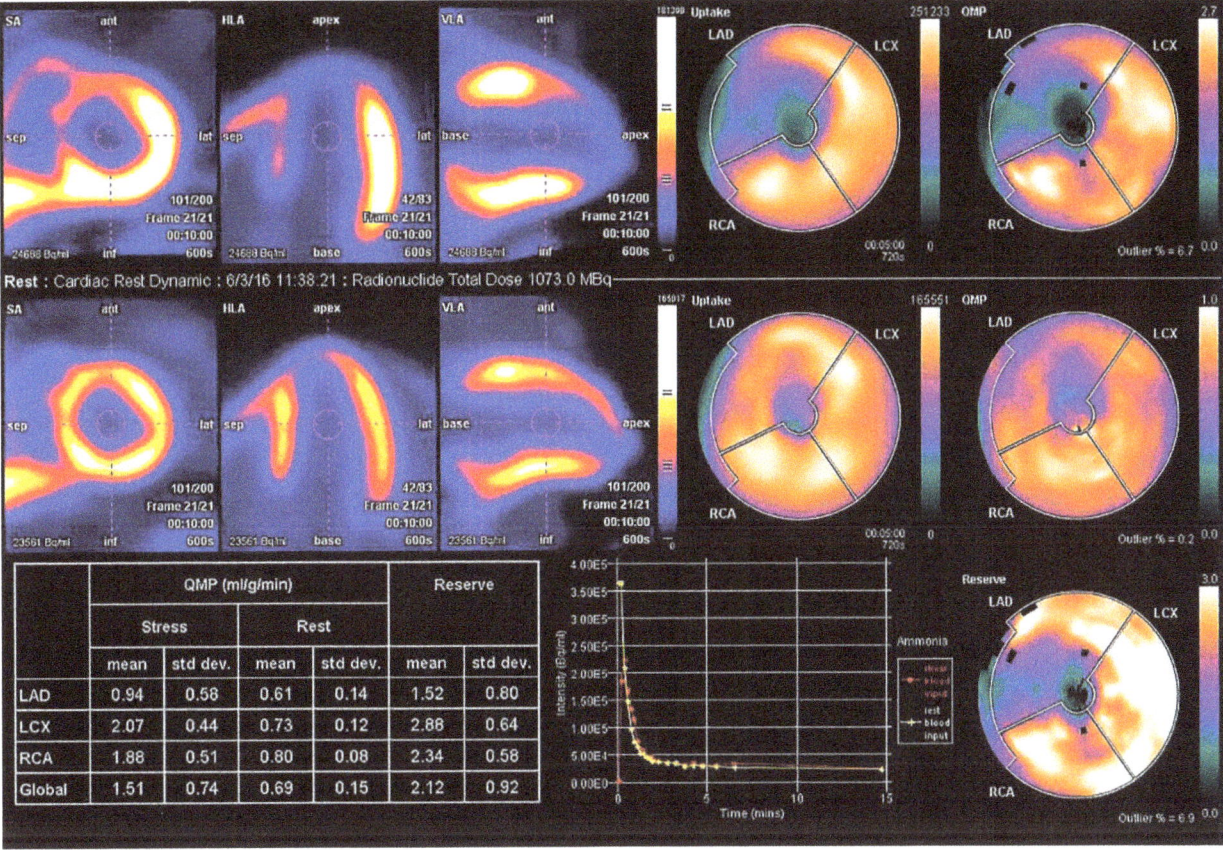

Fig. 8: Low CFR values noted in the left anterior descending artery (LAD) territory indicating disease in the LAD

different scanners remains a matter of concern. The integrated scanner also makes it more difficult and expensive to integrate the rapid changes in technology, especially CT. By contrast, a combined device may fit into 1 room and needs 1 operating team and does not require positioning of the patient into 2 different scanners.

Multicentric trials and prospective studies are required to establish the patient category, who would benefit most from both prognostic and diagnostic point of view.

Radiation Dosimetry

Radiation hygiene has always of concern with SPECT, PET- and/or CT-based imaging. Although deterministic effects do not occur within the dose range hybrid cardiac PET/CCTA protocols, stochastic effects demand scrutiny when subjecting the patients to these procedures and developing practices which cause least radiation exposure should always be the concern.

Hybrid cardiac imaging with CTA and SPECT-MPI has been reported to expose patients to excessively high radiation doses up to 41.5 mSv, which has prevented the acceptance and widespread use of this technique until now. New low-dose CTA acquisition protocols with prospective ECG triggering have recently been introduced and shown to offer a tremendous reduction in radiation dose to an average of 2.1 mSv at maintained accuracy, making this technique most suitable for hybrid imaging.[32,33]

Initially, coronary CT angiography with retrospective gated reconstructions was associated with a relatively high effective dose of 12–21 mSv. The latest helical dual-source and axial volumetric CT scanners allow for performing 'single-beat' coronary CT angiography at an effective dose of 5 mSv or even lower. Hybrid imaging with prospectively triggered CTA inconjunction with a stress only SPECT-MPI protocol achieves a reduction in radiation dose for hybrid imaging to 5.4 mSv.[34] Increased temporal resolution -256 and 320 slice scanners - 1 mSv. High-pitch protocols using dual-source CT scanners even enable CCTA scans to be performed within the sub-mSv range, although such devices fused with PET (or SPECT) technology are not yet available.[35] Tracers utilized for perfusion PET are accompanied by relatively favorable dosimetry, e.g. H_2O_{15} and 13 NH_3 convey an effective dose equivalent below 1 mSv. Similarly, introduction of solid-state detectors based on cadmiumzinc-telluride alloy have similarly reduced doses for SPECT.[36]

CONCLUSION

Hybrid cardiac imaging may allow easy noninvasive assessment of coronary plaque burden, its pathophysiological relevance and biological plaque activity, endothelial health, identification of flow limiting coronary stenosis providing individual risk estimates on which further management would be based. Hybrid cardiac SPECT and PET/CCTA may act as a "one stop shop" investigation allowing for a comprehensive evaluation of patients of suspected CAD.

REFERENCES

1. Topol Ej, Nissen SE. Our preoccupation with coronary luminology. The dissociation between clinical and angiographic findings in ischemic heart disease. Circulation. 1995;92(8):2333-42.
2. Silber S, Albertsson P, Aviles FF, Camici PG, et al. Guidelines for percutaneous coronary interventions. The task force for percutaneous coronary interventions of the European Society of Cardiology. Eur Heart J. 2005;26(8):804-7.
3. Gaemperli O, Schepis T, Valenta I, et al. Cardiac image fusion from stand alone SPECT and CT: clinical experience. J Nuc Med. 2007;48(5):696-703.
4. Martinez-Moller A, et al. Artifacts from misaligned CT in cardiac perfusion PET/CT studies: Frequency, effects, and potential solutions. J Nucl Med. 2007;48:188-93.
5. McCord ME, et al. Misalignment between PET transmission and emission scans: Its effect on myocardial imaging. J Nucl Med. 1992;33:1209-14.
6. Loghin C, Sdringola S, Gould KL. Common artifacts in PET myocardial perfusion images due to attenuation-emission misregistration: Clinical significance, causes, and solutions. J Nucl Med. 2004;45:1029-39.
7. Parkash R, deKemp RA, Ruddy TD, et al. Potential utility of rubidium 82 PET quantification in patients with 3-vessel coronary artery disease. J Nucl Cardiol. 2004;11:440-9.
8. Dorbala S, Vangala D, Sampson U, et al. Value of vasodilator left ventricular ejection fraction reserve in evaluating the magnitude of myocardium at risk and the extent of angiographic coronary artery disease: A 82Rb PET/CT study. J Nucl Med. 2007;48:349-58.
9. Klocke FJ, Baird MG, Lorell BH, et al. ACC/AHA/ASNC guidelines for the clinical use of cardiac radionuclide imaging—Executive summary: A report of the American College of Cardiology/American Heart Association Task Force on Practice Guidelines (ACC/AHA/ASNC Committee to revise the 1995 guidelines for the clinical use of cardiac radionuclide imaging). J Am Coll Cardiol. 2003;42:1318-33.
10. Di Carli MF, Dorbala S, Meserve J, et al. Clinical myocardial perfusion PET/CT. J Nucl Med. 2007;48:783-93.
11. Haberl R, Becker A, Leber A, et al. Correlation of coronary calcification and angiographically documented stenoses in patients with suspected coronary artery disease: Results of 1,764 patients. J Am Coll Cardiol. 2001;37:451-7.
12. Berman DS, Wong ND, Gransar H, et al. Relationship between stress-induced myocardial ischemia and atherosclerosis measured by coronary calcium tomography. J Am Coll Cardiol. 2004;44:923-30.
13. Bellasi A, Lacey C, Taylor AJ, et al. Comparison of prognostic usefulness of coronary artery calcium in men versus women (results from a meta- and pooled analysis estimating all-cause mortality and coronary heart disease death or myocardial infarction). Am J Cardiol. 2007;100:409-14.
14. Hoffmann U, Bamberg F, Chae CU, Nichols JH, Rogers IS, Seneviratne SK, et al. Coronary computed tomography angiography for early triage of patients with acute chest pain: The ROMICAT (rule out myocardial infarction using computer assisted tomography) trial. J Am Coll Cardiol. 2009;53:1642-50.
15. Schenker MP, Dorbala S, Hong EC, et al. Interrelation of coronary calcification, myocardial ischemia, and outcomes in patients with intermediate likelihood of coronary artery disease: A combined positron emission tomography/computed tomography study. Circulation. 2008;117:1693-700.
16. Van Werkhoven JM, et al. Prognostic value of multislice computed tomography and gated single-photon emission computed tomography in patients with suspected coronary artery disease. J Am Coll Cardiol. 2009;53:623-32.
17. Rozanski A, Gransar H, Wong ND, et al. Clinical outcomes after both coronary calcium scanning and exercise myocardial perfusion scintigraphy. J Am Coll Cardiol. 2007;49:1352-61.
18. Uebleis C, Becker A, Griesshammer I, et al. Stable coronary artery disease: Prognostic value of myocardial perfusion SPECT in relation to coronary calcium scoring—long-term follow-up. Radiology. 2009;252:682-90.
19. Chang SM, Nabi F, Xu J, et al. The coronary artery calcium score and stress myocardial perfusion imaging provide independent and complementary prediction of cardiac risk. J Am Coll Cardiol. 2009;54:1872-82.
20. Danad I, Raijmakers PG, Appelman YE, Harms HJ, de Haan S, van den Oever ML, et al. Hybrid imaging using quantitative H215O PET and CT-based coronary angiography for the detection of coronary artery disease. J Nucl Med. 2013;54:55-63.
21. Kajander S, Joutsiniemi E, Saraste M, Pietila M, Ukkonen H, Saraste A, et al. Cardiac positron emission tomography/computed tomography imaging accurately detects anatomically and functionally significant coronary artery disease. Circulation. 2010;122:603-13.
22. Mollet NR, Cademartiri F, van Mieghem CA, Runza G, McFadden EP, Baks T, et al. High-resolution spiral computed tomography coronary angiography in patients referred for diagnostic conventional coronary angiography. Circulation. 2005;112:2318-23.
23. Di Carli MF, Hachamovitch R. New technology for noninvasive evaluation of coronary artery disease. Circulation. 2007;115:1464-80.
24. Schuijf JD, Wijns W, Jukema JW, Atsma DE, de Roos A, Lamb HJ, et al. Relationship between noninvasive coronary angiography with multi-slice computed tomography and myocardial perfusion imaging. J Am Coll Cardiol. 2006;48:2508-14.
25. Gaemperli O, Schepis T, Koepfli P, Valenta I, Soyka J, Leschka S, et al. Accuracy of 64-slice CT angiography for the detection of functionally relevant coronary stenoses as assessed with myocardial perfusion SPECT. Eur J Nucl Med Mol Imaging. 2007;34:1162-71.
26. Santana CA, Garcia EV, Faber TL, et al. Diagnostic performance of myocardial perfusion imaging (MPI) and computerised tomography coronary angiography. J Nucl Cardiol. 2009;16:201-11.
27. Rispler S, Keidar Z, Ghersin E, et al. Integrated single-photon emission computerised tomography and computed

tomography coronary angiography for the assessment of hemodynamically significant coronary artery lesions. J Am Coll Cardiol. 2007;49(10):1059-67.
28. Fox K, Garcia MA, Ardissino D, et al. Guidelines on the management of stable angina pectoris: executive summary: the Task Force on the Management of Stable Angina Pectoris of the European Society of Cardiology. Eur Heart J. 2006;27(11):1341-81.
29. Boden WE, O'Rourke RA, Teo KK, et al. Optimal medical therapy with or without PCI for stable coronary disease. Engl J Med. 2007;356(15):1503-16.
30. Pattynama PM, De Roos A, Van der Wall EE, Van Voorthuisen AE. Evaluation of cardiac function with magnetic resonance imaging. Am Heart J. 1994;128:595-607.
31. Reichek N. Magnetic resonance imaging for assessment of myocardial function. Magn Reson Q. 1991;7:255-74.
32. Husmann L, Valenta I, Gaemperli O, et al. Feasibility of low-dose coronary CT angiography: First experience with prospective ECG-gating. Eur Heart J. 2008;29:191-7.
33. Husmann L, Valenta I, Kaufmann PA. Coronary angiography with lowdose computed tomography at 1.4 mSv. Herz. 2008;33:75.
34. Husmann L, Herzog BA, Gaemperli O, et al. Diagnostic accuracy of computed tomography coronary angiography and evaluation of stress only single-photon emission computed tomography/computed tomography hybrid imaging: Comparison of prospective electrocardiogram triggering vs. retrospective gating. Eur Heart J. 2008;30:600-7.
35. Achenbach S, Marwan M, Ropers D, Schepis T, Pflederer T, Anders K, et al. Coronary computed tomography angiography with a consistent dose below 1 mSv using prospectively electrocardiogram-triggered high-pitch spiral acquisition. Eur Heart J. 2010;31:340-6.
36. Herzog BA, Buechel RR, Katz R, Brueckner M, Husmann L, Burger IA, et al. Nuclear myocardial perfusion imaging with a cadmium-zinc-telluride detector technique: optimized protocol for scan time reduction. J Nucl Med. 2010;51:46-51.

16 Role of Coronary Flow Reserve in Coronary Artery Disease

Ashwani Sood, Abhiram GA, BR Mittal

INTRODUCTION

The elucidation of changing trends in cardiovascular disease requires an in-depth evaluation of the well-recognized risk factors in addition to the ever-emerging risk factors. The cardiovascular disease accounted for around 17.3 million deaths in 2008 with an estimated 41% deaths alone due to ischemic heart disease.[1]

With ever-increasing burden of cardiac morbidity and mortality, specifically in the low and middle income countries, early diagnosis of coronary artery disease (CAD) would play a pivotal role in prevention of disease-related deaths and complications. A significant proportion of attributable deaths (~6%) is because of elevated blood glucose values with impaired fasting glycemia and diabetes contributing to accelerated atherosclerosis and the highest hazard ratios.[2-4]

Logical systematic use of imaging techniques provides substantial information in both suspected as well as diagnosed CAD resulting in optimization of patient management. The better availability of positron emission tomography (PET) scanners is an attractive diagnostic capability in comparison to invasive techniques such as coronary angiography.[4,5]

DIAGNOSIS OF CORONARY ARTERY DISEASE

The diagnosis of CAD is based on systematic history and detailed physical examination even if patient is planned for noninvasive techniques with exceptions in certain emergency situations. The widely available, versatile noninvasive electrocardiogram (ECG) recording is used as the initial test as it unravels a multitude of clinical scenarios ranging from arrhythmias to electrolyte imbalances as well as ischemic changes in the myocardium.

Additional ECG tests like exercise ECG, may lead to evident but nonspecific ST-T wave changes, paving the way for further noninvasive testing. Patients unable to exercise due to co-morbid conditions or physical limitation may show suboptimal results on physical stress tests and need to be tested with pharmacological agents. Patients incapable to do exercise for optimum duration ultimately end up with poor prognosis.[6]

Imaging Modalities

Echo evaluation is warranted in certain cases of suspected CAD for diagnosis of primary pericardial or valvular disease leading to chest pain. Echo provides excellent information regarding the chambers and functional capabilities of the heart. Transitory wall motion abnormalities detected on instantaneously obtained images during stress testing using dobutamine may signal the presence of CAD. Supplementary data regarding the chamber size, functional capability in the form of ejection fraction, number of segments showing wall motion abnormality, make it an invaluable tool, although it is predominantly operator-dependent.[7]

Cardiac magnetic resonance imaging (MRI) is challenging because of the rapid motion of the heart and coronary arteries. Assessment of the structure and function through cardiac perfusion imaging can be done with MRI, although its cost and availability limits its widespread usage. It provides excellent spatial resolution and can be used for perfusion and viability studies of the myocardium. Image quality may be restricted due to artefacts and motions errors.[6,7]

Detection of obstructive CAD by coronary CT in intermediate risk patients is well established and possesses a high negative predictive value. The functional significance of a coronary stenosis detected on CT is relatively difficult to determine and, thus, has unreliable usefulness for lesion-specific, ischemia. Fractional flow reserve (FFR) derived from coronary computed tomographic angiography (CCTA) images is emerging as a novel noninvasive method to evaluate lesion-specific ischemia. Coronary calcium quantification techniques give information regarding the severity and prognosis of CAD.[8-10]

Nuclear Medicine Techniques

SPECT Myocardial Perfusion Imaging

Stress single photon emission computed tomography (SPECT) myocardial perfusion imaging is well-established technique for identification and analysis of the extent of CAD burden. Radiotracers such as thallium and technetium are widely used with exercise stress testing or pharmacological agents. Meta-analyses have shown the sensitivity and specificity to be 87% and 73%, respectively.[11] With the use of functional parameters facilitated by the use of gating techniques and incorporation of attenuation correction techniques, there has been improved performance of the myocardial SPECT perfusion imaging. The newer solid state techniques and additional CT systems have comparable capabilities in comparison to PET imaging.

Limitations of SPECT, Invasive Coronary Angiography and CT Angiography

In spite of its widespread availability, SPECT has an in-built shortcoming in the form of collimators concealing the detectors leading to reduced count rate with diminishing sensitivity. The tracers used in SPECT imaging have longer physical decay leading to higher radiation burden. The artefactual defects within the myocardium can occur due to overlap of liver/bowel activity over the ventricular wall particularly in physically inactive patients. The attenuation by diaphragm and dense breast tissues is better overcome in PET studies by CT attenuation correction software. The CT component in the PET imaging systems is well equipped to perform diagnostic CT scans providing valuable additional diagnostic information.[12,13] Viability imaging combined with perfusion scan, calculation of mismatch and scar scores, can be incorporated into clinical practice to assess improvement in myocardial function post-intervention.[14]

Studies comparing the noninvasive to invasive modalities for identifying the CAD burden are in general agreement. For advanced lesions, noninvasive as well as invasive testing is comparably effective in assessing the disease. Normal myocardial perfusion image (MPI) study in many instances shows no significant luminal stenosis on invasive angiography although atherosclerotic lesions with positive remodeling may be picked up on multidetector computed tomography (MDCT) with no significant flow limitation.[9,15] Invasive coronary angiography is the reference gold standard technique for evaluation of coronary artery disease for decades now and continues to remain so. The additional potential of it being a therapeutic modality as and when indicated makes it a powerful theranostic tool. However, the dependency for visual appraisal of lesions on the operating physician contributes to its drawback with inexperienced hands.

In some cases, the discrepant findings are due to differential patterns of vessel involvement (eccentric or circumferential) or due to poor contrast administration techniques. The supplementary use of FFR and intravascular ultrasound (IVUS) technique to characterize the plaque is definitely possible, although the risks of contrast reactions and major complications in terms of stroke and arrhythmias should be definitively weighed upon. Invasive coronary angiography remains the cornerstone for coronary tree imaging with its superior temporal and spatial resolution, nonetheless its role in determining the functional significance of stenosis similar to CT angiography, is very limited. The probability of causing a procedural risk with re-stenosis in a nonflow limiting anatomical lesion and the angiographic ambiguity of findings stenoses in asymptomatic individuals led to evaluation with functional parameters namely FFR and CFR. Estimation of functional significance of lesions leads to identification of such lesions causing symptoms thereby directly influencing the therapeutic strategies.[13,16,17]

CT angiography has many confounding questions in numerous scenarios. The low-grade lesions with outward positive remodeling and without considerable luminal compromise, are known to be harbinger of potential acute coronary syndromes. The spatial resolution of CT imaging is approximately half in comparison to the conventional angiography and temporal resolution is quite hindered inexplicably by the translational movements of the coronary arteries.[9]

Fractional flow reserve (defined as the ratio of maximum blood flow in a stenotic artery to maximum blood flow in the same artery) is an excellent parameter as it recognizes the purposeful lesions within the coronary arteries, being useful in angiographically intermediate stenoses. Stenoses with FFRs 0.75 or 0.80 have been shown to induce ischemia and, hence, are defined as functionally significant. The usefulness of FFR is restricted in cases of acute MI and technical limitations like submaximal hyperemia and concerns related to the catheter and guidewire make it a difficult proposition in everyday settings.[10,18-20] FFR applicability in the multivessel CAD is questionable with perceptible usefulness in single vessel disease. In contrast, the coronary flow reserve assesses multi-vessel disease in a better way as it is a ratio and compares the maximum achievable blood flow post-hyperemia to that at rest.[19]

Coronary Flow Reserve

Coronary flow reserve (CFR) is defined as a ratio of maximal (stimulated) to baseline (resting) coronary blood flow. CFR measurement has ample role in the effective judgment of the consequences of epicardial coronary stenoses as well as to examine the integrity of the microvascular circulation.

Methods to Measure CFR[4,13,18-22]

A PET approach for the assessment of regional myocardial blood flow (MBF) in mL/g/min involves the intravenous injection of perfusion positron-emitting tracer. Dynamic acquisition of images of the radiotracer passing through the central circulatory system to its extraction and retention in the left ventricular myocardium, are performed. Numerous methods, both invasive and noninvasive methods, have been used to measure CFR, albeit few fit the criteria of being inexpensive, available at all times and reproducible in several settings. The inert gases to thermodilution techniques, angiography to the fast-paced CT, have all been tried and tested in a host of backgrounds. The coronary flow is extremely heterogeneous due to multiple complex interacting and signaling pathways and the PET reasonably gives credence to heterogeneity in flow while calculating the coronary reserve.[23]

Intracoronary Doppler has been considered in the same sitting with the invasive coronary angiography (ICA) but is expensive and associated with risks because of its invasive nature. Transthoracic Doppler echocardiography is a relatively economical technique but only regional flow velocity in the left anterior descending artery (LAD) (middle and distal segments) is better measured and calculation of absolute coronary flow is difficult. CFR computation can be either in terms of flow, velocity or pressure in the coronary bed. Doppler catheterization and coronary sinus thermodilution measures the flow; whilst the velocity and pressure are measured by echo and the pressure-tipped sensor. The PET technique calculates the flow per 100 g of LV myocardium with assessment of designated territories.

CFR Using PET[4,5,13,20,24]

The linear relationship between tracer uptake and coronary perfusion leads to identification of even minor stenosis. The PET scans use different tracers for noninvasive qualitative as well as quantitative evaluation for regional blood flow in the myocardium. ^{15}O water, $^{13}NH_3$ and ^{82}Rb are the major ones with others like ^{62}Cu PTSM and ^{68}Ga-labeled albumin microspheres, ^{94m}Tc-teboroxime used in many different studies. Newer ^{18}F labeled tracers like ^{18}F-flurpiridaz are gaining ground due to their high extraction fraction at higher flow rate. ^{82}Rb has a short physical half-life and is generator produced, while $^{13}NH_3$ and ^{15}O require cyclotron for their production. ^{15}O water is an ideal tracer for quantification but is not readily available and short half-life restricts the semiquantitative analysis. $^{13}NH_3$ uptake exhibits a linear relationship with myocardial blood flow up to very high flow rates and it provides excellent spatial resolution. CFR is measured by the ratio obtained of the myocardial blood flow at peak hyperemia to that of at rest. The anatomical corollary of CFR is the noninvasive FFR based on the newer models of fluid dynamics, which is calculated by CT.

Technical Aspects[20,24]

Standard list mode acquisition having specific set of parameters in dynamic phase imaging, postsingle bolus intravenous administration of radiopharmaceutical is well-established technique for determining CFR. The tracer counts plotted as time activity curves obtained from arterial and myocardial tissue region of interests (ROIs) serve as inputs for calculation using the tracer kinetic model. The diffusion of tracer across two different compartments over a definite time interval (defined in terms of rate of tracer uptake) is calculated using kinetic model equations and the absolute MBF at stress and rest is automatically computed using software tools. The tracer kinetic model varies from being one compartmental for ^{15}O to three compartmental for $^{13}NH_3$.

Clinical Significance of CFR[5,9,10,13,14,16-21,25]

Multiple studies have been evaluated retrospectively to define the role of PET for accuracy in the diagnosis of CAD. The studies performed compared ^{82}Rb with ^{99m}Tc SPECT agents incorporating CT attenuation correction with the reference ICA have shown the higher sensitivity and specificity with PET than that with SPECT. The SPECT-MPI assesses the functional severity in coronary artery in relation to each other based on an assumption that the maximal perfused area is normal which is not so in a multitude of cases with multivessel pathology.

The immense potential of the cardiac PET ultimately led to the exploration of value of the imaging parameters for diagnosis and prognosis of coronary artery disease. CFR is an established diagnostic parameter in multivessel epicardial stenosis unraveling the balanced ischemia noted in stress SPECT-MPI **(Figs 1A and B)**. CFR is evaluated not only against perfusion parameters, but also on the basis of functional parameters such as the ejection fraction, calculated both at stress and rest. The stress-induced wall motion abnormalities with associated LV dysfunction and transient ischemic dilatation are comparatively determined better in PET imaging, the reason being of the simultaneous quick acquisition in poststress period. CFR scores over the SPECT-MPI on this very aspect being dependent on the maximum achievable blood flow to the baseline blood flow instead of inter-vessel perfusion status **(Figs 2A to C)**.

Study done by Zaidi et al. has shown that a normal MPI with a CFR value greater than 2 provides an assurance for a period of 3 years with no significant acute coronary syndrome risk where those with normal MPI and CFR <1.5 have a substantial increase in the hazard ratios and need to go for more aggressive forms of therapy, including stenting if required. The CFR calculation in patients with relatively normal MPI helps in detection of subclinical CAD with excellent prognosis in them if intervened earlier.

The CFR using dynamic imaging and compartmental modeling evaluates hyperemic and resting flows in multivessel

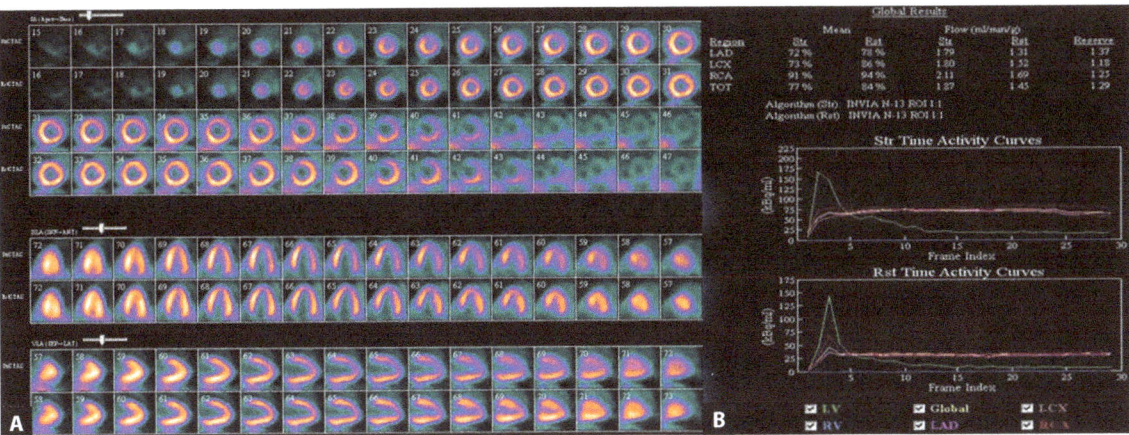

Figs 1A and B: A 60-year-old male patient with h/o long-standing diabetes of 8 years, underwent stress $^{13}NH_3$ cardiac PET; the cross-sectional images show normal perfusion within all walls of the LV myocardium (A). The time-activity curves show global reduction in the CFR (<2.0) along all the three vascular territories indicating that the normal perfusion images were actually reflecting the balanced ischemia (B)

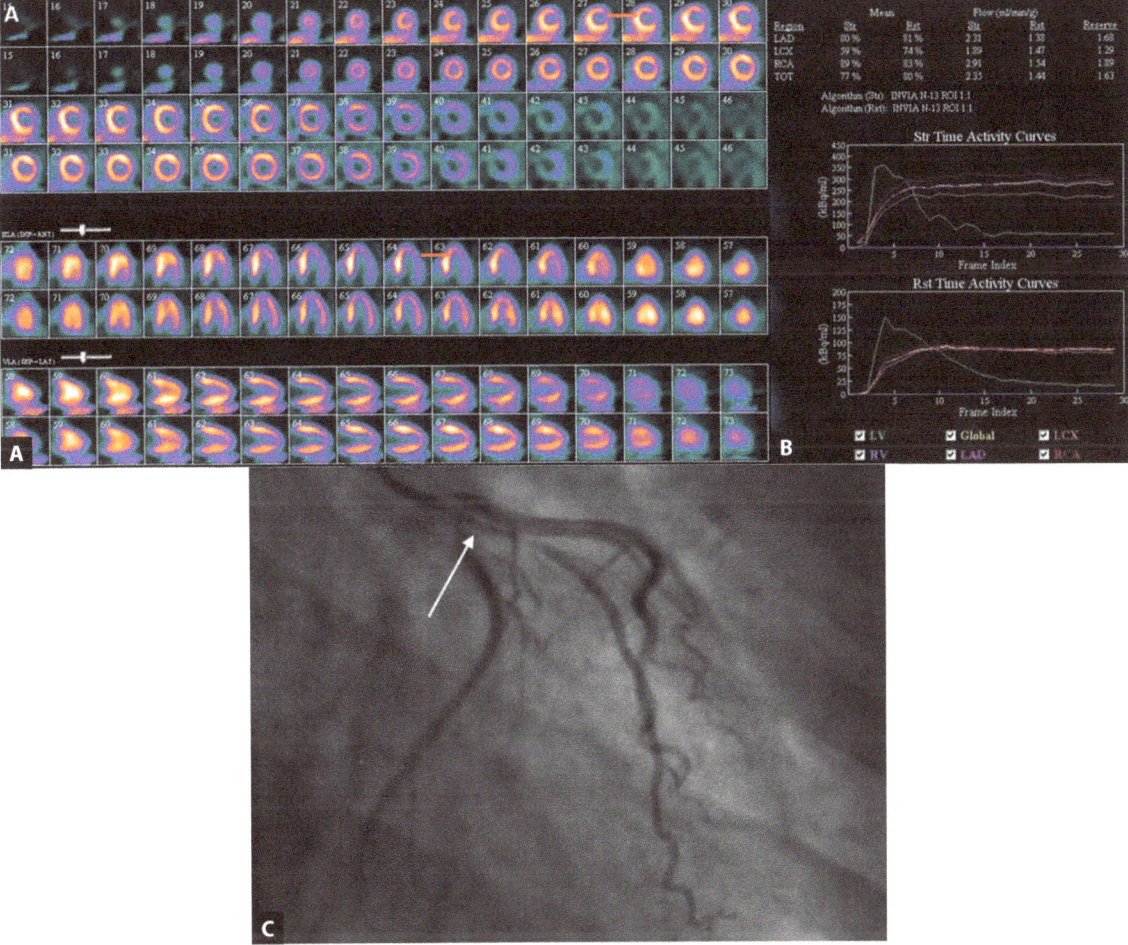

Figs 2A to C: A 59-year-old male diabetic patient underwent stress $^{13}NH_3$ cardiac PET; the cross-sectional stress perfusion images depict perfusion defect in anterolateral wall with reversibility in rest images in the left circumflex arterial territory (A). The time-activity curves show reduction in global CFR (<2.0) with severe reduction of CFR (1.29) in left circumflex artery territory (B). Subsequent invasive coronary angiography showed plaque causing significant stenosis in the left circumflex as well ramus intermedius arteries (C)

disease excellently while the FFR depends on the proximal to distal pressure difference. The testing of CFR is better than with coronary CT in practice because the CFR reflects the blunted response in a chronic ischemic scenario due to stenosis. The relationship between CFR and FFR is complex as CFR reflects the flow changes across the entire vascular bed, whereas FFR echoes changes in flow along a single lesion. Alterations in CFR have been shown in the conditions like dyslipidemia, smoking, hypertension, diabetes and the metabolic syndrome, and have also been shown to improve after treatment of these conditions. The microvascular disease of vessels leads to significant compromise in the blood flow to the myocardium, and diabetes being a CAD equivalent with its ever-rising incidence, needs early evaluation and timely therapeutic intervention. The quantitative CFR estimates from cardiac PET during stress reflects hyperemic reactivity to vasodilator agents which can be compromised in early stages of microvascular disease. Coronary circulatory dysfunction identified early helps in providing interventions in a timely fashion preventing further vascular complications like myocardial infarction.

Difficulties in Performing and Limitations of CFR[5,20,21,24]

The ever-increasing availability of PET, although makes it easier to perform cardiac studies, is still limited to the tertiary care centers. The availability of radiopharmaceuticals and the need for on-site cyclotron in case of $^{13}NH_3$ makes the modality a costly affair. Nevertheless overcoming these confines, studies related to CFR have led to a better understanding of direct influence of CFR on clinical decision making in two cohorts of people—one with universal myocardial oxygen deficiency with normal extramural arteries and the other with segmental ischemia with narrowing in one of the extramural arteries. Although the optimal cut-off values are not yet fully elucidated and clarified in clinical settings, quantification in larger populations may lead to its greater significance and practical applicability as a decision tool. The value of utility in clinical settings has to be determined in large scale randomized studies with focus on cut-off values to differentiate between epicardial narrowing and small-vessel disease. Postintervention CFR indices in patients and their comparison to preintervention values may provide additional prognostic utility. Achieving maximal dilatation of highest levels with optimized protocols will go a long way in incorporating the CFR as a part of evaluating apparatus for clinical management. Although the integrated physiology is well reflected in myocardial blood flow and CFR measurement, this limits the specificity of the test.

Future Prospects in CFR Measurement[26,27]

The CFR calculation using PET is well known and with the advent of newer modified gamma cameras using semiconductor detectors, calculation of CFR has been brought out with cadmium zinc telluride (CZT) gamma cameras. The technology combines a multi-pinhole collimator block interfaced with a multi-detector array of pixelated CZT modules enabling faster imaging with the automated software technique. The results have shown to be comparable with the values of CFR obtained with ammonia perfusion PET. The CZT cameras provide higher temporal and spatial resolution and with their ever-increasing availability, they provide a viable option for CFR in near future.

Conclusion

The assessment of blood flow within a vascular territory in absolute terms leads to more accurate stratification of CAD and thereby significantly improving the therapeutic strategy. The use of high-resolution PET scanner imaging with coronary flow reserve quantification unmasks the patients with multi-vessel and subclinical CAD, thereby helps in guiding decisions of lifestyle modifications and preventive medical therapy. The newer generation imaging modalities have given hope for better characterization and understanding of the complex pathophysiology of the coronary vasculature.

REFERENCES

1. Mendis S, Puska P, Norrving B. Global atlas on cardiovascular disease prevention and control. Geneva: World Health Organization in collaboration with the World Heart Federation and the World Stroke Organization; 2011.
2. Hata J, Kiyohara Y. Epidemiology of Stroke and Coronary Artery Disease in Asia. Circ J. 2013;77:1923-32.
3. Wong N. Epidemiological studies of CHD and the evolution of preventive cardiology. Nat Rev Cardiol. 2014;11:276-89.
4. Schindler T, Schelbert H, Quercioli A, Dilsizian V. Cardiac PET imaging for the detection and monitoring of coronary artery disease and microvascular health. JACC Cardiovasc Imaging. 2010;3:623-40.
5. Cassar A, Holmes D, Rihal C, Gersh B. Chronic coronary artery disease: diagnosis and management. Mayo Clinic Proceedings. 2009;84:1130-46.
6. Mieres JH, Makaryus AN. Noninvasive cardiac imaging. Am Fam Physician. 2007;75:1219-28.
7. Yoon Y, Choi J, Kim J, et al. Noninvasive diagnosis of ischemia-causing coronary stenosis using CT angiography. JACC: Cardiovasc Imaging. 2012;5:1088-96.
8. Klocke FJ, Baird MG, Lorell BH, et al. ACC/AHA/ASNC guidelines for the clinical use of cardiac radionuclide imaging—executive summary: a report of the American College of Cardiology/American Heart Association Task Force on Practice Guidelines (ACC/AHA/ASNC Committee to Revise the 1995 Guidelines for the Clinical Use of Cardiac Radionuclide Imaging). Circulation 2003;108:1404-18.
9. Ronald Mastouri, Stephen G Sawada, Jo Mahenthiran. Current noninvasive imaging techniques for detection of coronary artery disease. Expert Rev Cardiovasc Ther. 2010;8:77-91.
10. Schuijf JD, van Werkhoven JM, Pundziute G, et al. Invasive versus noninvasive evaluation of coronary artery disease. JACC Cardiovasc Imaging. 2008;1:190-9.

11. Pijls NH, Sels JW. Functional Measurement of Coronary Stenosis. J Am Coll Cardiol. 2012;59:1045-57.
12. Tonino PA, Fearon WF, De Bruyne B, et al. Angiographic versus functional severity of coronary artery stenoses in the FAME study fractional flow reserve versus angiography in multivessel evaluation. J Am Coll Cardiol. 2010;55:2816-21.
13. Schelbert HR. FFR and Coronary Flow Reserve: Friends or Foes? JACC Cadiovasc Imaging. 2012;5:203-6.
14. Pizzuto F, Voci P, Mariano E, Emilio Puddu P, Sardella G, Nigri A. Assessment of flow velocity reserve by transthoracic Doppler echocardiography and venous adenosine infusion before and after left anterior descending coronary artery stenting. J Am Coll Cardiol. 2001;38:155-62.
15. Daimon M, Watanabe H, Yamagishi H, et al. Physiologic assessment of coronary artery stenosis by coronary flow reserve measurements with transthoracic Doppler echocardiography: comparison with exercise thallium-201 single-photon emission computed tomography. J Am Coll Cardiol. 2001;37:1310-5.
16. Kaufmann P. Myocardial blood flow measurement by PET: technical aspects and clinical applications. J Nucl Med. 2005;46:75-88.
17. Hoffman J. Problems of Coronary Flow Reserve. Ann Biomed Engi. 2000;28:884-96.
18. Mc Ardle B, Dowsley T, Cocker M, et al. Cardiac PET: metabolic and functional imaging of the myocardium. Semin Nucl Med. 2013;43:434-48.
19. Hagemann CE, Ghotbi AA, Kjær A, Hasbak P. Quantitative myocardial blood flow with Rubidium-82 PET: a clinical perspective. Am J Nucl Med Mol Imaging. 2015;5:457-68.
20. Slomka P, Berman DS, Alexanderson E, Germano G. The role of PET quantification in cardiovascular imaging. Clin Transl Imaging. 2014;2:343-58.
21. Schindler TH, Quercioli A, Valenta I, Ambrosio G, Wahl RL, Dilsizian V. Quantitative assessment of myocardial blood flow-clinical and research applications. Semin Nucl Med. 2014; 44:274-93.
22. Nissen SE. Limitations of Computed Tomography Coronary Angiography. J Am Coll Cardiol. 2008;52:2145-7.
23. Nakansihi R, Budoff MJ. Noninvasive FFR derived from coronary CT angiography in the management of coronary artery disease: technology and clinical update. Vasc Health Risk Manag. 2016;12:269-78.
24. Nakazato R, Heo R, Leipsic J, Min JK. CFR and FFR assessment with PET and CTA: strengths and limitations. Curr Cardiol Rep. 2014;16;484.
25. Johnson N, Kirkeeide R, Gould K. History and Development of Coronary Flow Reserve and Fractional Flow Reserve for Clinical Applications. Interventional Cardiol Clinics. 2015;4:397-410.
26. Bocher M, Blevis IM, Tsukerman L, Shrem Y, Kovalski G, Volokh L. A fast cardiac gamma camera with dynamic SPECT capabilities: design, system validation and future potential. Eur J Nucl Med Mol Imaging. 2010;37:1887-902.
27. Nkoulou R, Fuchs TA, Pazhenkottil AP, et al. Absolute myocardial blood flow and flow reserve assessed by Gated SPECT with Cadmium-Zinc-Telluride detectors using 99mTc-tetrofosmin: head-to-head comparison with ^{13}N-Ammonia PET. J Nucl Med. 2016. jnumed.115.165498.

17 Nuclear Medicine in Assessment of Cardiac Dyssynchrony

Anirban Mukherjee, Chetan D Patel

INTRODUCTION TO CARDIAC DYSSYNCHRONY

Dyssynchrony literally means lack of synchrony. When pertaining to the heart, it reflects a state of electrical and/or mechanical incoordination between various cardiac chambers or myocardial segments within a chamber. assessment of the intraventricular and interventricular dyssynchrony has been the focus of investigation by various imaging modalities. Dyssynchrony can also be subdivided into systolic (during contraction) and diastolic (during relaxation).[1,2] The consequence of this incoordination leads to reduced pumping efficiency of the heart with ultimate end results of heart failure. Although echocardiography is the most commonly used modality, nuclear medicine techniques have demonstrated tremendous promise because of their objectivity and reproducibility in assessment of cardiac dyssynchrony.

NUCLEAR MEDICINE TECHNIQUES IN ASSESSMENT OF CARDIAC DYSSYNCHRONY

Equilibrium Radionuclide Angiography

Equilibrium radionuclide angiography (ERNA) is a well-established imaging modality and provides a relatively simple, reproducible and noninvasive method to assess ventricular function and wall motion, in particular, left ventricular ejection faction (LVEF).[3] Since the early 1980s, gated ERNA has used phase image analysis for the assessment of dyssynchronous cardiac contraction.[4] The phase image analysis is based on the first Fourier harmonic fit of the blood pool time versus radioactive curve to measure the magnitude and sequence of ventricular contraction in each pixel of the image. A phase angle is assigned b/w 0°–360° depending on the relative time delay from the R-wave to the start of the cardiac cycle for each pixel. A phase histogram is constructed corresponding to the sequence of ventricular contraction during cardiac cycle. Mean and Standard deviation (SD) of phase histogram is calculated for each ventricle separately. Intraventricular dyssynchrony is measured by standard deviation of the mean phase angle (SD mPA) for left ventricle (LV) and right ventricle (RV) and interventricular dyssynchrony is calculated as the difference between LV and RV mean phase angles (LV-RVmPA), in milliseconds (ms) and/or degree (°).[5]

Although softwares are available for assessment of cardiac dyssynchrony using ERNA, these are not standardized and different centers have used different softwares. At our center, we standardized vendor provided software and established the normal values of synchrony in our population from which the cut-off values of dyssynchrony were proposed **(Table 1, Figs 1 and 2)**.[6]

There are limited studies on assessment of cardiac dyssynchrony using Gated Blood Pool Spect (GBPS). Since, planar ERNA is limited due to the two-dimensional nature of the technique this may be overcome with phase analysis of GBPS, which has the potential to more accurately quantify dyssynchrony in three-dimension with high reproducibility.[7]

Table 1 Proposed cut off values of dyssynchrony on ERNA[6]

Left intraventricular dyssynchrony (SD LVmPA)	>27.1 ms, >13.2°
Right intraventricular dyssynchrony (SD RVmPA)	>68.7 ms, >33.1°
Interventricular dyssynchrony (LV-RV mPA)	>47.3 ms, >22.1°

Abbreviations: LV, left ventricle; RV, right ventricle; mPA, mean phase angle; SD, standard deviation; ms, milli second

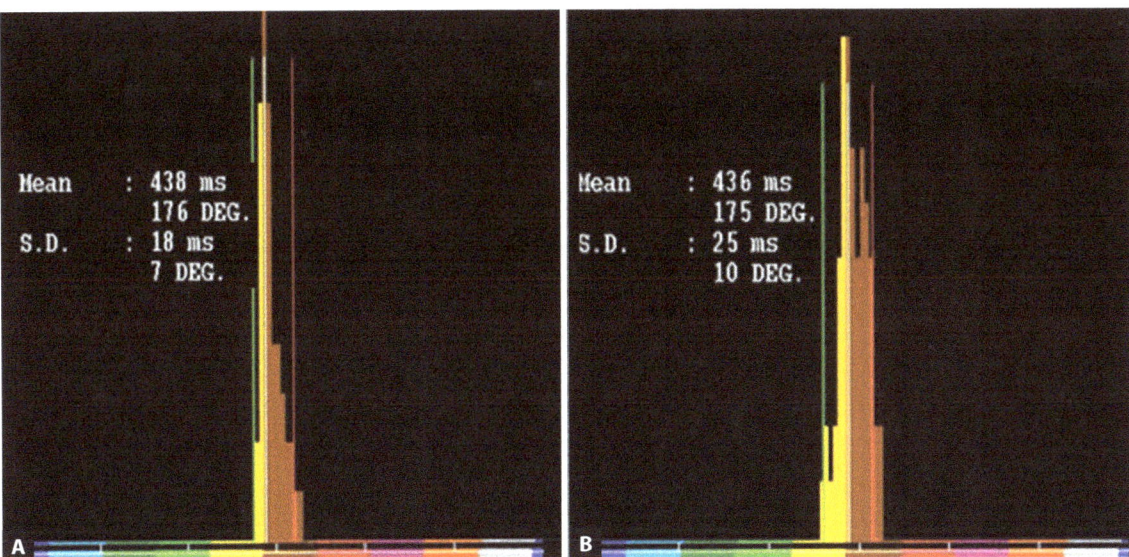

Figs 1A and B: Normal phase histogram of ERNA showing phase distribution of the left ventricle (A) and right ventricle (B). Intra-left ventricular synchrony (SD LVmPA-7°/18 ms), intra-right ventricular synchrony (SD RVmPA-10°/25 ms) and interventricular synchrony (LV-RVmPA -1°/2 ms

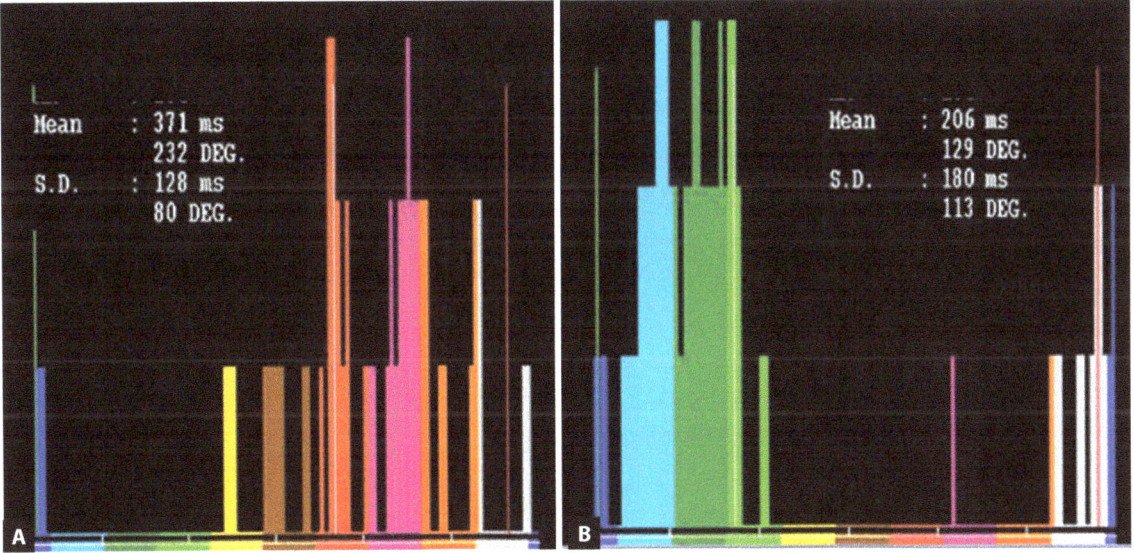

Figs 2A and B: Phase histogram of LV (A) and RV (B) on ERNA showing intra-left ventricular dyssynchrony (SD LVmPA-80°/128 ms), intra-right ventricular dyssynchrony (SD RVmPA-113°/180 ms) and inter-ventricular dyssynchrony (LV-RVmPA -103°/165 ms)

Gated Myocardial Perfusion SPECT

In 2005, Chen et al. developed a diagnostic tool for the assessment of LV mechanical dyssynchrony using phase analysis of gated myocardial perfusion SPECT (GMPS). Phase analysis of GMPS has shown several advantages such as simplicity, widespread availability, superior reproducibility, applicability to retrospective data and ability to simultaneously assess LV perfusion, function, and mechanical dyssynchrony.[8] In GMPS, Fourier analysis converts regional myocardial counts which relates to regional wall thickening into a continuous function to calculate a phase angle for each region. Phase angles of all regions of LV are obtained, to generate a phase distribution.[8]

Quantitative softwares for assessment of cardiac dyssynchrony on GMPS are commercially available providing objective parameters for assessment of intraventricular dyssynchrony and the normal values of synchrony have been established by many centers.[8-11] The two parameters commonly used to assess cardiac dyssynchrony on GMPS are phase standard deviation (PSD) and phase histogram bandwidth (PHB). At our center we have established the normal values of

Table 2 Normal values of synchrony parameters on GMPS[10]

	Range	Mean	SD
Phase standard deviation (PSD) (in degrees)			
Men			
Stress	9.2–25.2	14.3	4.7
Rest	3.6–18.2	8.9	2.9
Women			
Stress	4.7–20.8	11	4
Rest	3.3–16.5	7.7	2.7
Phase histogram bandwidth (PHB) (in degrees)			
Men			
Stress	23–72	40.1	11.9
Rest	20–54	30.6	7.6
Women			
Stress	16–70	34.7	12.6
Rest	12–52	25.3	8.6

Table 3 Cut-off values for presence of dyssynchrony on GMPS[10]

	Value (in degrees)
Phase standard deviation (PSD)	
Men	
Stress	23.7
Rest	14.7
Women	
Stress	19
Rest	13.1
Phase histogram bandwidth (PHB)	
Men	
Stress	63.9
Rest	45.8
Women	
Stress	59.9
Rest	42.5

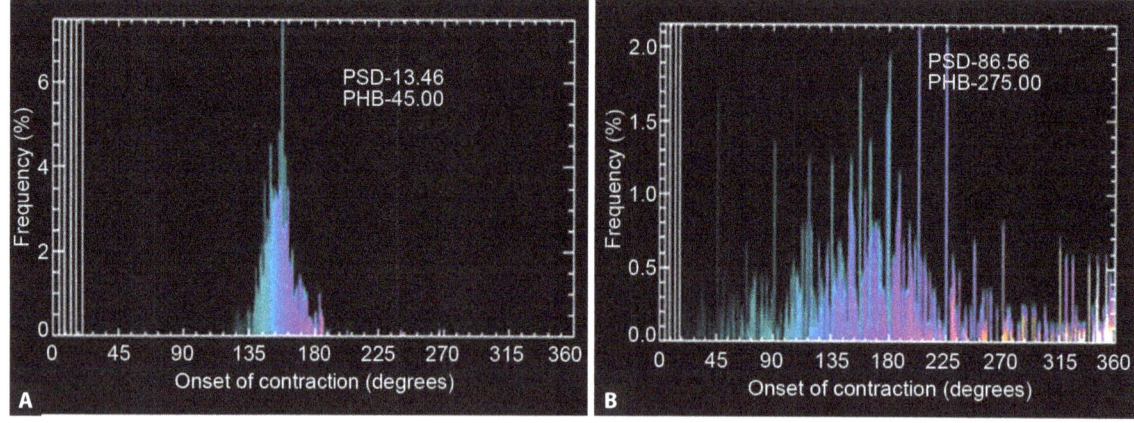

Figs 3A and B: Normal phase histogram on GMPS (A) and phase histogram in presence of intra-left ventricular dyssynchrony (B)

synchrony from which the cut-off values of dyssynchrony based on PSD and PHB parameters were proposed in our population **(Tables 2 and 3) (Figs 3A and B)**.[10]

Cardiac Positron Emission Tomography

Phase analysis with positron emission tomography (PET) perfusion tracers have been evaluated and like GMPS both PSD and PHB can be measured to assess cardiac dyssynchrony.[12,13] Cooke et al.[12] described normal values of PSD and PHB with Rb-82 PET **(Table 4)**. Even phase analysis of gated 18F-Fluorodeoxyglucose (18F-FDG) PET was been evaluated for assessment of LV dyssynchrony and compared with GMPS.[14] A significant correlation between SPECT and FDG PET derived dyssynchrony parameters, PHB ($r = 0.88$, $p < 0.001$) and PSD ($r = 0.88$, $p < 0.001$) was observed.

CLINICAL UTILITY OF ASSESSMENT OF CARDIAC MECHANICAL DYSSYNCHRONY

Prediction of Response to Cardiac Resynchronization Therapy

Cardiac resynchronization therapy (CRT) has emerged as an exciting treatment option for the subset of drug refractory heart

Table 4 Regadenoson stress and rest ^{82}Rb PET normal values[12]

	Stress	Rest
Phase SD (In degrees)		
Men	15.0 ± 7.0	22.7 ± 13.2
Women	13.2 ± 7.7	16.6 ± 14.3
Histogram bandwidth (In degrees)		
Men	38.1 ± 13.3	50.8 ± 18.7
Women	32.0 ± 13.5	44.0 ± 44.9

failure (HF) patients.[15] The American College of Cardiology/American Heart Association/Heart Rhythm Society guidelines recommend CRT in patients with end-stage drug-refractory HF (NYHA class II–IV), depressed LVEF (≤35%), and prolonged QRS duration (≥150 ms).[16] However, using these conventional criteria for selection of patients for CRT, it was noted that 20–40% of patients did not respond to CRT.[17,18]

Due to high device cost and associated procedural complications, it is important to refine the selection criteria and to define an objective parameter which can accurately predict the response to therapy prior to device implantation. Mechanical cardiac dyssynchrony has been recognized as an additional and essential criterion for response to CRT.[19,20] Many studies have showed the utility of ERNA and GMPS in prediction of CRT response.[21-27]

Dauphin et al.[21] studied the value of interventricular (IV) and intra-left ventricular dyssynchrony (ILVD) on ERNA for predicting CRT response in 74 patients with both ischemic and nonischemic dilated cardiomyopathy. They found that IVD was significantly higher in responders compared to nonresponders at baseline. Subsequent receiver operating characteristic (ROC) curve analysis showed that an IVD value of 25.5° was associated with a sensitivity of 91.4% and a specificity of 84.4% to predict CRT response. They concluded that in patients with wide QRS, IVD can predict response to resynchronization therapy. In another study, Toussiant et al.[22] noted that significant IVD at baseline combined with LVEF >15% have a sensitivity of 79% and a positive predictive value of 83% to predict an improvement of LVEF of >5% during follow-up. In contrast, Mukherjee et al.[23] noted that both ILVD and IVD were significantly larger in responders versus nonresponders. ROC curve analysis showed an optimal sensitivity of 95% and specificity of 80% at cut-off value of 30° for ILVD and an optimal sensitivity of 81% and specificity of 80% at cut-off value of 23° for IVD for prediction of response to CRT. However, on multivariate analysis, ILVD was found to be most important independent predictor for response to CRT.

There are limited studies on ERNA that have evaluated the role of right ventricular dyssynchrony in prediction of response to CRT. Burri et al.[24] found that patients with RV dysfunction have a lower likelihood of response to CRT. In agreement, Mukherjee et al.[25] found that patients with RV dyssynchrony had a lower response rate to CRT (43%) compared with the patients without RV dyssynchrony (89%).

Henneman et al.[26] first investigated the clinical utility of mechanical dyssynchrony assessed on GMPS in prediction of response to CRT. They obtained cut-off value of 43° for PSD and 135° for PHB for prediction of response to CRT. Mukherjee et al.[27] in a study of 32 nonischemic dilated cardiomyopathy patients noted that responders had significantly higher dyssynchrony indices of PSD (64 ± 17° vs 39 ± 13°; P<.01) and PHB (215 ± 64° vs 110 ± 44°; P<.01) compared to nonresponders. ROC curve analysis demonstrated that the maximum accuracy for prediction of CRT response was obtained with values of 128° for PHB and 43° for PSD (86% sensitivity and 80% specificity for both parameters). Recently, there has been a lot of interest in using imaging modalities especially GMPS to guide LV lead placement in CRT. The rationale is to identify the site of latest mechanical activation which is viable, where the lead can be placed to improve the success rate of CRT.[28,29]

Coronary Artery Disease

Association between coronary artery disease (CAD) and dyssynchrony has been the focus of interest. Several studies have demonstrated the relation of ILVD with myocardial ischemic and/or scar burden, relation of poststress ILVD with stress-induced ischemia and CAD extent.[30-32] Chen et al.[30] observed association between stress-induced ischemia and early poststress ILVD. The authors suggested that stress-induced myocardial ischemia caused dyssynchronous contraction in the ischemic region, leading to deterioration in LV synchrony and this pattern may aid the diagnosis of CAD. Huang et al.[31] observed that patients with multivessel disease (MVD) had significantly more global and territorial dyssynchrony at early poststress than at rest on Thallium-201 study. Gimelli et al.[32] on Tc99m-tetrofosmin study, observed higher prevalence of MVD disease in patients with ILVD at rest than those without dyssynchrony.

Assessment of cardiac dyssynchrony in patients with CAD can have prognostic value. Zafrir et al.[33] in a study group of 787 patients followed for mean duration of 18.3 ± 6.2 months observed that ILVD can predict cardiac death together with NYHA class, in patients with LV dysfunction. In another study, Uebleis et al.[34] in 135 patients with known CAD found that ILVD is an independent predictor of death. More data is needed regarding this aspect to firmly establish the prognostic value of dyssynchrony in CAD patients.

Other Clinical Applications

Assessment of cardiac dyssynchrony has also been used in other clinical subsets. Studies have shown its role in evaluation of patients with permanent pacemakers,[35] in prognostication and risk stratification of patients of non-ischemic cardiomyopathy.[36] Implantable cardiac defibrillator[37] and end stage renal disease.[38]

CONCLUSION

Accurate and reproducible assessment of cardiac dyssynchrony can be performed with nuclear imaging techniques. Phase analysis of ERNA and GMPS has gained considerable attention in prediction of response to CRT. Studies in literature have also shown the utility of nuclear medicine assessed cardiac dyssynchrony in CAD. With further research in this field, cardiac dyssynchrony can become a valuable asset in varied clinical settings.

REFERENCES

1. Owen CH, Esposito DJ, Davis JW, et al. The effects of ventricular pacing on left ventricular geometry, function, myocardial oxygen consumption, and efficiency of contraction in conscious dogs. Pacing Clin Electrophysiol. 1998;21:1417-29.
2. Auricchio A, Abraham WT. Cardiac resynchronization therapy: current state of the art—cost versus benefit. Circulation. 2004;109:300-7.
3. Strauss HW, Zaret BL, Hurley PJ, et al. A scintiphotographic method for measuring left ventricular ejection fraction in man without cardiac catheterization. Am J Cardiol. 1971;28:575-80.
4. Frais M, Botvinick E, Shosa D, et al. Phase image characterization of localized and generalized left ventricular contraction abnormalities. J Am Coll Cardiol. 1984;4:987-98.
5. Botvinick EH, Dunn R, Frais M, et al. The phase image: Its relationship to patterns of contraction and conduction. Circulation. 1982;65:551-60.
6. Singh H, Singhal A, Sharma P, et al. Quantitative assessment of cardiac mechanical synchrony using equilibrium radionuclide angiography. J Nucl Cardiol. 2013;20:415-25.
7. Harel F, Finnerty V, Gregoire J, et al. Comparison of left ventricular contraction homogeneity index using SPECT gated blood pool imaging and planar phase analysis. J Nucl Cardiol. 2008;15:80-5.
8. Chen J, Garcia EV, Folks RD, et al. Onset of left ventricular mechanical contraction as determined by phase analysis of ECG gated myocardial perfusion SPECT imaging: Development of a SPECT myocardial perfusion imaging diagnostic tool for assessment of cardiac mechanical dyssynchrony. J Nucl Cardiol. 2005;12:687-95.
9. Romero-Farina G, Aguadé-Bruix S, Candell-Riera J, et al. Cut-off values of myocardial perfusion gated-SPECT phase analysis parameters of normal subjects, and conduction and mechanical cardiac diseases. J Nucl Cardiol. 2015;22:1247-58.
10. Mukherjee A, Singh H, Patel C, et al. Normal values of cardiac mechanical synchrony parameters using gated myocardial perfusion single-photon emission computed tomography: Impact of population and study protocol. Indian J Nucl Med. 2016;31:255-9.
11. AlJaroudi W, Jaber WA, Grimm RA, et al. Alternative methods for the assessment of mechanical dyssynchrony using phase analysis of gated single photon emission computed tomography myocardial perfusion imaging. Int J Cardiovasc Imaging. 2012;28:1385-894.
12. Cooke CD, Esteves FP, Chen J, et al. Left ventricular mechanical synchrony from stress and rest 82Rb PET myocardial perfusion ECG-gated studies: differentiating normal from LBBB patients. J Nucl Cardiol. 2011;18:1076-85.
13. AlJaroudi W, Alraies MC, Menon V, et al. Predictors and incremental prognostic value of left ventricular mechanical dyssynchrony response during stress-gated positron emission tomography in patients with ischemic cardiomyopathy. J Nucl Cardiol. 2012;19:958-69.
14. Pazhenkottil AP, Buechel RR, Nkoulou R, et al. Left ventricular dyssynchrony assessment by phase analysis from gated PET-FDG scans. J Nucl Cardiol. 2011;18:920-5.
15. Cleland JGF, Daubert JC, Erdmann E, et al. The effect of cardiac resynchronization on morbidity and mortality in heart failure. N Engl J Med. 2005;352:1539-49.
16. Yancy CW, Jessup M, Bozkurt B, et al. 2013 ACCF/AHA guideline for the management of heart failure: a report of the American College of Cardiology Foundation/American Heart Association Task Force on Practice Guidelines. J Am Coll Cardiol. 2013;62:147-239.
17. Abraham WT, Fisher WG, Smith AL, et al. Cardiac resynchronization in chronic heart failure. N Engl J Med. 2002;346:1845-53.
18. Fox DJ, Fitzpatrick AP, Davidson NC. Optimization of cardiac resynchronization therapy: addressing the problem of 'nonresponders'. Heart. 2005;91:1000-2.
19. Bax JJ, Bleeker GB, Marwick TH, et al. Left ventricular dyssynchrony predicts response and prognosis after cardiac resynchronization therapy. J Am Coll Cardiol. 2004;44:1834-40.
20. Leclercq C, Faris O, Tunin R, et al. Systolic improvement and mechanical resynchronization does not require electrical synchrony in the dilated failing heart with left bundle-branch block. Circulation. 2002;106:1760-3.
21. Dauphin R, Nonin E, Bontemps L, et al. Quantification of ventricular resynchronization reserve by radionuclide phase analysis in heart failure patients-a prospective long-term study. Circ Cardiovasc Imaging. 2011;4:114-21.
22. Toussaint JF, Lavergne T, Kerrou K, et al. Basal asynchrony and resynchronization with biventricular pacing predict long-term improvement of LV function in heart failure patients. Pacing Clin Electrophysiol. 2003;26:1815-23.
23. Mukherjee A, Patel CD, Naik N, et al. Quantitative assessment of cardiac mechanical dyssynchrony and prediction of response to cardiac resynchronization therapy in patients with non-ischaemic dilated cardiomyopathy using equilibrium radionuclide angiography. Europace. 2016;18:851-7.
24. Burri H, Domenichini G, Sunthorn H, et al. Right ventricular systolic function and cardiac resynchronization therapy. Europace. 2012;12:389-94.
25. Mukherjee A, Patel CD, Roy A, et al. Interplay between right ventricular mechanical dyssynchrony and cardiac resynchronization therapy in patients with nonischemic dilated cardiomyopathy. Nucl Med Commun. 2016;37:1016-23.
26. Henneman MM, Chen J, Dibbets P, et al. Can LV dyssynchrony as assessed with phase analysis on gated myocardial perfusion SPECT predict response to CRT? J Nucl Med. 2007;48:1104-11.
27. Mukherjee A, Patel CD, Naik N, et al. Quantitative assessment of cardiac mechanical dyssynchrony and prediction of response to cardiac resynchronization therapy in patients with nonischaemic dilated cardiomyopathy using gated myocardial perfusion SPECT. Nucl Med Commun. 2015;36:494-501.
28. Lin X, Xu H, Zhao X, et al. Repeatability of left ventricular dyssynchrony and function parameters in serial gated myocardial perfusion SPECT studies. J Nucl Cardiol. 2010;17:811-6.
29. Sommer A, Kronborg MB, Poulsen SH, et al. Empiric versus imaging guided left ventricular lead placement in cardiac

resynchronization therapy (Imaging CRT): study protocol for a randomized controlled trial. Trials. 2013;14:113.
30. Chen CC, She TY, Chang MC, et al. Stress-induced myocardial ischemia is associated with early post-stress left ventricular mechanical dyssynchrony as assessed by phase analysis of 201Tl gated SPECT myocardial perfusion imaging. Eur J Nucl Med Mol Imaging. 2012;39:1904-9.
31. Huang W, Huang C, Lee C, et al. Relation of early post-stress left ventricular dyssynchrony and the extent of angiographic coronary artery disease. J Nucl Cardiol. 2014;21:1048-56.
32. Gimelli A, Liga R, Giorgetti A, et al. Determinants of left ventricular mechanical dyssynchrony in patients submitted to myocardial perfusion imaging: A cardiac CZT study. J Nucl Cardiol. 2016;23:728-36.
33. Zafrir N, Nevzorov R, Bental T, et al. Prognostic value of left ventricular dyssynchrony by myocardial perfusion-gated SPECT in patients with normal and abnormal left ventricular functions. J Nucl Cardiol. 2014;21:532-40.
34. Uebleis C, Hellweger S, Laubender RP, et al. Left ventricular dyssynchrony assessed by gated SPECT phase analysis is an independent predictor of death in patients with advanced coronary artery disease and reduced left ventricular function not undergoing cardiac resynchronization therapy. Eur J Nucl Med Mol Imaging. 2012;39:1561-9.
35. Singh H, Patel CD, Sharma G, et al. Comparison of left ventricular systolic function and mechanical dyssynchrony using equilibrium radionuclide angiography in patients with right ventricular outflow tract versus right ventricular apical pacing: A prospective single-center study. J Nucl Cardiol. 2015;22:903-11.
36. Goldberg AS, Alraies MC, Cerqueira MD, et al. Prognostic value of left ventricular mechanical dyssynchrony by phase analysis in patients with non-ischemic cardiomyopathy with ejection fraction 35-50% and QRS<150 ms. J Nucl Cardiol. 2014;21:57-66.
37. Aljaroudi WA, Hage FG, Hermann D, et al. Relation of left-ventricular dyssynchrony by phase analysis of gated SPECT images and cardiovascular events in patients with implantable cardiac defibrillators. J Nucl Cardiol. 2010;17:398-404.
38. Aggarwal H, Aljaroudi WA, Mehta S, et al. The prognostic value of left ventricular mechanical dyssynchrony using gated myocardial perfusion imaging in patients with end-stage renal disease. J Nucl Cardiol. 2014;21:739-46.

INVASIVE

18 Is Optical Coherence Tomography Ready to Replace Intravascular Ultrasound in Percutaneous Coronary Intervention?

Debabrata Dash

INTRODUCTION

Optical coherence tomography (OCT), an optical analog of intravascular ultrasound (IVUS) is an emerging catheter-based intravascular imaging modality for diagnostic and interventional procedures. It produces images with 10-times improved resolution compared with IVUS, at the expense of lower penetration into the tissue.[1] The high resolution of OCT imaging enables it to serve as an "optical biopsy" facilitating detailed plaque characterization and measurement of details that remained elusive for angiography and IVUS. Even if this modality emerged in cardiology as a research tool, it has the potential to become a standard routine tool for diagnostic application and guidance of percutaneous coronary intervention (PCI). The author analyses in depth its use for assessment of lesion severity, characterization of acute coronary syndrome (ACS), guidance of intracoronary stenting and evaluation of long-term results.

ROLE OF OPTICAL COHERENCE TOMOGRAPHY BEFORE PERCUTANEOUS CORONARY INTERVENTION

Plaque Composition and Lesion Severity

The OCT details coronary plaque morphology and identify thrombus, calcification intimal rupture, lipid rich plaque and fibrous cap thickness.[2] The presence, depth, and circumferential extent of calcification can affect percutaneous coronary intervention (PCI) result negatively.[3,4] IVUS identifies calcium but fails to measure the thickness.[5] OCT on the other hand, can measure superficial calcific components with a thickness of < 1.0–1.3 mm, affecting important decisions regarding interventionist's strategy, such as avoidance of direct stenting, use of bioabsorbable vascular scaffold (BVS), and use of scoring balloons or rotational atherectomy. The ability of OCT to precisely assess calcium accumulation and arc of circumference of within the arterial wall may significantly impact the final PCI result.

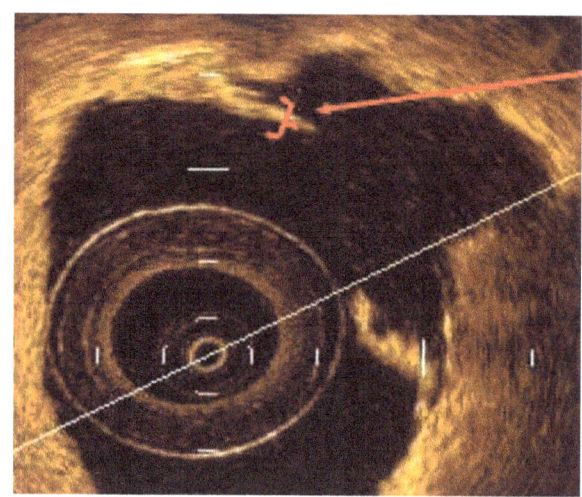

Fig. 1: Optical coherence tomography depicting thin cap fibroatheroma

As OCT identifies lipid pool with greater accuracy than IVUS. Suggesting how to treat the lesion and where to land the stent to avoid immediate ischemic complications. The identification of normal or "less diseased" reference vessel for accurate stent placement is of pivotal importance in PCI. Placing a stent over thin cap fibroatheroma (TCFA) **(Fig. 1)** is associated with periprocedural myocardial infarction, whereas disruption of such cases may lead to increased risk of neoatherosclerosis and stent thrombosis as demonstrated by OCT and pathological studies.[5,6] Even frequency of no-reflow increases according to lipid pool and fibrous cap thinning as suggested by OCT.[7] Avoidance of landing a stent within a TCFA or a calcified plaque reduces the rate of edge dissections, stent thrombosis and plaque embolization.[8,9]

The OCT allows clear delineation between the lumen and vessel wall. It has been validated in vitro and in vivo for

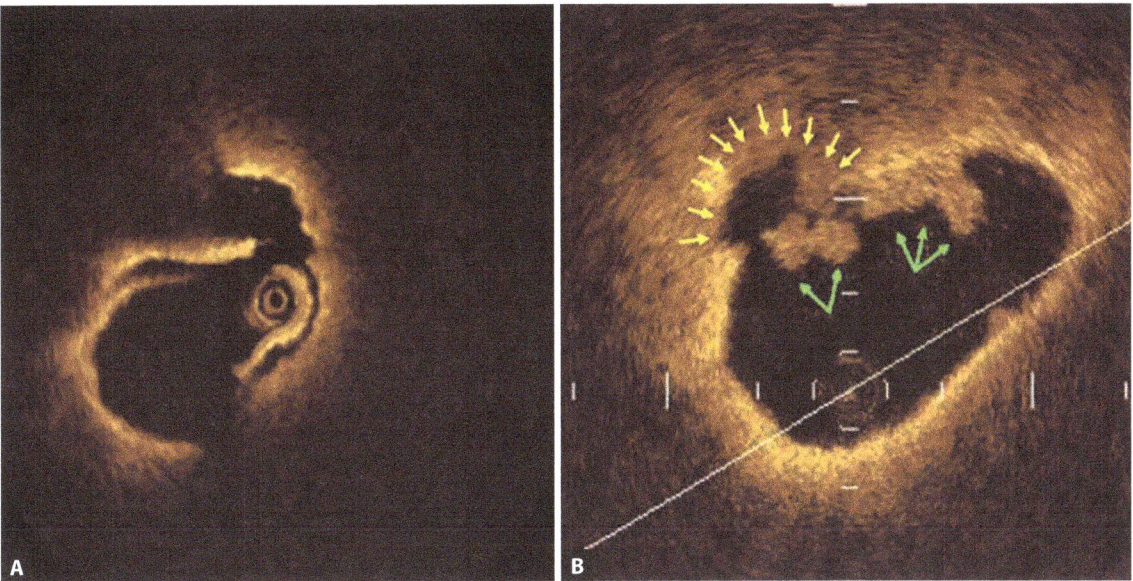

Figs 2A and B: Optical coherence tomography depicting. (A) Plaque rupture; (B) Plaque erosion

lumen measurements, demonstrating higher accuracy[10,11] and reproducibility[12] than IVUS. The very soft neointimal plaque could be missed by IVUS thereby making OCT a superior modality for evaluating in-stent restenosis. It could unravel the prevalent mechanism of restenosis (incomplete expansion vs intimal proliferation) due to the ability to visualize struts deep in the vessel wall.

Ambiguous Angiographic Lesions

The OCT may help in clarifying ambiguous lesions with angiographic haziness in ACS. It often detects ruptures plaques with thrombus attached to the site of plaque rupture.[13] Under these circumstances, the decision to proceed with treatment can stem more from morphological plaque features than from absolute measurement of minimal lumen area (MLA).[13] Misinterpretation of the culprit lesion could be the cause of additional early adverse ischemic syndromes in ACS.

Lesion Progression and Vulnerability

The OCT can identify lesions at risk of lesion progression and future adverse events. It detects lipid-rich TCFA combined with microvessels and foamy macrophages. Combined angiographic and OCT images with additional mathematic computation of flow velocity and shear stress may possibly allow better prediction of plaque evaluation.[14]

Acute Coronary Syndrome and Primary Percutaneous Coronary Intervention

The OCT is superior to IVUS in providing useful insights into pathophysiology of ACS, differentiating between plaque rupture/erosion **(Figs 2A and B)** and calcified nodules.[13] The effectiveness of thrombus removal and any further need for thrombus aspiration can be easily identified by this imaging modality. The remaining thrombus also may increase the risk of subsequent stent failure (e.g. stent thrombosis, late acquired incomplete stent apposition owing to clot reabsorption, and neoatherosclerosis). In addition, enhanced vessel constriction makes it difficult to choose the appropriate stent sizing and length. In this setting, stent length and size should be measured by accurate lumen measurements by OCT.

Bifurcation Lesions

Plaque distribution, carina geometry, and bifurcation angle have a great impact on PCI strategy selection and rate of side branch occlusion after stenting. Even if spared from lesion involvement, an elongated carina may obstruct side branch after main branch stenting. This type of "eyebrow" carina detectable on the longitudinal view and 3D reconstruction by OCT,[15-17] should prompt the interventionists to protect the side branch with another wire. It can also help navigate wire recrossing of the side branch, thereby avoiding stent distortion.

Left Main Disease

With the exceptions of ostial lesions, OCT enables quick evaluation of shaft and left main bifurcation disease. It evaluates extension of the disease into left anterior descending and/or left circumflex arteries, plaque type, the anatomic type of carina and degree of lesion involvement, size difference between left main and distal landing zone.[18] Post-PCI, it detects with greater accuracy than IVUS the presence of dissection, stent malapposition, underexpansion and size mismatch.

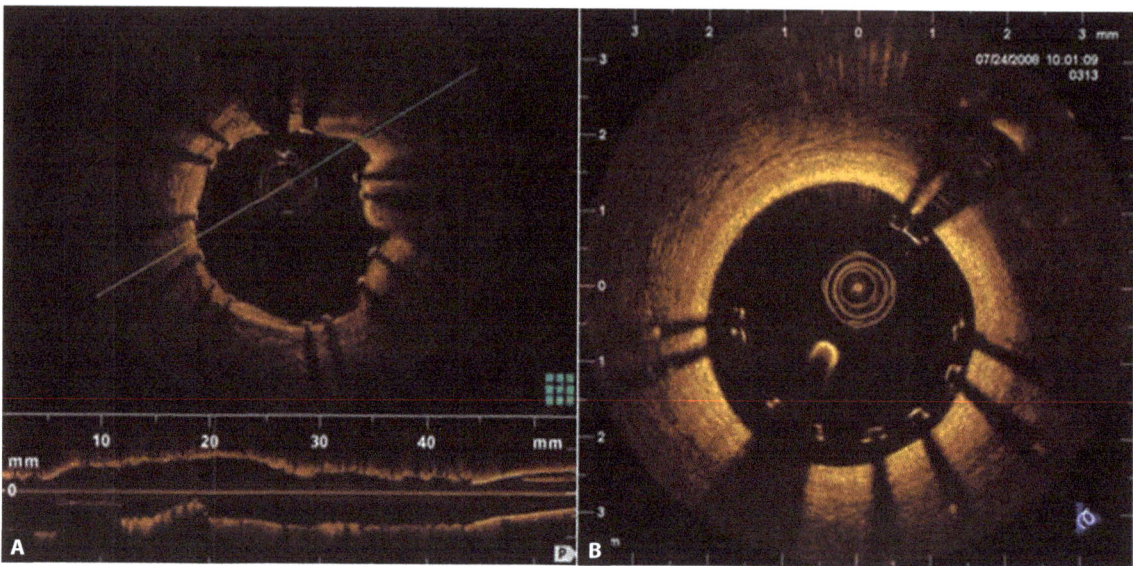

Figs 3A and B: Optical coherence tomography. (A) Stent underexpansion; (B) Incomplete stent apposition

Implantation of Bioabsorbable Vascular Scaffold

The OCT played a significant role in the development of bioabsorbable vascular scaffold (BVS) technology and in providing proof of the scaffold's biological and mechanical characteristics.[19] Unlike metallic stent, light is not attenuated by polymeric struts of BVS making them transparent on OCT imaging. BVS dimensions progressively increase without a change in lumen area between 1 and 3 years, and there is complete strut reabsorption at 3 to 5 years. The lesion preparation is of paramount importance owing to the reduced device expandability, because postdilatation is limited to balloons no more than 0.5 mm larger than BVS diameter. OCT has been recommended for BVS size selection and optimization, particularly in complex settings (i.e. calcified lesions, bifurcations, chronic total occlusions, ostial involvement), because a substantial stent underexpansion cannot be accommodated with overstretched diameter beyond its designated diameter.

OPTICAL COHERENCE TOMOGRAPHY IN ASSESSMENT OF STENTING

The OCT identifies the details such as stent underexpansion, incomplete stent apposition (ISA) **(Figs 3A and B)**, uneven stent strut distribution, intrastent thrombus, and dissections at the edges and inside the stent with the accuracy unmatched by IVUS **(Table 1)**.[20] It can measure minimal stent area (MSA) and lumen area of the reference vessel semiautomatically, allowing quick and accurate assessment of the expansion and sizing of the stent. ISA correlates with thrombus detection and late/very late stent thrombosis (L/VLST). ISA may delay neointimal healing of the stent[21-23] and incomplete endothelialization of the struts is a common morphological finding in fatal cases of L/VLST.[24,25] OCT is capable of detecting subclinical dissections, micro-dissections and other forms of vascular injury, like wire perforations, that remain unnoticed by IVUS. Recent data indicated that residual intrastent thrombus is related to periprocedural myocardial infarction in a multivariate logistic regression analysis.[5]

POSTINTERVENTION ASSESSMENT

The IVUS has classically used extensively to quantify neointimal hyperplasia (NIH) months after PCI. However, drug-eluting stents inhibit neointimal proliferation to such an extent (average late lumen loss in modern second-generation stents is as low as 0.1–0.2 mm) that it may not be detectable by IVUS as it lacks the axial resolution to evaluate it. On the other hand, the superior resolution of OCT allows for the visualization and measurement of thin layers of tissue growth covering stents **(Table 1)**. Several studies points to delayed intimal healing as the underlying mechanism in cases of stent thrombosis.[24,25] Percent neointimal volume to assess neointimal hyperplasia is delineated with greater accuracy by OCT as compared to IVUS. The absolute ISA volume or maximal ISA area, or maximal strut-vessel distance per strut are better predictors of the neointimal reaction to malappostion.[22] OCT also enables strut by strut analysis which is beyond the capability of IVUS. The neointimal healing response after PCI tends to decrease ISA areas and volume over time up to 24 months in different stents,[26-28] although one study has reported exactly the opposite in sirolimus eluting stent between 24 and 48 months.[29]

Table 1 Comparative technical summary of IVUS and OCT for diagnostic and interventional purposes

Features	OCT	IVUS
Axial resolution (um)	10–20	100–200
Lateral resolution (um)	20–90	200–300
Rotation speed (Hz)	16–160	30
Pull-back speed (mm/sec)	1–20	0.5–1
Tissue penetration (mm)	1–3	10
Scan diameter-field of view (mm)	7–11	15
Necrotic core	+++	+
TCFA	+++	–
Thrombus	+++	+
Stent expansion/sizing	+++	+++
Stent apposition	+++	++
Vascular injury	+++	++
PCI guidance	+	++
Stent restenosis/NIH	++	+++
Stent coverage	+++	–

The usefulness of each imaging technique has been graded from not useful (-) to very useful (+++), according to the rational explained.
Abbreviations: IVUS, intravascular ultrasound; NIH, neointimal hyperplasia; PCI, percutaneous coronary intervention; OCT, optical coherence tomography; TCFA, thin cap fibroatheroma

OCT quantifies quite accurately neointimal hyperplasia and determines if it is homogeneous, heterogeneous or layered.[30] This could help in better understanding of the mechanism of in-stent restenosis.

ARTIFACTS

Both IVUS and OCT experience artifacts during image acquisition. Certain artifacts are shared by both, whereas others are unique to their respective imaging technique. OCT's smaller profile and simplified rotational mechanisms make it less prone to mechanical artifacts. A study using a phantom model found that OCT experienced less nonuniform rotational distortion than IVUS, particularly in more tortuous vessel.[31]

WILL OPTICAL COHERENCE TOMOGRAPHY REPLACE INTRAVASCULAR ULTRASOUND?

In spite of tremendous advantages, OCT- the "new kid on the block", has also some shortcomings. Flushing is necessary to clear the blood to visualize the vessel wall. Predilation may be necessary before PCI to allow static blood to be flushed from the lumen. Alternatively, some interventionalists forgo pre-PCI imaging and only perform poststent OCT, so that the potential advantage of pre-PCI assessment and stent sizing is lost. There is lack of data on OCT predictors of stent failure, OCT criteria for stent sizing and optimization, and the clinical benefits of OCT-guided stent implantation. OCT has a limited penetration depth, an evident shortcoming for the assessment of total vessel size and vascular remodeling, and is inferior to IVUS in a progression-regression trials. The interpretation of pseudomicroscopic OCT images is quite difficult. Moreover, the discrimination between lipidic and calcific plaque components could be quite challenging as both can have low image intensity.[32] The author feels that OCT is not yet ready to replace IVUS. OCT stent studies continue to focus on mechanisms of stent failure (restenosis and thrombosis), long-term comparisons of different stent platforms (extent of tissue coverage and malapposition) and qualitative analysis of the composition of neointimal tissue. There are few clinical studies attempted to assess the utility of the OCT, either diagnostically or during stent-implantation procedures. The paradigms for IVUS guidance and criteria for optimization do not translate directly to OCT. Much work needs to be done to define the best OCT-guided stent sizing strategy and the appropriate endpoints for OCT-guided stent optimization.[20,33]

CONCLUSION

The OCT is a recently introduced high-resolution imaging modality having unique features that provide in-depth information regarding the vascular biology. It has established itself as an excellent tool for atherosclerosis characterization, especially in the detection of vulnerable plaques, and assessment of vascular response to intracoronary devices. The plethora of detailed structural information along with great potential for technology and software development makes OCT an outstanding tool for clinical decision making, guiding and optimizing PCI. Whether these beneficial advantages will translate into an improvement in patient-related outcomes is an issue to be determined in large prospective randomized studies. As of today, OCT is not ready, does not completely eliminate the need for IVUS imaging technologies and unlikely to replace IVUS in spite of superior resolution. OCT and IVUS are likely to be important and complementary imaging techniques *(rather than one being a substitute for the other)*. Moreover, fusion of both imaging modalities they could even be better and has considerable future potential.

REFERENCES

1. Huang D, Swanson EA, Lin CP, et al. Optical coherence tomography. Science. 1991;254:1178-81.
2. Prati F, Regar E, Mintz GS, et al. Expert review document on methodology and clinical applications of OCT. Physical principles, methodology of image acquisition and clinical application for assessment of coronary arteries and atherosclerosis. Eur Heart J. 2010;31:401-15.

3. Martin-Yuste, Barros A, Leta R, et al. Factors determining success in percutaneous revascularization of chronic total coronary occlusion: multidetector computed tomography analysis. Rev Esp Cardio. 2012;65:334-40.
4. Tenaglia AN, Buller CE, Kisslo KB, et al. Intracoronary ultrasound predictors of adverse outcomes after coronary artery interventions. J Am Coll Cardio. 1992;20:1385-94.
5. Porto I, Di Vito L, Burzotta F, et al. Predictors of periprocedural (type IVa) myocardial infarction, as assessed by frequency-domain optical coherence tomography. Circ Cardiovasc Interv 2012;5:89-96. S1-6.
6. Jonner M, Finn AV, Farb A, et al. Pathology of drug-eluting stents in humans: delayed healing and late thrombotic risk. J Am Coll Cardiol. 2006;48:193-202.
7. Tanaka A, Imanishi T, Kitabata H, et al. Lipid-rich plaque and myocardial perfusion after successful stenting in patients with non-ST segment elevation acute coronary syndrome: an optical coherence tomography study. Eur Heart J. 2009;30:1348-55.
8. Chamie D, Bezerra HG, Attizzani GF, et al. Incidence, predictors, morphological characteristics, and clinical outcomes of stent edge dissections detected by optical coherence tomography. JACC Cardiovasc Interv. 2013;6:800-13.
9. Mintz GS, Nissen SE, Anderson WD, et al. ACC Clinical Expert Consensus Document on standards for the acquisition, measurement and reporting of intravascular ultrasound studies: a report of the American College of Cardiology Task Force on Clinical Expert Consensus Documents (Committee to Develop a Clinical Expert Consensus Document on Standards for the Acquisition, Measurement and Reporting of Intravascular Ultrasound Studies [IVUS]). J Am Coll Cardiol. 2001;37:1478-92.
10. Gonzalo N, Serruys PW, Garcia-Garcia HM, et al. Quantitative ex vivo and in vivo comparison lumen dimensions measured by optical coherence tomography and intravascular ultrasound in human coronary arteries. Rev Esp Cardiol. 2009;62:615-24.
11. Kawase Y, Hoshini K, Yoneyama R, et al. In vivo volumetric analysis of coronary stents using optical coherence tomography with a novel balloon occlusion-flushing catheter: a comparison with intravascular ultrasound. Ultrasound Med Biol. 2005;31:1343-9.
12. Gonzalo N, Garcia-Garcia HM, , Serruys PW, et al. Reproducibility of quantitative optical coherence tomography for stent analysis. Euro Intervention. 2009;5:224-32.
13. Prati F, Regar E, Mintz GS, et al. Experts OCT Review Document. Expert review document part 2: methodology, terminology and clinical applications of OCT for the assessment of interventional procedures. Eur Heart J. 2012;33:2513-20.
14. Uemura S, Ishigami K, Soeda T, et al. Thin-cap fibroatheroma and microchannel findings in optical coherence tomography correlate with subsequent progression of coronary atheromatous plaques. Eur Heart J. 2012;33:78-85.
15. Di Mario C, Ikavou I, van der Gissen WJ, et al. Optical coherence tomography for guidance in bifurcation lesion treatment. Euro Intervention. 2006;6(Suppl J):99-106.
16. Farooq V, Serruys PW, Heo JH, et al. New insights into the coronary artery bifurcation hypothesis-generating concepts utilizing 3-dimensional optical frequency domain imaging. JACC Cardiovasc Interv. 2011;4:921-31.
17. Karanasos A, Tu S, van der Heide E, et al. Carina shift as a mechanism for side-branch compromise following main vessel intervention: insights from three-dimensional optical coherence tomography. Cardiovasc Diagn Ther. 2012;2:173-7.
18. Fujino Y, Bezerra HG, Attizani GF, et al. Frequency-domain optical coherence tomography assessment of unprotected left main coronary artery disease-a comparison with intravascular ultrasound. Catheter Cardiovasc Interv. 2013;82:E173-183.
19. Mattesini A, Secco GG, Dall' Ara G, et al. ABSORB biodegradable stents versus second-generation metal stents: a comparison study of 100 complex lesions treated under OCT guidance. JACC Cardiovasc Interv. 2014;7:741-50.
20. Waksman R, Kitabata H, Prati F, et al. Intravascular ultrasound versus optical coherence tomography. J Am Coll Cardiol. 2013;62:S32-S40.
21. Ozaki Y, Okumara M, Ismail TF, et al. The fate of incomplete stent apposition with drug-eluting stents: an optical coherence tomography-based natural history study. Eur Heart J. 2010;31:1470-6.
22. Gutierrez-Chico J, Wykrzykowska JJ, Nuesch E, et al. Vascular tissue reaction to acute malapposition in human coronary arteries: sequential assessment with optical coherence tomography. Circ Cardiovasc Interv. 2012;5:20-9.
23. Gutiérrez-Chico JL, Regar E, Nüesch E, et al. Delayed coverage in malapposed and side-branch struts with respect to well-apposed struts in drug-eluting stents: in vivo assessment with optical coherence tomography. Circulation. 2011;124:612-23.
24. Finn AV, Joner M, Nakazawa G, et al. Pathological correlates of late drug-eluting stent thrombosis: strut coverage as a marker of endothelialization. Circulation. 2007;115:2435-244.
25. Virmani R, Guagliumi G, Farb A, et al. Localized hypersensitivity and late coronary thrombosis secondary to a sirolimus-eluting stent: should we be cautious? Circulation. 2004;109:701-5.
26. Kume T, Akasaka T, Kawamoto T, et al. Assessment of coronary intima media thickness by optical coherence tomography: comparison with intravascular ultrasound. Circ J. 2005;69:903-7.
27. Gutiérrez-Chico JL, van Geuns RJ, Koch KT, et al. Paclitaxel-coated balloon in combination with bare metal stent for treatment of de novo coronary lesions: an optical coherence tomography first-in-human randomised trial, balloon first vs. stent first. Euro Intervention. 2011;7:711-722.
28. Gutiérrez-Chico JL, Jüni P, García-García HM, et al. Long-term tissue coverage of a biodegradable polylactide polymer-coated biolimus-eluting stent: comparative sequential assessment with optical coherence tomography until complete resorption of the polymer. Am Heart J. 2011;162:922-31.
29. Takano M, Yamamoto M, Mizuno M, et al. Late vascular responses from 2 to 4 years after implantation of sirolimus-eluting stents: serial observations by intracoronary optical coherence tomography. Circ Cardiovasc Interv. 2010;3:476-83.
30. Gonzalo N, Serruys PW, Okamura T, et al. Optical coherence tomography patterns of stent restenosis. Am Heart J. 2009;158:284-93.
31. Kawase Y, Suzuki Y, Ikeno F, et al. Comparison of nonuniform rotational distortion between mechanical IVUS and OCT using a phantom model. Ultrasound Med Biol. 2007;33:67-73.
32. Jennifer Huisman J, Hartmann M, and von Birgelen C. Ultrasound and light: friend or foe? On the role of intravascular ultrasound in the era of optical coherence tomography. Int J Cardiovasc Imaging. 2011;27:209-14.
33. Dash D. Application of intravascular ultrasound in the era of optical coherence tomography. EC Cardiology. 2015;2.1:90-3.

19 Association of Coronary Stenosis and Plaque Morphology with Fractional Flow Reserve and Outcomes

Jagat Narula

The Fractional Flow Reserve Versus Angiography for Multivessel Evaluation (FAME) trial[1,2] demonstrated that in patients with stable ischemic heart disease, an fractional flow reserve (FFR)-guided strategy to identify hemodynamically significant lesions requiring percutaneous coronary intervention (PCI) can safely defer revascularization in lower-risk lesions and reduce the number of procedures and rates of future urgent revascularization due to unstable angina or myocardial infarction (MI) compared with lesion selection by angiography alone. The FAME2 trial[3,4] extended these findings and demonstrated that deferring PCI in lesions with an abnormal FFR results in high rates of progressive ischemic symptoms, unstable angina, and MI, which require revascularization within 1–2 years. These outcomes could be prevented by PCI.[1-4] Although FFR identifies hemodynamically significant lesions likely to produce ischemia-related symptoms, less clear is why FFR might predict the subsequent risk for acute coronary syndrome (ACS) resulting from plaque rupture and coronary thrombosis, which is usually caused by lipid-rich plaques with distinct histological features.[5-13] These observations prompted us to explore whether plaque features of vulnerability and their physiologic properties are associated, causing a relevant pressure gradient across the lesion detectable by FFR.

SEVERITY OF LUMINAL STENOSIS AND FRACTIONAL FLOW RESERVE

Ischemia is best defined as an inadequate supply of oxygen relative to myocardial demand. The most widely used tests to assess ischemia are myocardial perfusion imaging (MPI) (noninvasive) and FFR (invasive). Myocardial perfusion imaging and FFR use the abnormal blood flow in the affected vessels as a surrogate marker for ischemia. In turn, this abnormal blood flow is related to relative or complete inability of the vessel to dilate on stress. Although the detection of ischemia is likely to be indicative of a severe epicardial coronary artery stenosis,[14] this association is not perfect.[2,15,16] Some severely stenotic lesions may not result in detectable ischemia (stenosis without ischemia [SWOI]), whereas other lesions with only a mild to moderate degree of angiographic stenosis may induce ischemia (ischemia without significant stenosis [IWOS]).[17] In the FAME study,[1,18] more than one-third of lesions with an angiographic 50–70% angiographic diameter stenosis demonstrated an FFR of 0.80 or less whereas one-fifth of lesions with a 71–90% angiographic diameter stenosis demonstrated an FFR greater than 0.80 (SWOI) **(Fig. 1A)**. In a separate prospective study of 1000 patients with 1129 coronary lesions,[15] more than one-half of lesions with greater than 50% angiographic diameter stenosis had an FFR greater than 0.80, whereas 1 in 7 lesions with less than 50% angiographic diameter stenosis had an FFR of 0.80 or less (IWOS) **(Fig. 1B)**. Among lesions with 50–70% luminal stenosis, approximately half had an FFR of 0.80 or less, whereas the other half had a normal FFR and no lesion-specific ischemia. These observations emphasize the importance of identifying factors beyond luminal stenosis that might contribute to inducible ischemia.

Some cases of IWOS may be explained by the inability of angiography to discriminate the true lesion severity with accuracy owing to diffuse disease or other artifacts.[19] Microvascular disease can result in inducible ischemia as detected by an abnormal MPI finding or abnormal coronary flow reserve in the absence of a severe epicardial coronary artery stenosis, which explains some cases of IWOS. Unlike coronary flow reserve, however, FFR is derived from the epicardial pressure gradient on vasodilator-induced maximal coronary flow and excludes microcirculatory resistance. Therefore, FFR is largely independent of changes in the basal flow and status of the microcirculation or systemic

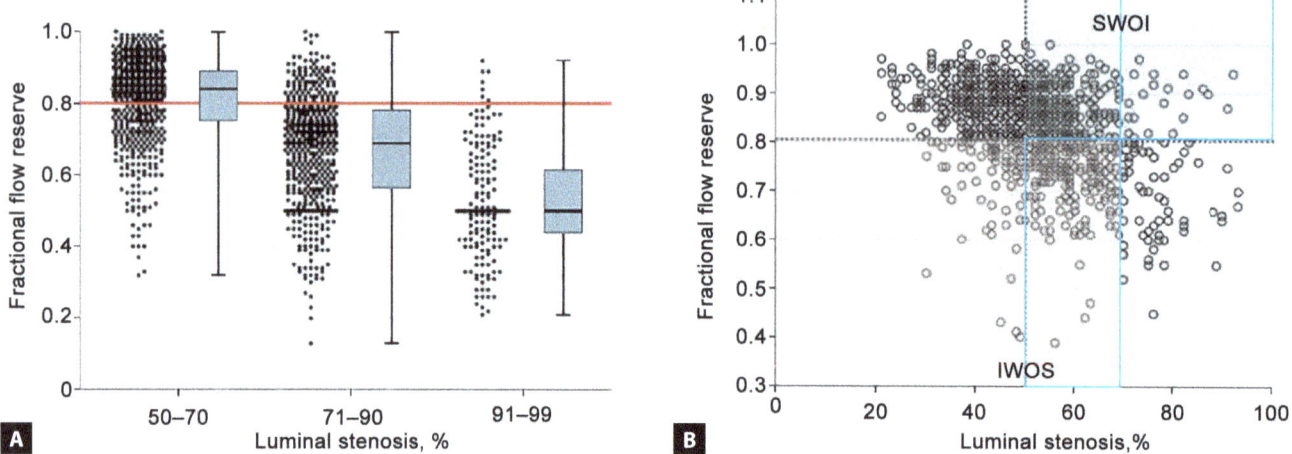

Figs 1A and B: Correlation between the degree of luminal stenosis by coronary angiography and ischemia detected by fractional flow reserve (FFR). (A) In the Fractional Flow Reserve Versus Angiography for Multivessel Evaluation (FAME) trial, among the 623 lesions with 50–70% stenosis, 218 (35.0%) had an FFR of 0.80 or less (FFR-verified ischemia without significant stenosis [IWOS]). Among 520 lesions with 71–90% stenosis, 104 (20.0%) demonstrated an FFR of greater than 0.80 (FFR-verified stenosis without ischemia [SWOI]). Boxes indicate first and third quartiles; horizontal lines in boxes, median; whiskers, minimum and maximum data distribution (modified from Tonino et al.[18]); (B) In a prospective study of 1000 patients (Study of the Natural History of FFR Guided Percutaneous Coronary Intervention[16] [IRIS FFR]), 343 of 605 coronary lesions (56.7%) with less than 50% angiographic stenosis had an FFR of greater than 0.80 (FFR-verified SWOI), whereas 75 of 461 lesions (16.3%) with less than 50% luminal stenosis had an FFR of 0.80 or less (FFR-verified IWOS). Using a cut point for a severe stenos is diameter of 70%, a large proportion of lesions with less than 70% angiographic diameter stenosis had an FFR of 0.80 or less. Among lesions with 50–70% angiographic diameter stenosis, approximately half were positive for FFR and half were negative for FFR (i.e. no predictive value). Data points indicate degree of stenosis and corresponding FFR (modified from Park et al.[15])

hemodynamics,[20] and microvascular disease cannot explain FFR-positive IWOS. On the other hand, some cases of MPI-verified SWOI may be explained by short lesion length, redundancy of the arterial supply through collateral vessel formation, and a limited myocardial territory supplied by the diseased artery. As regards FFR, features such as lesion length, entrance angle, exit angle, size of the reference vessel, and absolute flow relative to the territory supplied are important in determining focal hemodynamic responses to hyperemia and might explain the discrepancy between the epicardial luminal narrowing and FFR-based physiologic significance of the lesion in many cases.[21,22] Regardless of the causes, angiography is recognized as a suboptimal method to assess the ischemic potential of an epicardial coronary stenosis.

PLAQUE MORPHOLOGY AND FRACTIONAL FLOW RESERVE

Although the factors discussed above explain IWOS and SWOI in some cases, they do not explain the discrepancy in many others. Recent reports have linked the presence of lipid-rich plaques to the presence of FFR-verified ischemia demonstrated to be independent of the degree of luminal narrowing.[23,24] In a concomitant study of radiofrequency intravascular ultrasonography (IVUS) and FFR[25] performed in coronary arteries with 50–70% angiographic diameter stenosis, only the lipid-rich plaque type correlated with a reduced FFR; the FFR was concomitantly lower in increasingly larger necrotic cores. These results were confirmed in a larger study of 407 coronary lesions in 252 patients who underwent coronary computed tomographic angiography (CTA), computed tomography-based FFR assessment, and invasive angiography and FFR assessment.[23] The presence of a large plaque volume, large low attenuation plaque volume, and higher positive remodeling index were found to be strongly predictive of reduced FFR regardless of the degree of stenosis on multivariable analysis. Low-attenuation plaques (considered a CTA surrogate for necrotic core) with a positive remodeling index (termed 2-feature-positive plaque [2FPP]) have been reported to be associated with major adverse coronary events.[5,26] In another recent study of 484 coronary vessels,[24] comparison of coronary CTA-defined plaque characteristics and luminal stenosis and FFR assessed from CTA with invasive angiography and invasive FFR revealed that large low-attenuation plaques (volume >30 mm^3 on CTA) constituted the strongest lesion characteristic predictive of invasive FFR. Large low-attenuation plaques yielded diagnostic improvement for detecting lesion-specific ischemia by invasive FFR beyond degree of stenosis and other lesion characteristics, including lesion length.[24] In studies performing CTA and MPI concurrently,[23,27] the presence of

2FPP was associated with greater than 5% total myocardial ischemia burden, and conversely the presence of significant ischemia had a high positive predictive value for detecting 2FPP. The extent of luminal stenosis was not different between plaques that caused significant ischemia and those that did not; both demonstrated mean luminal stenosis of 75%.[27] Therefore, large lipid-rich, positively remodeled plaque (i.e. 2FPP), and not only the stenosis severity, demonstrates a strong likelihood of inflicting myocardial ischemia.

This association between large necrotic cores and low FFR (independent of luminal stenosis) cannot be readily explained by the currently recognized determinants of physiologic lesion severity. Fractional flow reserve is presumed to measure the net physiologic effects of a coronary stenosis by maximally dilating the distal arteriolar bed with the administration of adenosine. Although the reduced FFR in the absence of severe stenosis (IWOS) cannot be explained by adenosine-mediated arteriolar dilatation, nitroglycerin (invariably given before adenosine administration) may not induce dilatation at the site of a plaque containing a large necrotic core with extraluminal expansion and positive remodeling. If a lipid-rich plaque is associated with local inability of the stenotic vascular segment to dilate to the same extent as the rest of the vessel (possibly owing to a maximally stretched vessel similar to the glagovian limit[28]), the result would be a relative pressure drop at the time of maximal hyperemia. This process could underlie some of the unexplained cases of IWOS. On the other hand, luminally stenotic plaques without large necrotic cores and without outwardly stretched vessels (e.g. fibrotic or fibrocalcific plaques) may retain locally vasodilatory potential and at least partially explain SWOI.[29-31] If this explanation is valid, then the absence of ischemia may signal the presence of preserved vasodilatory capacity, which may also indicate that the plaque is unlikely to contain a large necrotic core.

Local oxidative stress and vascular inflammation have also been proposed to contribute to impaired vasodilator capacity.[30,31] The lipid rich necrotic core, a hallmark of the vulnerable plaque, inflicts local oxidative stress[32] and thus could play a contributory role.[17] The relationship between plaque composition (fibrous, fibrofatty, fatty, or calcific as identified by IVUS radiofrequency spectral analysis) and the vasodilatory potential of the local epicardial coronary artery evaluated by acetylcholine challenge suggested that only the presence of anecrotic core was associated with impaired vasodilator responses.[29]

FRACTIONAL FLOW RESERVE AND SUBSEQUENT CLINICAL EVENTS

In the last decade, the identification of the hemodynamic significance of coronary artery lesions has become increasingly important. The FAME and FAME 2 studies demonstrated that revascularization guided by FFR is superior to angiography-guided therapy and optimum medical therapy (OMT).[1,4] In the FAME trial[1] **(Flow chart 1A)**, the reduction in rates of major adverse cardiac events at 1 and 2 years with FFR-guided therapy compared with angiography-guided therapy was driven by a significant decrease in the incidence of MI and the need for urgent revascularization.[1,2] Analyses of the results of the FAME study[2] **(Flow chart 1A)** demonstrate that the superiority of the FFR-guided therapy most likely emerges from safe deferral of FFR-negative lesions to OMT, decreasing unnecessary procedures and their consequent complications **(Flow chart 1B)**. The FAME study also demonstrates that, compared with angiography-driven therapy, the FFR-guided strategy decreases the likelihood of MI by one-third (6.1% vs 9.9%) and urgent revascularization in a setting of MI by two-fifths (7.3% vs 12.7%). In the FAME2 trial **(Flow chart 1B)**, deferring PCI of stenotic lesions with an FFR of 0.80 or less resulted in higher rates of urgent revascularization (16.0% vs 4.0%) and postprocedure death or MI (8.2% vs 6.5%) compared with PCI for such lesions.[3,4] In that study,[3,4] the main difference in outcomes emerged from the need for urgent revascularization in the OMT group. As a result, it is currently believed that all FFR-positive lesions should be treated with revascularization. However, the rates of death and MI were not significantly different between the 2 groups in the FAME 2 study[4]; there was an 8.2% chance of death or MI in 2 years in the FFR-positive lesions treated with OMT alone, compared with 6.5% rate in the OMT group[4] **(Flow chart 1B)**. Therefore, we can conclude from these observations that (1) lesions with negative FFR findings can be treated safely with OMT alone and (2) although lesions with positive FFR findings are at higher risk for future events, whether all FFR-positive lesions need revascularization remains unclear.

In FAME and FAME2, an FFR-based strategy resulted in reduced rates of MI (and the composite outcome of death or MI), especially in the postprocedural period, and in reduced rates of new-onset ACS. This result raises an important issue. Although FFR identifies hemodynamically significant lesions likely to produce ischemia-related symptoms, how does FFR also predict the likelihood of ACS and MI that usually result from plaque rupture and coronary thrombosis?

PLAQUE MORPHOLOGY: A LINK BETWEEN FRACTIONAL FLOW RESERVE AND CLINICAL OUTCOMES

Examining the outcomes of different types of stenoses in the FAME trials allows formulation of a hypothesis regarding their possible underlying composition **(Fig. 3)**. As mentioned before, plaques with large necrotic cores should be predictive of ischemia and ACS. Conversely, despite luminal narrowing, the absence of ischemia (reflecting preserved vasodilatory capacity or SWOI) indicates plaques without large necrotic cores. This finding suggests that ischemia may be a sensitive

Flow charts 1A and B: Utility of fractional flow reserve (FFR) in differentiating high-risk vs low-risk plaques and identifying those lesions in need of revascularization. The Fractional Flow Reserve Versus Angiography for Multivessel Evaluation (FAME) and FAME 2 trials have demonstrated that percutaneous coronary intervention (PCI) may be safely deferred in lesions with FFR of greater than 0.80, and conversely those lesions with FFR of 0.80 or less have an improved prognosis with PCI. In the FAME trial, among 513 with deferred angiography and severe lesions (FFR >0.80) in the FFR group, only 1 myocardial infarction (MI; 0.2%) occurred and only 16 (3.1%) urgent revascularizations among 513 lesions were needed during the 2-year follow-up, compared with 49 MIs (9.9%) and 63 urgent revascularizations (12.7%) in the angiography-guided group of patients. In the FAME 2 trial, in which lesions with FFR of 0.80 or less were randomized to PCI with optimum medical therapy (OMT) vs OMT alone, the rates of postprocedural MI, total urgent revascularizations, and urgent revascularizations owing to MI were significantly higher in the OMT group compared with the PCI + OMT group and compared with the outcomes in a parallel registry OMT group of patients in whom the FFR was greater than 0.80 in all lesions. However, the rates of death and MI were not significantly different between the 2 groups[4]; an 8.2% chance of death or MI in 2 years was found in the FFR-positive lesions treated with OMT alone, not significantly different from the 6.5% rate in the OMT group (developed from the FAME and FAME 2 studies[1-4])

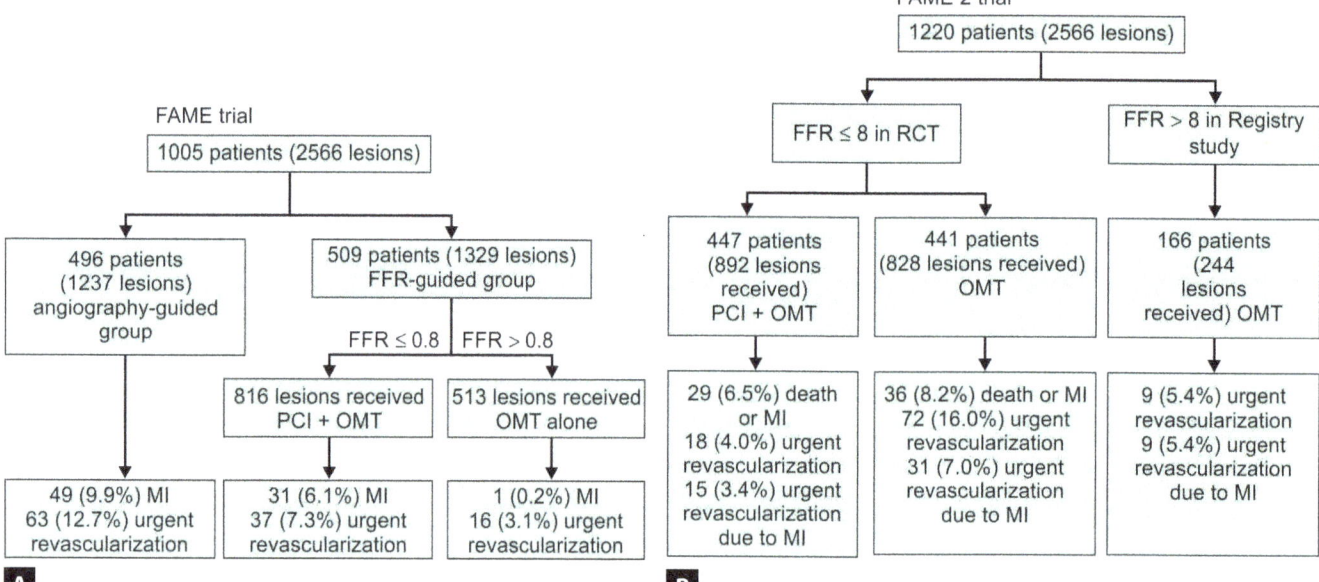

but not specific surrogate for the presence of a positively remodeled plaque with a large necrotic core and that the lack of ischemia indicates absence of such lipid-rich plaques with a normal vasodilator response.[27] Therefore, in the FAME trial, an FFR value of greater than 0.80 in 104 lesions with angiographic stenosis severity of 71–90% might suggest the absence of large necrotic core–carrying 2FPP in that subgroup. Conversely, the 218 plaques with intermediate luminal stenosis (50–70% by angiography) with an FFR of 0.80 or less probably indicates large-volume 2FPP or longer lesions in which the severity could not be determined accurately by angiography **(Fig. 2)**.

Because an abnormal FFR indicates a very severe stenosis or a plaque with a large lipid burden or both, treating all FFR-positive stenoses with PCI will lead to the revascularization of most plaques with features of vulnerability independent of the degree of luminal narrowing. On the other hand, treating all stenoses with a normal FFR with OMT alone appears to be safe, because such stenoses would have little, if any, large lipid-rich 2FPP **(Figs 3A and B)**. The study by Motoyama et al.[26] demonstrated that 2FPP was associated with the highest (22.5% for 27 months) event rate; events were more likely to occur in those with larger volumes, bigger necrotic cores, and a greater positive remodeling index. This more severe 2FPP, which might be associated with impaired local vasodilator capacity, would likely cause ischemia or FFR positivity. In the study by Motoyama et al.[26] plaque without a positive remodeling index or low attenuation plaque had a very low (<0.5% during 27 months) event rate. The long-term follow-up of these patients in a subsequent study[33] indicated that the 10-year event rates in positively remodeled stenosis with lipid-rich 2FPP is 9-fold higher than in the luminally stenotic lesions without 2FPP.[33] Similarly, among patients treated with OMT in the Providing Regional Observations to Study Predictors of Events in the Coronary Tree (PROSPECT) study,[13] ACS events during 3 years occurred in only 5 of 1650 plaques (0.3%) that by radiofrequency IVUS had a plaque burden of less than 70%, a lumen area of greater than 4.0 mm², and no thin-cap fibroatheroma.

We therefore propose that the benefit of FFR-guided therapy is based on the association of local vasodilator reserve and features of plaque vulnerability, that is, the extent of vascular remodeling, plaque volume, and size of the necrotic core. Fractional flow reserve is thus able to identify lesions indirectly with a low risk for plaque rupture and coronary thrombosis that may be treated effectively with OMT alone, while also

Chapter 19: Association of Coronary Stenosis and Plaque Morphology with Fractional Flow Reserve...

Angiographic diameter stenosis severity, %	FFR	No of lesions (% in subgroup) (% in entire cohort)	Possible histologic feature
Normal	>0.80	0	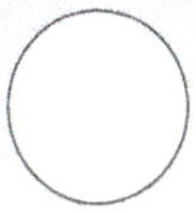
50–70	>0.80	402 (65) [33]	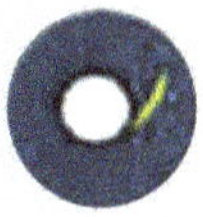 2FNP with moderate luminal stenosis
50–70	≤0.80	218 (35) [18]	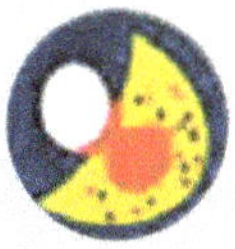 2FPP with moderate luminal stenosis
71–90	>0.80	104 (20) [8]	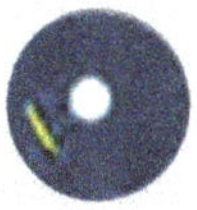 2FNP with moderate to severe luminal stenosis
71–90	≤0.80	409 (80) [33]	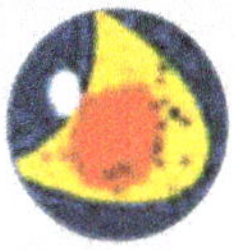 2FPP with moderate to severe luminal stenosis
			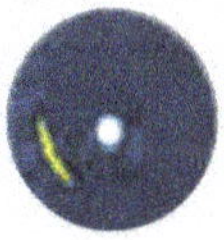 2FNP with severe luminal stenosis

Histological features:
1. Coronary artery lumen
2. Fibrous part of the plaque (entire navy blue area)
3. Necrotic core (entire yellow cell leakage (red dots), macrophages (black stars), and intraplaque hemorrhage (4)

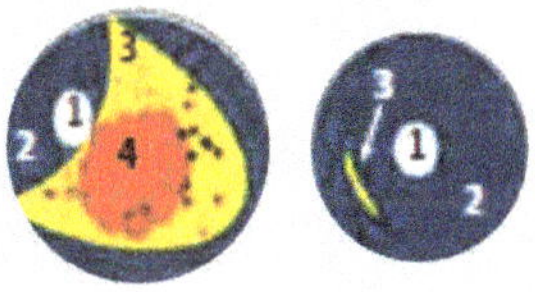

Fig. 2: Coronary stenosis severity, fractional flow reserve (FFR), and underlying pathologic features. The various groups of lesions in the Fractional Flow Reserve Versus Angiography for Multivessel Evaluation (FAME) trial are categorized according to their degree of luminal stenosis and FFR value. The possible underlying histological plaque features in each subgroup are postulated using the concepts developed in the text. Specifically, the likelihood of the presence of positively remodeled large-volume 2-feature–positive plaque (2FPP, with a positive remodeling index and a necrotic core) is represented in different groups of lesions according to the following observations: (1) The presence of large-volume 2FPP strongly predicts FFR-verified ischemia. (2) FFR-verified ischemia is a sensitive tool for detecting large-volume 2FPP. (3) Large-volume 2FPP is unlikely to be present in the FFR-negative subgroup; therefore, most plaques in the FFR-negative subgroup likely consist of nonatheromatous fibrotic lesions and less likely are associated with severe degree of luminal narrowing or long lesion length. (4) In the absence of significant luminal narrowing, FFR-verified ischemia is likely owing to the presence of large-volume (necrotic core) 2FPP. Lesion length and plaque volume are not depicted but may have a modulating effect on these considerations. (5) In the presence of a severe luminal stenosis (e.g. angiographic diameter stenosis, >70%), an FFR of greater than 0.80 suggests a normal vessel's ability to dilate, which further argues against the presence of large-volume 2FPP (or long lesion length). Most plaques in this subgroup are therefore likely fibrous, not lipid-rich lesions, and have short lesion length. (6) In the presence of severe luminal narrowing, an FFR of 0.80 or less could be owing to the presence of lipid-rich 2FPP or a fibrous, long-length lesion. The criteria in this figure do not detect 1-feature–positive plaques, which may be represented in either category and may have an intermediate prognosis between 2FPP and plaque with no high-risk features. 2FNP indicates 2-feature–negative plaque; black and red dots, red blood cells leaked from incompetent vessels (developed from the FAME and FAME 2 studies[1-4])

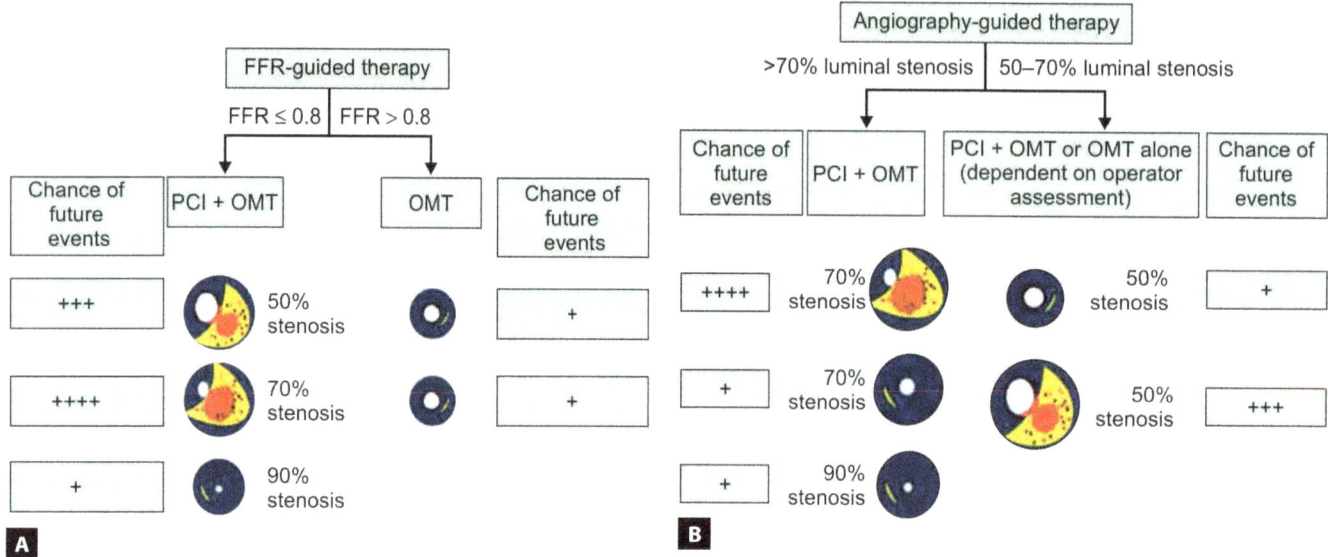

Figs 3A and B: Differences in fractional flow reserve (FFR) and angiography-guided therapies by plaque type. Based on the possible histological characteristics of each plaque type presented in Figure 4, the differences in FFR-guided treatment vs angiography-guided treatment are depicted. The chance of future events with each approach is estimated (range, + to ++++) based on plaque morphology-related prognostic data from prospective studies.[4,6] With FFR-guided therapy, nearly all high-risk lesions (including vulnerable plaques) are treated with percutaneous coronary intervention (PCI) plus optimum medical therapy (OMT), whereas lesions that are at low risk for future events are treated with OMT alone. In the angiography-guided therapy group, some lesions with angiographic diameter stenosis of 50–70% will be treated with PCI, whereas others will receive OMT alone, depending on the operator's assessment of the lesions' severity (which is known to have wide variability). Up to 35% of lesions in this subgroup in the Fractional Flow Reserve Versus Angiography for Multivessel Evaluation (FAME) trial had an FFR of 0.80 or less. Therefore, the angiography-guided approach will leave some high-risk lesions with vulnerable features that do not undergo revascularization. This finding may in part explain the paradoxically increased rate of urgent revascularization during follow-up with angiography-guided therapy despite the greater use of initial PCI in addition to more frequent stent-related thrombosis and restenosis events. Moreover, angiography-guided therapy will lead to revascularization of many lesions that may safely be deferred to OMT alone, which increases the risk for periprocedural complications Graphics for the possible histological features are described in Figure 2

identifying probably most lesions at high risk for future ACS and those producing unacceptable degrees of angina owing to extreme luminal compromise.

CONCLUSION

Normal vasodilatory capacity is a prerequisite for lack of a significant pressure drop during hyperemia. Hence, a coronary stenosis with a normal FFR has a low likelihood of having plaques with high-risk features. This finding makes FFR a reliable tool to detect sizable vulnerable plaques independent of the severity of luminal narrowing. The deferral of FFR-negative lesions to OMT is therefore safe and avoids unnecessary revascularization and stent procedures, reduces periprocedural complications, and results in fewer late stent-related events (thrombosis and restenosis) compared with a more liberal angiography-guided approach. In essence, FFR may be considered a security checkpoint that prevents most plaques with vulnerable features from going undetected **(Fig. 4)**.

The combination of ischemia testing (e.g. MPI and invasive or noninvasive FFR) with plaque composition assessment (e.g. CTA, radiofrequency IVUS, and optical coherence tomography) to guide revascularization decisions may further improve risk stratification and patient outcomes compared with either strategy alone. As tools to assess plaque composition become prospectively validated to predict subsequent major adverse cardiac events, which was demonstrated with radiofrequency IVUS in the PROSPECT study,[13] future trials should be performed to compare the utility of FFR alone versus plaque composition assessment alone versus a combined approach in guiding revascularization decisions for patients with stable coronary artery disease and those with stabilized ACS.

ARTICLE INFORMATION

Accepted for publication: February 12, 2016.

Published online: April 20, 2016.
doi:10.1001/jamacardio.2016.0263.

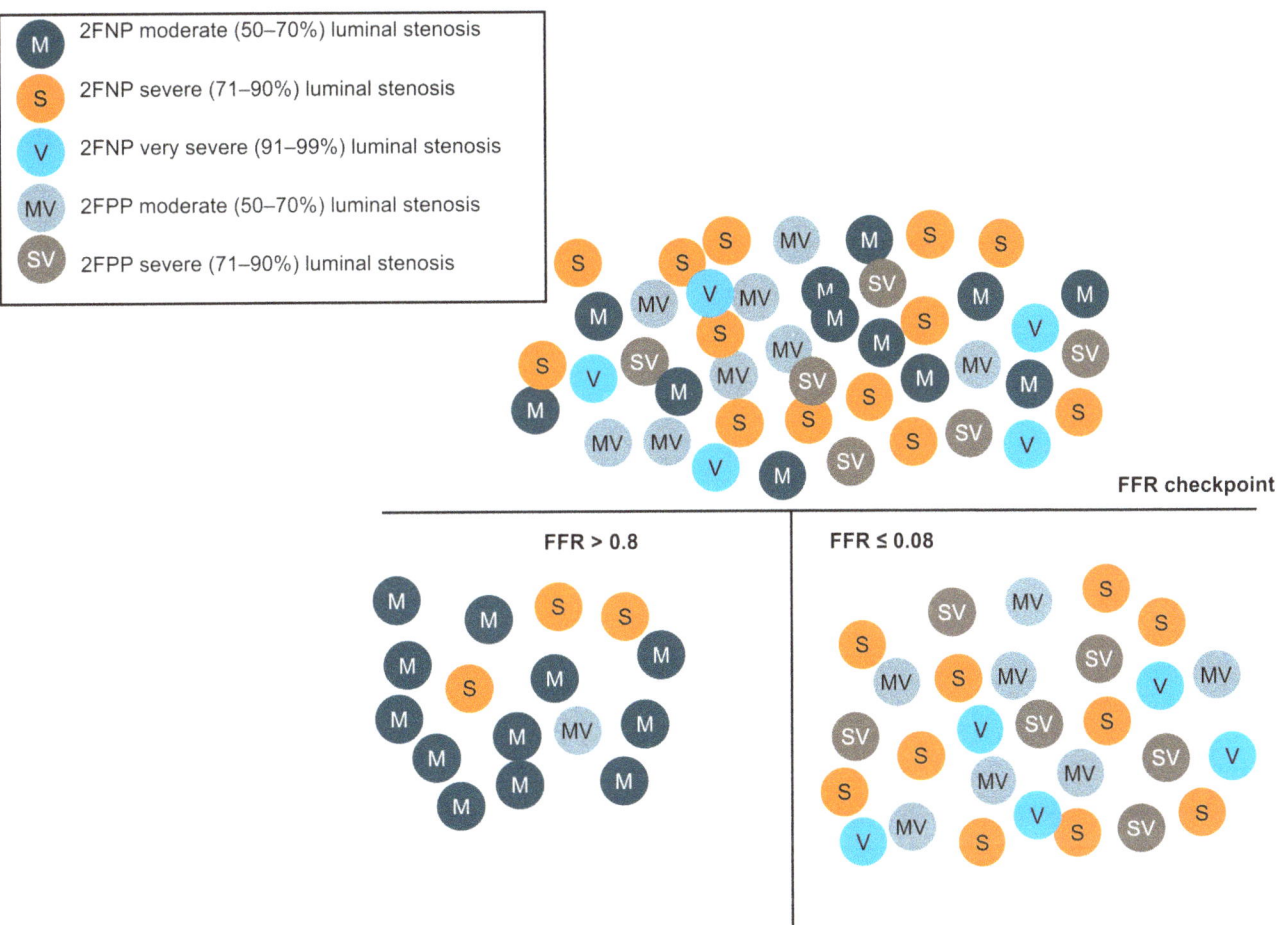

Fig. 4: Fractional flow reserve (FFR) as a security check point for detecting plaques at high risk for future events. Detection of ischemia is a sensitive (but not specific) measure for detecting large-volume 2-feature–positive plaque (2FPP, with a positive remodeling index and a necrotic core), independent of the angiographic degree of luminal stenosis. FFR-guided therapy thus may be considered a check point that leaves very few large lipid-rich 2FPP—those with highest risk for future events—to medical therapy alone. On the other hand, FFR leads to revascularization of most lipid-rich 2FPP (moderate [MV] and severe [SV] vulnerable lesions) and plaque with a severe degree of luminal stenosis without features of vulnerability (severe [S] and very severe [V] nonvulnerable lesions). 2FNP indicates 2-feature–negative plaque; M, moderate nonvulnerable lesions.

Author contributions: Drs Ahmadi and Narula had full access to all the data in the study and take responsibility for the integrity of the data and the accuracy of the data analysis.
Study concept and design: Ahmadi, Narula.
Acquisition, analysis, or interpretation of data: Ahmadi, Stone, Serruys, Wong, Nørgaard, O'Gara, Chandrashekhar, Narula.
Drafting of the manuscript: Ahmadi, Stone, Leipsic, Narula.
Critical revision of the manuscript for important intellectual content: All authors.
Statistical analysis: Ahmadi, Shaw, Narula.
Administrative, technical, or material support: Ahmadi, Narula.
Study supervision: Leipsic, Narula.

Conflict of interest disclosures: All authors have completed and submitted the ICMJE Form for Disclosure of Potential Conflicts of Interest and none were reported.

JAMA Cardiology Published online April 20, 2016.

Copyright 2016 American Medical Association. All rights reserved.

REFERENCES

1. Tonino PA, De Bruyne B, Pijls NH, et al. FAME Study Investigators. Fractional flow reserve versus angiography for guiding percutaneous coronary intervention. N Engl J Med. 2009;360(3):213-24.

2. Pijls NH, Fearon WF, Tonino PA, et al. FAME Study Investigators. Fractional flow reserve versus angiography for guiding percutaneous coronary intervention in patients with multivessel coronary artery disease: 2-year follow-up of the FAME (Fractional Flow Reserve Versus Angiography for Multivessel Evaluation) study. J Am Coll Cardiol. 2010;56(3):177-84.
3. De Bruyne B, Pijls NH, Kalesan B, et al. FAME 2 Trial Investigators. Fractional flow reserve–guided PCI versus medical therapy in stable coronary disease [published correction appears in N Engl J Med. 2012;367(18):1768]. N Engl J Med. 2012;367 (11):991-1001.
4. De Bruyne B, Fearon WF, Pijls NH, et al. FAME 2 Trial Investigators. Fractional flow reserve–guided PCI for stable coronary artery disease. N Engl J Med. 2014;371(13):1208-17.
5. Motoyama S, Kondo T, Sarai M, et al. Multislice computed tomographic characteristics of coronary lesions in acute coronary syndromes. J AmColl Cardiol. 2007;50(4):319-26.
6. Maurovich-Horvat P, Hoffmann U, Vorpahl M, Nakano M, Virmani R, Alkadhi H. The napkin-ring sign: CT signature of high-risk coronary plaques? JACC Cardiovasc Imaging. 2010;3(4):440-4.
7. Nishio M, Ueda Y, Matsuo K, et al. Detection of disrupted plaques by coronary CT: comparison with angioscopy. Heart. 2011;97(17):1397-402.
8. Otsuka K, Fukuda S, Tanaka A, et al. Napkin-ring sign on coronary CT angiography for the prediction of acute coronary syndrome. JACC Cardiovasc Imaging. 2013;6(4):448-57.
9. Rogers IS, Tawakol A. Imaging of coronary inflammation with FDG-PET: feasibility and clinical hurdles. Curr Cardiol Rep. 2011;13(2):138-44.
10. Rosa GM, Bauckneht M, Masoero G, et al. The vulnerable coronary plaque: update on imaging technologies. Thromb Haemost. 2013;110(4):706-22.
11. Prati F, Regar E, Mintz GS, et al. Expert's OCT Review Document. Expert review document on methodology, terminology, and clinical applications of optical coherence tomography: physical principles, methodology of image acquisition, and clinical application for assessment of coronary arteries and atherosclerosis. Eur Heart J. 2010;31 (4):401-15.
12. Tearney GJ, Yabushita H, Houser SL, et al. Quantification of macrophage content in atherosclerotic plaques by optical coherence tomography. Circulation. 2003;107(1):113-9.
13. Yabushita H, Bouma BE, Houser SL, et al. Characterization of human atherosclerosis by optical coherence tomography. Circulation. 2002;106(13):1640-5.
14. Gould KL, Lipscomb K, Calvert C. Compensatory changes of the distal coronary vascular bed during progressive coronary constriction. Circulation. 1975;51(6):1085-94.
15. Park SJ, Kang SJ, Ahn JM, et al. Visual-functional mismatch between coronary angiography and fractional flow reserve. JACC Cardiovasc Interv. 2012;5(10):1029-36.
16. Layland J, Oldroyd KG, Curzen N, et al. FAMOUS–NSTEMI investigators. Fractional flow reserve vs angiography in guiding management to optimize outcomes in non-ST-segment elevation myocardial infarction: the British Heart Foundation FAMOUS-NSTEMI randomized trial. Eur Heart J. 2015;36(2):100-11.
17. Ahmadi A, Kini A, Narula J. Discordance between ischemia and stenosis, or PINSS and NIPSS: are we ready for new vocabulary? JACC Cardiovasc Imaging. 2015;8(1):111-4.
18. Tonino PA, Fearon WF, De Bruyne B, et al. Angiographic versus functional severity of coronary artery stenoses in the FAME study Fractional Flow Reserve versus Angiography in Multivessel Evaluation. J Am Coll Cardiol. 2010;55(25):2816-21.
19. Yamashita T, Colombo A, Tobis JM. Limitations of coronary angiography compared with intravascular ultrasound: implications for coronary interventions. Prog Cardiovasc Dis. 1999;42(2):91-138.
20. de Bruyne B, Bartunek J, Sys SU, Pijls NH, Heyndrickx GR, Wijns W. Simultaneous coronary pressure and flow velocity measurements in humans: feasibility, reproducibility, and hemodynamic dependence of coronary flow velocity reserve, hyperemic flow versus pressure slope index, and fractional flow reserve. Circulation. 1996;94(8):1842-9.
21. Kern MJ, Samady H. Current concepts of integrated coronary physiology in the catheterization laboratory. J Am Coll Cardiol. 2010; 55(3):173-85.
22. Johnson NP, Kirkeeide RL, Gould KL. Coronary anatomy to predict physiology: fundamental limits. Circ Cardiovasc Imaging. 2013;6(5):817-32.
23. Park HB, Heo R, ó Hartaigh B, et al. Atherosclerotic plaque characteristics by CT angiography identify coronary lesions that cause ischemia: a direct comparison to fractional flow reserve. JACC Cardiovasc Imaging. 2015;8(1):1-10.
24. Gaur S, Øvrehus KA, Dey D, et al. Coronary plaque quantification and fractional flow reserve by coronary computed tomography angiography identify ischaemia-causing lesions [published online January 12, 2016]. Eur Heart J. doi:10.1093 /eurheartj/ehv690.
25. Tanaka S, Noda T, Segawa T, et al. Relation between functional stenosis and tissue characterization of intermediate coronary plaques in patients with stable coronary heart disease. J Cardiol. 2010;55(3):296-302.
26. Motoyama S, Sarai M, Harigaya H, et al. Computed tomographic angiography characteristics of atherosclerotic plaques subsequently resulting in acute coronary syndrome. J Am Coll Cardiol. 2009;54(1):49-57.
27. Shmilovich H, Cheng VY, Tamarappoo BK, et al. Vulnerable plaque features on coronary CT angiography as markers of inducible regional myocardial hypoperfusion from severe coronary artery stenoses. Atherosclerosis. 2011;219(2):588-95.
28. Glagov S, Weisenberg E, Zarins CK, Stankunavicius R, Kolettis GJ. Compensatory enlargement of human atherosclerotic coronary arteries. N Engl J Med. 1987;316(22):1371-5.
29. Lavi S, Bae JH, Rihal CS, et al. Segmental coronary endothelial dysfunction in patients with minimal atherosclerosis is associated with necrotic core plaques. Heart. 2009;95(18):1525-30.
30. Lavi S, McConnell JP, Rihal CS, et al. Local production of lipoprotein-associated phospholipase A2 and lysophosphati-dylcholine in the coronary circulation: association with early coronary atherosclerosis and endothelial dysfunction in humans. Circulation. 2007;115(21):2715-21.
31. Lavi S, Yang EH, Prasad A, et al. The interaction between coronary endothelial dysfunction, local oxidative stress, and endogenous nitric oxide in humans. Hypertension. 2008;51(1):127-33.
32. Naghavi M, Libby P, Falk E, et al. From vulnerable plaque to vulnerable patient: a call for new definitions and risk assessment strategies: part I. Circulation. 2003;108(14):1664-72.
33. Motoyama S, Ito H, Sarai M, et al. Plaque characterization by coronary computed tomography angiography and the likelihood of acute coronary events in mid-term follow-up. J Am Coll Cardiol. 2015;66(4):337-46.

Section 2

Clinical Cardiology

Emerging Therapies
- PCSK9 Inhibitors: Will they be the Next Wonder Drug after Statins?
- Fighting the Devil of Stroke in Atrial Fibrillation: The New Weapons in the Armory

Coronary Artery Disease
- Management of Prehospital Phase of Acute Myocardial Infarction
- STEMI Care in India and the Real World: Pharmacoinvasive Approach
- Bioresorbable Vascular Scaffold
- Statin Intolerance
- Sudden Cardiac Death: How to Predict and Prevent it?
- New Gadgets Knocking at the Door: Leadless Pacemakers, Subcutaneous Implantable Cardioverter Defibrillators, Wearable Defibrillators
- Echocardiographic Evaluation of Left Atrial Clot and its Utility in Clinical Practice
- Clinical Applications of Nuclear Cardiology Procedures and its Future Directions
- Cardiac Positron Emission Tomography Perfusion Tracers: Current Status and Future Directions

EMERGING THERAPIES

20. PCSK9 Inhibitors: Will they be the Next Wonder Drug after Statins?

PC Manoria, Pankaj Manoria, Piyush Manoria, SK Parashar

INTRODUCTION

A new revolutionary era has begun after statin era in 2015 with approval of two proprotein convertase subtilisin/Kexin type 9 (PCSK9) inhibitors, evolucumab and alirocumab. Statins which we have been using for last 25 years has decreased cardiovascular (CV) events by 30–35%. It has shown benefit across all levels of low-density lipoprotein cholesterol (LDL-C), in fact they are now being designated as CV risk reducing agent and should be used in all patients with CV disease and those at high risk of it. However statins have limitations that there is substantial residual atherogenic risk, muscle toxicity, diabetogenecity and relative inefficacy in patients with high high-density lipoprotein cholesterol (HDL-C) levels.

Statin therapy has become an integral part of therapy both for secondary prevention and high risk patients for primary prevention. However, they have limitations that at best they can decrease cardiovascular events (CVE) by 30–35% **(Fig. 1)**, in addition they have muscle toxicity, are diabetogenic and there is relative inefficacy in patients with high HDL-C.

RESIDUAL ATHEROGENIC RISK POSTSTATIN THERAPY

In patients on optimum statin therapy, 60–65% of cardiovascular events (CVE) will continue to occur and therefore attempts have been made to reduce the residual atherogenic risk. There are several determinants of this residual risk like low HDL-C, high triglyceride (TG), TG-rich lipoproteins (Lps), Lp(a) and other risk factors for cardiovascular disease (CVD).

Low HDL-C as a Determinant of Residual Atherogenic Risk

Trials like TNT[1] have shown that low HDL-C is one of the important predictor of residual atherogenic risk in patients on high dose statins. Likewise, the meta-analysis of 14 studies[2] also

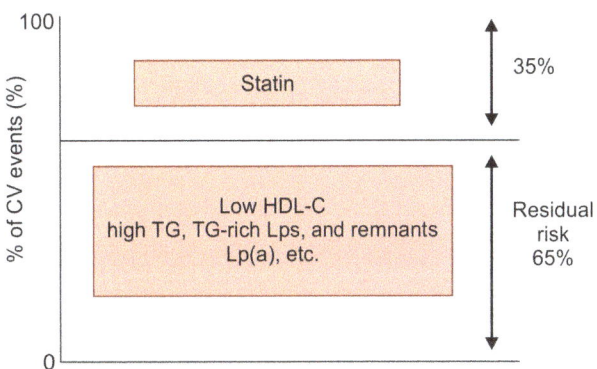

Fig. 1: Reduction of CV events by intensive statin therapy

Table 1 Trials of HDL-C elevation on top of intensive statin therapy

Niacin
• AIM HIGH (2011)[3]
• HPS-2 THRIVE (2013)[4]
CETP inhibitors
• ILLUMINATE (2007)[5]
• dal-OUTCOMES (2012)[6]
• ACCELERATE
Ongoing trials
• REVEAL

showed that low HDL-C is an important risk factor for CVD in patients on statins. Based on this, several trials were designed to reduce residual atherogenic risk in patient on intensive statin therapy by increasing HDL-C.

But despite a sound theoretical basis all trials of HDL elevation[3-6] on top of intensive statin therapy till date have been flop trials **(Table 1)**.

Niacin has failed to show benefit in the AIM HIGH and HPS-2 THRIVE studies. The CETP inhibitors were introduced as block buster for elevating HDL-C but despite marked elevation of HDL-C in blood with these agents, all trials till date has been negative. Only one trial, REVEAL is ongoing and the result is likely to be released after 2–3 years.

HIGH TRIGLYCERIDES AS A DETERMINANT OF RESIDUAL ATHEROGENIC RISK

There is no outcome data of lowering of triglycerides (TG) on top of statins. The ACCORD LLA Trial[7] which was carried out to see the benefits of fibrates on top of statins was negative. However the sub-group analysis of ACCORD LLA[8] with TG above 200 mg/dL and low HDL did show a benefit but the sub-group analysis is only hypothesis generating and has to be tested in a large randomized trial. Somehow TG has not been properly investigated particularly in Indian context to document the benefit of lowering it in the high risk sub-group.

Thus the treatment of dyslipidemia which started with targeting LDL-C and then moved on further to target HDL-C and TG but these attempts were unsuccessful. Interestingly with PCSK9 inhibitors, the target has again shifted back to LDL-C.

PCSK9

Serum proprotein convertase subtilisin/kexin 9 (PCSK9) is a protein that regulates LDL-C levels in the blood by regulating LDL receptors (LDL-R). It is secreted from the liver, goes into the blood, circulates back to liver and directly binds to LDL receptors increasing their degradation and thereby reducing the rate at which LDL-C is removed from circulation[9] and thus increasing LDL-C levels in blood. Thus PCSK9 seems to be an important regulator or LDL metabolism.

PCSK9 is also affected by genetic mutation and has fascinating genetic data. There are two types of mutation:

Loss-of-function Mutation (Table 2)

The more common 'loss-of-function' mutations have low LDL-C throughout their life and this provides atheroprotection.[10-12] It is also a good argument to treat patients sooner to lower LDL-C levels to observe greater beneficial effects to prevent the development of cardiovascular disease.

The first suggestion that impaired PCSK9 activity might lower CVD events stems from a study in 2006 looking at mutations in the gene. Even in high-risk populations, mutations resulting in loss of function of PCSK9 resulted in not only LDL-C reduction but also even greater reductions in CVD events.

Gain-of-function Mutation

The rare PCSK9 'gain-of-function' mutation[13] is an autosomal dominant trait that cause familial hypercholesterolemia (FH) and predispose to atherosclerotic cardiovascular disease. There are now numerous confirmed mutations for gain of function, all associated with high LDL-C.

It is not surprising that the gain-of-function mutations escaped us for so long because these mutations account for less than 0.2% of all mutations. You have to look very hard to find them. In fact, it is the gain-of-function mutation that helped us understand PCSK9, but it is the loss-of-function mutation that paved the way for all the new developments. Even a small difference in LDL first seen in a child actually translates into a huge decrease in coronary disease.

Both statins and ezetimibe[14] increase secretion of PCSK9, which could attenuate their efficacy by reducing the amount of cholesterol cleared from circulation. This explains the limitation of statin therapy and may be the best explanation regarding the classic rule of 6 observed with statin therapy. This rule refers to the fact that every time the statin dose is doubled, there is only an approximately 6% complementary decrease in LDL-C levels.

Therefore, the combination of PCSK9 inhibition with a statin would be a sensible and logical approach and will cause a dramatic decrease in LDL-C levels.

PCSK9 Inhibition

PCSK9 inhibition is emerging as an important therapeutic option for modulating LDL cholesterol. Its inhibition can be achieved by gene silencing, small peptides or monoclonal antibodies (Mabs). PCSK9 Mabs[15] are commonly used to inhibit PCSK9. They bind specifically to human PCSK9, and prevent its interaction with LDL-R, thereby decreasing LDL-C. PCSK9 Mabs is an injectable medication administered subcutaneously. They are currently being evaluated in various trials. Three PCSK9 Mabs, i.e. alirocumab (Regeneron/Sanofi Product REGN727/SAR236553), evolocumab (Amgen Product AMG 145), and bococizumab (Pfizer Product RN 316) have been evaluated in various trials.

Table 2 PCSK9 loss-of-function mutations

	PCSK9 mutation	LDL-C reduction, %	CHD-risk reduction, %	Hazard ratio (95% CI)
Dallas Heart Study	Y142X or C679X	40	N/A	
ARIC	Y142X or C676	28	88	0.11 (0.02–0.81)
	R46L	15	47	0.50 (0.31–0.79)
Benn et al	R46L	13	130	0.70 (0.58–0.86)

Table 3 Trials of PCSK9 inhibitor evolocumab in the PROFICIO Global Programme

PHASE II STUDIES				
S.No.	Trial	Nu	Drug	Subset
1.	MENDEL[16]	405	Evolocumab	Monotherapy
2.	GAUSS[17]	160	Evolocumab	Statin-intolerant
3.	LAPLACE-TIMI 54[18]	600	Evolocumab	Combination therapy
4.	RUTHERFORD[19]	168	Evolocumab	Heterozygous (HeFH)
5.	OSLER[20]	1104	Evolocumab	
PHASE III STUDIES				
6.	MENDEL-2[21]	614	Evolocumab	Monotherapy
7.	GAUSS-2[22]	307	Evolocumab	Statin-intolerant
8.	LAPLACE-2[23]	1899	Evolocumab	Combination therapy
9.	RUTHERFORD-2[24]	331	Evolocumab	Heterozygous FH
10.	DESCARTES[25]	901	Evolocumab	Combination therapy
11.	TESLA[26]	49	Evolocumab	Homozygous familial hypercholesterolemia (HoFH)
12.	TAUSSIG (ongoing)[27]	61	Evolocumab	Homozygous familial hypercholesterolemia
13.	YUKAWA (ongoing)[28]	404	Evolocumab	High CV Risk
14.	GLAGOV (ongoing)	910	Evolocumab	Looking at atherosclerosis regression by IVUS

Evolocumab

This has already been approved for clinical use and is available commercially as 1 mL pen containing 140 mg. It is given in doses of 140 mg biweekly/420 mg. monthly SC. It was tested in the PROFICIO Global Program which had 14 trials and roughly 30,000 patients **(Table 3)**. Most of the trials have been completed but FOURIER outcome trial is still ongoing. Most of these trials have shown significant reduction in LDL-C by 40–60% on top of statins. There is also consistent and robust reduction in other lipoproteins. The Lp(a) is reduced by approximately 25%, triglyceride and non HDL-C are also decreased. The HDL-C and apo-A1 are increased.

Alirocumab

This is approved for clinical use in USA and is commercially available as 1 mL pen containing 75 or 150 mg. It is given in doses in 150 mg biweekly SC. It was evaluated in ODYSSEY Global Programme which included 11 trials and roughly has 22,000 patients **(Table 4)**.

The various trials of alirocumab in the ODYSSEY Global Programme are outlined below:

ODYSSEY FH STUDIES[29]: FH I, FH and HIGH FH: The primary objective of these three studies is to demonstrate the efficacy and safety of alirocumab as an add-on therapy in patients with hereditary familial hyperlipidemia (HeFH)

Table 4 ODYSSEY Global Programme

ODYSSEY Global Programme phase 2/3 (11 Trials) Alirocumab 150 mg biweekly SC 22,000 patients		
• FH I, FH II and HIGH FH • COMBO I and II • MONO	• ALTERNATIVE • OPTIONS I AND II • LONG-TERM	ODYSSEY OUTCOME Trial

who are not adequately controlled with their lipid-modifying therapy.

ODYSSEY Combo I and Combo II[30]: The primary objective of these two studies is to demonstrate the safety and efficacy of alirocumab as an add-on therapy in patients with primary hypercholesterolemia at high cardiovascular risk who are not adequately controlled with their lipid-modifying therapy.

ODYSSEY MONO[31]: The primary objective of this study is to demonstrate the safety and efficacy of alirocumab as monotherapy in comparison with ezetimibe in patients with primary hypercholesterolemia.

ODYSSEY ALTERNATIVE[32]: The primary objective of this study is to demonstrate the safety and efficacy of alirocumab in comparison with ezetimibe in patients with primary hypercholesterolemia (heFH and non-familial hypercholesterolemia) who are unable to tolerate statins.

Table 5 SPIRE Trials

SPIRE-1	BOCOCIZUMAB Bococizumab 150 mg biweekly SC	SPIRE-2

ODYSSEY OPTIONS I and OPTIONS II: The primary objective of these studies is to evaluate the safety and efficacy of alirocumab as an add-on therapy in patients with primary hypercholesterolemia at high cardiovascular risk or with heFH who are not adequately controlled on statins, in comparison to several second line lipid lowering strategies.

ODYSSEY LONG-TERM[33]: The primary objective of this study is to evaluate the long-term safety and tolerability of alirocumab in patients with hypercholesterolemia at high cardiovascular risk or patients with heFH inadequately controlled with their current lipid-modifying therapy.

Bococizumab

This is being evaluated in two outcome trials SPIRE-1 and SPIRE-2 **(Table 5)**. It is given in doses of 150 mg biweekly SC.

The SPIRE-1 is evaluating the PCSK9 inhibitor, bococizumab's (RN316), compared to placebo, in reducing the occurrence of major cardiovascular events, including cardiovascular death, myocardial infarction, stroke, and unstable angina requiring urgent revascularization, in high risk subjects who are receiving background lipid lowering therapy and have cholesterol laboratory values of LDL-C>70 mg/dL (1.8 mmol/L) and <100 mg/dL (2.6 mmol/L) or non-HDL-C > 100 mg/dL (2.6 mmol/L) and <130 mg/dL (3.4 mmol/L).

The SPIRE-2 Trial is evaluating the PCSK9 inhibitor, bococizumab's compared to placebo, in reducing the occurrence of major cardiovascular events, including cardiovascular death, myocardial infarction, stroke and unstable angina requiring urgent revascularization in high risk subjects who are receiving background lipid lowering therapy and have cholesterol laboratory values of LDL-C > 100 mg/dL (2.6 mmol/L) or non-HDL-C >130 mg/dL (3.4 mmol/L).

Side Effects

PCSK9 inhibitors have excellent safety compared to statins. The side effects are seen in only minority of patients[34] and includes itching, swelling, pain or bruising at the injection site, nasopharyngitis and flu are common side effects of the drug. One patient had leukocytoclastic vasculitis which resolved with steroids.

There do not seem to be any muscle side effects or an effect on creatine kinase, nor does there seem to be any signal on the liver. Cognitive adverse events (CAEs)[35] like amnesia and memory impairment have been reported from data in OSLER Trial and ODYSSEY long-term but they are seen only in <1% of patients. The EBBINGHAUS Trial is ongoing to assess the effect of PCKS9 inhibitor on cognitive health in high risk cardiovascular subjects. The results are expected in September 2017. These agents do not have diabetogenic effects. The discontinuation rate is only 7%. From a safety point of view, these monoclonal antibodies seem to be better than most currently available drugs for lowering LDL-C that we have.

In fact, an injectable therapy might actually promote better adherence than tablets. If a patient receives an injection once every 2 or 4 weeks, adherence is better but there is an issue of cost. After 2.5 years of experience with these medications, nothing unpleasant has come out. In the past 10 years trials of several classes of drugs have completely failed, so this is a big breath of relief.

Are there any off-target Effects?

The circulating levels of PCSK9 seem to play no other significant role other than to modulate the recycling of the LDL receptor. There are also about 3 or 4 patients who have a double mutation, and they have no detectable PCSK9. LDL levels are around about 14–15 mg, or less than 0.5 mmol. Those who have been women have had normal reproductive endocrine function and normal lifestyles. There does not seem to be any downside to inhibition of PCSK9 in the plasma.

There are now well over 5000 patients who have been exposed to PCSK9 antibodies for 3–12 months in randomized placebo-controlled trials, which is more exposure than the first statin had by the time it got into the market. We are seeing a cleaner safety profile of a well-tolerated drug, and an efficacy that is greater than the highest dose of the most effective statin. There are LDL reductions in the range of 55–65% with a good safety profile. There is no such thing as a drug without any side effects, but at the moment, serious side effects appear unlikely and rare with this class. Obviously, we have to wait and see, but no one is seeing cause for concern at this stage.

CLINICAL APPROVAL IN EUROPE AND USA

Europe

The European Medicines Agency in July 2015 approved evolocumab as an adjunct to diet in patients with elevated cholesterol levels who are unable to reach their recommended LDL-C goal despite taking an optimal dose of statin. Patients deemed statin intolerant or those in whom a statin is contraindicated would also be eligible for treatment with evolocumab. The committee has also made it available for treatment of patients with homozygous familial hypercholesterolemia.

USA

The USA FDA has approved alirocumab injection (Praluent, Sanofi and Regeneron Pharmaceuticals) on July 24, 2015. The drug has been approved for treatment of patients with

Table 6 Indications of PCSK9

1.	Failure to achieve LDL-C goals despite optimal doses of statins in high CV risk individuals
2.	Statin intolerance
3.	Familial hypercholesterolemia

familial hypercholesterolemia (FH), clinical atherosclerotic cardiovascular disease in conjunction with maximally tolerated statin therapy and diet modification failing to reach LDL targets and statin intolerance.

Where will this Class of Agents Fit in ?

The indications of PCSK9 are outlined in **Table 6**.

OSLER and ODYSSEY LONG-TERM Trials

Two recent trials, the OSLER[20] and ODYSSEY LONG-TERM[33] completed recently have shown interesting results. The Open-Label Study of Long-Term Evaluation against LDL Cholesterol (OSLER) Trial **(Fig. 2)** examined the long-term effects of evolocumab as an extension of the open label, randomized controlled OSLER 1 and 2 Trials and included 4,465 patients. Eligible patients had completed either of the trials without suffering any adverse events that required discontinuation of study drug. Participating patients were randomized to the PCSK9 inhibitor plus standard therapy versus standard therapy alone without placebo control. Approximately 70% of patients were receiving background statin therapy. The majority of patients were Caucasian with approximately 80% having other cardiovascular risk factors including hypertension, diabetes, metabolic syndrome, current cigarette use, or family history of premature coronary artery disease or familial hypercholesterolemia. Throughout the 48–56 week trial period, study patients had regular visits while the standard care group was contacted only by telephone.

The incidence of adverse events, the primary endpoint, was more common in the evolocumab group (69.2% vs 64.8%). However, serious adverse events were similar (7.5% in each group). Percent reduction in LDL-C was a secondary endpoint. Baseline LDL-C was 120 mg/dL before the initial randomization into the parent studies and was reduced by 61% to a mean of 48 mg/dL, which is consistent with previous findings regarding the percent reduction. An important point is that although the levels of LDL-C were driven very low, adverse neurocognitive events did not correlate with the level of LDL-C despite occurring more frequently in the evolocumab group (0.9% vs 0.3% in the standard-therapy group). A key endpoint of clinical significance to address the above questions was the adjudicated incidence of cardiovascular events, including death, myocardial infarction, unstable angina requiring hospitalization, coronary revascularization, stroke, transient ischemic attack, and heart failure requiring hospitalization. These cardiovascular events occurred in a 1% of the evolocumab group versus 2% of the standard therapy group (HR 0.47, p = 0.0003).[36]

The ODYSSEY LONG TERM Trial **(Fig. 3)** enrolled 2,341 high-risk patients with heterozygous familial hypercholesterolemia, known coronary artery disease, or coronary artery disease risk equivalent in a randomized, double-blind, placebo-controlled trial. Eligible patients had LDL-C levels above 70 mg/dL and were currently taking either high-dose statins or maximum tolerated dosages. Other lipid lowering therapies were also allowed and all patients were instructed on the Therapeutic Lifestyle Changes or equivalent diet. The majority (93%) of patients were Caucasian with nearly 18% having heterozygous familial hypercholesterolemia. Mean LDL-C at baseline was 122.7 mg/dL in the alirocumab group versus 121.9 in the placebo group.

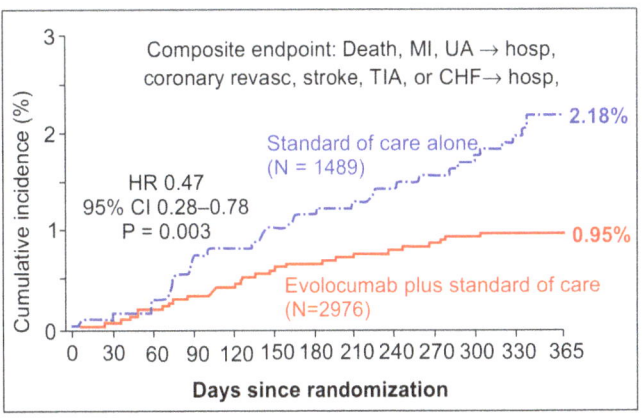

Fig. 2: Cardiovascular outcomes in OSLER trials

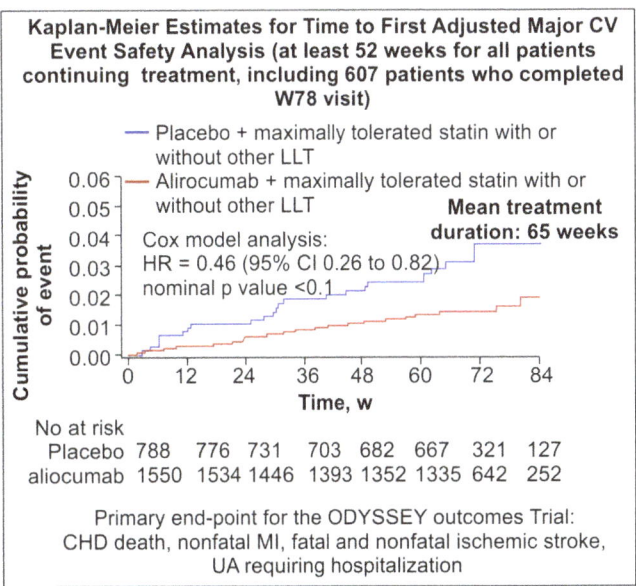

Fig. 3: ODYSSEY LONG-TERM study

Table 7 Ongoing outcome trials of PCSK9 inhibitors

S.No.	Trial	Drug
1.	ODYSSEY	Alirocumab
2.	FOURIER	Evolocumab
3.	SPIRE	
	• SPIRE-1	Bococizumab
	• SPIRE-2	Bococizumab

The primary endpoint, change in LDL-C levels from baseline to 24 weeks, was positive. LDL-C levels were reduced by 61% in the alirocumab group to a mean of 48 mg/dL compared to an increase of 0.8% in the placebo group. This degree of change is consistent with previous studies. Importantly, as was seen in the OSLER Trial, no effect was seen in levels of fat-soluble vitamins or cortisol as a result of the significantly decreased LDL-C levels. The safety endpoints included adverse events as well as adjudicated cardiovascular events and were not significantly different between the two groups.

Adjudicated cardiovascular events occurred in 4.6% of the alirocumab group versus 5.1% of the control group (p = 0.02). A post-hoc analysis of cardiovascular events that included a composite of death from coronary heart disease, nonfatal myocardial infarction, fatal or nonfatal ischemic stroke, or unstable angina requiring hospitalization showed lower rates with alirocumab than with placebo (1.7% vs 3.3%, HR 0.52, p = 0.02).[37]

Taken together, current studies show promise for the future clinical application of PCSK9 inhibitors. Certainly the role of PCSK9 in cardiovascular disease has come a long way since the gene was discovered in 2003.

Three outcome studies, i.e. FOURIER, ODYSSEY and SPIRE-1 and 2 are ongoing which will decide the fate of these agents **(Table 7)**. The trials are likely to be completed in 2017.

CONCLUSION

The future of PCSK9 inhibitors seems bright and hopefully we are now heading for another revolutionary era after statins. They are safe drugs with no major side effects and are not diabetogenic. They may prove to be the next wonder drug after statins.

REFERENCES

1. Fruchart JC, Sacks F, Hermans MP, et al. The Residual Risk Reduction Initiative: a call to action to reduce residual vascular risk in patients with dyslipidemia. Am J Cardiol. 2008;102(10 Suppl): 1K -34K.
2. Baigent C, Keech A, Kearney PM, et al. Efficacy and safety of cholesterol lowering treatment: prospective meta-analysis of data from 90,056 participants in 14 randomised trials of statins. Lancet. 2005;366:1267-78.
3. The AIM-HIGH Investigators. Niacin in Patients with Low HDL Cholesterol Levels Receiving Intensive Statin Therapy. N Engl J Med. 2011;365:2255-67.
4. HPS2-THRIVE randomized placebo-controlled trial in 25 673 high-risk patients of ER niacin/laropiprant: trial design, pre-specified muscle and liver outcomes, and reasons for stopping study treatment. HPS2-THRIVE Collaborative Group. EUR Heart J. 2013;34(17):1279-91.
5. Barter PJ, Caulfield Mark, Eriksson Mats, et al. for the ILLUMINATE Investigators. Effects of Torcetrapib in Patients at High Risk for Coronary Events. N Engl J Med. 2007;357(21):2109-22.
6. Schwartz GC, et al. for the dal-OUTCOMES Investigators. Effects of Dalcetrapib in Patients with a Recent Acute Coronary Syndrome. N Engl J Med. 2012;367:2089-99.
7. The ACCORD Study Group. Effects of combination lipid therapy in type 2 diabetes mellitus. N Engl J Med. 2010;362(17):1563-74.
8. Hegele RA, Ginsberg HN, et al. The polygenic nature of hyper-triglyceridaemia: implications for definition, diagnosis, and management. N Engl J Med. 2010;363:692-4.
9. Yamamoto T, Lu C, Ryan RO. A two-step binding mode of PCSK9 interaction with the low density lipoprotein receptor. J Biol Chem. 2011;286:5464-70.
10. Cohen J, et al. Low LDL cholesterol in individuals of African descent resulting from frequent nonsense mutations in PCSK9 Nat Genet. 2005;37:161-5.
11. Cohen J, et al. Sequence Variations in PCSK9, Low LDL, and Protection against Coronary Heart Disease. N Engl J Med. 2006;354:1264-72.
12. Been M, et al. PCSK9 R46L, low-density lipoprotein cholesterol levels, and risk of ischemic heart disease: 3 independent studies and meta-analyses. J Am Coll Cardiol. 2010;55:2833-42.
13. Abifadel M, Varret M, Rabes JP, et al. Mutations in PCSK9 cause autosomal dominant hypercholesterolemia. Nat Genet. 2003;34:154-6.
14. Ason B, Tep S, Davis HR Jr, et al. Improved efficacy for ezetimbie and rosuvastatin by attenuating the induction of PCSK9. J Lipid Res. 2011;52:679-87.
15. Marais DA, Blom DJ, Petrides F, Goueffic Y, Lambert G. Proprotein convertase subtilisin/ kexin type 9 inhibition. Curr Opin Lipidol, 2012;23:511-7.
16. Koren MJ, Scott R, Kim JB, et al. Efficacy, safety and tolerability of a monoclonal antibody to proprotein convertase subtilisin/kexin type 9 as monotherapy in patients with hypercholesterolaemia (MENDEL): a randomized, double-blind, placebo-controlled, phase 2 study. Lancet. 2012;380:1995-2006.
17. Sullivan D, Olsson AG, Scott R. Effect of a Monocional Antibody to PCSK9 on Low-Density Lipoprotein Cholesterol Levels in Statin-Intolerant Patients The GAUSS Randomized Trial. JAMA. 2012;308:2497-506.
18. Giugliano RP, Desai NR, Kohli P, et al. Efficacy, safety, and tolerability of a monoclonal antibody to proprotein convertase subtilisin/kexin type 9 in combination with a statin in patients with hypercholesterolaemia (LAPLACE-TIMI 57); a randomized, placebo- controlled, dose-ranging, phase 2 study. Lancet. 2012;380:2007-17.
19. Raal F, Scott R, Somaratne R, Bridges I, Li G, Wasserman SM, et al. Low-density lipoprotein cholesterol-lowering effects of AMG 145, a monoclonal antibody to proprotein convertase subtilisin/

kexin type 9 serine protease in patients with heterozygous familial hypercholesterolemia: the Reduction of LDL-C with PCSK9 inhibition Heterozygous Familial Hypercholesterolemia Disorder (RUTHERFORD) randomized trial. Circulation. 2012;126:2408-17.
20. Sabatine MS, Giugliano RP, et al. Efficacy and Safety of Evolocumab in Reducing Lipids and Cardiovascular Events N Engl J Med. 2015;372:1500-9.
21. Koren MJ, Lundqvist P, et al. Anti-PCSK9 monotherapy for hypercholesterolemia. The MENDEL-2 Randomized, Controlled Phase III Clinical Trial of Evolocumab. J Am Coll Cardiol. 2014;63(23):2531-40.
22. Stroes E, Colquhoun D. Anti-PCSK9 Antibody Effectively Lowers Cholesterol in Patients With Statin Intolerance The GAUSS-2 Randomized, Placebo-Controlled Phase 3 Clinical Trial of Evolocumab. J Am Coll Cardiol. 2014;63(23):2541-8.
23. Robinson JG, Nedergaard BS, et al. Effect of evolocumab or ezetimibe added to moderate-or high-intensity statin therapy on LDL-C lowering in patients with hypercholesterolemia: the LAPLACE-2 Randomized Clinical Trial. JAMA. 2014; 311(18):1870-82.
24. Raal FJ, Stein EA, et al. PCSK9 inhibition with evolocumab (AMG 145) in heterozygous familial hypercholesterolaemia (RUTHERFORD-2): a randomized, double-blind, placebo-controlled trial. Lancet. 2014;385:331-40.
25. Blom DJ, Hala T, et al. A 52-week placebo-controlled trial of evolocumab in hyperlipidemia. NEJM. 2014;371(19):1809-19.
26. Raal FJ, Honarpour N, et al. Inhibition of PCSK9 with evolocumab in homozygous familial hypercholesterolaemia (TESLA Part B): a randomised, double-blind, placebo-controlled trial. Lancet. 2015;385:341-50.
27. Bruckert E, Blaha V, et al. Trial Assessing Long-Term Use of PCSK9 Inhibition in Patients with Genetic LDL Disorders (TAUSSIG): Efficacy and Safety in Patients with Homozygous Familial Hypercholesterolemia Receiving Lipid Apheresis. Circulation. 2014;130:A17016.
28. Kiyosue A, Honarpour N, et al. Effect of evolocumab (AMG 145) in hypercholesterolemic, statin-treated, Japanese patients at high cardiovascular risk: results from the phase III YUKAWA 2 study. J Am Coll Cardiol. 2015;65(10-S):A1369.
29. Kastelein JJ, Robinson JG, et al. Efficacy and safety of alirocumab in patients with heterozygous familial hypercholesterolemia not adequately controlled with current lipid-lowering therapy: design and rationale of the ODYSSEY FH studies. Cardiovasc Drugs Ther. 2014;28:281-9.
30. Cannon Cp, Carious B, et al. Efficacy and safety of alirocumab in high cardiovascular risk patients with inadequately controlled trial. Eur Heart J. 2015;36:1186-94.
31. Kohli P, Desai NR, et al. Design and rationale of the LAPLACE-TIMI 57 trial: a phase II, double-blind, placebo-controlled study of the efficacy and tolerability of a monoclonal antibody inhibitor of PCSK9 in subjects with hypercholesterolemia on background statin therapy. Clin Cardiol. 2012;35:385-91.
32. Moriarty PM, Jacobson, et al. Efficacy and safety of alirocumab, a monoclonal antibody to PCSK9, in statin-intolerant patients: design and rationale of ODYSSEY ALTERNATIVE, a randomized phase 3 trial. J Clin Lipidol. 2014;8:554-61.
33. Robinson JG, Farnier M, et al. Efficacy and safety of alirocumab in reducing lipids and cardiovascular events. N Eng J Med. 2015;372:1489-99.
34. MS Sabatine, RP Giugliano, et al. Efficacy and safety of evolocumab in reducing lipids and cardiovascular events. N Engl J Med. 2015;372:1500-9.
35. K Richardson, M Schoen, et al. Statins and cognitive function: a systematic review. Ann Intern Med. 2013;159:688-97.
36. MS Sabatine, RP Giugliano, et al. Efficacy and safety of evolocumab in reducing lipids and cardiovascular events. N Engl J Med. 2015;372:1500-9.
37. Robinson JG, Farnier M, Krempf M, et al. Efficacy and safety of alirocumab in reducing lipids and cardiovascular events. N Engl J Med. 2015;372:1489-99.

21
Fighting the Devil of Stroke in Atrial Fibrillation: The New Weapons in the Armory

PC Manoria, Pankaj Manoria, Piyush Manoria, SK Parashar

INTRODUCTION

Atrial fibrillation (AF) is the most common cardiac arrhythmia encountered in clinical practice, and its prevalence is progressively increasing round the globe. It accounts for 1/3 of all strokes and is the leading cause of embolic stroke. The risk of stroke is 5 times in nonvalvular AF and 17 times with valvular AF.

Stroke is a devastating complication of atrial fibrillation. Prevention is the best solution, and indeed this is possible with optimum oral anticoagulation.

Stroke is a devastating complication of AF due to several reasons outlined in **Table 1**. However, stroke can be prevented in vast majority of patients by optimum anticoagulation.

The site of thrombus formation for stroke in AF is in left atrium/appendage. In nonvalvular AF, 90% of times the clot is in the left atrial appendage and this is the basis of left atrial appendage closure device in this condition.

It is important to bear in mind that the risk of stroke is same in all types of atrial fibrillation, i.e. paroxysmal, persistent and permanent.

For nearly 60 years, vitamin K antagonist (VKA) like warfarin was the only available option for prevention of stroke. However, warfarin has several limitations:

Warfarin has several limitations such as narrow therapeutic range, unpredictable pharmacokinetics and pharmacodynamics due to frequent drug to food and drug-to-drug interactions, wide fluctuation of international normalized ratio (INR), repeated monitoring of INR with dosage adjustments, slow onset and slow offset action.

1. It has a very narrow therapeutic range, i.e. the difference between therapeutic and toxic dose is very less and an INR of 2-3 is required for optimum anticoagulation[1] but patients are often outside the therapeutic range.[2] If the INR drops below 2, the risk of stroke increases 2 times, 3 times and 7 times for INR 1.7, 1.5 and 1.3 respectively.[3] If it gets elevated above 3, the bleeding risk is increased (**Fig. 1**).[4,5] The patient on warfarin is therefore always walking on a tight rope to keep balance between safety and efficacy of the drug.
2. The pharmacokinetics and pharmacodynamics of warfarin are variable and unpredictable due to high frequency of drug-to-drug and drug-to-food interactions,[6,7] which may enhance or reduce the anticoagulant effect of VKA. Thus the same dose may produce different therapeutic response in different individuals and also in same individuals over different periods. This requires frequent INR estimations, repeated dose adjustments and visits to doctors. The patients on warfarin often do not have TTR above the recommended value of 65%.
3. There is wide fluctuation of INR in patients on warfarin therapy and this is an important predisposing factor for development of intracranial hemorrhage which is potentially fatal.
4. It has a slow onset and a slow offset of action.
5. It has also teratogenicity and genetic polymorphism to *CYP2C9/VKORC1* genes.

Table 1 Salient features of stroke in patients with atrial fibrillation

- Large hemispheric infarct which may kill the patient.
- Persistent neurological disability with poor functional recovery
- Longer duration of hospitalization
- 30-day mortality 24%
- Hemorrhagic transformation more common
- No warning signs
- Not amenable to lytic therapy
- Increased recurrence rate

Chapter 21: Fighting the Devil of Stroke in Atrial Fibrillation: The New Weapons in the Armory

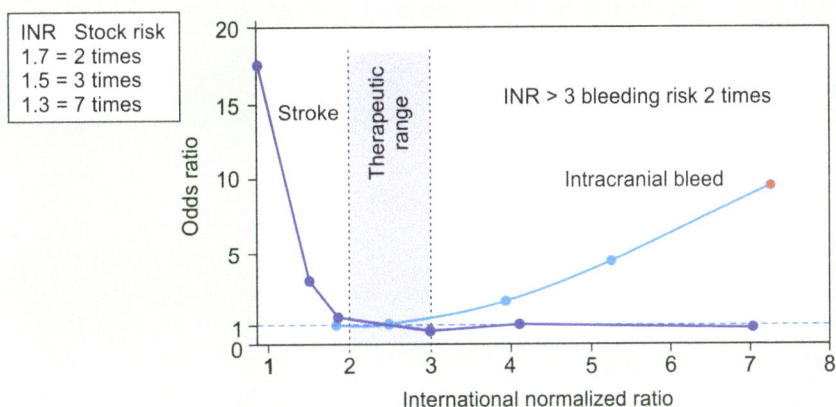

Fig. 1: Narrow therapeutic range of warfarin and relationship of INR to risk of stroke and bleeding

Due to above limitations of VKAs, there has been an ongoing search for better options and currently, we have four new weapons in the armory to fight the devil of stroke in atrial fibrillation **(Table 2)**. The term novel oral anticoagulant (NOAC) is not appropriate as these agents are commercially available, and currently they are designated as target specific oral anticoagulants (TSOACs).

All these drugs have been approved for commercial use in USA, Europe and several other countries. However, in India except only three drugs dabigatran, rivaroxaban and apixaban are available.

The beauty of new oral anticoagulants is that they are user friendly both for the patients and the doctor because of predictable pharmacokinetics, no drug to food interaction, minimal drug-to-drug interactions and no drug monitoring or dosage adjustments.

The beauty of TSOACs is that they are user-friendly drugs due to several reasons outlined in **Table 3**.

In addition, they have several other advantages also. They reduce the risk of intracranial hemorrhage by 50% which is an important cause of mortality in patients on VKAs. Besides this, they also decrease hemorrhagic stroke and fatal bleeds. In terms of reduction of ischemic stroke, most of the new agents are non-inferior but dabigatran 150 mg twice daily is superior to warfarin.

The pharmacokinetics of new OACs is outlined in **Table 4**.
The clinical profile of new OACs are outlined in **Table 5**.
Dabigatran, Rivaroxaban and Apixaban were evaluated in landmark trials Randomized evaluation of long-term anticoagulant therapy (RE-LY)[8], rivaroxaban once daily oral direct factor xa inhibition compared with vitamin K antagonism for prevention of stroke and embolism trial in atrial fibrillation (ROCKET-AF)[9] and Apixaban for reduction in stroke and other thromboembolic events in atrial fibrillation (ARISTOTLE)[10] trials respectively. The comparative data of above three trials is exhibited in **Table 6**.

Table 2 New TSOACs for preventing stroke in atrial fibrillation

Drug	Class	Trial	US FDA approval
Dabigatran	Direct factor IIa inhibitor	RELY	October 2010
Rivaroxaban	Direct factor Xa inhibitor	ROCKET AF	November 2011
Apixaban	Direct factor Xa inhibitor	ARISTOTLE	December 2012
Edoxaban	Direct factor Xa inhibitor	ENGAGE TIMI 56	January 2015

Table 3 Advantages of new TSOACs over VKAs

Rapid onset and offset of action
Predictable pharmacokinetics
Fixed dosing
No need for routine monitoring
Minimal drug-to-drug interaction
No drug to food interaction
Safety profile comparable or better than warfarin
Non-inferior or superior than warfarin

WHEN TO USE NEW ORAL ANTICOAGULANTS?

The TSOACs are a boon to patients of atrial fibrillation who have oscillating INRs with warfarin.

The newer agents can be used in following subsets of patients:
1. New patients of atrial fibrillation.
2. Patients on warfarin with oscillating INRs with poor control.

Table 4 Pharmacokinetics of new oral anticoagulants

Parameter	Dabigatran Etexilate	Rivaroxaban	Apixaban	Edoxaban
Mechanism of action	Selective direct FIIa inhibitor	Selective direct FXa inhibitor	Selective direct FXa inhibitor	Selective direct Xa inhibitor
Oral bioavailability (%)	6.5	80–100	50	62
Half-life, hour	12–17	5–13	8–15	6–11
Renal elimination (%)	85	66 (36 unchanged and 30 inactive metabolites)	27	50 of absorbed drug
Time to maximum inhibition, hour	0.5–2	1–4	1–4	1–2
Potential metabolic drug interactions	*Inhibition of P-gp*: Verapamil—reduce dose; Dronedarone avoid	Potent Inhibitors of *CYP3A4* and P-gp*: Avoid	Potent inhibitors of *CYP3A4* and P-gp*: Avoid	Potent inhibitors of P-gp*: Reduce dose
	Potent inducers of P-gp†: avoid	Potent inducers of CYP3A4‡ and P-gp: Use with caution	Potent inducers of CYP3A4 ‡and P-gp† use with caution	Potent inducers of P-gp†: Avoid

P-gp inhibitors include verapamil, amiodarone, dronedarone, quinidine, and clarithromycin.
*Potent inhibitors of *CYP3A4* include antifungals (e.g. ketoconazole, intraconazole, voriconazole, posaconazole), chloramphenicol, clarithromycin, and protease inhibitors (e.g. ritonavir, atanazavir).
† P-gp inducers include rifampicin, St. John's wort (Hypercium perforatum), carbamazepine, and phenytoin.
‡Potent *CYP3A4* inducers include phenytoin, carbamazepine, Phenobarbital, and St. John's wort.
Abbreviations: CYP, cytochrome P450 isoenzyme; F, factor; P-gp, P-glycoprotein.

3. High risk of intracranial hemorrhage like patients with severe hypertension.
4. Lower risk patients who are receiving aspirin instead of warfarin because of hassles of lifelong monitoring of INR and food restriction may be benefited by apixaban which is much more effective than aspirin in reducing stroke risk in this subset of patients with the bleeding risk equivalent to aspirin.

LIMITATIONS OF NEW ORAL ANTICOAGULANTS

The newer oral anticoagulants have several limitations.

The TSOACs have limitations that they require monitoring in patients with renal dysfunction and cannot be used in end-stage renal disease, lack of availability of validated tests for monitoring and increased GI bleeds with dabigatran and rivaroxaban.

Renal Dysfunction

All newer OAC are excreted through kidneys **(Table 7)**.

Therefore these drugs are contraindicated in patients with end stage CKD with creatinine excretion < 30 mL/min/ patients on hemodialysis. They can be used in patient with mild (creatinine clearance 50–80 mL/min.) and moderate renal failure (creatinine clearance 30–50 mL/min.) with great caution. Renal function monitoring and dosage adjustment is necessary. Lower dosages of dabigatran (110 mg bid/75 mg bid In USA) rivaroxaban (15 mg od) apixaban (2.5 mg bid) should be used. It is important to remember that patients with renal insufficiency are a high-risk group both for development of stroke as well as bleeding.

Monitoring Anticoagulant Effect

There are no validated tests to monitor anticoagulant effects of newer agents. The effect of dabigatran can be monitored by dilute thrombin time but this is not easily available. A qualitative idea about the anticoagulant effect of dabigatran can be obtained by measuring activated partial thromboplastin time (aPTT). If the value is >80 seconds at trough, there is higher risk of bleed.

Antidote

The good news is that the antibody to dabigatran, Idarucizumab has been approved for clinical use in USA and Europe by US FDA and EMA in October 2015. The approval came after the

Table 5 Clinical profile of warfarin with dabigatran, rivaroxaban and apixaban

Parameter	Warfarin	Dabigatran	Rivaroxaban	Apixaban
Dose adjustment	Frequently required	Not required	Not required	Not required
Monitoring	Frequent by INR	No monitoring	No monitoring	No monitoring
Therapeutic range	Narrow	Wide	Wide	Wide
TTR	Difficult to maintain	Easy	Easy	Easy
Measurement of anticoagulant activity	INR	Thrombin time aPTT >80 seconds at trough implies high risk of bleeding	Anti Xa activity	Anti Xa activity
Antidote	Vitamin K	Idarucizumab, a specific antidote is available in Europe and USA but not as yet in India	No specific antidote available but is in late stages of development PCC and recombinant factor VIIa can be used	No specific antidote available but is in late stages of development PCC and recombinant factor VIIa can be used
Dialysability	Not excreted through kidneys	Yes	No (highly bound to protein)	No (highly bound to protein)
Approved for use	All subsets of atrial fibrillation	Non-valvular atrial fibrillation only	Non-valvular atrial fibrillation only	Non-valvular atrial fibrillation only
Myocardial infarction	↓	↑	Not ↑	Not ↑

Abbreviations: aPTT, activated partial thromboplastin time; PCC, prothrombin concentrate complex; PCC 50 μg/kg in a single dose reverses rivaroxaban-induced prolongation of prothrombin time but whether it attenuates rivaroxaban-induced bleeding is unknown. It has little effect on dabigatran-induced prolongation of activated partial thromboplastin time in volunteers.

reverse AD trial. The antidote produces complete and rapid reversal of anticoagulant effect of dabigatran. Normalization of dilute thrombin time/ecarin clotting time is achieved in 100% within minutes of drug administration. It is administered in dosage of 2.5 mg two boluses 15 minutes apart. It is safe and well tolerated, and does not produce any prothrombotic effects. The antidote to dabigatran is likely to be available in India in future.

Antidote to factor Xa inhibitors, Andexanet alfa is also in late stages of development it has been successfully tested against Rivaroxaban and Apixaban in Phase III study and is being tested against edoxaban. It immediately and significantly reverses anticoagulant effect of above anticoagulants.

Although time and again, we say that one of the advantages of warfarin is that we have antidote to it. But the reality is that even when given intravenously, it takes 8–12 hours to act and therefore cannot be utilized in life-threatening bleeds. Such bleeds with warfarin are treated with Fresh Frozen Plasma/Prothrombin complex concentrate/Recombinant factor VIIa.

Treatment of Bleeding with Newer Agents

The bleeding with dabigatran can now be easily tackled with its antidote. Till antidote to dabigatran is available in India, bleeding following their use can be treated by general measures such as charcoal filtration, if the drug is ingested 2 hours before and dialysis (only dabigatran is dialyzable). Prothrombin Complex Concentrate/Recombinant Factor VIIa is also useful in bleeding due to TSOACs. Unlike warfarin one of the advantages of newer agents is that the half life of TSOACs is very short.

Gastrointestinal Bleed

Dabigatran 150 mg twice daily and Rivaroxaban 20 mg daily is associated with increased gastrointestinal (GI) bleed. Apixaban 5 mg/day and dabigatran 110 mg twice daily is not associated with increased GI bleed. These drugs do not cause lesions in GI tract. The bleeding occurs from pre-existing lesions and they increase pre-existing microscopic bleeding. Patients with prior GI bleed or at risk of GI bleed should undergone endoscopy prior to initiating therapy. NSAIDs should be avoided while using these drugs.

Increased Myocardial Infarction

There is a non-significant trend towards increased acute myocardial infarction with dabigatran therapy in the RE-LY trial. The difference could be due to warfarin effectiveness in reducing MI due to inhibition of factor VIIa and tissue factor complex which contribute to stabilizing coronary

Table 6 Comparison of trials of TSOACs for prevention of stroke in AF

Parameter	Rely		Rocket AF	Aristotle
Agent	Dabigatran		Rivaroxaban	Apixaban
Control	Warfarin		Warfarin	Warfarin
Number	18113		14269	18201
Mean $CHADS_2$ Score	2.1		3.5	2.1
$CHADS_2 > 3$	32%		86%	30%
Median age	72		73	70
INR-TTR	68%		55%	62%
Dose	150 mg bid /110 mg bid		20 mg daily or 15 mg daily in patient with CC* 30–49 mL/min	5 mg bid or 2.5 mg bid for patients with high bleeding risk♣
Stroke /Systemic embolism	150 mg bid	110 mg bid		
a. ITT	↓35%	↓10% (NI)	↓12% (NI)	↓21%
b. OT	↓44%		↓21%	
Ischemic stroke	↓	±	±	±
Hemorrhagic stroke	↓	↓	↓	↓
Major Bleeding	(NI)♠	↓20%	(NI)	↓31%
Intracranial bleeding	↓60%	↓69%	↓33%	↓58%
GI hemorrhage	↑	±	±	±
Mortality	-	-	-	↓11%
Discontinuation rates	21%		25%	

*Creatinine clearance
♣Any two of the following—Age ≥ 80 years, weight < 60 kg, or serum creatinine ≥ 1.5 mg/dL).
♠Noninferior.

Table 7 Renal excretion of new OACs

Drug	Renal excretion
Dabigatran	80%
Rivaroxaban	66%
Apixaban	25%
Edoxaban	50%

atherosclerotic plaques. But coronary artery disease is not a contraindication for these drugs. The use of rivaroxaban and apixaban is not associated with an increase in AMI.

Which Patient should Continue with Warfarin?

The TSOACs are approved for use only in non-valvular atrial fibrillation. Warfarin still remains the only drug for valvular atrial fibrillation, financial constraints and intolerance to TSOACs.

Even after availability of TSOACs, warfarin will continue to be used in the following indications:

1. Patients who are already on long-term warfarin with well-controlled INRs and handling the monitoring without problem will drive uncertain overall advantages from switching to new oral anticoagulants. These patients should be allowed to continue warfarin.
2. Warfarin may still be needed in patients with:
   a. Intolerance to new anticoagulants
   b. Indications for which new anticoagulants have yet not been approved.
   c. Financial constraints.

For initiating oral anticoagulant (OAC) therapy for prevention of stroke, one has to calculate the risk of stroke by $CHADS_2$[11,12] **(Tables 8 and 9)** and CHA_2DS_2 VASC[13-16] scores **(Table 10)** and the bleeding risk by HAS-BLED score[17] **(Table 11)**.

The $CHADS_2$ has the limitation that it is not sensitive for prediction of stroke when the score is low, i.e. 0 to 1 and under such circumstances CHA_2DS_2-VASc should be utilized.

The $CHADS_2$ score is simple but has the limitation that it is not sensitive for prediction of stroke when the score is low, i.e. 0–1. A score of 0 is associated with a stroke risk of 1.9% per year. Therefore with low $CHADS_2$ score, more sensitive CHA_2DS_2-VASc score should be utilized as this is predictive of stroke even with low scores.

The HAS-BLED is the most validated score for assessing the bleeding risk.

A high bleeding risk is not a contraindication for OAC and the risk benefit ratio is still in favor of the patient. In this subset, TSOACs should be preferred but if warfarin is used the INR should be kept between 2.0 and 2.5 with frequent monitoring. However, a vigilant watch should be kept for detection of bleeding in early stages. Drugs with rapidly acting antidote should be preferred.

NICE Guidelines 2014

The SAMe-TT_2R_2 scoring system of NICE Guidelines 2014 can be utilized to predict as to which patients of atrial fibrillation will have good INR and TTR control

Table 8 $CHADS_2$ score

Parameter	Score
Cardiac failure	1
Hypertension	1
Age ≥ 75 years	1
Diabetes mellitus	1
Stroke or TIA (previous history)	2

Abbreviation: TIA, transient ischemic attack

Table 9 Estimation of stroke risk in AF using $CHADS_2$

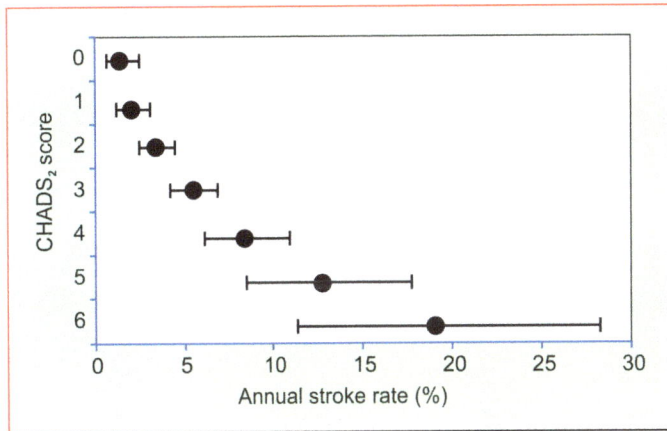

$CHADS_2$ score	Patients (n = 1733)	Adjusted stroke rate (%/year)
0	120	1.9
1	463	2.8
2	523	4.0
3	337	5.9
4	220	8.5
5	65	12.5
6	5	18.2

Table 10 Stroke risk assessment with CHA_2DS_2-VASc

CHA_2DS_2-VASc criteria	Score
Congestive heart failure/left ventricular dysfunction	1
Hypertension	1
Age ≥75 years	2
Diabetes mellitus	1
Stroke/transient ischemic attack/TE	2
Vascular disease (prior myocardial infarction, peripheral artery disease or aortic plaque)	1
Age 65–74 years	1
Sex category (i.e. female gender)	1

Total score	Patients (n = 7329)	Adjusted stroke rate (%/year)*
0	1	0.0
1	422	1.3
2	1230	2.2
3	1730	3.2
4	1718	4.0
5	1159	6.7
6	679	9.8
7	294	9.6
8	82	6.7
9	14	15.2

*ACC/AHA/HRS Guidelines, 2014
Score 0: No antithrombotic therapy or low dose aspirin (former preferred Class IIa)
Score 1: Either low dose aspirin or OAC (latter preferred Class IIb)
Score 2: Only OAC (Class I: Warfarin /dabigatran/rivaroxaban /apixaban)

Table 11 Bleeding risk assessment on anticoagulation—HAS-BLED

HAS-BLED risk criteria	Score
Hypertension	1
Abnormal renal or liver function (1 point each)	1 or 2
Stroke	1
Bleeding	1
Labile INRs	1
Elderly (e.g. age >65 years)	1
Drugs or alcohol (1 point each)	1 or 2

Abbreviation: INR, international normalized ratio

HAS-BLED total score	N	Number of bleeds	Bleeds per 100 patient-years*
0	798	9	1.13
1	1286	13	1.02
2	744	14	1.88
3	187	7	3.74
4	46	4	8.70
5	8	1	12.5
6	2	0	0.0
7	0	–	–
8	0	–	–
9	0	–	–

*P value for trend = 0.007

Table 12 Scoring system of NICE guidelines, 2014

Parameters	SAMe-TT$_2$R$_2$ score
S	*Sex*: Female
A	*Age*: < 60 years
M	Medical history (more than two co-morbidities)
T	Treatment (interacting drugs, e.g. amiodarone for rhythm control)
T	Tobacco use (doubled)
R	Race (doubled)

Score	Interpretation
0 to 2	Warfarin (Anticipated INR control and TTR good)
> 2	TSOACs (Anticipated INR control and TTR bad)

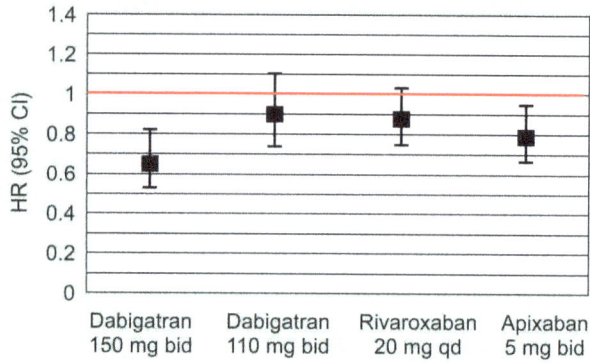

Fig. 2: Comparable primary efficacy endpoints of stroke or systemic embolism

with warfarin. If the score < 2 it can be anticipated that warfarin will be an appropriate drug but if the score > 2, TSOACs should be used.

The NICE Guidelines released in July 2014 has given a new score, SAMe-TT$_2$R$_2$[18] **(Table 12)** for predicting who will have good INR and TTR control on warfarin. If the score is 0–2, the anticipated INR and TTR control is good but if the score is > 2 the patients should not be prescribed warfarin and therapy should be initiated with newer agents.

COMPARISON OF TSOACs

In the absence of head-to-head trial with new agents, it is very difficult to comment on superiority or inferiority of any drug but the results of landmark trials can be utilized to decide as to which agent may be more appropriate for a given subset of patient of atrial fibrillation.

The hazard ratio for primary efficacy endpoints of stroke or systemic embolism is displayed in **Figure 2**, and primary safety endpoint of major bleeding is shown in **Figure 3**. Based on these HR ratios, dabigatran is most effective in reduction of ischemic stroke and apixaban produces minimal bleeding

There is no doubt that the new agents have distinct advantages over warfarin and are poised to be game changers in prevention of stroke in atrial fibrillation. Currently, cost is a major issue but this is likely to be resolved with increasing use of these drugs.

The superiority or inferiority of new agents cannot be judged by the existing landmarks trials because the patients included in these trials have different CHADS$_2$ and HAS-BLED scores and the TTR are also different. It seems unlikely that in future any head-to-head trial will be conducted.

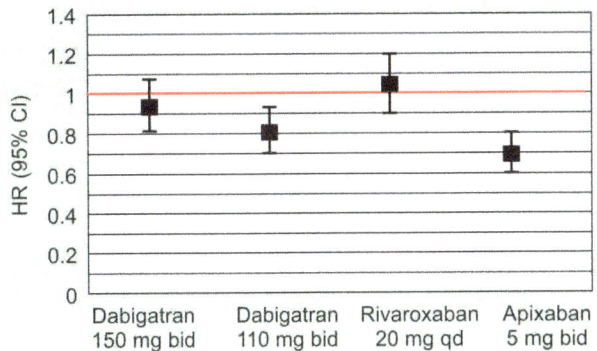

Fig. 3: Comparable primary safety endpoints of major bleeding

CONCLUSION

Thus TSOACs are useful addition to the drug armamentarium for prevention of stroke. With approval of antidote to dabigatran (idarucizumab), the drug will be used more widely and with greater safety. For prevention of stroke most of them are non-inferior but dabigatran 150 mg. twice daily is superior to warfarin. They are user friendly both for patients and physicians/cardiologists. In addition, they produce 50% reduction in the intracranial bleeds, which, is potentially a lethal complication. No doubt, they are costly, but if the patient is properly explained the advantages of these drugs, many of them opt for it.

REFERENCES

1. Fuster V, Ryden LE, Cannom DS, et al. ACC/AHA/ESC 2006 Guidelines for the Management of Patients with Atrial Fibrillation: a report of the American College of Cardiology/American Heart Association Task Force on Practice Guidelines and the European Society of Cardiology Committee for Practice Guidelines (Writing Committee to Revise the 2001 Guidelines for the Management of Patients with Atrial Fibrillation): developed in collaboration with the European Heart Rhythm Association and the Heart Rhythm Society. Circulation. 2006;114:e257-54.
2. Samsa GP, Matchar DB, Goldstein LB, et al. Quality of anticoagulation management among patients with atrial fibrillation: results of a review of medical records from 2 communities. Arch Intern Med. 2000;160:967-73.
3. Hylek EM, Go AS, Chang Y, et al. Effect of intensity of oral anticoagulation on stroke severity and mortality in atrial fibrillation. N Engl J Med. 2003;349:1019-26.
4. Hylek EM, Singer DE. Risk factors for intracranial hemorrhage in outpatients taking warfarin, Ann Intern Med. 1994;120:897-902.
5. Hylek EM, Skates SJ, Sheehan MA, Singer DE. An analysis of the lower effective intensity of prophylactic anticoagulation for patients with non-rheumatic atrial fibrillation. N Engl J Med. 1996;335:540-6.
6. Du Breuil AL, Umland EM. Outpatient management of anticoagulation therapy. Am Fam Physician. 2007;75:1031-42.
7. Holbrook AM, Pereira JA, Labiris R, et al. Systematic overview of warfarin and its drug and food interactions. Arch Intern Med. 2005;165:1095-106.
8. Connolly SJ, Ezekowitz Md, Yusuf S, et al. Dabigatran versus warfarin in patients with atrial fibrillation. NEJM. 2011;361:1139-51.
9. Patel RM, Mahaffey KW, Garg J, et al. Rivaroxaban versus warfarin in nonvalvular atrial fibrillation. NEJM. 2011;365:883-91.
10. Granger CB, Alexander JH, McMurray JJ, et al. Apixaban versus warfarin in patients with atrial fibrillation. NEJM. 2011;365:981-92.
11. Gage BF, et al. Validation of clinical classification schemes for predicting stroke: results from the national registry of atrial fibrillation. JAMA. 2001;285:2864-70.
12. Gage BF, et al. Validation of Clinical Classification Schemes for Predicting Stroke Results From the National Registry of Atrial Fibrillation. JAMA. 2001;285(22):2864-70.
13. Lip GY, et al. Refining Clinical Risk Stratification for Predicting Stroke and Thromboembolism in Atrial Fibrillation using a novel risk factors-based approach: The Euro Heart Survey on Atrial Fibrillation. Chest. 2010;137(2):263-72.
14. Lip G, et al. Identifying patients at high risk for stroke despite anticoagulation: A comparison of contemporary stroke risk stratification schemes in an anticoagulated atrial fibrillation cohort. Stroke. 2010;41:2731-38.
15. Camm J, et al. Guidelines for the management of atrial fibrillation. The Task Force for the Management of Atrial Fibrillation of the European Society of Cardiology (ESC). Eur Heart J. 2010;31:2369-429.
16. Hart RG, Pearce LA, Aguilar MI, et al. Meta-analysis: antithrombotic therapy to prevent stroke in patients who have nonvalvular atrial fibrillation. Ann Intern Med. 2007;146:857-67.
17. Pisters R, et al. A novel user-friendly score (HAS-BLED) to assess 1-year risk of major bleeding in patients with atrial fibrillation: the Euro Heart Survey. Chest. 2010;138:1093-100.
18. Apostolakis S, Sullivan RM, Olshansky B, Lib GYH. Factors affecting quality of anticoagulation control among patients with atrial fibrillation on warfarin. The SAMe-TT$_2$R$_2$ Score. Chest. 2013;144(5):1565.

CORONARY ARTERY DISEASE

22 Management of Prehospital Phase of Acute Myocardial Infarction

AK Pancholia

INTRODUCTION

The prompt delivery of high quality coronary care to patients following acute coronary syndromes is of paramount importance. This is especially so in acute myocardial infarction (AMI) with ST-elevation on the presenting electrocardiogram, as 26% of patients died before reaching the hospital (**Fig. 1**) while the rapid restoration of patency of the infarct-related artery improves survival.[1] Although the medical and technologic revolution in the last three decades has improved clinical outcome in patients sustaining acute ST-elevation myocardial infarction (STEMI), residual morbidity and mortality remain major health concerns. Delay in initiating treatment after AMI may be categorized into two phases: patient delay, i.e. the time between symptom onset and call for help and healthcare system delay which encompasses the response to patient call, transport to the institution, and the time to appropriate treatment following arrival at hospital.

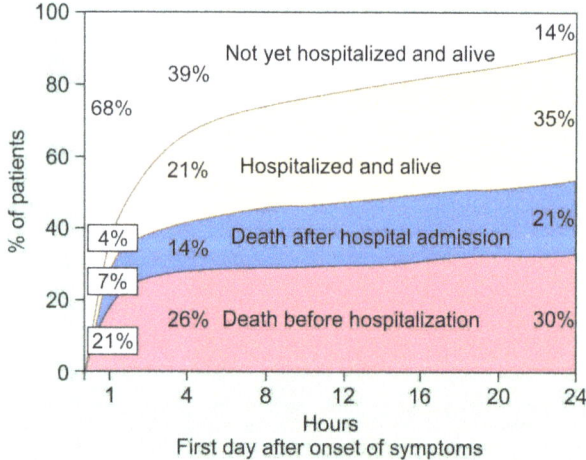

Fig. 1: Survival in the first day after acute myocardial infarction

Over the years various methods have been proposed to reduce these delays. Provision of out-of-hospital mobile coronary care in the community with staff trained in the recognition and management of acute myocardial ischemia/infarction reduces transport and hospital delay times. The efficacy and safety of such prehospital initiated treatment has been demonstrated in many early studies.[2,3] Patients with ST-segment elevation on the initial ECG and suitable for fibrinolytic therapy have been studied out-of-hospital.[4,5-11] A small number of randomized trials have also compared the efficacy of prehospital initiated fibrinolytic therapy with therapy first commenced in-hospital.[4,5,8-12] These studies have demonstrated consistently a reduced pain to needle time with prehospital treatment, with an average gain of 1 hour.[13,14] A physician-staffed prehospital coronary care unit in addition to providing early fibrinolytic therapy has the advantage of prompt identification and treatment of the early complications of acute myocardial ischemia/infarction.

PATHOPHYSIOLOGY AND IMPACT OF TIME

Abrupt coronary obstruction leads to transmural ischemia within the area at risk determined by the coronary anatomy. The jeopardized myocardium develops irreversible changes starting in the subendocardium and progressing outwards. This progression of necrosis has been termed the 'wavefront phenomenon'.[15] In anesthetized dogs, infarct size increases with duration of coronary occlusion for up to 6 hours. After 6 hours, reperfusion has no effect on infarct size. The temporal and spatial progression of necrosis across the ventricular wall represents a fundamental pathophysiological phenomenon. Indirect evidence suggests that in humans average infarct size without reperfusion therapy is about 20% of the left ventricle. If thrombolytic treatment is started 1 hour after onset, 70% of jeopardized myocardium is salvaged, but it is 0% when thrombolysis initiated 5 hours after onset.[16,17]

Limited benefit following myocardial reperfusion in acute myocardial infarction may result from an underestimation of occlusion time. On the other hand, coronary occlusion may be intermittent despite the presence of continuous pain. Intermittent spontaneous reperfusion may prevent or limit myocardial damage and benefit may then follow from relatively late therapeutic interventions.[18]

DELAYS IN PROVIDING TREATMENT FOR CARDIAC EMERGENCIES

Delays in providing treatment depends on four factors:
1. Patient decision time
2. Doctor decision time
3. Dispatching
4. Ambulance response interval.

Patient Decision Time

The interval from the onset of symptoms until medical assistance is sought varies widely. Despite widespread public education, reports on patient delays have demonstrated only small trends to shorter time intervals.[19] Decision time is not closely related to knowledge of heart symptoms. Symptoms are often interpreted incorrectly[20] because of psychological defence mechanisms such as denial[21] or displacement and rationalization;[22] but responses are influenced by severity of pain,[23] the emotional reactions to it,[24] and the degree of left ventricular dysfunction.[25]

Doctor Decision Time

Although call-to-needle times can be very short when general practitioners give thrombolytics prehospital,[26] many studies have shown that the involvement of the majority who do not themselves give thrombolytic therapy in the management of myocardial infarction results in substantial delay in definitive treatment given after arrival in hospital.[27,28] Calling a general practitioner alone in response to a cardiac arrest may be even less appropriate in countries where few are equipped for defibrillation.

Dispatching

The dispatcher has four decisions to make: (1) whether or not to send an ambulance; (2) if an ambulance is to be sent the type of ambulance to be deployed; (3) how much urgency is needed; (4) whether advice should be given to the caller on actions to be taken meanwhile. The first of these is the most difficult even for experienced medical dispatchers, because the quality of information is frequently too poor for any safe decision not to send an ambulance.[29] Many ambulances are dispatched to patients whose complaints turn out not to have been urgent.[30] Many ambulance control centers send vehicles in response to all requests for help whilst others use algorithms to assess the urgency and priority of calls.

Ambulance Response Interval

The ambulance response interval (which measures the duration from call to arrival at the patient's side) of the first or only tier is in general the shortest of all the delays. In some countries, a time limit is set whereby 95% of all ambulance journeys must be completed within 15 minutes and 80% within 10 minutes. In others, strict time criteria are being set for selected cases based on the information received and using systems of prioritized despatch. Both of these approaches are in line with the concepts of early defibrillation for cardiac arrest and early reperfusion for acute myocardial infarction.

PREHOSPITAL ECGs IN PATIENTS WITH STEMI: WHAT ARE THE BENEFITS? (BOX 1)

Multiple studies have demonstrated the benefits of prehospital ECGs for decreasing door-to-drug time and door-to-balloon time in patients with STEMI.[31] The direction and magnitude of the time savings are clinically relevant, resulting in an approximately 10-minute decrease in door-to-drug time and 15- to 20-minute decrease in door-to-balloon time.[31,32] However, these time savings may not reflect the full potential of prehospital ECGs to decrease delays in reperfusion therapy. In fact, studies have shown further reductions in door-to-balloon time when prehospital ECGs are used to activate the catheterization laboratory while the patient is enroute to the hospital.[33-39] For patients transported by EMS without prehospital ECG, delay from symptom onset to reperfusion therapy, which reflects the overall period of ischemic injury, can be divided into four time intervals: (a) symptom onset to EMS arrival, (b) EMS arrival to hospital arrival, (c) hospital arrival to ECG, and (d) ECG to reperfusion. Prehospital ECG programs, if effectively implemented and coordinated with hospital systems of care, would be expected to decrease the latter 3 time intervals. The second interval is composed of time from first medical contact by EMS to hospital door, and EMS personnel may behave with more urgency if a diagnosis of STEMI has been made in the field. The third interval is essentially eliminated with a prehospital ECG. The fourth

---

BOX 1 Benefits of prehospital ECG

- Recognize AMI
- Identify reperfusion candidates
- *Earlier the better:* Time is muscle
- Reduce time to thrombolysis
- Reduce time to PCI
- Prehospital thrombolysis

Abbreviations: AMI, acute myocardial infarction; PCI, percutaneous coronary infarction

interval can be decreased by advanced notification of the hospital to receive and evaluate the patient, to activate the catheterization laboratory while the patient is en-route, or to bypass the emergency department and transport the patient directly to the catheterization laboratory. Scholz and colleagues reported the impact of prehospital ECGs on these time intervals from 114 patients with STEMI treated within an integrated system of care.[40] The system consisted of acquiring a prehospital ECG by emergency responders, transmitting the prehospital ECG to a fax machine at the percutaneous coronary intervention (PCI) hospital cardiac intensive care unit, activating the catheterization laboratory en-route if STEMI was diagnosed, and bypassing the emergency department when the catheterization laboratory team was on-site. The time spent at the scene decreased from 25 to 19 minutes, time spent in the emergency department decreased from 14 to 3 minutes, time from arterial access to balloon decreased from 21 to 11 minutes, door-to-balloon time decreased from 54 to 26 minutes, and first medical contact to balloon time decreased from 113 to 74 minutes. It is concluded that systematic, quarterly feedback on performance to cardiology, emergency department, and EMS stakeholders was an important component in improving prehospital and hospital processes of care.[40]

CURRENT GUIDELINES FOR PREHOSPITAL ECGs AMONG PATIENTS WITH ST-SEGMENT–ELEVATION MYOCARDIAL INFARCTION

American Heart Association national guidelines,[41-43] as well as other consensus and scientific statements,[44-46] recommend that emergency medical services (EMS) acquire and use prehospital ECGs to evaluate patients with suspected acute coronary syndrome. Despite these recommendations, prehospital ECGs are used in fewer than 10% of patients with ST-segment–elevation myocardial infarction (STEMI),[47] and this rate has not substantially changed since the mid-1990s. Furthermore, even when a prehospital ECG is acquired, the information is often not effectively translated into action and coordinated with hospital systems of care to decrease delays in reperfusion therapy.

The Chain of Survival for Cardiac Arrest

In no medical emergency is time such a decisive determinant of outcome as in circulatory arrest. The 'chain of survival' concept clearly describes the important links involved.[48,49] The chain is usually regarded as having four links.

Early Access

Immediate access to an ambulance dispatch center is a primary requirement because any delay in calling the ambulance service inevitably decreases the prospects of survival. The initial contact should not be with a physician, unless he/she has the role of first tier in the EMS and has a defibrillator. The caller's description of the problem should influence the degree of priority that is accorded preferably by the use of one of the evaluated algorithm systems: the dispatcher should be alerted by any suggestion of impaired consciousness and should not be reassured by the statement that the victim is breathing, as gasping may continue for minutes after circulatory arrest. Convulsion and vasovagal collapse may cause confusion.

Early Cardiopulmonary Resuscitation (CPR)

It has been estimated that at any point in time between collapse and first defibrillation, bystander CPR at least doubles the chance of survival,[50,51] with the possible exception of the first few minutes.[51]

Early Defibrillation

In most instances, ventricular fibrillation is the initial rhythm associated with circulatory arrest. As time passes, the waveform of ventricular fibrillation loses amplitude and frequency until no deflections can be detected. Electrical defibrillation is the only effective therapy for ventricular fibrillation, and the interval between the onset of the arrhythmia and the delivery of the first defibrillating shock is the main determinant of successful defibrillation and survival. The possibility of successful defibrillation decreases by more than 5% per minute from the time of collapse. To achieve early defibrillation, it is mandatory that people other than doctors be permitted to defibrillate. In particular, all first tier ambulances should be equipped with defibrillators, and ambulance personnel should be proficient in their use.[52] Nonmedical ambulance personnel can be trained in defibrillation in as little as 8–10 hours, provided they have good training in basic life support.

Automated External Defibrillation

The automated external defibrillator (AED) can be employed by persons with a limited training targeted to use of the equipment, but without sufficient knowledge for a reliable diagnosis of ventricular fibrillation.[53] This makes it possible to bring the defibrillator to locations with large crowds such as stadiums, airports, shopping malls, and railway stations, where trained first aid personnel can employ them rapidly and in locations where EMS intervention is almost impossible such as airplanes or cruise ships.

Early Advanced Care

In many instances, CPR and defibrillation alone do not achieve or sustain resuscitation, and advanced cardiac life support is necessary further to improve the prospect of survival. In some systems, endotracheal intubation and intravenous medication are not provided out of hospital, while in others advanced life support is available from the first tier of the ambulance service, or more commonly by a second tier. Transportation to the hospital intensive care unit should not be allowed to interrupt appropriate advanced care.

TREATMENT OF ACUTE CORONARY SYNDROMES IN THE PREHOSPITAL PHASE

General Measures for Patients without Overt Complications

Pain relief: Pain should be relieved as quickly as possible. This is a priority because pain will increase anxiety and the resulting sympathetic stimulation will aggravate myocardial ischemia. Pain should, therefore, be controlled adequately as soon as possible. Opioids such as morphine (or diamorphine where its use is permitted) should be administered intravenously and titrated until pain is adequately relieved. Subcutaneous and intramuscular injections should be avoided. Nitrates and intravenous beta-blockers that may be given for other reasons can contribute to pain relief by improving the underlying ischemia. Anxiolytics, in particular benzodiazepines, may be given if anxiety is perceived as a major component of the patient's distress.

Treatment of early nausea, vomiting, hypotension, and bradycardia: These common features of the initial phase of acute heart attacks may be due to excess vagal tone and/or the side effects of analgesics, nitrates, and beta-blockers. Antiemetic drugs such as metoclopramide may be used to counter nausea and vomiting. Bradycardia (with or without hypotension) despite the relief of pain and nausea may be improved by the administration of atropine. Persisting hypotension is likely to reflect severe myocardial damage.

Aspirin administration: Aspirin significantly improves the prognosis of patients with suspected acute myocardial infarction or unstable angina.[54] The efficacy of aspirin in reducing cardiovascular death seems to be similar in patients treated early and late.[55] Thus, aspirin (150 to 300 mg, preferably) should be given to all patients with acute coronary syndromes in the absence of clear contraindications irrespective of the delay between presumed onset of symptoms and first evaluation. Since antiplatelet activity may be obtained within 30 minutes antithrombotic protection should not be delayed until arrival in hospital. Aspirin is simple to administer, it does not require specific monitoring, and as a single dose it is well tolerated. The additive effect of aspirin and fibrinolytics on cardiovascular mortality and the preventive effect of aspirin on the 'excess' of recurrence of myocardial infarction with thrombolysis was observed when aspirin was given immediately before the infusion of fibrinolytic agents. If fibrinolytic therapy is given in the prehospital phase, aspirin should be administered concomitantly to help prevent early reocclusions. Heparin was the reference antithrombotic treatment for the acute phase of myocardial infarction, but the risk of major bleeding was significantly increased by 50%. Heparin as an adjunctive treatment to streptokinase and aspirin has not been shown to improve mortality in two large trials, but it did increase the risk of bleeding.[56,57]

Prehospital beta-blockade: The efficacy of beta-blocking agents in preventing death and reinfarction after myocardial infarction is well established. Many trials and meta-analyses[58-61] have assessed the value of starting intravenous beta-blockade early after the onset of symptoms. A meta-analysis of the trials available to early 1985 showed a 13% reduction in total short-term mortality ($P<0.02$), a 20% reduction in reinfarction ($P<0.02$), and a 15% reduction in ventricular fibrillation or cardiac arrest ($P<0.05$) and the two subsequent large trials[58,59] were consistent with this evidence. In addition, intravenous beta-blockade reduces ischemic pain and tachyarrhythmias. Despite these results, experience of beta-blockade in the early phase of myocardial infarction is limited. No evidence of a mortality benefit from early beta-blockade as compared with delayed beta-blockade was seen in one randomized trial, but the study was not powered for showing differences in mortality. The ESC task force consider there is no strong indication for systematic use of beta-blockade before hospital admission.

Prophylactic use of oral or intravenous nitrates: More than 80,000 patients with acute myocardial infarction have been involved in 22 studies comparing early intravenous or oral nitrates with control groups. Two large studies, GISSI-3[62] and ISIS 4,[63] contributed most of the patients and reported no mortality benefit. A meta-analysis[63] showed only a 5.5% reduction of mortality ($P = 0.03$). This translates into a saving of 3.8 deaths per 1000 treated. Whether this benefit is sufficient to justify routine use of nitrates is debatable, particularly with the added uncertainties of the prehospital phase. Nitrates may be deleterious in cases of right ventricular ischemia or infarction which may complicate inferior left ventricular changes. Persistent pain or the presence of heart failure may of course be valid indications for their use for patients with these specific conditions, but they are not at present recommended for routine administration.

Prophylactic use of ACE inhibitors: Long-term use of ACE inhibitors started a few days after myocardial infarction has been established as an effective treatment to reduce mortality and reinfarction in patients with clinical signs of heart failure or with an impaired ejection fraction. Early treatment with ACE inhibitors is considered relatively safe, although it increases the risk of hypotension, cardiogenic shock, and renal dysfunction.[63] Because of these side effects and of the lack of information on the early prehospital phase, the ESC Task Force do not recommend the prophylactic prehospital use of ACE inhibitors.

Prophylactic use of antiarrhythmic therapy: Lidocaine has been advocated to prevent ventricular fibrillation in patients with acute myocardial infarction. Several studies have been performed to test the efficacy of prophylactic lidocaine for this indication. Meta analyses[64,65] have shown a reduction of approximately 35% in the incidence of ventricular fibrillation but also a nonsignificant trend to an increase in mortality. Studies restricted to the prehospital phase have included data on 7386 patients, but these have not provided any evidence for a reduction in mortality as a result of prophylactic antiarrhythmic therapy. With current knowledge routine use of lidocaine or other prophylactic antiarrhythmics in the prehospital phase cannot be recommended.

REPERFUSION THERAPY: PREHOSPITAL THROMBOLYSIS

Current Guidelines

All guidelines are based on the results of RCTs comparing primary PCI (PPCI) and thrombolysis, as well as on observational data from registries. As most guidelines were published a few years ago, the most recent data have obviously not been taken into account. All agree that time is critical and reperfusion should be initiated as soon as possible.[66-68] The American Heart Association (AHA) and the American College of Cardiology (ACC) favor the use of PHT over PCI, placing the emphasis on the time factor rather than on the method of reperfusion. AHA/ACC guidelines state that PHT should be performed only following the confirmation of STEMI on a 12-lead ECG, interpreted by a physician on site or after transmission to a specialist. A reperfusion checklist should also be completed to ensure that the patient has no contraindications to thrombolytics and to identify high-risk patients who would benefit more from PPCI. PHT should be performed within 30 minutes of the arrival of the emergency services. If PHT cannot be administered and the patient is subsequently transported to a hospital that has no PCI facility, the door-to-needle time (arrival at the hospital to the administration of thrombolytic, DN) should be 30 minutes. If, however, the hospital can offer PCI, the door-to-balloon time (arrival to PCI, DB) should be 90 minutes.[66,69] The recent update of the ACC/AHA guidelines[66] insists that patients presenting to a hospital with PCI capability should be treated with PPCI within 90 minutes of first medical contact (level of evidence A). In patients presenting to a hospital without PCI capability and who cannot be transferred to a hospital center and undergo PCI within 90 minutes of first medical contact, fibrinolytic therapy should be administered within 30 minutes of hospital presentation unless contraindicated (level of evidence B). The goal is to organize systems of care such that the total ischemic time be 120 minutes. The goals for each management step are the following: time from symptom onset to first call to emergency medical service (EMS): 5 minutes, with 1 minutes EMS dispatch; EMS on scene within 8 minutes, ECG on scene and consider prehospital fibrinolytic therapy by EMS if capable and time to lytic therapy 30 minutes; if transportation to a hospital without PCI capability, DN time 30 minutes; if transportation to a hospital with PCI capability, EMS-to-balloon time 90 minutes (if patient self-transport: DB time 90 minutes). In its most recent guidelines,[67] the European Society of Cardiology (ESC) recommends reperfusion by PPCI, if performed by an experienced operator within 120 minutes of the first medical contact or within 90 minutes of first medical contact if the patients present within 2 hours of the onset of symptoms and have a large myocardial area at risk and a low bleeding risk. PPCI should be used in patients with contraindications to thrombolysis and is the preferred treatment for patients in shock. Otherwise, thrombolysis should be administered as soon as possible. If thrombolysis fails (based on the lack of sufficient ST-segment resolution), rescue PCI should be performed within a reasonable time delay (up to 12 hours after symptom onset). If thrombolysis is successful (50% ST-segment resolution at 60–90 minutes, reperfusion arrhythmias, disappearance of chest pain), coronary angiography is recommended in the absence of contraindications. To avoid an early PCI during the prothrombotic period following fibrinolysis, on the one hand, and to minimize the risk of reocclusion, on the other hand, a time window of 3–24 hours following successful fibrinolysis is recommended.[67] In contrast, facilitated PCI (using thrombolytics or GP IIb/IIIa inhibitors before primary angioplasty) is not recommended.

PREREQUISITES FOR PREHOSPITAL THROMBOLYSIS

It is important to know the structure of the prehospital thrombolysis program. The program includes:
- Well-equipped cardiac ambulances.
- Ability to perform 12 lead ECG in ambulances.
- Trained medics and paramedics to interpret ECGs.
- ECG transmission facility to a specialized center.
- Capability to treat cardiac and cerebrovascular emergencies in ambulances.
- Availability of bolus dose—thrombolytic agents.
- Facility to provide awareness and education program directed at the general population on disease manifestation and strategies to reduce ambulance service time.

CHOICE OF THROMBOLYTIC AGENTS FOR PREHOSPITAL THROMBOLYSIS

The National Institute for Clinical Excellence supports reperfusion with fibrinolytics, recommending prehospital thrombolysis (PHT) using the newer agents, reteplase and tenecteplase, whose bolus application simplifies administration. Time is crucial here too and therapy should be initiated within 12 hours of symptom onset.[70] The European Resuscitation Council guidelines state: thrombolysis is indicated in the absence of contraindications if PCI is not possible within 90 minutes, or if symptom duration is 3 hours and delay to PCI 60 minutes. PCI is indicated, if available within 90 minutes (60 minutes, if presenting within 3 hours of symptom onset) if thrombolytics are contraindicated, the patient is in cardiogenic shock, severe left ventricular failure, or presents later than 3 hours. All guidelines stress that a network for STEMI management should be developed on a national and/or regional level, with continuous monitoring to show how reperfusion strategies work in real-life situations.

PREHOSPITAL VERSUS IN-HOSPITAL THROMBOLYSIS

However, as documented in a meta-analysis of six randomized trials, PHT is significantly superior to in-hospital thrombolysis (IHT) in terms of hospital mortality and it saved 45 minutes compared with IHT, which could potentially preserve myocardial tissue and improve outcomes[71] **(Fig. 2)**.

COMPARISON OF THROMBOLYSIS WITH PERCUTANEOUS CORONARY INTERVENTION IN RANDOMIZED CONTROLLED TRIALS[5]

Randomized controlled trials (RCTs) have shown PPCI to be more effective than fibrinolysis for STEMI when performed by an experienced team within 90 minutes of first medical contact.[72-74] Keeley et al. evaluated 23 trials comparing PPCI with thrombolysis using streptokinase or a fibrin-specific agent. Regardless of the thrombolytic agent, PPCI was more effective, even if transfer to centers with appropriate facilities was necessary.[72-74] Comparison of angioplasty and prehospital thrombolysis in acute myocardial infarction (CAPTIM), compared PHT and PPCI. Patients who received thrombolysis within 2 hours of symptom onset showed a strong trend towards lower 30 days mortality than those who had undergone PPCI. Beyond 2 hours, the difference between the groups was almost reversed in favor of PPCI.[75] The findings from CAPTIM are consistent with those from PRAGUE-2, which showed that within 3 hours of symptom onset, mortality rates were almost identical, but in patients randomized after 3 hours, mortality following thrombolysis was much higher.[76] The investigators concluded that if STEMI patients can be transferred within 20–30 minutes, they should receive PPCI. If this cannot be performed within 60 minutes, thrombolysis can be administered up to 3 hours after onset. Beyond 3 hours, thrombolysis should not be used, and patients should be transferred for PPCI. Likewise, in the Primary Coronary Angioplasty vs. Thrombolysis (PCAT)-2 Trialists Collaborative Group meta-analysis,[77] 30-day mortality doubled in the fibrinolysis group as the time delay increased from 1 to 6 hours. The re-infarction rate was also higher in this group and increased with the time delay (not observed in the PPCI group). Thus, the time delay to reperfusion remains central to the choice of strategy.[77] Another important point is the role of subsequent PCI after PHT. In CAPTIM, 70% of patients in the thrombolysis group underwent PCI before day 30, with 26% requiring rescue PCI. Therefore, the actual comparison in this trial was between PPCI and PHT followed by PCI if thrombolysis failed.[75] Furthermore, the role of systematic PCI within 24 hours of thrombolysis was tested in the Grupo de Analisis de la Cardiopatia Isquemica Aguda (GRACIA-1) trial[78] and in the CARESS-in-AMI trial.[79] In both instances, the policy of systematic PCI following thrombolysis yielded better results than conservative management. The WEST (Which Early ST-elevation myocardial infarction Therapy) study extended this concept and compared tenecteplase alone with tenecteplase and mandatory PCI within 24 hours and PPCI with a loading dose of clopidogrel. The results suggested that rapidly applied pharmacological reperfusion with follow-up (rescue and routine) PCI within 24 hours produced equivalent results to PPCI.[80]

Registry Data

Inclusion and exclusion criteria of RCTs imply that only ideal situations are represented. Registry data provide a more realistic view of treatment strategies and outcomes in unselected populations. Consequently, results of registries and trials often differ. Björklund et al. demonstrated a 1 year mortality of 8.8% for STEMI patients treated with fibrinolytics in a RCT, in contrast

Study	Number of patients	Odds ratio (95% CI)	Favors prehospital thrombolysis	Favors in-hospital thrombolysis
MITI. 1993	360	0.69 (0.30–1.57)		
EMIP. 1993	5469	0.86 (0.72–1.03)		
GREAT. 1991	311	0.56 (0.25–1.23)		
Roth et al. 1990	116	0.80 (0.17–3.77)		
Schofer et al. 1990	78	0.46 (0.04–5.31)		
Castaigne et al. 1989	100	0.74 (0.14–3.86)		
Overall	6434	0.83 (0.70–0.98)		

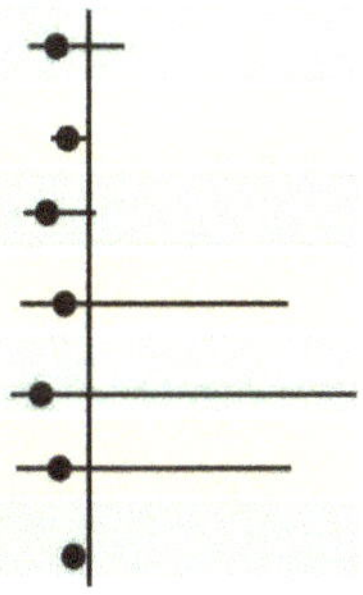

Fig. 2: Prehospital versus in-hospital thrombolysis

to 20.3% for patients not included in the trial but treated at a trial hospital, and 19.0% for patients treated in a nontrial hospital (P, 0.001 for both). Thus, less critically ill patients are preferentially selected for inclusion in RCTs.[81]

French Registries

The first nationwide French registry, in 1995, showed equivalent results for 1 year mortality with intravenous thrombolysis and PPCI. However, PHT and IHT were not analysed separately, as PHT was seldom used in France at that time.[82] In the USIC 2000 Registry, reperfusion was selected according to several criteria, including the time to reach a catheterization laboratory and the availability of the specialist team. In contrast to RCTs, the USIC 2000 results favored PHT.[83] This may have been influenced by the large proportion of patients who underwent rapid coronary angiography, similar to that found in CAPTIM, and much higher than in trials such as DANAMI-2,[84] which found PCI to confer a higher survival advantage than IHT if performed within 2 hours of symptom onset.

Vienna Registry (Fig. 3)

The results of the Vienna STEMI registry, which included 1053 acute STEMI patients admitted to hospital, were similar to those of CAPTIM.[75,85] PHT, when initiated within 2 hours of symptom onset, showed a (not statistically significant) trend towards reduced mortality compared with PPCI. Only a small number of patients underwent PPCI within 2 hours. As in other registries and CAPTIM, the advantage of PHT was lost as times to administration increased. Overall, PPCI was associated with an increased survival benefit over PHT. However, because 91% underwent coronary angiography (rescue or systematic) while in hospital, the results are not strictly those of PHT alone, rather a combination of thrombolysis and angiography with or without mechanical intervention. The conclusion reflected trial results: within 2 hours of symptom onset, thrombolysis should be administered, preferably prehospital, if PPCI cannot be performed within 90 minutes of the first medical contact.

Swedish Registry

In the large RIKS-HIA (Register of Information and Knowledge about Swedish Heart Intensive Care Admissions), PHT had better outcomes than IHT, but patients who received PPCI had lower mortality and re-infarction rates and shorter hospital stays.[86] Comparing 30 days and 1 year results between the ambulance-managed PHT patients and the primary angioplasty group shows that both reperfusion methods yield very similar mortality figures: 5.4 versus 4.9% at 30 days and 7.2 versus 7.6% at 1 year, respectively. Time delay to reperfusion appeared very important in the thrombolysis groups, as mortality increased sharply beyond 2 hours. The difference was less dramatic for PPCI. Overall, time delay was central to the benefit incurred by any type of reperfusion, but loss of benefit with increasing delay was less pronounced with PPCI. Therefore, the authors concluded that, within 2 hours of symptom onset, patients should receive PHT only if PPCI is not available within 4 hours. This conclusion, however, did not take into account the results of PHT in ambulance-transported patients.

International GRACE Registry

The Global Registry of Acute Coronary Events (GRACE) followed 44,372 STEMI and non-STEMI patients from 1999 until 2005, looking for improvement in outcomes when evidence-based treatment guidelines were followed.[87] The proportion of STEMI patients eligible for any kind of reperfusion therapy did not change significantly over the study period, but the proportion undergoing PPCI increased by 37%, whereas pharmacological reperfusion decreased by 22%. Correspondingly, in-hospital mortality and cardiogenic shock decreased. However, recommended adjuvant pharmacological treatment increased markedly throughout the study. The decrease in mortality can be attributed to increased experience in invasive treatment strategies and more efficient prehospital management, but also to the effect of improved adjuvant therapies. The GRACE registry, therefore, shows that the implementation of guidelines is central to the provision of improved patient care.

Indian Perspective

In todays practice, evidence-based medicine is mandatory. However, we must review each modality of therapy from an Indian perspective. Reperfusion therapy of AMI should necessarily have a geographical referral system. This means that the patient will be treated by the nearest quality controlled

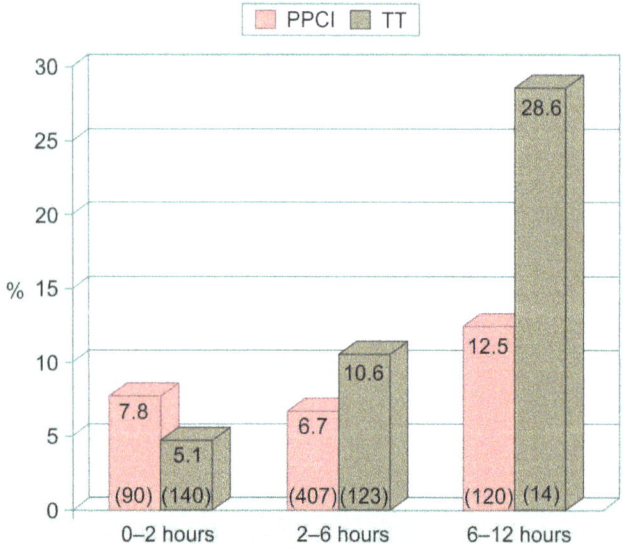

Fig. 3: Vienna STEMI registry

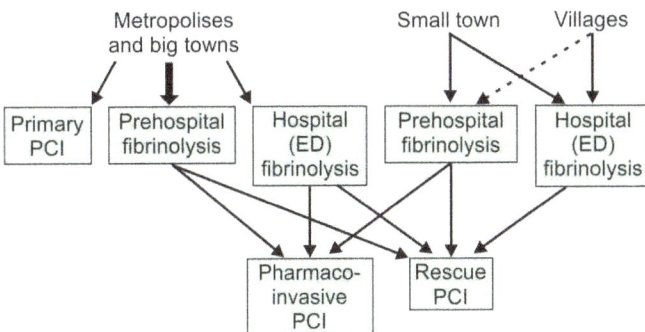

Flow chart 1: Proposed model of STEMI management in next decade in India

CCU or prehospital ambulance service. A particular emergency medical care service whether CCU or ambulance service should be marked for a given population in the vicinity of the service. A routinely available ambulance service with the paramedic staff is not geared to provide prehospital thrombolysis today. City-based major institutions should provide emergency satellite units to achieve the time benefit required in treating AMI. Implementation of prehospital thrombolysis in India will require support, interest and participation of hospital administrators, dedicated community leaders, physicians, cardiologists and appropriate structuring and resourcing of emergency medical services. Applying evidence based medicine without quality control protocols can be more dangerous than not abiding by the therapy guidelines. This rule applies also to in-hospital thrombolysis and primary PCI.[88] The proposed model of STEMI management in next decade in India has been given in **Flow chart 1**.

CONCLUSION

Exercising the opportunities in prehospital cardiac care could substantially enhance patient outcomes. With the current EMS capabilities, the ideal prehospital system should include prehospital diagnosis by clinical symptoms and prehospital ECG with initiation of fibrinolysis or triage to the appropriate medical institution for rapid institution of definitive therapy. At a minimum, we should aim for a dedicated response system to achieve an increase in inhospital state of readiness to reduce time-to-reperfusion. Extension of these advances to other cardiac emergencies, including sudden cardiac death, high-risk non-STEMI acute coronary syndromes, and stroke, will continue to improve the outcomes in these common potentially catastrophic conditions. There are no longer logical reasons to delay response to these calls for action, because time is elapsing, and with it, needless morbidity and mortality are occurring in our patients.

REFERENCES

1. The GUSTO Angiographic Investigators. The effects of tissue plasminogen activator, streptokinase, or both on coronary artery patency, ventricular function, and survival after acute myocardial infarction. N Engl J Med. 1993;329:1615-22.
2. Pantridge JF, Geddes JS. A mobile intensive care unit in the management of myocardial infarction. Lancet. 1967;2:271.
3. Pantridge JF, Adgey AAJ. Pre-Hospital Coronary Care. The mobile coronary care unit. Am J Cardiol. 1969;24:666-73.
4. Castaigne AD, Hervé C, Duval-Moulin A-M et al. Prehospital use of APSAC: Results of a Placebo-Controlled Study. Am J Cardiol. 1989;64:30A-3A.
5. The European myocardial infarction project group. Prehospital thrombolytic therapy in patients with suspected acute myocardial infarction. N Engl J Med. 1993;329:383-9.
6. Barbash GI, Roth A, Hod H, et al. Improved survival but not left ventricular function with early and prehospital treatment with tissue plasminogen activator in acute myocardial infarction. Am J Cardiol. 1990;66:261-6.
7. The Thrombolysis Early in Acute Heart Attack Trial Study group. Very early thrombolytic therapy in suspected acute myocardial infarction. Am J Cardiol. 1990;65:401-7.
8. McNeill AJ, et al. A double blind placebo controlled study of early and late administration of recombinant tissue plasminogen activator in acute myocardial infarction. Br Heart J. 1989;61:316-21.
9. Great Group. Feasibility, safety, and efficacy of domiciliary thrombolysis by general practitioners: Grampian region early anistreplase trial. Br Med J. 1992;305:548-53.
10. Schofer J, Büttner J, Geng G, et al. Prehospital thrombolysis in acute myocardial infarction. Am J Cardiol. 1990;66:1429-33.
11. BEPS Collaborative group. Prehospital thrombolysis in acute myocardial infarction: The Belgian Eminase Pre hospital Study (BEPS). Eur Heart J. 1991;12:965-7.
12. Weaver WD, et al., for the Myocardial Infarction Triage and Intervention Project Group. Prehospital-initiated vs hospital-initiated thrombolytic therapy. The Myocardial Infarction Triage and Intervention Trial. JAMA. 1993;270:1211-6.
13. Morrison LJ, Verbeek PR, McDonald AC, et al. Mortality and prehospital thrombolysis for acute myocardial infarction. A Meta-analysis. JAMA. 2000;283:2686-92.
14. Boersma E, Maas ACP, Deckers JW, et al. Early thrombolytic treatment in acute myocardial infarction: reappraisal of the golden hour. Lancet. 1996;348:771-5.
15. Reimer KA, et al. The wavefront phenomenon of ischemic cell death. 1. Myocardial infarct size vs duration of coronary occlusion in dogs. Circulation. 1977;56:786-94.
16. Weaver WD. Time to thrombolytic treatment: factors affecting delay and their influence on outcome. J Am Coll Cardiol. 1995; 25(Suppl):3S-9S.
17. Boersma E, Maas ACP, Deckers JW, Simoons ML. Early thrombolytic treatment in acute myocardial infarction: reappraisal of the golden hour. Lancet. 1996;348:771-5.
18. Lesnefsky EJ, et al. Increased left ventricular dysfunction in elderly patients despite successful thrombolysis: the GUSTO-I angiographic experience. J Am Coll Cardiol. 1996;28:331-7.
19. Blohm MB, et al. An evaluation of the results of media and educational campaigns designed to shorten the time taken by patients with acute myocardial infarction to decide to go to hospital. Heart. 1996;76:430-4.
20. Meischke H, et al. Reasons patients with chest pain delay or do not call 911. Ann Emerg Med. 1995;25:193-7.
21. Hackett TP, Cassem NH. Factors contributing to delay in responding to the signs and symptoms of acute myocardial infarction. Am J Cardiol. 1969;24:651-8.

22. Gilchrist IC. Patient delay before treatment of myocardial infarction. Br Med J. 1973;I:535-7.
23. Rawles JM, et al. Association of patient delay with symptoms, cardiac enzymes, and outcome in acute myocardial infarction. Eur Heart J. 1990;11:643-8.
24. Kenyon LW, et al. Psychological factors related to prehospital delay during acute myocardial infarction. Circulation. 1991;84:1969-76.
25. Trent RJ, et al. Delay between the onset of symptoms of acute myocardial infarction and seeking medical assistance is influenced by left ventricular function at presentation. Br Heart J. 1995;73:125-8.
26. Rawles J, Sinclair C, Waugh N. Call-to-needle times in Grampian: the pivotal role of the general practitioner in achieving early thrombolysis (Abstr). Heart. 1996;75(Suppl 1).
27. Birkhead JS on behalf of the joint audit committee of the British Cardiac Society and cardiology committee of the Royal College of Physicians of London. Time delays in provision of thrombolytic treatment in six district hospitals. Br Med J. 1992;305:445-8.
28. Bleeker JK, Simoons ML, Erdman RAM, et al. Patient and doctor delay in acute myocardial infarction: a study in Rotterdam, the Netherlands. Br J Gen Pract. 1995;45:181-4.
29. Leprohon J, Patel VL. Decision-making strategies for telephone triage in emergency medical services. Med Decis Making. 1995;15:240-53.
30. Sramek M, Post W, Koster RW. Telephone triage of cardiac emergency calls by dispatchers. A prospective study of 1386 emergency calls. Br Heart J. 1994;71:440-5.
31. Canto JG, et al. The prehospital electrocardiogram in acute myocardial infarction: is its full potential being realized? National Registry of Myocardial Infarction 2 Investigators. J Am Coll Cardiol. 1997;29:498-505.
32. Curtis JP, et al. The pre-hospital electrocardiogram and time to reperfusion in patients with acute myocardial infarction, 2000-2002: findings from the National Registry of Myocardial Infarction-4. J Am Coll Cardiol. 2006;47:1544-52.
33. Bradley EH, et al. Achieving door-to-balloon times that meet quality guidelines: how do successful hospitals do it? J Am Coll Cardiol. 2005;46:1236-41.
34. Bradley EH, Herrin J, et al. Strategies for reducing the door-to-balloon time in acute myocardial infarction. N Engl J Med. 2006;355:2308-20.
35. Bradley EH, Curry LA, et al. Achieving rapid door-to-balloon times: how top hospitals improve complex clinical systems. Circulation. 2006;113:1079-85.
36. Swor R, et al. Prehospital 12-lead ECG: efficacy or effectiveness? Prehosp Emerg Care. 2006;10:374-7.
37. Gross BW, et al. An approach to shorten time to infarct artery patency in patients with ST-segment elevation myocardial infarction. Am J Cardiol. 2007;99:1360-3.
38. Dhruva, et al. ST-Segment Analysis Using Wireless Technology in Acute Myocardial Infarction (STAT-MI) trial. J Am Coll Cardiol. 2007;50:509-13.
39. Nallamothu BK, Bradley EH, Krumholz HM. Time to treatment in primary percutaneous coronary intervention. N Engl J Med. 2007;357:1631-8.
40. Scholz KH, et al. Contact-to-balloon time and door-to-balloon time after initiation of a formalized data feedback in patients with acute ST-elevation myocardial infarction. Am J Cardiol. 2008;101:46-52.
41. Antman EM, et al. ACC/AHA guidelines for the management of patients with ST-elevation myocardial infarction–executive summary: a report of the American College of Cardiology/American Heart Association Task Force on Practice Guidelines (Writing Committee to Revise the 1999 Guidelines for the Management of Patients With Acute Myocardial Infarction). Circulation. 2004;110:588-636.
42. ECC Committee, Subcommittees and Task Forces of the American Heart Association. 2005 American Heart Association Guidelines for Cardiopulmonary Resuscitation and Emergency Cardiovascular Care. Circulation. 2005;112(Suppl IV):IV-1–IV-203.
43. Antman EM, et al. 2007 Focused Update of the ACC/AHA 2004 Guidelines for the Management of Patients With ST-Elevation Myocardial Infarction: a report of the American College of Cardiology/American Heart Association Task Force on Practice Guidelines: developed in collaboration with the Canadian Cardiovascular Society, endorsed by the American Academy of Family Physicians: 2007 Writing Group to Review New Evidence and Update the ACC/AHA 2004 Guidelines for the Management of Patients With ST-Elevation Myocardial Infarction, Writing on Behalf of the 2004 Writing Committee. Circulation. 2008;117:296-329.
44. Emergency department: rapid identification and treatment of patients with acute myocardial infarction: National Heart Attack Alert Program Coordinating Committee, 60 Minutes to Treatment Working Group. Ann Emerg Med. 1994;23:311-29.
45. Dracup K, et al. The physician's role in minimizing prehospital delay in patients at high risk for acute myocardial infarction: recommendations from the National Heart Attack Alert Program: Working Group on Educational Strategies to Prevent Prehospital Delay in Patients at High Risk for Acute Myocardial Infarction. Ann Intern Med. 1997;126:645-51.
46. Hutter AM Jr, Weaver WD. 31st Bethesda Conference: emergency cardiac care: task force 2: acute coronary syndromes: section 2A: prehospital issues. J Am Coll Cardiol. 2000;35:846-53.
47. Canto JG, et al. The prehospital electrocardiogram in acute myocardial infarction: is its full potential being realized? National Registry of Myocardial Infarction 2 Investigators. J Am Coll Cardiol. 1997;29:498-505.
48. Ahnefeld FW. Die Wiederbelebung bei Kreislaufstillstand. Verhandlungen Deutsche Gesellschaft fu¨r Innere Medizin. 1968;74:279-87.
49. Cummins R, Ornato JP, Thies WH, Pepe PE. Improving survival from sudden cardiac arrest: the 'chain of survival' concept. A statement for health professionals from the Advanced Cardiac Life Support Subcommittee and the Emergency Cardiac Care Committee, American Heart Association. Circulation. 1991;83:1832-47.
50. Herlitz J, et al. Effect of bystander initiated cardiopulmonary resuscitation on ventricular fibrillation and survival after witnessed cardiac arrest outside hospital. Br Heart J. 1994;72:408-12.
51. Bossaert L, Van Hoeyweghen R and Cerebral Resuscitation Study Group. Bystander cardiopulmonary resuscitation (CPR) in out-of-hospital cardiac arrest. Resuscitation. 1989;17(Suppl):S55-S69.
52. Stults KR, Brown DD, Schug VL, Bean JA. Prehospital defibrillation performed by emergency medical technicians in rural communities. N Engl J Med. 1984;310:219-23.

53. European Resuscitation Council guidelines for the use of automated external defibrillators by EMS providers and first responders. A statement from the Early Defibrillation Task Force, with contributions from the Working Groups on Basic and Advanced Life Support, and approved by the Executive Committee of the European Resuscitation Council. Resuscitation. 1998;37:91-4.
54. Antiplatelet Trialists' Collaboration. Collaborative overview of randomised trials of antiplatelet therapy-I: prevention of death, myocardial infarction, and stroke by prolonged antiplatelet therapy in various categories of patients. Br Med J. 1994;308: 81-1-6.
55. ISIS-2 (Second International Study of Infarct Survival) Collaborative Group. Randomised trial of intravenous streptokinase, oral aspirin, both, or neither among 17 187 cases of suspected acute myocardial infarction: ISIS-2. Lancet. 1988;ii:349-60.
56. ISIS-3 (Third International Study of Infarct Survival) Collaborative Group. ISIS-3: a randomised comparison of streptokinase vs tissue plasminogen activator vs anistreplase and of aspirin plus heparin vs aspirin alone among 41 299 cases of suspected acute myocardial infarction. Lancet. 1992;339:753-70.
57. Gruppo Italiano per lo Studio della Sopravvivenza nell'Infarto miocardico. GISSI-2: a factorial randomised trial of alteplase versus streptokinase and heparin versus no heparin among 12 490 patients with acute myocardial infarction. Lancet. 1990;336:65-71.
58. ISIS-I (First International Study of Infarct Survival) Collaborative Group. Randomised trial of intravenous atenolol among 16 027 cases of suspected acute myocardial infarction: ISIS-I. Lancet. 1986;ii: 57-66.
59. The MIAMI Trial Research Group. Metoprolol in acute myocardial infarction (MIAMI). A randomised placebocontrolled international trial. Eur Heart J. 1985;6:199-226.
60. Borzak S, Gheorghiade M. Early intravenous beta-blocker combined with thrombolytic therapy for acute myocardial infarction: the thrombolysis in myocardial infarction (TIMI-2) trial. Prog Cardiovasc Dis. 1993;36:261-6.
61. Yusuf S, Peto R, Lewis J, Collins R, Sleight P. Beta blockade during and after myocardial infarction: an overview of the randomized trials. Progr Cardiovasc Dis. 1985;27:335-71.
62. Gruppo Italiano per lo Studio della Sopravvivenza nell'Infarto miocardico. GISSI-3: effects of lisinopril and transdermal glyceryl trinitrate singly and together on 6-week mortality and ventricular function after acute myocardial infarction. Lancet. 1994;343: 1115-22.
63. ISIS-4 (Fourth International Study of Infarct Survival) Collaborative Group. ISIS-4: a randomised factorial trial assessing early oral captopril, oral mononitrate, and intravenous magnesium sulphate in 58 050 patients with suspected acute myocardial infarction. Lancet. 1995;345:669-85.
64. MacMahon S, et al. Effects of prophylactic lidocaine in suspected acute myocardial infarction: an overview of results from the randomized, controlled trials. JAMA. 1988;260:1910-6.
65. Hine LK, Laird N, Hewitt P, Chalmers TC. Meta-analytic evidence against prophylactic use of lidocaine in acute myocardial infarction. Arch Intern Med. 1989;149:2694-8.
66. Antman EM, Hand M, Armstrong PW, Bates ER, Green LA, Halasyamani LK, et al. 2007 Focused Update of the ACC/AHA 2004 Guidelines for the Management of Patients with ST-Elevation Myocardial Infarction: a report of the American College of Cardiology/American Heart Association Task Force on Practice Guidelines: developed in collaboration with the Canadian Cardiovascular Society endorsed by the American Academy of Family Physicians: 2007 Writing Group to Review New Evidence and Update the ACC/AHA 2004 Guidelines for the Management of Patients With ST-Elevation Myocardial Infarction, Writing on Behalf of the 2004 Writing Committee. Circulation. 2008;117: 296-329.
67. Van de Werf F, Bax J, et al. The Task Force on the management of ST-segment elevation acute myocardial infarction of the European Society of Cardiology. Management of acute myocardial infarction in patients presenting with persistent ST-segment elevation. Eur Heart J; 2008.
68. Bassand JP, et al. Implementation of reperfusion therapy in acute myocardial infarction. A policy statement from the European Society of Cardiology. Eur Heart J. 2005;26:2733-41.
69. Lee K, Woodlief L, Topol E, Weaver D, Betriu A, Col J, Simoons M, Aylward P, Van der Werf F, Califf R, for the GUSTO-I Investigators Predictors of 30-day mortality in the era of reperfusion for acute myocardial infarction. Results from an international trial of 41 021 patients. Circulation. 1995;91:1659-68.
70. National Institute for Clinical Excellence. Technology Appraisal Guidance; http:// www.nice.org.uk/nicemedia/pdf/52_ Thrombolysis_full_guidance.pdf (2002).
71. Morrison L, Verbeek P, McDonald A, Sawadsky B, Cook D. Mortality and prehospital thrombolysis for acute myocardial infarction. A meta-analysis. JAMA. 2000;283:2686-92.
72. Keeley E, Boura J, Grines C. Primary angioplasty versus intravenous thrombolytic therapy for acute myocardial infarction: a quantitative review of 23 randomised trials. Lancet. 2003;361: 13-20.
73. Pinto D, et al. Hospital delays in reperfusion for ST-elevation myocardial infarction. Implications when selecting a reperfusion strategy. Circulation. 2006;114:2019-25.
74. Otterstad J, Brosstad F. Results from clinical trials on ST-elevation myocardial infarction in a historic perspective with some pathophysiological aspects. Scand Cardiovasc J. 2003;37:316-23.
75. Steg G, et al. for the Comparison of Angioplasty Prehospital Thrombolysis In acute Myocardial infarction (CAPTIM) Investigators Impact of time to treatment on mortality after prehospital fibrinolysis or primary angioplasty. Circulation. 2003;108:2851-6.
76. Widimsky P, et al. on behalf of the 'PRAGUE' Study Group Investigators Long distance transport for primary angioplasty vs immediate thrombolysis in acute myocardial infarction. Final results of the randomized national multicentre trial—PRAGUE-2. Eur Heart J. 2003;24:94-104.
77. Boersma E, the PCAT-2 Trialists' Collaborative Group. Does time matter? A pooled analysis of randomized clinical trials comparing primary percutaneous coronary intervention and in-hospital fibrinolysis in acute myocardial infarction. Eur Heart J. 2006;27:779-88.
78. Fernandez-Avile´s F, et al. Routine invasive strategy within 24 hours of thrombolysis versus ischaemia-guided conservative approach for acute myocardial infarction with ST-segment elevation (GRACIA-1): a randomised controlled trial. Lancet. 2004;364:1045-53.
79. Di Mario C et al. on behalf of the CARESS-in-AMI investigators Immediate angioplasty versus standard therapy with rescue angioplasty after thrombolysis in the Combined Abciximab REteplase Stent Study in Acute Myocardial Infarction (CARESS-

in-AMI): an open, prospective, randomised, multicentre trial. Lancet. 2008;371:559-68.
80. Armstrong P, WEST Steering Committee A comparison of pharmacologic therapy with/without timely coronary intervention vs. primary percutaneous intervention early after ST-elevation myocardial infarction: the WEST (Which Early ST-elevation myocardial infarction Therapy) study. Eur Heart J. 2006;27:1530-8.
81. Bjo¨rklund E, et al. Outcome of ST-elevation myocardial infarction treated with thrombolysis in the unselected population is vastly different from samples of eligible patients in a large-scale clinical trial. Am Heart J. 2004;148:566-73.
82. Danchin N, Vaur L, Gene`s N, Etienne S, Angio¨ı M, Ferrie`res J, Cambou JP. Treatment of acute myocardial infarction by primary coronary angioplasty or intravenous thrombolysis in the 'real world': one-year results from a nationwide French survey. Circulation. 1999;99:2639-44.
83. Danchin N, et al. for the USIC Investigators Impact of prehospital thrombolysis for acute myocardial infarction on 1-year outcome. Circulation. 2004;110:1909-15.
84. Andersen H, Nielsen T, et al. for the DANAMI-2 Investigators A comparison of coronary angioplasty with fibrinolytic therapy in acute myocardial infarction. New Engl J Med. 2003;349:733-42.
85. Kalla K, Christ G, et al. for the Vienna STEMI Registry Group Implementation of guidelines improves the standard of care. The Viennese Registry on Reperfusion Strategies in ST-Elevation Myocardial Infarction (Vienna STEMI Registry). Circulation. 2006;113:2398-405.
86. Stenestrand U, Lindba¨ck J, Wallentin L, for the RIKS-HIA Registry Long-term outcome of primary percutaneous coronary intervention vs prehospital and in-hospital thrombolysis for patients with ST-elevation myocardial infarction. JAMA. 2006;296:1749-56.
87. Fox K, et al. for the GRACE Investigators Decline in rates of death and heart failure in acute coronary syndromes, 1999-2006. JAMA. 2007;297:1892-1900.
88. Sathe S, et al. Prehospital thrombolysis. API-Medicine update; 2010.

23
STEMI Care in India and the Real World: Pharmacoinvasive Approach

HK Chopra

INTRODUCTION

The principal clinical syndromes that result are acute ST elevation myocardial infarction (STEMI), deep vein thrombosis, pulmonary embolism, acute ischemic stroke, acute peripheral arterial occlusion, and occlusion of indwelling catheters. Of these, acute myocardial infarction (AMI) accounts for maximum number of morbidity and mortality. Over the last century, pharmacoinvasive approach has gained prominence in the management of STEMI and has helped hundreds of physicians in reanalyzing coronary vessel occlusions. This chapter reviews major milestones in the history of pharmacoinvasive approach in STEMI.

DEVELOPMENT OF THROMBOLYTIC THERAPY

The Discovery of Streptokinase

The first thrombolytic streptokinase was discovered by Dr William Smith Tillett in 1933 by sheer serendipity. He was Associate Professor of Medicine and Director of the Biological Division at Johns Hopkins University, at that time. He observed that streptococci agglutinated in test tubes that contained human plasma but not in those that contained human serum. He hypothesized that the agglutination of streptococci is caused by fibrinogen in plasma that is deficient in serum. The fibrinogen probably is adsorbed onto the surface of streptococci, rendering the plasma devoid of free fibrinogen. In order to prove his hypothesis, Tillett devised a simple experiment. He took oxalated human plasma containing fibrinogen, which would not clot due to calcium depletion. He added calcium to the control test tubes, and hemolytic streptococci and calcium to the rest of the test tubes, hoping that the hemolytic streptococci would adsorb the fibrinogen and prevent the formation of a clot. However, the results of this experiment were uniformly negative: there was clot formation in all the tubes, regardless of the presence of streptococci. Dejected with the results of this experiment, he left the tubes in the tray without cleaning.

After some time, to his surprise, he found that there was clot lysis in the tubes containing streptococcal cultures. This led him to conclude that the streptococci had synthesized a fibrinolytic agent that was responsible for dissolving the clots. **(Table 1)**. This was the probable mechanism for clot lysis, rather than adsorption of fibrinogen as he had earlier presumed. He confirmed these findings on larger scale and on 27 June 1933, Tillett and Garner submitted their findings as 'Fibrinolytic activity of hemolytic streptococci'.

The agent was termed as streptococcal fibrinolysin which was crude and impure, thus could not be used clinically.[1,2]

Mechanism of Action of Streptokinase

In 1941, Milstone reported the existence of a substance, normally present in plasma that was required for dissolution of the clot. He termed it the "lytic factor." Christensen and Kaplan independently determined that the lytic factor was a proteolytic enzyme normally present in plasma as an inactive precursor. The streptococcal substance (fibrinolysin) activates the proteinase precursor, converting it to an active enzyme in a manner analogous to the conversion of trypsinogen to trypsin by enterokinase. The active serum proteinase then lyses the fibrin clot. Christensen and MacLeod proposed the term "streptokinase" in 1945 to replace the term fibrinolysin originally applied to the streptococcal component of the system. They further suggested the name "plasminogen" for the inactive form of the serum proteinase and "plasmin" for the active enzyme.[2]

Source for Streptokinase

Evans reported the discovery of fibrinolytic properties in certain strains of *Streptococcus equisimilis*.[3] Christensen reported that the strain *S. equisimilis* H46A can act as a commercial source

Table 1 Milestones of fibrinolysis research

Year	Investigator	Observation
1933	Tillett and Garner	Fibrinolytic principal in hemolytic streptococcal broth
1941–1945	Milestone, Tagnon, Christensen	Precursor of plasmin converted by streptococcal agent to active enzyme
1948–54	Mullertz, Williams, Sobel, et al. Lack, Ratnoff, et al.	Fibrinolytic inhibitors and activators (t-PA, UK, Staphylokinase)
1949	Sol Sherry	Successfully used fibrinous, purulent, and sanguineous pleural exudations, hemothorax, and tuberculous meningitis
1953	Kline, Mullertz	Purification of plasminogen
1961	Guest and Celander	Urokinase
1981	Rijken and Collen	Activator purified from melanoma line
1983	Pennica, et al.	Cloning and expression of rt-PA
1990s	Meta-analysis	Recombinant mutant derivatives of rt-PA

for streptokinase as it does not produce erythrogenic toxins, is less fastidious in its growth requirements than are most other group A strains and could be grown on semisynthetic media. This was a discovery of immense importance as till date, the commercial streptokinase used for thrombolytic therapy, is derived from *S. equisimilis* (Lancefield Group C).

Human Studies on Streptokinase

In late 1949, Tillett and Sherry successfully used streptokinase to treat fibrinous, purulent, and sanguineous pleural exudations, hemothorax, and tuberculous meningitis.[4,5] In these studies, streptokinase was associated with few side effects such as a pyrogenic reaction with associated malaise, headache, arthralgia, and occasionally nausea and febrile responses.[6] This was probably due to impurities in the existing formulation. Later on, further purification of streptokinase was taken up by Lederle Laboratories. The first report on intravascular thrombolysis in humans came up in 1956 by EE Cliffton at the Cornell University Medical College, New York, who used streptokinase in 40 patients with intravascular thrombosis of diverse etiology. His study was associated with nonuniform canalization results and frequent bleeding complications. Despite this fact, he must be credited with the first use of thrombolytic agents for the treatment of pathological thrombi, as well as with the first catheter-directed administration of a thrombolytic agent.

In late 1958, Fletcher and associates performed new studies regarding an intravenous approach to the treatment of STEMI patients. Their patients were infused with streptokinase in massive doses and for prolonged periods after MI. Except for the development of a hemorrhagic diathesis in a few patients, there were no significant complications, and the mortality rate was significantly lower in patients who had received streptokinase, in comparison with other treatments. This proved that streptokinase infusion via the intravenous route was a promising therapeutic approach to STEMI.[7,8]

After the success of intravascular thrombolysis with streptokinase, Ruegsegger and colleagues successfully dissolved intracoronary clots for the 1st time in various animal models. With serial angiography, they clearly showed dissolution of clots in high proportion of animals. An important finding of this study was that the heart muscle could not be saved from death if more than a few hours passed between clotting and lysis which has now emerged as the concept of golden hour in the management of STEMI. The earlier thrombolysis resulted in smaller area of infarction as compared to controls in this study.[9]

In spite of the success spurts, the production of streptokinase in the US was stopped due to the inefficiency in production of less pyrogenic preparations. It still remained the drug of choice in Europe and Australia for several decades. However, in the US, the focus was shifted to another thrombolytic molecule, urokinase.

Several small scale trials conducted on streptokinase during 1960s and 1970s failed to establish the therapeutic superiority of streptokinase till 1979 when the European Cooperative Study Group for Streptokinase Treatment in Acute Myocardial Infarction published its findings from a large scale trial. The trial conducted in 2,388 patients found that the overall mortality rates within 6 months of streptokinase therapy after AMI were significantly lower (p <0.01) in the streptokinase group (15.6%) than in the control group (30.6%).[10] In 1980s, several trials demonstrated that use of streptokinase within 1.5 to 3 hours of infarction was associated with high reperfusion rates. Still, these results were not sufficient to establish practice guidelines.

Intracoronary Use of Streptokinase: Post-1979 intracoronary streptokinase use in few STEMI patients, which is associated with cardiac complication like reperfusion arrhythmis in 80%

patients. Despite the more effective clot lysis, intracoronary administration fell to an equal footing with intravenous administration due to the associated side effects.

There was no clear protocol design for use of streptokinase in STEMI, but the observation made was that when streptokinase was administered within 1.5–3 hours of symptom onset, reperfusion rate as high as 90% was achieved, and with delay in treatment, the prognosis worsened. Intravenous streptokinase in evolving STEMI was published for the first time from India in a Pilot Observational Study.[11]

Finally, in 1986, a landmark trial, GISSI (Gruppo Italiano per la Sperimentazione della Streptochinasi nell'Infarto Miocardico) in 11,806 patients in 176 coronary care units dissipated the confusion. There was a significant difference in mortality rates between the streptokinase group and the nonstreptokinase group (controls) at 12 months (17.2% in the streptokinase group vs 19.0% in controls, $p = 0.008$; relative risk, 0.90), especially in the 0–3 and 3–6 hours groups (relative risks, 0.89 and 0.87, respectively). Thus, GISSI succeeded in firmly establishing the efficacy of intravenously administered streptokinase.[12] Intravenous Streptokinase in STEMI 6–36 months follow up published in India.[13] This was followed by many clinical trials to reinforce the benefit of streptokinase. Large multicenter trials like GUSTO (Global Utilization of Streptokinase and Tissue Plasminogen Activator for Occluded Coronary Arteries), GISSI-2 (Gruppo Italiano per so Studio della Sopravvienza nell'Infarto Miocardico), and ISIS-3 (Third International Study of Infarct Survival Collaborative Group) compared the efficacy of tissue plasminogen activator (t-PA) with that of streptokinase. GUSTO shows no difference in mortality at the end of 30 days.[14] GISSI-2 reported similar mortality rates at 6 months, while ISIS-3 found no significant difference in mortality rates in patients treated with t-PA or streptokinase. The development of antibodies against streptokinase is the major concern for reuse of streptokinase. Although, t-PA has become a popular thrombolytic agent today, streptokinase continues to be choice of thrombolytic agent in millions suffering from AMI due to the cost benefit.

Urokinase

The most commonly employed urokinase has been of tissue-culture origin, manufactured from human neonatal kidney cells. A recombinant form of urokinase (rUK) was tested in a single trial of patients with acute myocardial infarction (MI) and in two multicenter trials of patients with peripheral arterial occlusion. It had a higher molecular weight and a shorter half-life than its low molecular-weight counterpart. Despite these differences, however, the clinical effects of the two agents have been quite similar. McNamara and Fischer were the first to describe the use of urokinase for local thrombolytic treatment, using a high-dose protocol featuring graded, stepwise reductions in dose as the infusion progressed.[15]

Tissue-type Plasminogen Activator

In early 1947, it was reported that fibrinokinase present in animal tissue can activate plasminogen, many authors tried purification and characterization of plasminogen activators from sources like pig heart, ovaries and human post mortem vascular perfusates. The first highly purified form of t-PA was obtained from uterine tissue (about 1 mg of t-PA from 5 kg tissue). t-PA has been purified from the culture fluid of a stable human melanoma cell line (Bowes, RPMI-7272). D Pennica (1982) from the Department of Molecular Biology of Genentech Inc. initiated the cloning and expression of the t-PA gene (Sixth Congress on Fibrinolysis in Lausanne, Switzerland). The recombinant t-PA (rt-PA) was shown to be indistinguishable from the natural activator isolated from human melanoma cell culture, with respect to biochemical properties.

Alteplase (tPA and rtPA)

Tissue plasminogen activator (tPA), originally developed in the mid-1980s after molecular cloning techniques were used to express human (tPA) DNA. Alteplase is a naturally occurring fibrinolytic agent produced by endothelial cells and is intimately involved in the balance between intravascular thrombogenesis and thrombolysis. Natural tPA is a single chain (527 amino acid) serine protease, and in contrast to most serine proteases (e.g., urokinase), the single-chain form has significant activity. tPA exhibits significant fibrin specificity. In plasma, the agent is associated with little plasminogen activation. At the site of the thrombus, however, the binding of tPA and plasminogen to the fibrin surface induces a conformational change in both molecules, greatly facilitating the conversion of plasminogen to plasmin and dissolution of the clot. tPA also manifests the property of fibrin affinity, that is, it binds strongly to fibrin. Other fibrinolytic agents, such as prourokinase, do not demonstrate fibrin affinity.

A predominantly single-chain form of rtPA was eventually approved for the indications of acute MI and massive pulmonary embolism. rtPA has been studied extensively in the setting of coronary occlusion.[16]

In the GUSTO-I study of 41,000 patients with acute MI; rtPA was more effective than streptokinase in achieving vascular patency. Alteplase demonstrates statistically significant reduction in 30 days mortality compared with streptokinase. Despite a slightly greater risk of intracranial hemorrhage with rtPA, overall mortality was significantly reduced (GUSTO Investigators, 1993). COBALT trial was carried out to test the hypothesis that double dose alteplase is equivalent to accelerated dose of alteplase (n = 7169). The 30 days mortality was higher in double bolus group than in accelerated group, therefore, accelerated alteplase over period of 90 min remains the preferred choice. Alteplase is approved by the FDA in treatment of STEMI (2002), Pulmonary Embolism (2002), and Ischemic Stroke (1996).

Reteplase (rPA)

Reteplase was developed as a third-generation recombinant tissue type plasminogen activator. It consists of only the kringle-2 and protease domain of the t-PA molecule. Reteplase is similar to alteplase but the modification provides a longer half-life (13–16 min). The fibrin affinity of reteplase is low compared to Alteplase which improves its penetration into the clot. Due to higher penetration inside the thrombi additional fibrinolytic activity is achieved which helps in rapid reperfusion leading to less bleeding episodes.

Reteplase was developed with the goal of avoiding the necessity of a continuous intravenous infusion, thereby simplifying ease of administration. Reteplase produced in *Escherichia coli* cells, is nonglycosylated, demonstrating a lower fibrin-binding activity and a diminished affinity to hepatocytes. This latter property accounts for a longer half-life than rtPA, potentially enabling bolus injection versus prolonged infusion. Reteplase has been studied in several small trials, and its safety and efficacy appear to be similar to alteplase.[17] Reteplase was approved by FDA in the year 1996 for treatment of STEMI.

Several trials have been conducted to prove the efficacy of the reteplase in management of AMI. GUSTO-III trial compared the double bolus reteplase against accelerated infusion of alteplase. The observation proves reteplase efficacy as equal to accelerated alteplase. In RAPID-1, 2 trials, the angiography patency was assessed post-AMI. The angiography findings shows higher rate of patency and greater thrombolysis in myocardial infarction (TIMI)-3 flow with reteplase than alteplase. INJECT trial (the International Joint Efficacy Comparison of Thrombolytics) compared the mortality rate following randomization with reteplase vs streptokinase. The mortality rate was lower with reteplase compared with streptokinase. Reteplase has longer half-life, higher and faster thrombolytic patency than alteplase, lower hemorrhagic risk than alteplase. It is given as a bolus without weight adjustment.

Tenecteplase (TNK-tPA)

This molecule was bioengineered in an effort to lengthen the duration of bioavailability of tPA. Three regions in kringle-1 and the protease portion of tPA, which mediated hepatic clearance, fibrin specificity, and resistance to plasminogen activator inhibitor were identified. These three sites were modified to create TNK-tPA, a novel molecule with a greater half-life and fibrin specificity. The longer half-life of TNK-tPA allowed successful administration as a single bolus, in contrast to the infusion required for rtPA. In addition, TNK-tPA manifests greater fibrin specificity than rtPA, resulting in less fibrinogen depletion. In studies of acute coronary occlusion, TNK-tPA performed at least as well as rtPA, concurrent with greater ease of administration.[17] It received US FDA approval for the management of acute MI in the year 2000. The first biosimilar tenecteplase (Elaxim) was indigenously developed in India by Gennova Biopharmaceuticals at Pune. Several clinical trials have been conducted to establish efficacy of tenecteplase. Efficacy for clot lysis of single bolus tenecteplase was studied in thrombolysis in myocardial infarction (TIMI) 10 A and 10 B trials while safety was assessed in ASSENT 1(Assessment of the Safety of a New Thrombolytic). The results of these studies suggest that body weight adjusted single bolus dose of tenecteplase is equivalent to 90 min regime of alteplase.

Indigenous tenecteplase has convincing evidence supporting its utility in Indian STEMI patients. In STEPP-AMI study, the primary end-point occurred in 11.1% in pharmacoinvasive (PI) group and in 3.9% in primary PCI (PPCI) group, p = 0.07 (RR = 2.87; 95% CI 0.92 to 8.97). The infarct-related artery patency at angiogram was 82.2% in PI group and 22.6% in PPCI group (p < 0.001).[15] The Indian registry on use of indigenous tenecteplase in 15222 STEMI patients revealed that overall rate for achieving clinically successful thrombolysis (CST) by TNK was 95.43%.[18]

Prehospital Thrombolysis

Prehospital thrombolysis (PHT) plays important role in early and effective management of STEMI. The American Heart Association (AHA) and the American College of Cardiology (ACC) favor[19,20] the use of pre-hospital thrombolysis over percutaneous coronary intervention (PCI). CAPTIM trial reports that prehospital thrombolysis within 2 hours of symptom onset is superior to PCI.[21]

Advantages of Newer Agents Over the Older Agents

Alteplase was found to have a more favorable mortality results than streptokinase in GUSTO study. It had better thrombolytic/fibrinolytic action than urokinase. The disadvantages were higher bleeding risk and lack of resistance to plasminogen activator inhibitor (PAI-1). Reteplase although was more potent than alteplase was associated with higher bleeding risk. The advantage associated with reteplase was that it could be given in form of bolus injection rather than continuous infusion. With the introduction of tenecteplase, we now have a thrombolytic that can be given as a bolus injection, is more fibrin-specific and resistant to plasminogen activator inhibitor.

TRENDS IN THROMBOLYSIS FOR STEMI

Although the first thrombolytic was discovered in 1933. The clinical use of thrombolytics in the management of acute MI was delayed till 1980s. This was due to the controversies in the pathogenesis of MI. It was earlier thought that coronary thrombosis is a consequence rather than cause of myocardial infarction. This confusion was resolved in 1980, when DeWood and his colleagues showed that 87% of patients presenting within 4 hours of acute MI had total coronary occlusion.

He showed the angiographic evidence for coronary thrombosis in STEMI patients for the first time and was able to retrieve the thrombus using Fogarty catheter in 88% of these patients. DeWood's paper led to credence to the concept of endogenous fibrinolysis and ushered the era of fibrinolytics.[22]

By the end of 1980s, large randomized trials had been conducted in this area. The meta-analyses of these trials suggested that the sooner the thrombolytic given after the onset of chest pain, the greater the survival benefit. This led to the concept of 'golden hour' in myocardial thrombolysis which was later lengthened to a period of three hours. The findings of GREAR trial suggested that modest delays in the treatment may be detrimental as myocardial cell death starts within minutes of symptom onset and prehospital thrombolysis is effective in saving lives.[23]

Prehospital Thrombolysis

Although, primary PCI within first 6 hours of chest pain is suggested as the most preferred therapy for STEMI, it is not feasible in routine clinical settings due to delays in transfer, unavailability of catheterization facility and scarcity of skilled personnel (Kushner et al, 2009). Five-year follow-up of a multicentric trial CAPTIM shows that prehospital fibrinolysis with immediate transfer for rescue angioplasty, if needed, is associated with similar mortality as compared to P-PCI if managed within 6 hours of onset of chest pain and prehospital thrombosis improved long-term mortality when administered within first 2 hours.[20] Major breakthroughs in treatment of STEMI have been summarized in **Table 2**.

Pharmacoinvasive Approach for STEMI

Thrombolytic therapy despite its convenience, has certain limitations owing to the risk of reocclusion, failure of thrombolysis which can increase the mortality in STEMI patients. Thrombolysis at the site of a ruptured atherosclerotic plaque provides a further nidus for rethrombosis and occlusion. Immediate thrombolysis followed by angioplasty is likely to reduce the chances of reocclusion due to rethrombosis or residual thrombus. This hypothesis led to emergence of pharmacoinvasive therapy that combined the benefits of both thrombolysis and PCI.

Facilitated PCI

The initial trials of facilitated PCI (i.e. preceded by thrombolytics) (ASSENT-4 and FINESSE) evaluated the benefits of thrombolysis immediately followed by PCI. However, these were not associated with consistent mortality benefits in all patient groups. Full dose tenecteplase followed by immediate PCI in ASSENT-4 was associated with increased risk of thrombosis. This was probably due to restricted use of clopidogrel and Gp IIb/IIa inhibitors in ASSENT-4 trial. On the other hand, FINESSE trial was associated with increase in the bleeding events as compared to PPCI despite using similar dose of heparin.[23]

Pharmacoinvasive Approach

Multiple trials evaluated the effect of immediate thrombolysis followed by PCI after a gap of 2-24 hours. This enabled PCI at a later stage with full dose Gp IIb/IIIa inhibitors, heparin and antiplatelet without increased risk of bleeding. These trials include GRACIA-2, FAST-MI, TRANSFER-AMI and WEST. The largest randomized clinical trial so far, TRANSFER-AMI (n = 1059) showed that thrombolysis using tenecteplase, aspirin and LMW heparin followed by PCI within 6 hours was associated with lower ischemic complications as compared to standard thrombolysis followed by rescue PCI, if necessary. The other three trials have shown efficacy of pharmacoinvasive strategy as comparable to PPCI.[22]

The 1-year results from STREAM confirm that mortality rates were low, and that a PI strategy resulted in a similar mortality as PPCI. The composite end-point of death, shock, congestive heart failure, and reinfarction was numerically lower in the PI arm at 30 days.[25]

The 5-year survival data from FAST-MI study shows that crude five-year survival rate was 65% in patients without reperfusion therapy, 88% for patients with fibrinolysis and 84% for those with PPCI. Direct comparison of the two reperfusion techniques showed a nonsignificant trend favoring fibrinolytic treatment (HR 0.73, 0.50-1.06; p = 0.10).[26]

Reasons for Superiority of Pharmacoinvasive Approach

- Most feasible and effective reperfusion strategy in clinical settings with lack of immediate availability of PCI
- Immediate thrombolysis in this strategy can be more conveniently achieved now with the availability of newer thrombolytics like tenecteplase
- Widens the window between thrombolysis and PCI that allows greater time for transfer of patients to PCI-capable hospitals
- The time gap between thrombolysis and PCI allows liberal use of GP IIb/IIIa inhibitor, clopidogrel and heparin without inadvertent increased risk of bleeding

Hence, pharmacoinvasive strategy has been recommended more strongly for high-risk STEMI patient than nonhigh-risk AMI patient in STEMI guidelines.

A scenario not infrequently encountered in our practice is given below. A 45-year-old normotensive and non-diabetic male shopkeeper had chest and upper abdominal pain beginning early in the morning. The pain initially was intermittent and temporarily subsided. Our patient attributed the discomfort to upper gastrointestinal discomfort and he had some home available remedies for gastric discomfort.

Table 2 Major breakthroughs in the treatment of STEMI

Year	Author	Treatment
1912	James Herrick	Importance of rest in MI management
1923	Wearn	Rest, hydric restriction, digitalis use for pulmonary congestion
1928	Parkinson and Bedford	Morphine use to relieve pain, rest for long time
1946	Wright IS	Use of warfarin in treatment of coronary thrombosis with MI
1949	Tillett and Sherry	Streptokinase use in humans (fibrinous pleural adhesions)
1957	Cliffton	Plasmin (fibrinolysin) in human thrombotic disease
1958	Fletcher, et al.	Streptokinase in patients with acute MI
1959	Ruegsegger and colleague	Lysis of artificial clots in man by streptokinase
1959	McLean J	The discovery of heparin
1960	Bernard Lown	Intense fluid replacement, use of O_2, early mobility
1961	Desmond Julian	Coronary care unit
1963, 1967	Shumway NE, et al.	Heart transplant
1965	James Black	Described beta blocker propranolol
1966	Schmutzler, et al.	IV Streptokinase in AMI
1971	John Vane	Discovery of antiplatelet activity of aspirin
1979	Rentrop, et al., Schroder, et al.	Intracoronary and intravenous streptokinase for acute MI
1981	Weimar, et al.	t-PA for human thrombosis (deep vein thrombosis)
1981	Chazov E, et al.	Administration of fibrinolysin in AMI
1984	Willam Ganz, et al.	Intravenous streptokinase in evolving acute myocardial infarction
1984	Chopra HK, et al.	Intravenous streptokinase in AMI
1984	van de Werf, et al.	Recombinant t-PA in acute MI
1985	William Ganz, et al.	The effect of rate of IV STK in AMI
1986–88	GISSI, ISIS-2, ASSET, AIMS	Survival benefit with IV streptokinase, rt-PA vs. placebo in acute MI
1988	ISIS-2	Aspirin became mainstay treatment
1988	Pfeffer MA, et al.	Development of ACE inhibitors
1988	TIMI trial	Early open artery theory
1988	Sabatine MS, et al, ISIS-2	Anticoagulants to fibrinolytics
1990	Chopra HK, et al.	IV streptokinase in AMI 6–36 months follow-up
1993	Braunwald E, et al, GUSTO	Thrombolytic trials
1994	Grines CL, et al	Primary PCI
2002	Zhao Z-Q, et al.	Postconditioning
2008	NINDS, Hacke, et al.	Recombinant t-PA in ischemic stroke
2011	Shah VK, et al.	Stem cell therapy
2011	Ishikawa K, et al.	Gene therapy
2012	Brodie BR, et al.	Aspiration thrombectomy prior to coronary stenting
2012	Soler-Botija C, et al.	Tissue engineering
2013	Iyengar SS, et al.	Pharmacologic reperfusion therapy with TNK in STEMI
2014	Dalal JJ, et al.	Consensus statement of pharmacoinvasive approach in STEMI
2015	Thomas Alexander, et al.	*CSI Forum:* Consensus Statement *Framework for a National STEMI Program:* Consensus document developed by STEMI India, Cardiological Society of India and Association Physicians of India

Four hours later, after reaching his workplace, the pain returned in a severe form and associated with vomiting. He reached out to the local general practitioner, who evaluated him and administered injectable ranitidine and antiemetics. There was temporary improvement and he went back to his office. He applied for leave and reached home. On the way home, he had an episode of fainting and was rushed to the hospital in the nearby town which was 40 km away. He was admitted and evaluated to have extensive ST-elevation anterior wall myocardial infarction (STEMI) with qRBBB. He was thrombolyzed with streptokinase with a window period of 14 hours. He seemed to be stable. Later in the night, the patient developed acute pulmonary edema and required intravenous diuretics, nitroglycerin and morphine. Next day morning, the patient was referred to a PCI-capable center, which was 50 km away. He underwent an angiogram that showed an occluded proximal left anterior descending artery and an ejection fraction of 20-25%. He underwent rescue PCI and stenting to proximal LAD with nonmedicated stent. The procedure was complicated by no flow and hypotension, for which adjunctive pharmacotherapy along with intra-aortic balloon pump were used. He remained in CCU for 7 days and was later discharged with an ejection fraction of 20-25%. The patient was discharged on multiple medications. One month after his acute MI, the patient continued to have class III dyspnea with exertion and was unable to return to work. A follow-up echocardiogram demonstrated impaired left ventricular systolic function (EF–25%) with severe apical hypokinesis. He was advised an implantable cardiac defibrillator, which he could not afford.

The above scenario is fairly frequently seen by Indian cardiologists even in 2016. The case brings out glaring deficiencies at various levels in STEMI care in India. Individually, we have excellent hospitals, physicians, clinical cardiologists, and cardiac interventionists. Of late, we are having good ambulance services, at least in some states. However, we do not have ANY system in place for STEMI care across the country. The worldover dedicated STEMI programs are successfully implemented in many Western countries for nearly three decades. This commentary focuses on the possible systems that may be put in place to improve the acute care of STEMI across India. Most of the improvement in outcomes in Indian patients could be achieved by timely implementation of the proven therapies focusing the time window.

STEMI CARE IN INDIA: PROBLEMS AND SOLUTIONS

Indian ACS patients, for reasons not exactly clear, seem to present with higher percentage of STEMI. They are less likely to receive timely reperfusion therapy, invasive therapy and evidence-based medicines.[27] The above patient scenario brings forth a few major lacunae in STEMI care that include lack of dedicated STEMI care systems, lack of instantaneously available ECG facility at first point of medical contact, lack of patient awareness, lack of physician readiness, lack of equipped ambulance systems network for patient transport (Emergency Cardiac Services: ECS) and pay from pocket for even Emergency Medical Services (EMS). These are the major reasons for the excess mortality and poorer outcomes seen in Indian patients with STEMI.[27]

In a registry involving 50 cities, only 58.5% of patients with STEMI were thrombolyzed mostly with streptokinase and a minority received percutaneous coronary intervention (PCI). The average delay in presentation was >6 hours. The real situation in most parts of India is likely to lower as these registries have sampled data from tertiary care centers and some of the better developed states. The reported 30-day outcomes for patients with STEMI in the Create registry were death (8.6%), reinfarction (2.3%), and stroke (0.7%). Mortality benefits of PPCI lost if it is delayed more than 60 minutes as depicted in the Global Registry of Acute Coronary Event.[28] Importantly, the poor are marginalized in STEMI care and are less likely to receive thrombolytics, percutaneous coronary intervention and even lipid-lowering drugs. Consequently, the mortality was also higher for poor patients.[29]

In the Italian Registry of TNK in STEMI of 27,000 patients,[30] it has been shown the thrombolysis with TNK is easily, accessible, and available everywhere. Door-to-balloon time in PPCI exceeds 90 minutes practically. Then, PPCI does not reduce mortality consistently. Rapid diagnosis and early reperfusion are pillars of success in STEMI care. TNK is Class 1A recommendation for STEMI ACCP Guideline[31] and is recommended in pre-hospital thrombolysis protocol (Vienna STEMI Registry.[32] The Mayo Clinic STEMI Protocol[33] and The French FAST-MI registry.[34] The potential of TNK cannot be overemphasized. It is given a bolus dose with no hypertension, no allergic reactions, longer half-life, high fibrin specificity and simplified weight adjusted dose, with mostly very minor manageable bleeding. It is an agent of first choice for pre-hospital thrombolysis in STEMI. It has been shown in one of the studies that only 4% of transferred patients received PPCI within 90 min.[35] Prehospital thrombolysis is the strongest independent predictor of in-hospital survivor in the UK.[36]

A recently published Indian registry on STEMI consisting of 15,222 patients 722 centres treated with indigenous tenecteplase (TNK) has shown clinically successful thrombolysis in 96.5% of patients in less than three hours, 96% in three-to-six hours and 85.3% in more than six hours of STEMI.[37] Pharmacoinvasive therapy, including early administration of thrombolysis (TNK) followed by PCI within 3–24 hours after initiation of thrombolytic therapy regardless of success of thrombolysis. However, in case of thrombolytic failure, a rescue PCI should be instantaneously performed. Timely guided protocol for early thrombolysis with tenecteplase (Grade IA) at the level of physician, non-PCI capable centers/nursing homes with intensive care facility and subsequent access to PCI-capable centers improves STEMI outcome.[38] Such a strategy may be the preferred strategy in India as PPCI possible only in 10% of STEMI patients.[39]

There are significant barriers to effective STEMI care. They are at public awareness level, patient level, hospital/physician level and at the Government and societal levels. Patients often ignore symptoms, self-medicate and even when they decide to seek medical attention, they consult non-physicians in India. To overcome these barriers, organized patient education and awareness programs are urgently needed. Cardiological Society of India (CSI), Association of Physicians of India (API) and the Indian Medical Association (IMA) should join hands in these awareness programs. Such programs should not only use the traditional methods like public lectures, print materials, but should also focus on television, internet and social media. The public should be educated that for anyone beyond their teens, an ECG is a must for acute pain or discomfort from jaw to umbilicus, including upper limbs. Public should be educated about the significance of time, seeking immediate medical attention and timely reaching the 'right' hospital or physician for STEMI care.

Another most important barrier is at the level of hospital systems. For a country like India, wherein only less than 10% of STEMI patients receive PCI, primary PCI cannot and will not be the answer for every patient of STEMI. We should rely on thrombolysis, especially bolus agents like tenecteplase (TNK), and promptly shifting the patients to a PCI-capable center. Considering the efficacy, a strategy of prehospital thrombolysis should be ideally suited for Indian conditions. Considering the diverse Indian conditions, a combination of strategies could be more appropriate. For instance, primary PCI should be the preferred strategy in most of the hospitals, who are already offering 24 × 7 emergency PCI services and the patient can reach the available STEMI care PPCI-capable centers less than 90 min.[40] In case, there is a delay in access to PPCI-capable center due to lack of transfer facility, densely populated cities, traffic congestions, etc. Other cities and small district towns would have certified STEMI care physicians and hospitals. These hospitals should do the initial care, thrombolysis with TNK, management of complications and then should have an organized way of early transfer to nearby cities wherein early angiogram and PCI are possible. For rest of rural India, prehospital thrombolysis with TNK could be the ideal strategy. For these to become practical, we need to have **Integrated STEMI Care Systems**. We need to have emergency ambulances, equipped with a facility to do an ECG and transmit to a central station, wherein a cardiologist can ascertain STEMI. Upon confirmation of STEMI, the patient should receive aspirin and statin. These ambulances should also have medical and paramedical personnel who can assess sickness, administer a questionnaire to assess the suitability for thrombolysis with TNK. The patient should be taken in the ambulance that has facility to monitor rhythm and defibrillator. Automated algorithms can decide, based on the place, distance to a STEMI hospital or a PCI-capable center, whether to shift for primary PCI or to a hospital for thrombolysis or prehospital thrombolysis in the ambulance itself. Accordingly, the hospital should be activated and no time should be wasted at the hospital emergency. If prehospital thrombolysis is decided, the patient or relative may talk to a centrally stationed cardiologist and the medical personnel get a consent and administer the agent under cardiac monitoring inside the ambulance, while the patient is being shifted to a nearby hospital.

The above ambitious plan could only work if there is governmental participation and the STEMI care is integrated to the existing emergency care systems in India. The government should make emergency STEMI treatment at subsidized cost to all Indians, may be through medical insurance schemes. The Government should identify STEMI care centers in each city, district and rural areas and certify them. The information on the list of PCI-capable and other STEMI care centers should be widely and easily available. Government should also ensure the availability of thrombolytic, especially bolus agents like TNK at subsidized cost to the poor. Recently published STREAM Trial 2014 with 1-year mortality follow up data has shown that PPCI less than 60 minutes is not practical in most of the STEMI patients, thus, TNK followed by PCI in 24 hours is strongly recommended protocol.[40]

Therefore, Golden time window intervention of < 2 hours is most powerful predictor of salvaging jeopardized myocardium in STEMI and significantly reduces STEMI-inflicted morbidity and mortality. If TNK is given in <60 minutes, it may reduce infarct size from larger to smaller, transmural to subendocardial or may even abort MI, thus help improving subsequent PCI outcome by reducing thrombus burden and better TIMI flow. Time delay >90 minutes reduce the benefit of PPCI. Thus the objective of integrated TIMI care is to minimize time from chest discomfort to ECG <30 minutes (FMC), ECG to drug intervention <60 minutes, drug intervention to PCI < 90-120 minutes will definitely have STEMI-inflicted morbidity and mortality benefit in our country to create global impact. We must act locally to impact globally.

FUTURE DIRECTIONS FOR STEMI PROGRAM IN INDIA

CSI Forum

Consensus Statement: Framework for a National STEMI Program: Consensus document developed by STEMI INDIA, Cardiological Society of India (CSI) and Association Physicians of India:[41] Addressing some of these issues, STEMI India, a not-for-profit organization, Cardiological Society of India (CSI) and Association of Physicians of India (API) have developed a protocol of "systems of care" for efficient management of STEMI, with integrated networks of facilities. Leveraging newly-developed ambulance and emergency medical services, incorporating recent state insurance schemes for vulnerable populations to broaden access, and combining innovative, "state-of-the-art" information technology platforms with existing hospital infrastructure, are the crucial aspects of this system. A pilot program was successfully employed in the state of Tamil Nadu. The purpose of this statement is to describe the framework and methods associated with this program with an aim to improve delivery of reperfusion therapy for STEMI in India. This program can serve as model STEMI systems of care for other low-and-middle income countries.

REFERENCES

1. Tillett WS. The fibrinolytic activity of hemolytic streptococci in relation to the source of strains and to cultural reactions. J Bacteriol. 1935;29:111-30.
2. Sikri N, Bardia A. A history of streptokinase use in acute myocardial infarction. Tex Heart Inst J. 2007;34:318-27.
3. Evans AC. Studies on hemolytic streptococci: VIII. *Streptococcus equisimilis*. J Bacteriol. 1944;48:267-84.
4. Tillett WS, Sherry S. The effect in patients of streptococcal fibrinolysin (streptokinase) and streptococcal desoxyribonuclease on fibrinous, purulent, and sanguineous pleural exudations. J Clin Invest. 1949;28:173-90.
5. Sherry S, Tillett WS, Read CT. The use of streptokinase-streptodornase in the treatment of hemothorax. J Thorac Surg. 1950;20:393-417.
6. Hubbard WN Jr. The systemic toxic responses of patients to treatment with streptokinase streptodornase. J Clin Invest. 1951;30:1171-4.
7. Fletcher AP, Alkjaersig N, Sherry S. The maintenance of a sustained thrombolytic state in man. I. Induction and effects. J Clin Invest. 1959;38:1096-110.
8. Fletcher AP, Sherry S, Alkjaersig N, Smyrniotis FE, Jick S. The maintenance of a sustained thrombolytic state in man. II. Clinical observations on patients with myocardial infarction and other thromboembolic disorders. J Clin Invest. 1959;38:1111-9.
9. Ruegsegger P, Nydick I, Hutter RC, Freiman AH, Bang NU, Cliffton EE, Ladue JS. Fibrinolytic (plasmin) therapy of experimental coronary thrombi with alteration of the evolution of myocardial infarction. Circulation. 1959;19:7-13.
10. Streptokinase in acute myocardial infarction. European Cooperative Study Group for Streptokinase Treatment in Acute Myocardial Infarction. N Engl J Med. 1979;301:797-802.
11. Chopra KL, Chopra HK, Aggarwal KK, Parashar SK, et al. Intravenous streptokinase and oral nifedipine in evolving myocardial infarction—a pilot study. Indian Heart J. 1984;36(6):347-51.
12. Effectiveness of intravenous thrombolytic treatment in acute myocardial infarction. Gruppo Italiano per lo Studio della Streptochinasi nell'Infarto Miocardico (GISSI). Lancet. 1986;1:397-402.
13. Chopra KL, Chopra HK, Aggarwal KK, et al. IV Stk in AMI. 6-36 months follow up. HK Chopra (Ed). Indian Heart Journal. 1990;42(1):13-25.
14. The GUSTO Investigators. An international randomized trial comparing four thrombolytic therapies for acute myocardial infarction. N Engl J Med. 1993;329:673-82.
15. Ouriel K. A history of thrombolytic therapy. J Endovascular Ther. 2004;11(Suppl 2):128-33.
16. Cannon CP, McCabe CH, Gibson CM, et al. TNK-tissue plasminogen activator in acute myocardial infarction. Results of the thrombolysis in myocardial infarction (TIMI) 10A dose-ranging trial. Circulation. 1997;95:351-6.
17. Victor SM, Subban V, Alexander T, G BC, Srinivas A, S S. A prospective, observational, multicenter study comparing tenecteplase facilitated PCI versus primary PCI in Indian patients with STEMI (STEPP-AMI). Open Heart. 2014;1(1):e000133.
18. Iyengar SS, Nair T, Hiremath JS, Jadhav U, Katyal VK, Kumbla D, et al. Pharmacologic Reperfusion Therapy with Indigenous Tenecteplase in 15,222 patients with ST-elevation Myocardial Infarction—The Indian Registry. Indian Heart J. 2013;65(4):436-41.
19. O'Gara PT, Kushner FG, Ascheim DD, Casey DE Jr, Chung MK, de Lemos JA, et al. CF/AHA Task Force. 2013 ACCF/AHA guideline for the management of ST-elevation myocardial infarction: executive summary: a report of the American College of Cardiology Foundation/American Heart Association Task Force on Practice Guidelines. Circulation. 2013;127(4):529-55.
20. Bonnefoy E, Steg PG, Boutitie F, Dubien PY, Lapostolle F, Roncalli J, et al. Comparison of primary angioplasty and prehospital fibrinolysis in acute myocardial infarction (CAPTIM) trial: a 5-year follow-up. European Heart Journal. 2009;30:1598-606.
21. Maroo A, Topol EJ. The early history and development of thrombolysis in acute myocardial infarction. J Thromb Haemost. 2004;2:1867-70.
22. Gray D. Thrombolysis: Past, present and future. Postgraduate Med J. 2006;82:372-5.
23. Hanna EB, et al. The evolving role of glycoprotein IIb/IIIa inhibitors in the setting of percutaneous coronary intervention strategies to minimize bleeding risk and optimize outcomes. JACC Cardiovasc Interv. 2010;3(12):1209-19.
24. Cantor WJ. Routine early angioplasty after fibrinolysis for acute myocardial infarction. N Engl J Med. 2009;360(26):2705-18.
25. Sinnaeve PR, Armstrong PW, Gershlick AH, Goldstein P, Wilcox R, Lambert Y, et al. ST-segment-elevation myocardial infarction patients randomized to a pharmacoinvasive strategy or primary percutaneous coronary intervention: Strategic Reperfusion Early After Myocardial Infarction (STREAM) 1-year mortality follow-up. Circulation. 2014;130(14):1139-45.
26. Danchin N, Coste R, Ferrières J, Steg P, Cottin Y, Blanchard D, et al. Comparison of Thrombolysis Followed by Broad Use of Percutaneous Intervention with Primary Percutaneous Coronary Intervention for Myocardial Infarction (FAST-MI) ST-Segment Elevation Acute Myocardial Infarction: Data From the French Coronary Registry on Acute ST-Elevation (FAST-MI). Circulation 2008;118;268-76.
27. Xavier D, Pais P, Devereaux PJ, Xie C, Prabhakaran D, Reddy KS, Gupta R, Joshi P, Kerkar P, Thanikachalam S, Haridas KK, Jaison TM, Naik S, Maity AK, Yusuf S. CREATE registry investigators. Treatment and outcomes of acute coronary syndromes in India (CREATE): a prospective analysis of registry data, Lancet. 2008;371(9622):1435-42.
28. Nallamothu B, Fox KA, Kennelly BM, Van de Werf F, Gore JM, StegPG, Granger CB, Dabbous OH, Kline-Rogers E, Eagle KA. GRACE Investigators. Relationship of treatment delays and mortality in patients undergoing fibrinolysis and primary percutaneous coronary intervention. The Global Registry of Acute Coronary Events. Heart. 2007;93:1552-5.
29. Mehta Sameer, et al. STEMI Interventions - Future Perspectives, Excerpt from: Chapter 19, Cath Lab Digest. 2008;16(2).
30. Melandri G, et al. Italy Review of tenecteplase (TNKase) in the treatment of acute myocardial infarction. Vascular Health and Risk Management. 2009;5:249-56.
31. Jack Hirsh, Gordon Guyatt, Gregory W Albers, Robert Harrington, Holger J Schünemann. Antithrombotic and Thrombolytic Therapy: American College of Chest Physicians Evidence-based Clinical Practice Guidelines (8th Edn). Chest. 2008;133 (6_suppl):110S-112.
32. Kalla K, Christ G, Karnik R, Malzer R, Norman G, Prachar H, Schreiber W, Unger G, Glogar HD, Kaff A, Laggner AN,

Maurer G, Mlczoch J, Slany J, Weber HS, Huber K. Vienna STEMI Registry Group. Implementation of guidelines improves the standard of care: the Viennese registry on reperfusion strategies in ST-elevation myocardial infarction (Vienna STEMI registry). Circulation. 2006;113(20):2398-405. Epub 2006 May 15

33. Ting HH, Rihal CS, Gersh BJ, Haro LH, Bjerke CM, Lennon RJ, Lim CC, Bresnahan JF, Jaffe AS, Holmes DR, Bell MR. Regional systems of care to optimize timeliness of reperfusion therapy for ST-elevation myocardial infarction: the Mayo Clinic STEMI Protocol. Circulation. 2007;116(7):729-36. Epub 2007 Aug 1.

34. Cambou JP1, Simon T, Mulak G, Bataille V, Danchin N. The French registry of Acute ST elevation or non-ST-elevation Myocardial Infarction (FAST-MI): study design and baseline characteristics. Arch Mal Coeur Vaiss. 2007;100(6-7):524-34.

35. Nallamothu BK, Bates ER, Herrin J, Wang Y, Bradley EH, Krumholz HM. Times to treatment in transfer patients undergoing primary percutaneous coronary intervention in the United States: National Registry of Myocardial Infarction (NRMI)-3/4 analysis. Circulation. 2005;111:761-7.

36. Gale CP, Manda SOM, Batin PD, Weston CF, Birkhead JS, Hall AS. Predictors of in-hospital mortality for patients admitted with ST-elevation myocardial infarction: a real-world study using the Myocardial Infarction National Audit Project (MINAP) database. Heart. 2008;94:1407-12.

37. Iyengar SS, Nair T, Hiremath JS, Jadhav U, Katyal VK, Kumbla D, Sathyamurthy I, Jain RK, Srinivasan M, et al. Pharmacologic reperfusion therapy with indigenous tenecteplase in 15,222 patients with ST-elevation myocardial infarction: the Indian Registry. Indian Heart J. 2013;65(4):436-41.

38. Dalal JJ, Alexander T, Dayasagar V, Yengar SS, Kerkar PG, Mullasari A, Sathe SP, Wander GS, et al. 2013 Consensus Statement for Early Reperfusion and Pharmacoinvasive approach in patients presenting with chest pain diagnosed as STEMI (ST Elevation Myocardial Infarction) in an Indian Setting JAPI. 2014;62.

39. Mehta Sameer, Oliveros E, Reynbakh O, Kostela J, Ossa MM, Zhang T, Botelho R, Rodriguez D, Botero M, Thomas J, Para D, et al. Thrombolytic Therapy in STEMI Interventions. CSI Cardiology Update; 2014.

40. Peter R Sinnaeve, Paul W Armstrong, Anthony H Gershlick, Patrick Goldstein, Robert Wilcox, Yves Lambert, Thierry Danays, Louis Soulat, Sigrun Halvorsen, Fernando Rosell Ortiz, Katleen Vandenberghe, Anne Regelin, Erich Bluhmki, Kris Bogaerts. Frans Van de Werf. The STREAM investigators ST–Segment-Elevation Myocardial Infarction Patients Randomized to a Pharmacoinvasive Strategy or Primary Percutaneous Coronary Intervention Strategic Reperfusion Early After Myocardial Infarction (STREAM): 1-Year Mortality Follow-Up Circulation. 2014;130:1139-45.

41. Thomas Alexandera, Ajit S Mullasari, Zuzana Kaifoszova, Umesh N Khot, Brahmajee Nallamothu, Rao GV Ramana, Meenakshi Sharma, Kala Subramaniam, Ganesh Veerasekar, Suma M Victor, Kiran Chand, Deb PK, Venugopal K, Chopra HK, Santanu Guha, Amal Kumar Banerjee, Muruganathan Armugam A, Manotosh Panja, Gurpreet Singh Wander. CSI Forum: Consensus Statement Framework for a National STEMI Program: Consensus document developed by STEMI INDIA, Cardiological Society of India and Association Physicians of India Indian Heart Journal. 2015;67(5):497-502.

24. Bioresorbable Vascular Scaffold

MS Hiremath

INTRODUCTION

Advances in percutaneous coronary interventions (PCIs) have revolutionized the management of ischemic heart disease in the last century. But ever since the first PCI performed by Andreas Gruentiz in 1977, the most feared complication of the procedure was acute occlusion secondary to elastic recoil and intimal and medial dissection with superadded intramural hematoma.[1] Though balloon angioplasty (BA) results were highly unpredictable (restenosis rate 40%), majority of vessels tolerate the focal plaque dissection and heal sufficiently, modulated by lifestyle changes, preventive medicine and anti-atherosclerotic pharmacotherapy.[2]

Coronary stents were designed to create larger intimal lumen, seal dissection and resist recoil and late remodeling.[3,4] In STRESS and BENESTENT-1 trial use of balloon-expanding bare metal stent (BMS) was associated with 20–30% reduction in clinical and angiographic restenosis compared to BA. Over a period of time, BMS underwent modification in terms of design (thin strut, self-expanding/balloon expanding, open cell/close-cell), composition (stainless steel/cobalt chromium), leading to improvement in deliverability and reduction in stent thrombosis (ST) but in-stent restenosis (ISR) remain the major limitation.

With the advent of drug-eluting stent (DES), which maintained the mechanical advantage of BMS in terms of radial strength, local delivery of antiproliferative drug (paclitaxel/sirolimus/zotarolimus/everolimus/biolimus) at the site of implantation, significantly reduced the clinical and angiographic restenosis **(Fig. 1)**.

ISR of BMS is considered as a stable condition with early peak of intimal hyperplasia followed by a regression period beyond 1year, endothelialization of BMS is complete by 12 weeks.[5,6] Whereas antiproliferative drug from DES reduce neointimal formation, impeding smooth muscle cell proliferation and migration.[7,8] Delayed/incomplete endothelialization causing uncovered stent and local arterial

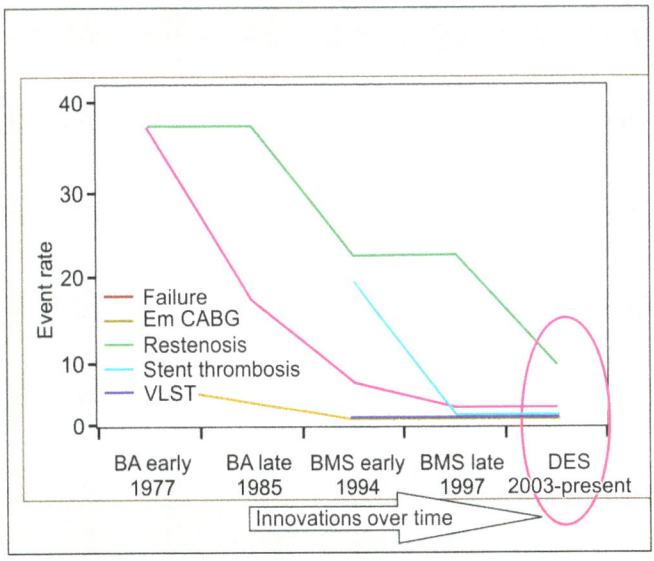

Fig. 1: Evolution of percutaneous coronary intervention (PCI) and its limitations
Abbreviations: VLST, very late stent; DES, drug-eluting stent

hypersensitivity to polymer leads to late and very-late stent thrombosis and late malapposition, acquired or persistent.[9] Incomplete endothelialization leading to uncovered struts leads to advanced neoatherosclerosis with neointimal rupture is an another cause of very late stent thrombosis.[10] Further advancement in DES design, i.e. biodegradable polymer when compared with durable polymer did not show any superiority in clinical trials.[11,12]

Thus the idea of fully dissolvable scaffolds which will eliminate problems with current DES has evolved over the years. Serruys et al.[13] demonstrated that after PCI, vessel lumen appear to stabilize after 3 months, so that scaffolding of vessel is only a transient need **(Tables 1 and 2)**.

Table 1 Advantages of bioresorbable scaffold

- Long length of vessel can be treated without formation of permanent metal jacket
- Provide scaffold only when needed during vessel healing
- Restore local vasomotion
- Will not interfere with MRI or CT imaging
- Will not preclude future surgical or percutaneous revascularization
- May afford new treatment option for unstable/vulnerable plaque
- Suitable for pediatric use
- Freedom from persistent side-branch obstruction by struts

Table 2 Characteristics of ideal BRS

- Should have moderate degradation rate over a predictable finite period, leaving no residua matrix
- Should be biocompatible, nontoxic
- Should have high tensile strength with low-profile, balloon-expandable design for easy deliverability
- Should not be thrombogenic and should not release any embolization during degradation
- Should have acceptable shelf-life

BRS in clinical use and in experimental development are based on 2 platforms: A. polymer-based, B. Metal-based

POLYMER BASED

Poly L–lactic acid (PLLA) is homopolymer of L-lactide, semicrystalline with slow degradation rate and high tensile strength. It undergoes degradation by hydrolysis which leads to formation of water soluble low molecular weight components metabolized into water and carbon dioxide via Kreb's cycle. Limitation of polymer-based bioresorbable scaffold (BRS) include potential for inflammation of a bulkier profile composed to metallic stents.

Collapse pressures of PLLA-based stents are nearly equal to that of stainless steel metal stents.[14]

METAL BASED

Magnesium is used for production of metal-based BRS. Electronegative charge that emerges during degradation of metal BRS is antithrombotic, in addition, due to its high mechanical strength it provides adequate radial strength even with thinner strut size compared to other BRS. Latest generation metal BRS provide radial support for 9–12 months.[15]

Intravascular ultrasound (IVUS) Everolimus-eluting Bioabsorbable scaffold (E-BVS) : This is a only commercially available BRS with backbone of high molecular weight PLLA with PDLAA coating serving as a bioabsorbable matrix for an everolimus eluting layer. Its highly deliverable and conformable stent by virtue of its thin stents and low profile material mounted on ML vision SDS balloon. The stent include two radiopaque platinum markers on end rings of stents for enhance visibility. Total absorption time enhanced time is about 2 years.

COHORT A

A Bioabsorbable Everolimus-eluting Coronary Stent System for Patients with Single De-novo Coronary Artery Lesions) trial: This was the BVS system first in human prospective open label trial enrolling patients with simple de nova coronary stenosis.[16,17]

The design of BVS revision 1.0 used in cohort A of the trial was circumferential out of phase zigzag loops and linkages either directly or by straight bridges.

There was good procedural success (29 out of 31 attempts) and good safety profile at end of 2 years with major adverse cardiac events (MACE) rate of 3.4% which remain unchanged over 5 years follow up. But intravascular ultrasound (IVUS) imaging at 6 reported 11–12% reduction in stents area which was more than metallic EES. In cohort B, BVS revision 1.1 was used (**Figs 2A and B**), which has different design and

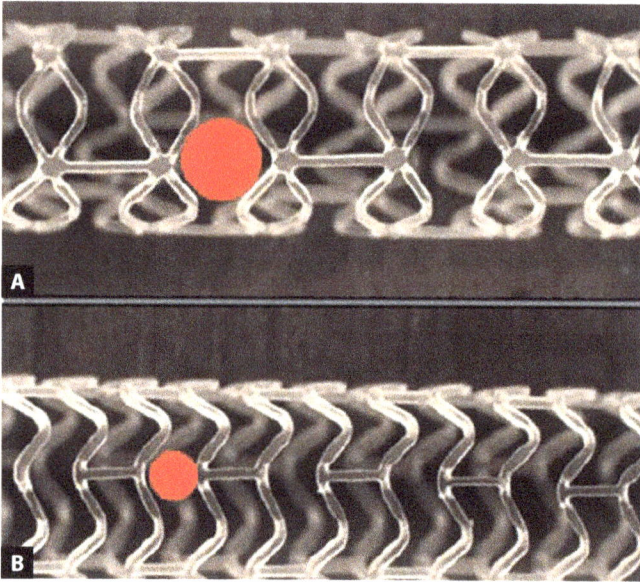

Figs 2A and B: Design of the different bioresorbable vascular scaffold (BVS). (A) BVS 1.0 design. The struts are distributed as circumferential out-of-phase zigzag hoops linked together by three longitudinal bridges between each hoop. The maximal circular unsupported surface area is drawn as a red circle; (B) BVS 1.1 design. The struts are arranged as in-phase zigzag hoops linked together by three longitudinal bridges. The strut distribution is more uniform and allows the maximal circular unsupported surface area (red circle) to be smaller than in the BVS 1.0

Table 3 Three years of ABSORB clinical data

Hierarchical	6 months (n = 30)	12 months (n = 29)*	24 months (n = 29)*	36 months (n = 29)*
Ischemia-driven TLR	0%	0%	0%	0%
By PCI	0%	0%	0%	0%
By CABG	0%	0%	0%	0%
Nonischemia-driven TLR% (n)	3.3%(1)**	3.4%(1)	3.4%(1)	3.4%(1)
Cardiac death	0%	0%	0%	0%
Noncardiac death	0%	0%	3.4%(1)	6.9%(2)
MI	3.3%(1)	3.4%(1)	3.4%(1)	3.4%(1)
Q-wave MI	0%	0%	0%	0%
Non Q-wave MI	3.3%(1)	3.4%(1)**	3.4%(1)	3.4%(1)**
Nonischemia-driven TVR (non-TLR)	6.7%(2)	6.9%(2)	6.9%(2)	6.9%(2)
Any TVR	10.0%(3)	10.3%(3)	10.3%(3)	10.3%(3)

Abbreviations: MACE, major adverse cardiac events; MI, myocardial infarction; TLR, target lesion revascularization; PCI, percutaneous coronary interventions; CABG, coronary artery bypass grafting; MI, myocardial infarction; TVR, target vessel revascularization.
*One patient withdraw consent and missed the 9, 12, 18 months and 2 and 3-year visits, but the vital status of the patients in the absence of cardiac event is known through the referring physician.
**This patient also underwent a TLR, not qualified as ID-TLR (DS = 42%) followed by postprocedural troponin qualified as a non-QMI and died from his Hodgkin's disease at 888 days postprocedure.

manufacturing process so as to enhance mechanical strength and durability allowing more uniform stent distribution and reduce maximal unsupported surface area. The polymer mass coating content amount of drug and stent thickness remained same. This allowed slower bioresorption process of BVS 1.1 compared to BVS 1.0 thereby eliminating late shrinkage higher inhibition of neointimal response.

Cohort B enrolled 101 patients from 12 centers with maximum of 2 de novo native coronary artery lesion with maximum diameter of 3.0 mm and length ≤14 mm with a percentage stenosis ≥ 50% and 100% and TIMI flow grade of >1. At 30 days, there was no occurrence of stent thrombosis no need for repeat procedure (ischemia driven target-lesion revascularization).

6-month follow-up with OCT showed late lumen loss of 0.19mm ± 0.18 mm with a limited relative decrease in minimal luminal areas of 5.4%. OCT follow-up showed that 96.8% of the stents were covered (uniform covered box appearance). Mean neointimal growth measured by OCT between and on top of the polymeric stents equals 1.25 mm or 16.9% of scaffold areas.[18]

At 12 months follow-up **(Table 3)**, angiographic late lumen loss was 0.27 mm ± 0.32 mm with relative decrease in minimal lumen area of 1.94%. OCT showed 96.69% of struts were covered. Two patients experienced periprocedural and iatrogenic myocardial infarction and 2 patients underwent revascularization; thus MACE rate was 7.1%.[18]

In recently published meta-analysis[19] showed inferior angiographic permanence of E-BVS compared to metallic EES at 10 month follow-up. By contrast, some studies have shown similar angiographic outcome (surveillance done at 12 months or later) when compared with metallic EES (p=0.12 for indevice and p=0.16 for insegment late lumen loss).[20] But whatever the angiographic outcome, overall revascularization rate was similar for E-BVS and metallic EES.[21] The same meta-analysis[19] showed high risk (2 times) of subacute stent thrombosis (between 1 and 30 days postprocedure) with E-BVS despite optimal compliance with dual antiplatelet regimen. Multicenter Comprehensive Analysis[22] showed that incidence of ST can be minimized by optimizing implantation technique.

Long-term angiographic follow-up will shed light on to the adaptive response of coronary vessel wall and its possible effect on clinical outcomes after BVS implantation.

E-BVS IMPLANTATION: TIPS AND TRAPS

By virtue of thicker struts (157 μm) and crossing profile (1.4 mm) in comparison to metallic stents, E-BVS are more difficult to deliver, especially in complex lesions. So, optimal lesion preparation prior to E-BVS implantation has been encouraged to facilitate their successful delivery and adequate expansion. Current-generation BVS have a relatively bulky profile with thick struts (157 × 191 μm) and lower radial force, and, as a consequence, have numerically higher acute recoil (6.7 ± 6.4% vs 4.3 ± 7.1%),[23] and more eccentric radial expansion (0.85 ± 0.08 vs 0.90 ± 0.06; p <0.001)[24] when compared to the XIENCE V® metallic stent (Abbott vascular). Taking these features and late lumen loss into account, aggressive lesion preparation with high-pressure

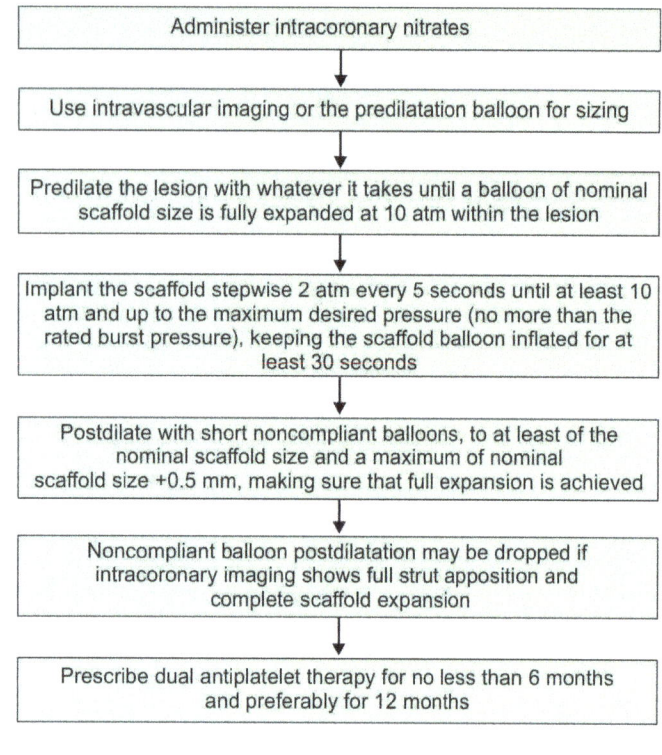

Flow chart 1: Practical operating protocol for new users of BVS[27]

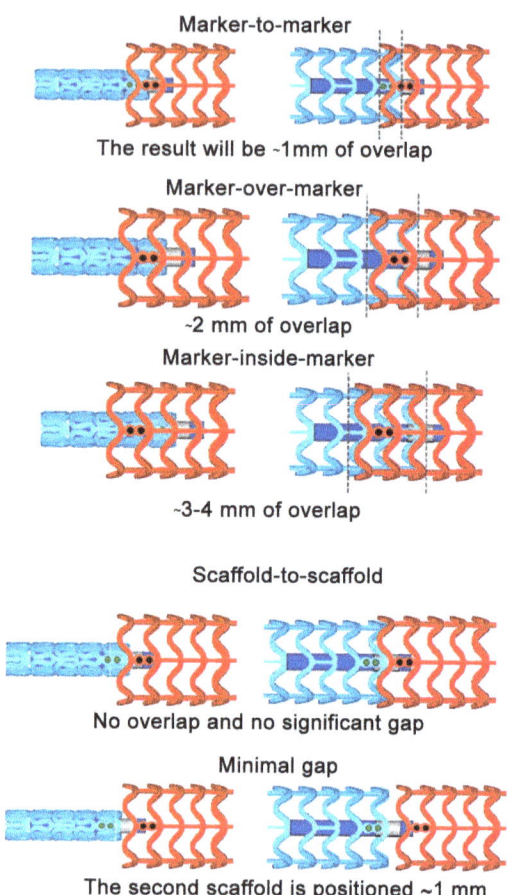

Fig. 3: BVS overlapping techniques

post-dilatation, especially in the setting of complex lesions, is strongly encouraged to achieve optimal procedural results **(Flow chart 1)**.[25,26]

As a general rule, BVS should not be implanted into lesions that cannot be adequately prepared with balloon inflations, particularly when the balloon used for predilatation cannot be fully expanded or when the result of dilation is unsatisfactory (i.e. residual stenosis >40%). The goal of lesion preparation is to facilitate scaffold delivery, reduce plaque shift, and, most importantly, to allow optimal scaffold expansion **(Fig. 3)**.[27]

The scaffold should cover ≥2 mm of the healthy vessel at either edge of the lesion. Deployment must occur gradually, pressurizing the delivery system in 2 atmosphere increments every five seconds until complete expansion of the scaffold. At this point, the inflation pressure must be maintained for at least 30 seconds. Due to the polymeric material, the BVS has a maximum scaffold expansion limit of 0.5 mm above its nominal diameter, which should be respected strictly during implantation. Upon scaffold deployment, one should aim to obtain <10% residual stenosis, full scaffold expansion and optimal wall apposition. Therefore, routine post dilatation for 10–30 seconds using a high-pressure noncompliant balloon is advisable unless intracoronary imaging confirms full expansion and apposition **(Figs 4A and B)**.[27]

Miyazaki T et al.[28] demonstrated that predilatation using a cutting balloon probably results in reduced elastic recoil, when compared to the use of a conventional balloon alone, leading to better deployment of a BVS at the site of the target lesion. The larger expansion index with the use of a cutting balloon also assist in BVS postdilatation. Though this study could not demonstrate that use of cutting translated into improved clinical outcomes with respect to ischemia-driven TLR. Thus use of cutting balloon may reduce acute recoil prior to BVS deployment, facilitate optimal sizing and result in improved radial concentric expansion of BVS, even in the setting of complex and calcified lesions.

Bifurcation Lesions

During bifurcation coronary interventions, side branch (SB) recrossing and fenestration, kissing balloon inflation are very difficult with BVS stent because of its bulky profile, thick struts and low radial strength. Single stent strategy is preferred. The classic kissing balloon inflation is not recommended due to the possibility of proximal strut fracture, kissing with minimal balloon overlap ("snuggle or mini-kissing") can be used. Second stent if required metallic stent is preferred. Techniques

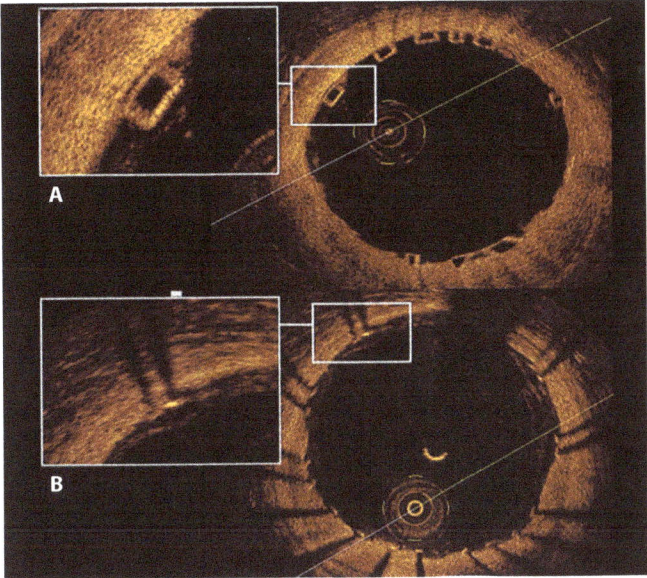

Figs 4A and B: Optical coherence tomography (OCT) imaging of the bioresorbable scaffolds and metallic platform stents. (A) Bioresorbable vascular scaffold imaged with OCT. The strut appearance is translucent and allows a perfect imaging of the vessel wall; (B) Metallic platform stent imaged with OCT. The metallic struts are opaque to the OCT light and produce the typical shadow into the vessel wall

with least strut layering should be preferred (i.e. T, T and small protrusion) when a second stent or scaffold is needed.[27]

Long Lesions

The relatively thick struts of BVS mandate keeping the overlap to a minimum to avoid delays in healing.[29] The scaffold edges fall within the 1 mm balloon markers on each end and the scaffold marker beads are placed approximately 1 mm from the scaffold end. There various overlap techniques described, but most commonly used are the "marker-to-marker" (~1 mm of overlap) and "scaffold-to-scaffold" (no overlap) techniques.[27]

Higher risk of subacute stent thrombosis with E-BVS seen in recent trials, example, the 6-month incidence of ScT was 2% in the GHOST-EU,[30] as high as 3% in the academic medical center single-center registry,[31] and in the BVS EXAMINATION trial,[32] rates at 1 month were 2.1% for BVS, 0.3% for DES, and 1.0% for bare-metal stents (p =0.06 for BVS vs DES). This have been attributed to implantation techniques rather than biomechanic properties of BVS. Following implantation strategies to reduce stent thrombosis are recommended[27] like predilation with noncompliant balloon up to the same size as the reference vessel diameter (RVD), BVS implantation only in case of full expansion of the noncompliant balloon, implantation of a BVS of the same size as the RVD at 10–12 atm, and postdilation with noncompliant balloons up to a maximum of 0.5 mm larger at 14–16 atm. When researchers implemented a BVS-specific implantation strategy, the 12-month stent thrombosis rates decreased from 3.3% to 1.0%, and this drop remained significant after adjusting for multivariable propensity score (hazard ratio: 0.19; 95% confidence interval: 0.05-0.70; $p = 0.012$).[22]

ROLE OF INTRAVASCULAR IMAGING IN BVS IMPLANTATION AND FOLLOW-UP

Anecdotal cases of BVS thrombosis following inadequate expansion and apposition of the BVS have indirectly supported an extensive application of intravascular imaging techniques.[33] In absence of clear evidence of benefit from large controlled trials, there is agreement among the authors that new users of BVS especially should have a low threshold for the use of imaging before and after BVS implantation.

Optical coherence tomography (OCT) preferred over intravascular ultrasound (IVUS) during BVS implantation. The monochromatic peak wavelength of OCT is differently reflected, refracted and absorbed by polymeric or metallic stents. Most of the OCT light energy is transmitted through polymeric struts such that only part of it is reflected at endoluminal and abluminal sides of struts generating a visible optical frame and the core of the strut is imaged as black square at baseline. As a consequence the vessel wall is easily imaged through the struts without any major shadowing **(Figs 5A to D)**.[34]

Porcine coronary artery model imaged with OCT compared with corresponding histology at regular intervals after E-BVS implantation.[35] At 2 years, 80.4% of struts were seen as preserved box appearance and by histology these structures appeared to be composed of proteoglycans with polymeric material being at such low level as to be no longer quantifiable by chromatography.

E-BVS FROM CLINICAL TRIALS TO CLINICAL PRACTICE

ISAR-ABSORB registry[36] analysed angiographic and clinical results of patients undergoing E-BVS implantation in real-world setting (76% had multivessel disease, 50% had ACC/AHA type B2/C lesion, 40% were acute coronary syndrome). At angiographic follow-up in-stent late loss was 0.26 ± 0.51 mm, and binary angiographic restenosis was 7.5%. At 12 months, the rate of death, myocardial infarction, or target lesion revascularization was 13.1%. Definite stent thrombosis occurred in 2.6%, target lesion revascularization rate at 12 months was 9.1%, which is higher than that observed in previous trials which included relatively simple lesion with stable coronary artery disease patients. Thus, demonstrating high antistenotic efficacy and satisfactory outcomes in terms of clinical efficacy. But observed stent thrombosis rate at 6 months was 2.0% and at 12 month was 2.6% which much higher than metallic EES (2 times). Most the cases of stent thrombosis occurred with 30 days of implantation, this suggests possible role of implantation technique rather than specific biochemical properties of the stent. Thus, refinement

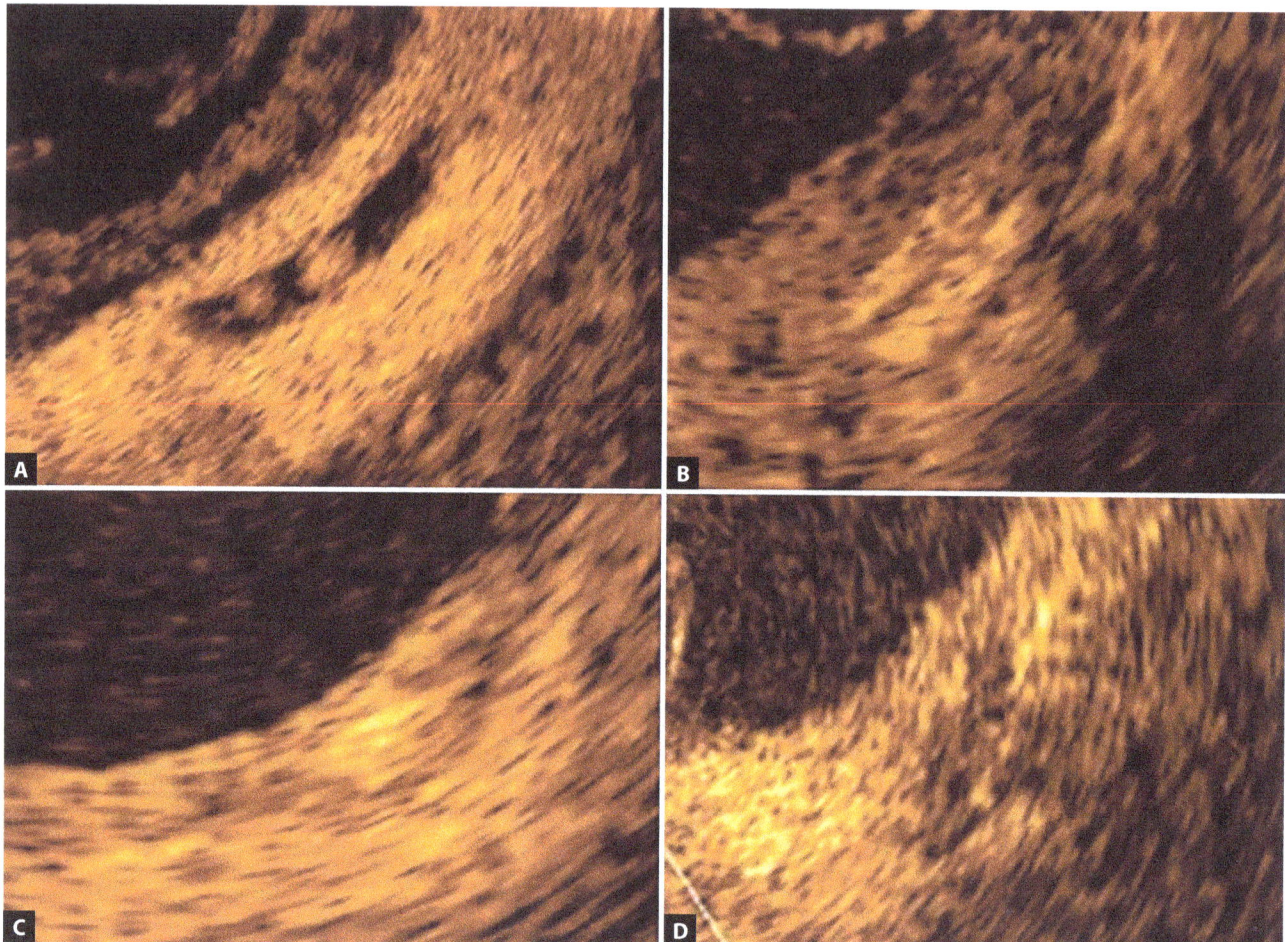

Figs 5A to D: Strut appearance of the bioresorbable vascular scaffold at follow-up. (A) Preserved box appearance: sharp defined, bright reflection borders with preserved box-shaped appearance; strut body shows low reflection; (B) Open box: luminal and abluminal long-axis borders thickened bright reflection; short-axis borders not visible; (C) Dissolved bright box: partially visible bright spot, contours poorly defined; no box-shaped appearance; (D) Dissolved black box: black spot, contours poorly defined, often confluent; no box-shaped appearance

of implantation technique are recommended[27] to reduce the rate of stent thrombosis over a period of time.

NONINVASIVE ASSESSMENT OF BVS

CT scan is an established method to noninvasively assess coronary calcification and de novo coronary stenosis. But presence of metallic stent precludes the use of CT scan due to artifact. Presence of radiolucent backbone of polylactide, MSCT could be used to assess changes in the lumen and vessels after E-BVS implantation. In the recent study,[37] the feasibility of quantitative assessment of coronary MSCT was 100%, whereas the noninvasive FFR assessment was possible in 72%. At 5 years, 18 patients underwent MSCT angiography. All scaffolds were patent, with a median minimal lumen area of 3.25 mm^2 (interquartile range: 2.20 to 4.30). Noninvasive FFR analysis was feasible in 13 of 18 scans, which yielded a median distal FFR of 0.86 (interquartile range: 0.82 to 0.94).

RESTORATION OF VASOMOTION

One of the most important hypothesized advantage of BRS was restoration of coronary vasomotion after period of stent resorption.[38] To study vasomotion either the endothelium independent vasoconstrictor methylergometrine maleate, or the endothelium dependent vasoactive agent acetylcholine is given. Follow-up studies[37] have shown complete restoration of vasomotion at the end of 2 years.

Other BRS in Trials (Tables 4A and B)

Current Limitations

BRS still have limited applications, and to date they do not outperform the current generation of high performance metallic drug-eluting devices. Its usefulness in complex scenario like left main stenosis, calcific vessel, diabetic patients is yet to be validated.

Chapter 24: Bioresorbable Vascular Scaffold   169

Table 4A Results for current existing bioresorbable scaffolds

Basic material			Poly-lactic acid						
Scaffold name	Igaki-Tamai stent	Absorb BVS 1.0	Absorb BVS 1.1	DESolve 1st generation	DESolve 2nd generation	Amaranth	ARTI8Z BRS	Xinsorb BRS	Acute BRS
Manufacturer	Kyoto Medical Planning Co Ltd, Kyoto, Japan	Abbott Vascular, Santa Monica, CA, USA	Abbott Vascular, Santa Monica, CA, USA	Elixir Medical Corp. Sunnyvale, CA, USA	Elixir Medical Corp. Sunnyvale, CA, USA	Amaranth Medical Inc, CA, USA	Arterial Remodeling Tech., France	Shandong HuaAn Biotech., Co. Ltd, China	OrbusNeich, Fort Lauderdale FL, USA
Composition	PLLA	PLLA	PLLA	PLLA	PLLA	PLLA	PLLA, PDLA	Poly-lactic acid, poly e-caprolactone, poly-glycolic acid	PLLA, L-lactic-co-e-caprolactone, PDLA
Design of the latest generation	Zigzag helical coil	Out-of-phase sinusoidal hoops with links	In-phase zigzag hoops, cross-linked by bridges	Tubularly arranged hoops, linked by bridges	Tubularly arranged hoops, linked by bridges	Zigzag hoops, linked by bridges	Creep-resistant hinge	—	Helically linked double ring
Thickness of strut, µm	170	150	150	150	150	—	—	150-170	150
Visualization	Gold radio-paque markers at both ends	Radiopaque metal markers at both ends	Radiopaque metal markers at both ends	2 platinum radiopaque markers	2 platinum radiopaque markers	—	—	2 radiopaque markers	Radiopaque markers
Special feature	Self-expandable when heated	—	—	Minor malapposition is self-corrected	Minor malapposition is self-corrected	Consists of multiple layers	—	Radial strength is comparable to that of DES	Dual elution
Anti-proliferative drug elution	No	Everolimus	Everolimus	Myolimus	Novolimus	No	No	Sirolimus	Abluminal side: sirolimus Luminal: CD34 + antibodies
Resorption time	3 yrs	Up to 3 yrs	Up to 3 yrs	1 yr	1 yr	1-2 yrs	1.5-2 yrs	—	—
Status	CE mark (for peripheral use)	CE mark (for coronary use); randomized-controlled trial BVS vs. DES) is currently enrolling patients	CE mark (for coronary use)	CE mark (for coronary use)		Clinical evaluation, new version under dev.	Clinical evaluation	30 patients enrolled in FiM study	Pre-clinical evaluation

Contd...

Contd...

Basic material	Poly-lactic acid							
	Igaki-Tamai FiM 50 patients 127 ± 17 mos	Cohort A 30 patients 5 yrs	Cohort B 101 patients 24 mos ABSORB Extend 250 patients 24 mos	DESolve FiM 15 patients 12 mos	DESolve Nx Study 126 patients 12 mos	Amaranth FiM 13 patients 6 mos	Pre-clinical results ARTDIVA FiM	Pre-clinical results
Trials (no. in cohort and duration)								
Imaging findings	Acute recoil 22 ± 7% MLD: 2.68 ± 0.43 mm post-procedural; 1.76 ± 0.74 mm at 6 mos; 2.22 ± 0.56 mm at 3 yrs Scaffold CSA: 5.44 mm² post-procedural; 3.64 mm² at 6 mos; 5.18 mm² at 3 yrs	Acute recoil 0.20 ± 0.21 mm MLD: 2.32 mm post-procedural; 1.89 mm at 6 mos; = 1.76 mm at 2 yrs LLL: 0.43 mm at 6 mos; 0.48 mm at 2 yrs	Cohort B findings Min. lumen area: 5.45 ± 1.08 mm² post-procedural; 5.12 ± 1.01 mm² at 6 mos; 5.13 ± 1.25 mm² at 2 yrs Mean lumen area: 6.53 ± 1.24 mm² post-procedural; 6.36 ± 1.18 mm² at 6 mos; 6.85 ± 1.78 mm² at 24 mos LLL: 0.16 ± 0.18 mm at 6 mos; 0.27 ± 0.20 mm at 2 yrs No evidence of late or very late scaffold recoil	Scaffold CSA 6.57 ± 0.68 mm² post-procedural; 6.80 ± 0.85 mm² at 6 mos LLL: 0.20 ± 0.10 mm	LLL: 0.21 ± 0.34 mm at 6 mos	LLL: 0.93 ± 0.41 mm	Acute recoil: 2.9% LLL: <0.3 mm at 3 and 6 mos	Acute recoil: 2.9% LLL: <0.3 mm at 3 and 6 mos	Acute recoil: 0.66 ± 4.32% No significant differences between the X Insorb BRS and concerning neointimal growth, MLD, and scaffold/stent area
Target lesion revascularization	16% at 1 year 16% at 3 yrs 18% at 5 yrs 28% at 10 yrs	0.0% (ID) 3.4% (non-ID)	Cohort B 6 cases (ID) ABSORB Extend 9.0%	1 case	1.6% at 6 mos 3.3% at 1 yr (both non-ID)	—	—	—
Major adverse cardiac events	50% at 10 yrs	3.4% (ID)	Cohort B 4.0% ABSORB Extend 7.3%	2 cases	3.3% at 6 mos 5.7% at 1 yr			

Table 4B Results for current existing bioresorbable scaffolds

Basic material	Magnesium			Others		
						Ideal BioStent
Scaffold name	AMS	DREAMS 1.0	DREAMS 2.0	REVA BRS	REVA ReZolve	
Manufacturer	Biotronik, Berlin, Germany	Biotronik, Berlin, Germany	Biotronik, Berlin, Germany	Reva Medical Inc., San Diego, CA, USA	Reva Medical Inc., San Diego, CA, USA	Xenogenics Corp., Canton, MA, USA
Composition	Magnesium and rare earth metals	Magnesium and rare earth metals	Magnesium and rare earth metals	Desaminotyrosine polycarbonate	Desaminotyrosine polycarbonate	Poly-lactic anhydride containing 2 salicylic acid molecules linked to 1 sebacic acid molecule
Design of the latest generation	4-crown design	6-crown design	6-crown design	Slide-and-lock ("ratchet")	Slide-and-lock ("ratchet")	Tube with laser-cut voids
Thickness of strut, μm	165	120	150	204	122	200
Visualization	Latest generation with radiopaque markers			Fully radiopaque	Fully radiopaque	–
Special feature	Electronegative charge that emerges during degradation process has an antithrombotic function					Polymer causes less inflammation
Antiproliferative drug elution	No	Paclitaxel	Sirolimus	Paclitaxel	Sirolimus	Sirolimus
Resorption time	2 mos	9–12 mos	–	2–3 years	2–3 years	15 mos
Status	Clinical evaluation	Clinical evaluation	Clinical evaluation	Clinical evaluation; CE trial ongoing	Clinical evaluation; CE trial ongoing	Clinical evaluation, pre-clinical evaluation of the thinner 2nd generation
Trials (no. in cohort and duration)	PROGRESS AMS 63 patients up to 28 mos	BIOSOLVE-46 patients up to 3 years	BIOSOLVE-II	FiM – 15 mos	RESTORE 26 patients 12 mos	FiM 11 patients 1.5 yrs
Imaging findings	In-scaffold lumen diameter: 2.47 ± −0.37 mm post-procedural; 1.38 ± 0.51 mm at 4 mos Degree of stenosis: 12.65 ± 5.53% post-procedural; 48.37 ± 17.0% at 4 mos LLL: 1.08 ± 0.49 mm at 4 mos	LLL: 0.65 ± 0.5 at 6 mos; 0.52 ± 0.39 mm at 12 mos MLD: 2.56 ± 0.35 mm Post-procedural; 1.95 ± 0.59 mm at 6 mos; 2.06 ± 0.47 mm at 12 mos Scaffold CSA: 7.29 ± 1.39 mm² post-procedural; 6.49 ± 2.11 mm² at 6 mos; 6.40 ± 20.4 mm² at 12 mos	–	–	Acute recoil: 3.8 ± 6.7% LLL 0.29 ± 0.33 mm at 12 mos	No evidence of stent recoil
Target lesion revascularization	39.7% at 4 mos 45.0% at 12 mos	4.7% at 12 mos	–	–	3 cases after 12 mos	–
Major adverse cardiac events	23.8% at 4 mos 26.7% at 12 mos	2 periprocedural target vessel myocardial infarctions	–	–	–	–

CONCLUSION

Most of randomized trials have studied E-BVS in simple de novo lesions in chronic stable angina, have showed results comparable to present metallic EES, same trend towards non-inferiority is seen in real world scenario. This device recently received US-FDA approval [The panel voted on the safety (9 yes, 1 nay), efficacy (10 yes, 0 nay), and risk/benefit profile (9 yes, 1 abstain) of absorb based on data from the ABSORB III study 12-month target vessel event rates with metallic EES are <5% in the context of recent clinical trials. A clinical trial of E-BVS compared with second generation DES could require over 20,000 patients to answer the question of relative superiority of E-BVS with respect to late stent thrombosis. Given the realities of clinical trials, such an investigation is unlikely. So equaling metallic EES's immediate and midterm outcomes should be the first goal of BRS, once this target is met unresolved issues like more complex implantation, duration of antiplatelet regimen has to be solved.

REFERENCES

1. Gruntzig A. Transluminal dilatation of coronary-artery stenosis. Lancet. 1978;1:263.
2. Ormiston JA, Stewart FM, Roche HG, et al. Late regression of the dilated site after coronary angioplasty. Circulation. 1997;96:468-74.
3. Serruys PW, Jaegere PD, Kiemeneij F, et al. A comparison of balloon-expandable-stent implantation with balloon angioplasty in patients with coronary artery disease. N Engl J Med. 1994;331:489-95.
4. Fischman DL, Leon MB, Baim DS, et al. A randomized comparison of coronary-stent placement and balloon angioplasty in the treatment of coronary artery disease. N Engl J Med. 1994;331:496-501.
5. Kimura T, Yokoi H, Nakagawa Y, et al. Three-year follow-up after implantation of metallic coronary-artery stents. N Engl J Med. 1996;334:561-7.
6. Komatsu R, Ueda M, Naruko T. Neointimal tissue response at sites of coronary stenting in humans. Circulation. 1998;98:224-3.
7. Atary JZ, Bergheanu SC, van der Hoeven BL, et al. Impact of sirolimus-eluting stent implantation compared to bare-metal stent implantation for acute myocardial infarction on coronary plaque composition at nine months follow-up: a virtual histology intravascular ultrasound analysis. Results from the Leiden MISSION! intervention study. Eurointervention. 2009;04:572.
8. Nakazawa G, Finn AV, Virmani R, et al. Coronary responses and differential mechanisms of late stent thrombosis attributed to first-generation sirolimus and paclitaxel-eluting stents. J Am Coll Cardiol. 2011;57(4):390-8.
9. Téphane Cook, Elena Ladich, et al. Correlation of intravascular ultrasound findings with histopathological analysis of thrombus aspirates in patients with very late drug-eluting stent thrombosis. Circulation. 2009;120:391-9.
10. Nakazawa G, Otsuka F, Nakano M, et al. The pathology of neoatherosclerosis in human coronary implants: bare-metal and drug-eluting stents. J Am Coll Cardiol. 2011;57(11):1314.
11. Byrne RA, Kastrati A, Massberg S, et al. Biodegradable polymer versus permanent polymer drug-eluting stents and everolimus-versus sirolimus-eluting stents in patients with coronary artery disease: 3-Year outcomes from a randomized clinical trial. J Am Coll Cardiol. 2011;58(13):1325-31.
12. Kang SH, Park KW, Do-Yoon Kan. Biodegradable-polymer drug-eluting stents vs. bare metal stents vs. durable-polymer drug-eluting stents: a systematic review and Bayesian approach network meta-analysis. European Heart. 2014;35(17):1147-58.
13. Serruys PW, Luijten HE, Beatt KJ. Incidence of restenosis after successful coronary angioplasty: a time-related phenomenon. A quantitative angiographic study in 342 consecutive patients at 1, 2, 3, and 4 months. Circulation. 1988;77:361-71.
14. Grizzi I, Garreau H, Li S, Vert M. Hydrolytic degradation of devices based on poly (DL-lactic acid) size-dependence Biomaterials. 1995;16(4):305-11.
15. Heublein B, Rohde R, Kaese V, Niemeyer M, et al. Biocorrosion of magnesium alloys: a new principle in cardiovascular implant technology? Heart. 2003;89:651-6.
16. Serruys PW, Ormiston JA, Onuma Y, et al. A bioabsorbable everolimuseluting coronary stent system (ABSORB): 2-year outcomes and results from multiple imaging methods. Lancet. 2009;373:897-910.
17. Serruys PW, Onuma Y, Ormiston JA, et al. Evaluation of the second generation of a bioresorbable everolimus drug-eluting vascular scaffold for treatment of de novo coronary artery stenosis: six-month clinical and imaging outcomes circulation. 2010;122:2301-12.
18. Serruys PW, Onuma Y, Dudek D, et al. Evaluation of the second generation of a bioresorbable everolimus-eluting vascular scaffold for the treatment of de novo coronary artery Stenosis:12-month clinical and imaging outcomes. J Am Coll Cardiol. 2011;58:1578-88.
19. Salvatore Cassese, Robert A Byrne, Gjin Ndrepepa, Sebastian Kufner. Everolimus-eluting bioresorbable vascular scaffolds versus everolimus-eluting metallic stents: a meta-analysis of randomised controlled trials. Lancet. 2016;387-10018:537.
20. Kimura T, Kozuma K, Tanabe K, et al. A randomized trial evaluating everolimus-eluting absorb bioresorbable scaffolds vs. everolimus-eluting metallic stents in patients with CAD: ABSORB Japan. Eur Heart J DOI: *http://dx.doi.org/10.1093/eurheartj/ehv435*.
21. Gao R, Yang Y, Han Y, et al. Randomized comparison of everolimus-eluting absorb bioresorbable vascular scaffolds vs. everolimus-eluting metallic stents in patients with coronary artery disease: The ABSORB China trial. J Am Coll Cardiol 2015; published online Oct 6. DOI:10.1016/j.jacc.2015.09.054.
22. Puricel S, Cuculi F, Weissner M, et al. Bioresorbable coronary scaffold thrombosis multicenter comprehensive analysis of clinical presentation, mechanisms, and predictors. J Am Coll Cardiol. 2016;67:921-31.
23. Onuma Y, Serruys PW, Gomez J, et al. ABSORB Cohort A and B investigators. Comparison of in vivo acute stent recoil between the bioresorbable everolimus-eluting coronary scaffolds (revision 1.0 and 1.1) and the metallic everolimus-eluting stent. Catheter Cardiovasc Interv. 2011;78:3-6.
24. Brugaletta S, Gomez-Lara J, Diletti R, Farooq V, van Geuns RJ, de Bruyne B, Dudek D, Garcia-Garcia HM, Ormiston JA, Serruys PW. Comparison of in vivo eccentricity and symmetry indices

between metallic stents and bioresorbable vascular scaffolds: insights from the ABSORB and SPIRIT trials. Catheter Cardiovasc Interv. 2012;79:219-28.
25. Basavarajaiah S, Naganuma T, Latib A, Colombo A. Can bioabsorbable scaffolds be used in calcified lesions? Catheter Cardiovasc Interv. 2014;84:48-52.
26. Naganuma T, Latib A, Panoulas VF, Sato K, Miyazaki T, Colombo A. Why do we need post-dilation after implantation of a bioresorbable vascular scaffold even for a soft lesion? JACC Cardiovasc Interv. 2014;7:1070-2.
27. Tamburino C, Latib A, van Geuns RJ, Sabate M, Mehilli J, Gori T, et al. Contemporary practice and technical aspects in coronary intervention with bioresorbable scaffolds: a European perspective. EuroIntervention. 2015;11:45-52.
28. Miyazaki T, Latib A, Ruparelia N, Colombo A, et al. The use of a scoring balloon for optimal lesion preparation prior to bioresorbable scaffold implantation: a comparison with conventional balloon predilatation. Euro Intervention. 2016;11:e1580-e1588.
29. Farooq V, Serruys PW, Heo JH, Gogas BD, Virmani R, et al. Intracoronary optical coherence tomography and histology of overlapping everolimus-eluting bioresorbable vascular scaffolds in a porcine coronary artery model: the potential implications for clinical practice. JACC Cardiovasc Interv. 2013;6:523-32.
30. Capodanno D, Gori T, Nef H, et al. Percutaneous coronary intervention with everolimus-eluting bioresorbable vascular scaffolds in routine clinical practice: early and midterm outcomes from the European multicentre GHOST-EU registry. Euro Intervention. 2015;10:1144-53.
31. Kraak RP, Hassell ME, Grundeken MJ, et al. Initial experience and clinical evaluation of the absorb bioresorbable vascular scaffold (BVS) in real-world practice: the AMC Single Centre Real World PCI Registry. EuroIntervention. 2015;10:1160-8.
32. Brugaletta S, Gori T, Low AF, et al. Absorb bioresorbable vascular scaffold versus everolimus eluting metallic stent in ST-segment elevation myocardial infarction: 1-year results of a propensity score matching comparison: the BVSEXAMINATION Study. J Am Coll Cardiol Intv. 2015;8:189-97.
33. Gori T, Schulz E, Münzel T. Immediate, acute, and subacute thrombosis due to incomplete expansion of bioresorbable scaffolds. JACC Cardiovasc Interv. 2014;7:1194.
34. Gomez-Lara J, Brugaletta L, Diletti R, et al. A comparative assessment by optical coherence tomography of the performance of the first and second generation of the everolimus-eluting bioresorbable vascular scaffolds. European Heart Journal. 2011;32:294-304.
35. Onuma Y, Serruys PW, Perkins L EL, et al. Intracoronary optical coherence tomography and histology at 1 month and 2, 3, and 4 years after implantation of everolimus-eluting bioresorbable vascular scaffolds in a porcine coronary artery model an attempt to decipher the human optical coherence tomography images in the ABSORB trial. Circulation. 2010;122:2288-300.
36. Hoppmann P, Kufner S, Cassese S, Wiebe J, Schneider S. Angiographic and clinical outcomes of patients treated with everolimus-eluting bioresorbable stents in routine clinical practice: Results of the ISAR-ABSORB registry. Catheter Cardiovasc Interv. 2016;87(5):822-9.
37. Onuma Y, Dudek D, Thuesen L. Five-year clinical and functional multislice computed tomography Angiographic Results After Coronary implantation of the fully resorbable polymeric everolimus-eluting scaffold in patients with de novo coronary artery disease the ABSORB Cohort A Trial. J Am Coll Cardiol Intv. 2013;6:999-1009.
38. Maier W, Windecker S, Kung A, et al. Exercise-induced coronary artery vasodilation is not impaired by stent placement. Circulation. 2002;105(20):2373-7.

25

Statin Intolerance

Peeyush Jain, (Col.) Viney Jetley

STATIN-MYOPATHY

Introduction

Statin-induced myopathy in real-world practice occurs in about 10% of patients. Its mechanism is uncertain. Myopathy is more common with statins metabolized by CYP3A4 and may not be dependent on statin dose or achieved low density lipoprotein cholesterol (LDL-C). Major non-statin risk factors for myopathy and rhabdomyolysis are concomitant gemfibrozil therapy and chronic kidney disease. Statin withdrawal is not necessary in asymptomatic mild rise in creatine kinase (CK). LDL-C lowering is difficult when statin-induced myalgia is severe but reduction in statin dose, switching over to a less lipophilic statin, or intermittent statin dosing ranging from once a week to alternate days may help. Outcomes of non-statin lipid lowering therapy in statin intolerant patients are not documented. Chinese Red Yeast Rice may offer an unconventional alternative but its effects on cardiovascular events are also not known. One promising therapy for the future is inhibition of proprotein convertase subtilisin/kexin 9 (PCSK9). There are no effective treatments for statin myopathy. Limited data on Coenzyme Q_{10} and vitamin D are not encouraging. Nevertheless, most cases of severe statin myopathy improve after statin withdrawal. Persistence of myopathy after withdrawal should lead to search for polymyositis, necrotic myopathy, or some other unrelated cause.

COMMON CONCERNS ASSOCIATED WITH LONG-TERM USE OF STATINS

Statins [3-hydroxy-3-methylglutaryl coenzyme A (HMG-CoA) reductase inhibitors] reduce cardiovascular (CV) morbidity and mortality in populations at risk and are safe in majority of patients.[1] Yet being in use for >2 decades, concerns about myopathy, elevated transaminases, new onset diabetes, dementia, cancer, and cataract continue to be raised.[2,3] Muscle-related symptoms are the most common side effect of statin therapy. Though myopathy is reversible in majority after statin withdrawal, CV risk reduction in severe statin intolerance remains challenging.

Clinical Manifestations of Statin Intolerance

Statin-induced muscle symptoms may manifest as muscle pain, tenderness, or weakness. Pain is typically aching or cramping, widespread or generalized, and may be exacerbated by exercise. Muscle weakness is usually proximal. Nocturnal leg cramps may occur. Rhabdomyolysis is rare. Subjective variations in symptoms may mislead clinicians to overlook the possibility of statin myopathy.[3-5]

For descriptive purposes, statin myopathy may be broadly classified into *myalgia* [muscle symptoms without creatine phosphokinase (CK) elevation], *myositis* (muscle symptoms with CK elevation), and *rhabdomyolysis* [muscle symptoms with marked CK elevations (>10 times upper limit of normal, ULN) with an elevated serum creatinine and occasional myoglobinuria]. Occasionally, CK elevation without myalgia may also occur.

Incidence of Statin Myopathy

A meta-analysis of 71,108 subjects in 18 randomized placebo-controlled primary and secondary prevention trials of statin monotherapy with 3,01,374 person years of follow-up concluded that the numbers need to harm (NNH) with statin therapy was 197 for any adverse event against the number needed to treat (NNT) of 27 to prevent one CV event. NNH for CK >10 times ULN or rhabdomyolysis was 3,400 and NNH for rhabdomyolysis was 7,428. The adverse event rate was highest with atorvastatin and lowest with fluvastatin.[6]

In another systematic review of 20 randomized trials, voluntary notifications, and case reports with 1,80,000 person years of follow-up, the incidence of muscle symptoms in cohort studies and randomized controlled trials was 11/1,00,000 patient years and the incidence of muscle symptoms and CK elevation >10 times ULN was 5/1,00,000 person years.[7] The incidence of rhabdomyolysis was 3.4/1,00,000 patient years. Incidence was higher with lovastatin, simvastatin, and atorvastatin [statins metabolized by cytochrome P450 3A4 (CYP3A4)] than pravastatin and fluvastatin.

The incidence of statin-induced myopathy in real-world practice is higher than reported in clinical trials as high risk patients like elderly and those with renal and hepatic impairment are generally excluded in the latter.[8] In the United States Food and Drug Administration (USFDA) Adverse Event Reporting System Database, recorded till 2002, myopathy was reported in 0.38 cases per million statin prescriptions.[9] However, these findings are likely an underestimation due to voluntary nature of reporting in such databases. Prediction of Muscular Risk in Observational Conditions (PRIMO), a managed care database in France found that 832 of 7,924 (10.5%) unselected patients treated with high-dose statin therapy reported myalgias during 1 year follow-up. The number of patients reporting muscle symptoms was highest in those receiving simvastatin (18.2%), followed by atorvastatin (14.9%), pravastatin (10.9%), and fluvastatin (5.1%).[10]

Mechanism of Statin Myopathy

The mechanism of statin myopathy is not known. It has been suggested that reduced synthesis of mevalonate following inhibition of HMG-CoA reductase reduces a number of isoprenoids besides inhibition of cholesterol synthesis. Isoprenoid deficiency may have varied effects including impairment of synthesis of ubiquinone (Coenzyme Q10, CoQ10). CoQ10 depletion has been proposed to predispose to myopathy due to abnormal mitochondrial energy production.[11] CoQ_{10} may also have antioxidant function at the level of mitochondria and lipid membranes.[12] Though statin treatment does reduce circulating CoQ10 levels, its effect on muscle CoQ10 content is not clear.[13,14] CoQ10 supplementation can raise its circulating levels but whether it prevents or improves myopathy is also not clear.[15]

Reduction in isoprenoid levels may also induce skeletal muscle apoptosis and myopathy in a dose-dependent manner.[16,17] Statins block the production of farnesyl pyrophosphate and this prevents the prenylation of GTP-binding proteins RacI, and RhoA and their translocation from cytosol to the membrane.[17] A reduction in the levels of the prenylated forms of these proteins leads to increased cytosolic calcium levels with subsequent activation of the proteolytic enzymes capase-3 and capase-9, which play a central role in cell death.[18] This is supported by an *in vitro* study in which statin-induced muscle apoptosis was prevented by supplementation with farnesyl pyrophosphate and geranylgeranyl pyrophosphate.[17]

In animal models, statins increase cytoplasmic calcium by increasing mitochondrial calcium permeability. It also increases calcium release from the sarcoplasmic reticulum by reducing calcium ATPase activity.[12,19] Increased cytoplasmic calcium levels have been shown to cause cramps, myalgias, and apoptosis.[20,21]

Statin myopathy may have genetic determinants. Study of the Effectiveness of Additional Reductions in Cholesterol and Homocysteine (SEARCH) trial hypothesized that genetic variants may affect statin blood levels.[22] In this trial, a genome-wide analysis demonstrated that myopathy was strongly associated with a single nucleotide polymorphism within intron 11 of *SLCO1B1* gene on chromosome 12. SLCO1B1 encodes the organ anion transporting polypeptide responsible for hepatic uptake of statins. In SEARCH trial, 60% of myopathy cases were associated with SLCO1B1 variants.

As many as 31 candidate genes have been associated with statin-induced myalgia. A recent investigation of genetic variants predictive of muscle side effects in statin-treated patients utilizing a physiogenomic approach validated 3 previously hypothesized candidate genes: COQ2 encoding para-hydroxybenzoate-polyprenyltransferase, which participates in the biosynthesis of CoQ10; ATP2B1 which encodes a calcium transporting ATPase involved in calcium homeostasis; and DMPK which encodes a protein kinase implicated in myotonic dystrophy.[23] Further understanding of such genetic markers could help in prediction of statin myopathy.

Predisposing Factors

Major risk factors for rhabdomyolysis are thought to be concomitant therapy with gemfibrozil and chronic kidney disease (CKD). But predisposition to statin-myopathy is lot more complex than these two factors and may be influenced by demographic and anthropometric characteristics, lifestyles, genetic factors, concomitant disorders and medications, and statin-related factors **(Table 1)**.

Statins metabolized by CYP3A4 (lovastatin, simvastatin, and atorvastatin) are 4 times more likely to cause myopathy, particularly rhabdomyolysis, than fluvastatin and pravastatin.[9] Most cases of myopathy manifest within first 3 months of initiation of statin treatment but may be delayed as much as 1 year.[25] In one study of 45 subjects with statin-induced myopathy, symptoms developed after a mean of 6.3 ± 9.8 months and persisted up to 2.3 ± 3.0 months after discontinuation.[26] It is generally believed that an increase in statin exposure increases the risk of myopathy[3] but in a review of atorvastatin trials, the reported frequency of myalgias was identical with low versus high doses (1.4% with 10 mg/day and 1.5% with 80 mg/day).[27] The rate of myopathy and rhabdomyolysis for simvastatin 80 mg/day has been reported to be about 4 times higher than that for atorvastatin 80 mg/day.[28] Retrospective analysis of Pravastatin or Atorvastatin Evaluation and Infection Therapy, (PROVE-IT) study and another meta-analysis suggest that adverse effects of statins are not related to achieved low density lipoprotein cholesterol (LDL-C).[29] In one meta-analysis, with 3,09,506 person-years of follow-up, there was

Section 2: Clinical Cardiology

Table 1 Risk factors for statin myopathy

Demographic features	Uncontrolled hypothyroidism
Elderly	Major recent surgery
Personal or family history of muscular symptoms or cramps	Elevated CK levels
Female gender	Hypoalbuminemia
? caribbean and black Africans	Renal insufficiency
Anthropometric characteristics	Medication affecting statin metabolism
Low body mass index	Amiodarone
Lifestyles	Cyclosporin
Excessive physical activity	Diltiazem
Excessive alcohol consumption	Gemfibrozil
Genetic factors	Macrolide antibiotics
Statin-related factors	Protease inhibitors
High dose	Systemic azole antifungals
Statins metabolized by CYP3A4	Verapamil
Lipophilic statins	Other concomitant medication
Concomitant disorders	Corticosteroids
Hepatic dysfunction	Fusidic acid[24]

no significant relationship between percent LDL-C lowering, absolute LDL-C reduction or achieved LDL-C levels, and rates of rhabdomyolysis.[30] While the combination of ezetimibe, bile-acid sequestering agents, niacin, and fenofibrate with moderate doses of statins appears to be reasonably safe, there is paucity of data related to long-term safety of combination therapy with high-dose statins.

Diagnosis

Statin intolerance should be considered in patients with muscle symptoms after elimination of other causes. Those with tolerable symptoms and CK elevation <5 times ULN may be followed clinically. Patients with severe myalgia and those with CK elevation >5 times ULN should stop statin. After CK has fallen in normal range, statin may be re-introduced to confirm intolerance.

LDL-C Reduction in Statin Intolerant Subjects

LDL-C reduction in presence of unacceptable symptoms and/or severe elevation of CK levels is difficult and there are no established guidelines to manage this situation. The following may be tried:

1. *Reduce the statin dose:* Though practiced commonly, no clinical trial has addressed to the feasibility and efficacy of such a strategy.

2. *Switch-over to another statin:* There are scarce data documenting the safety of another statin if a patient has not been able tolerate one statin. The available evidence indicates that this is unsuccessful in about half of the instances. In one study of 45 patients with statin myopathy, 37 were given another statin. Twenty one (57%) had recurrence of myalgia.[26] To minimize recurrence of statin myopathy with another statin, it may be worthwhile to change over (i) from a lipophilic statin to a hydrophilic statin or (ii) a CYPP450 dependent to a non-CYP450 dependent statin, or (iii) a high dose of a less potent statin to a lower dose of a more potent statin (iv) switch over to fluvastatin that is least likely to cause myopathy. A prospective open-label pilot study (n = 61), rosuvastatin 5–10 mg/day was generally well tolerated by statin-intolerant patients in short term.[31] A 12-week double-blinded, double-dummy trial of 199 statin intolerant patients found that fluvastatin 80 mg/day lowered LDL-C by 32.8% compared with 15.6% with ezetimibe (p < 0.0001) and the fluvastatin XL/ezetimibe combination lowered LDL-C by 46.1% with the incidence of muscle related symptoms 24% (ezetimibe), 17% (fluvastatin), and 14% (combination) and no instances of CK increases >10 times ULN.[32]

3. *Intermittent statin dosing* statins with long half life like atorvastatin and rosuvastatin may have lipid lowering effect beyond 24 hours. The rationale is that the adverse effects of statins may be related to the cumulative amount of drug ingested over time, and if so, the adverse effects may be attenuated by alternate-day dosing.[33] Thus, intermittent dosing, ranging from alternate day to once a week dosing may be justified for atorvastatin with a mean half-life of 14 hours which also has active metabolites with a half-life of 20–30 hours that contribute to 70% of its HMG CoA reductase activity.[34] Rosuvastatin also has a long half-life of 18 hours.[35]

Studies with alternate day atorvastatin
- Uncontrolled studies
  - In one study, 61 hypercholesterolemic patients received 10 mg atorvastatin every alternate days for 8 weeks that resulted in 23% reduction in LDL-C.[36]
  - In another study, 25 patients given alternate day atorvastatin (mean dose 18.8 mg) or rosuvastatin (mean dose 9.7 mg) had 43% reduction in LDL-C with atorvastatin and 28% reduction with rosuvastatin (p < 0.05 for both).[37]
- Controlled studies
  - Alternate day versus daily dosing of atorvastatin study (ADDAS) reported equal efficacy of 10 mg daily or alternate day 20 mg of atorvastatin.[38]
  - In another study of 61 patients there was an equal improvement in lipids after 3 months of 20 mg atorvastatin every day or every alternate day.[39]

Studies with alternate day rosuvastatin
- Rosuvastatin 2.5 mg and 5 mg on alternate days for 6 weeks in 2 atorvastatin intolerant patients resulted in

LDL-C reduction of 38% and 20% respectively without further myalgias.[40]
- In a retrospective analysis, 37 of 51 (72.5%) patients with statin intolerance were able to tolerate alternate day rosuvastatin, mean dose 5.6 mg, for 4 months that led to 34.5% reduction in mean LDL-C in patients who were able to tolerate rosuvastatin (p < 0.001), enabling approximately 50% to achieve their LDL-C goal.[41]
- Thirty-seven Chinese patients who were randomly given rosuvastatin 10 mg every other day (n = 19) or once-daily (n = 18) for 6 weeks had identical reduction in LDL-C (37.5% vs 36.9%, p > 0.05).[42]

Studies with twice weekly rosuvastatin
- In one study, 80% (32 of 40) patients intolerant to daily statins were able to tolerate 5–10 mg of rosuvastatin twice weekly for a mean of 8 weeks with 26% reduction in mean LDL-C.[43]

Studies with once a week rosuvastatin
- In one study, 8 patients intolerant to daily statin given 5–20 mg of rosuvastatin once a week registered 29% reduction in mean LDL-C.[44]

Combination therapy with intermittent statin dosing
- Fifty six statin intolerant patients were given ezetimibe 10 mg/day and atrovastatin 10 mg twice weekly was added after evaluating patients' response. By this strategy, there was 34% reduction in the mean LDL-C levels and 84% of the subjects were able to achieve target LDL-C.[45]

A recent review of 10 studies of varying regimens with atorvastatin and/or rosuvastatin concluded that at least 70% of statin intolerant patients were able to tolerate an intermittent dosing strategy without recurrence of previous treatment-limiting adverse effects. The LDL-C lowering varied from 12–38%, which is lower than daily dosing.[46] Another review of 17 studies (14 prospective and 3 retrospective) involving alternate-day statin dosing concluded that alternate-day statin therapy may limit adverse reactions and potentially increase compliance and positively affecting the lipids concurrently.[47] Yet, these conclusions are based on uncontrolled or small studies with brief follow-up. The efficacy of cardiovascular risk reduction cannot be determined from such trials and therefore large scale randomized trials are necessary to define the role of this strategy and an optimal regimen.

4. *Non-statin lipid lowering therapy*: Non-statin drugs like a bile acid sequestrant, ezetimibe, or nicotinic acid may be considered if the patient remains intolerant to alternative statin(s), dose reduction, or intermittent dosing. Colesevelam, a nonabsorbable water soluble hydrogel, reduces LDL-C by 15–19%, but there is no clinical trial data demonstrating its efficacy in statin intolerant patients.[48] Ezetimibe, a specific inhibitor of intestinal cholesterol absorption, reduces LDL-C by 15–20% with monotherapy.[49] In a series of 27 statin intolerant patients, ezetimibe was well-tolerated over 3 months and resulted in 26% reduction in LDL-C (p < 0.001).[50] In a retrospective analysis of 16 statin intolerant patients, a combination of colesevelam and ezetimibe reduced LDL-C by 42.2% and was well-tolerated.[51] In addition to increasing HDL-C and decreasing triglyceride levels, nicotinic acid leads to a modest reduction in LDL-C.[52] Even though there are no published data on its safety and efficacy in statin intolerant patients, coronary drug project, a large randomized controlled trial in pre-statin era, reported a significant decrease in coronary events.[53] Angiographic trials in the 80^s also demonstrated that a combination of niacin and colestipol slowed angiographic progression of coronary atherosclerosis.[54,55]

5. *Alternative therapies*: Chinese red yeast rice, made by fermenting the yeast, Monascus purpureus, over rice contains monacolin K, a natural form of lovastatin that reduces LDL-C by inhibiting HMG CoA reductase.[56] In a randomized placebo-controlled trial of 62 statin intolerant dyslipidemic patients (mean baseline LDL-C 163 mg/dL), red yeast rice reduced LDL-C by 21.3% after 6 months without increase in CK levels or myalgias.[57] LDL-C reduction was maintained up to 1 year in a study of 48 statin-intolerant patients with a combination of monacoline K, phytostanols, and benerine.[58] A community-based trial compared the tolerability of red yeast rice and pravastatin in patients unable to tolerate other statins. A total of 43 adults were randomly assigned to red yeast rice 2,400 mg twice daily (group 1) or pravastatin 20 mg twice daily (group 2) for 12 weeks. The incidence of treatment discontinuation due to myalgia was 5% in group 1 versus 9% in group 2 (p = 0.99). No difference was found in pain severity or muscle strength between the 2 groups. Thus, red yeast rice was as well tolerated as pravastatin in patients intolerant to other statins.[59] Another retrospective study identified 25 patients treated with red yeast rice for ≥4 weeks who had discontinued lipid lowering drug therapy due to myalgias (68%), gastrointestinal intolerance (16%), and/or elevated alanine aminotransferase levels (8%). In statin-intolerant patients, red yeast rice was found to reduce LDL-C by 19% during 74 ± 39 days of treatment and was well tolerated by 92% of the patients.[60] Monocolin K contents of various formulations of red yeast rice may vary substantially from brand to brand and batch to batch. The long-term effects of red yeast rice on cardiovascular events are also not known.

Prevention

It is difficult to predict, prevent, or control statin-myopathy. Few options are available, given a lack of understanding of its pathogenesis. Limited data are available on the role of CoQ_{10} or vitamin D supplementation. Fortunately, most cases resolve after statin-withdrawal when necessary.

Coenzyme Q_{10} (CoQ_{10}): In a double blind study in patients with myopathic symptoms (n = 18), 100 mg/day of CoQ_{10} for 4 weeks reduced myalgias by 40% (p < 0.001).[61] Another double-blinded study of 60 patients also found significant improvement in symptoms of statin-induced myopathy with CoQ_{10} supplementation (p < 0.001).[62] In another open-label study of 28 patients, administration of CQ_{10} for 6 months led to about 50% reduction in muscle pain and weakness (p < 0.0001).[63] These findings have not been substantiated by other studies and systematic reviews.[64-67] An ongoing placebo-controlled cross over trial of CoQ_{10} in patients with history of myalgia during statin treatment is currently underway to examine the extent and intensity of muscle pain during treatment with simvastatin.[68]

Vitamin D: An association between statin-related myopathy and vitamin D deficiency has been reported. It has been proposed that low CYP enzyme activity related to vitamin D deficiency may increase blood levels and hence, toxicity of CYP metabolized statins. As vitamin D deficiency has been proposed to predispose to toxicity of CYP metabolized statins, concurrent vitamin D may reduce dosage requirements, thereby reducing toxicity. A case series report suggested an association between vitamin D insufficiency and statin-induced myalgia that may be reversed with vitamin D supplementation while continuing statin therapy; 92% (35/38) of the patients with statin-induced myalgias and low vitamin D levels were rendered myalgia free after vitamin D supplementation for 3 months.[69] In a recent prospective study, 150 hypercholesterolemic patients with low serum 25-hydroxy (25-OH) vitamin D, unable to tolerate statin(s) because of myopathy, were restarted on statin therapy after 3 weeks of vitamin D supplementation. After a median of 8.1 months, 87% of previously intolerant patients were able to continue statins without myalgia.[70] However, in a recent pilot study of 93 statin-treated patients, 33% of whom reported myopathy, serum 25-OH vitamin D was not found to be a predictor of myopathy.[71] In another retrospective study of electronic database of 6,808 patients to whom statins were dispensed, no association was found between low 25-OH vitamin D levels and statin-induced myalgia or CK elevation.[72] Given the paucity of studies, their suboptimal quality, and contradictory findings, further study is needed to define the role of vitamin D deficiency in statin myopathy.[73]

Persistence of Myopathy After Statin Withdrawal

Persistence of neuromuscular symptoms and elevated CK levels after withdrawal of statin therapy is not uncommon and may be the result of statin-related myotoxicity or an underlying neuromuscular disorder. In a series of 52 consecutive patients with muscle weakness, myalgia, or both, along with elevated CK levels (mean 1000 U/L) that had persisted for > 3 months after discontinuation of statin therapy, 47 (90%) were found to have possible statin-induced myotoxicity with a good prognosis at the 6-month follow-up. Five patients (10%) presented with abnormalities on electromyography and muscle biopsy and received the diagnoses of paraneoplastic polymyositis, amyotrophic lateral sclerosis, Kennedy's disease, muscle phosphorylase *b* kinase deficiency, and necrotic myopathy of uncertain cause. It was suggested that patients with neuromuscular symptoms and elevated CK levels that persist after statin withdrawal should be systematically evaluated for an underlying neuromuscular disease. Electromyography was an excellent screening test to determine whether a muscle biopsy was needed. As some patients who are believed to have a statin-induced myopathy may have pre-existing myopathies, routine measurement of CK before the initiation of statin therapy should be helpful in making an earlier diagnosis of a neuromuscular disease.[74]

A Note on PCSK9 Inhibition and Statin Intolerance (Table 2)

Based on the results of RUTHERFORD-2 and TESLA Part B, evolocumab has recently been approved in several countries

Table 2 Clinical Trials of PCSK9 inhibitors in statin intolerant patients

GAUSS
In this study of 160 statin intolerant patients with a mean LDL-C of 193 mg/dL, EVOLOCUMAB 280, 350, 420 mg once in 4 w or EVOLOCUMAB 420 + ezetemibe, or ezetemibe alone, the magnitude of LDL-C reduction at 12 weeks was EVOLOCUMAB alone: 41% to 51%, EVOLOCUMAB + ezetemibe: 63%, and ezetemibe alone: 15%. The proportion of subjects achieving LDL-C <100 mg/dL was EVOLOCUMAB alone: 47% to 61%, EVOLOCUMAB + ezetemibe: 90%, and ezetemibe alone: 7%. Myalgia was reported by 3% on monotherapy, CK elevation >10 times was found in 2 patients and none developed significant elevation of hepatic transaminases.[75]
ODYSSEY Alternative
ODYSSEY ALTERNATIVE compared alirocumab with ezetimibe in patients at moderate to high cardiovascular risk with statin intolerance. Patients (n = 361) received single-blind (sc) and oral placebo for 4 weeks during placebo run-in. Patients reporting muscle-related symptoms during the run-in were to be withdrawn. Continuing patients were randomized to double-blind alirocumab, ezetimibe, or atorvastatin 20 mg/day for 24 weeks. Primary end point was percent change in LDL-C from baseline to week 24 for alirocumab vs ezetimibe. Alirocumab reduced mean LDL-C by 45.0% versus 14.6% with ezetimibe (p = 0.0001). Skeletal muscle-related events were less frequent with alirocumab versus atorvastatin (hazard ratio 0.6, p = 0.042).[76]
GAUSS-3
GAUSS-3 trial evaluated evolocumab in patients with high cholesterol who cannot tolerate statins. It met its co-primary endpoints of mean percent reductions from baseline in LDL-C at weeks 22 and 24, and the percent reduction from baseline in LDL-C at week.[77]

including US and EU as an adjunct to other therapies for treatment of adults with HeFH, HoFH or clinical atherosclerotic cardiovascular disease (ASCVD). Alirocumab is also approved as adjunct to diet and maximally tolerated statin therapy for the treatment of adults with HeFH ASCVD, who require additional lowering of LDL-C. It is noteworthy that at the time of writing, the effect of both evolocumab and alirocumab on cardiovascular morbidity and mortality has not been determined. US FDA has categorically not approved either evolocumab or alirocumab for statin intolerant patients but one phase II (GAUSS)[75] and two phase III studies (Odyssey Alternative and Gauss-3)[76,77] suggest that PCSK inhibitors may be of value in stain-intolerant subjects. A significant proportion of study subjects on PCSK9 inhibitors also report myalgias though discontinuation rates are low.

REFERENCES

1. Baigent C, Keech A, Kearney PM, et al. Cholesterol Treatment Trialists' (CTT) Collaborators. Efficacy and safety of cholesterol-lowering treatment: prospective meta-analysis of data from 90,056 participants in 14 randomised trials of statins. Lancet. 2005;366:1267-78.
2. Gotto AM Jr. Statins, cardiovascular disease, and drug safety. Am J Cardiol. 2006;97(8A):3C-5C.
3. Armitage J. The safety of statins in clinical practice. Lancet. 2007;370:1781-90.
4. Harper CR, Jacobson TA. The broad spectrum of statin myopathy: from myalgia to rhabdomyolysis. Curr Opin Lipidol. 2007;18:401-8.
5. Phillips PS, Haas RH. Statin myopathy as a metabolic muscle disease. Exp Rev Cardiovasc Ther. 2008;6:955-69.
6. Silva MA, Swanson AC, Gandhi PJ, Tataronis GR. Statin-related adverse events: a meta-analysis. Clin Ther. 2006;28:26-35.
7. Law M, Rudnicka AR. Statin safety: a systematic review. Am J Cardiol. 2006;97(8A):52C-60C.
8. Jacobson TA. Toward "pain-free" statin prescribing: clinical algorithm for diagnosis and management of myalgia. Mayo Clin Proc. 2008;83:687-700.
9. Davidson MH, Clark JA, Glass LM, Kanumalla A Statin safety: an appraisal from the adverse event reporting system. Am J Cardiol. 2006;97(8A):32C-43C.
10. Bruckert E, Hayem G, Dejager S, et al. Mild to moderate muscular symptoms with high-dosage statin therapy in hyperlipidemic patients—the PRIMO study. Cardiovasc Drugs Ther. 2005;19:403-14.
11. Klopstock T. Drug-induced myopathies. Curr Opin Neurol. 2008;21:590-5.
12. Owczarek J, Jasińska M, Orszulak-Michalak D. Drug-induced myopathies. An overview of the possible mechanisms Pharmacol Reports 2005;57:23-4.
13. Lamperti C, Naini AB, Lucchini V, et al. Muscle coenzyme Q10 level in statin-related myopathy. Arch Neurol. 2005;62:1709-12.
14. Laaksonen R, Jokelainen K, Sahi T, et al. Decreases in serum ubiquinone concentrations do not result in reduced levels in muscle tissue during short-term simvastatin treatment in humans. Clin Pharmacol Ther. 1995;57:62-6.
15. Marcoff L, Thompson PD. The role of coenzyme Q10 in statin-associated myopathy: a systematic review. J Am Coll Cardiol. 2007;49:2231-7.
16. Dirks AJ, Kimberly MJ. Statin-induced apoptosis and skeletal myopathy. Am J Physiol Cell Physiol. 2006;291:C1208–C1212.
17. Guijarro C, Blanco-Colio LM, Ortego M, et al. 3-Hydroxy-3-methylglutaryl coenzyme a reductase and isoprenylation inhibitors induce apoptosis of vascular smooth muscle cells in culture. Circ Res. 1998;83:490-500.
18. Mammen AL, Amato AA. Statin myopathy: a review of recent progress. Curr Opin Rheumatol. 2010;22:644-50.
19. Liantonio A, Giannuzzi V, Cippone V, et al. Fluvastatin and atorvastatin affect calcium homeostasis of rat skeletal muscle fibers in vivo and in vitro by impairing the sarcoplasmic reticulum/mitochondria Ca^{2+}-release system. J Pharmacol Exp Ther. 2007;321:626-34.
20. Mohaupt MG, Karas RH, Babiychuk EB, et al. Association between statin-associated myopathy and skeletal muscle damage CMAJ. 2009;181:E11-E18
21. Sirvent P, Mercier J, Vassort G, Lacampagne A. Simvastatin triggers mitochondria-induced Ca2+ signaling alteration in skeletal muscle. Biochem Biophys Res Commun. 2005;329:1067-75.
22. SEARCH Collaborative Group, Link E, Parish S, Armitage J, et al. SLCO1B1 variants and statin-induced myopathy--a genomewide study. N Engl J Med. 2008;359:789-99.
23. Ruaño G, Windemuth A, Wu AH, et al. Mechanisms of statin-induced myalgia assessed by physiogenomic associations. Atherosclerosis. 2011;218:451-6.
24. Magee CN, Medani SA, Leavey SF, et al. Severe rhabdomyolysis as a consequence of the interaction of fusidic acid and atorvastatin. Am J Kidney Dis. 2010;56:e11-5.
25. Molokhia M, McKeigue P, Curcin V, Majeed A. Statin induced myopathy and myalgia: time trend analysis and comparison of risk associated with statin class from 1991-2006. PLoS One. 2008;3:e2522.
26. Hansen KE, Hildebrand JP, Ferguson EE, et al. Outcomes in 45 patients with statin-associated myopathy arch. Intern Med. 2005;165:2671-6.
27. Newman C, Tsai J, Szarek M, et al. Comparative safety of atorvastatin 80 mg versus 10 mg derived from analysis of 49 completed trials in 14,236 patients. Am J Cardiol. 2006;97:61-7.
28. Davidson MH, Robinson JG. Safety of aggressive lipid management. J Am Coll Cardiol. 2007;49:1753-62.
29. Wiviott SD, Cannon CP, Morrow DA, et al. PROVE IT-TIMI 22 Investigators. Can low-density lipoprotein be too low? The safety and efficacy of achieving very low low-density lipoprotein with intensive statin therapy: a PROVE IT-TIMI 22 substudy. J Am Coll Cardiol. 2005;46:1411-6.
30. Alsheikh-Ali AA, Maddukuri PV, Han H, Karas RH. Effect of the magnitude of lipid lowering on risk of elevated liver enzymes, rhabdomyolysis, and cancer: insights from large randomized statin trials. J Am Coll Cardiol. 2007;50:409-18.
31. Glueck CJ, Aregawi D, Agloria M, et al. Rosuvastatin 5 and 10 mg/day: A pilot study of the effects in hypercholesterolemic adults unable to tolerate other statins and reach LDL cholesterol goals with nonstatin lipid-lowering therapies. Clin Ther. 2006;28:933-42.
32. Stein EA, Ballantyne CM, Windler E, et al. Efficacy and tolerability of fluvastatin XL 80 mg alone, ezetimibe alone, and the

combination of fluvastatin XL 80 mg with ezetimibe in patients with a history of muscle-related side effects with other statins. Am J Cardiol. 2008;101:490-6.
33. Marcus FI, Baumgarten AJ, Fritz WL, Nolan PE Jr. Alternative-day dosing with statins. Am J Med. 2013;126:99-104.
34. Lennernäs H. Clinical pharmacokinetics of atorvastatin. Clin Pharmacokinet. 2003;42:1141-60.
35. Martin PD, Mitchell PD, Schneck DW. Pharmacodynamic effects and pharmacokinetics of a new HMG CoA reductase inhibitor, rosuvastatin after morning or evening administration in healthy volunteers. Br J Clin Pharmacol. 2002;54:472-77.
36. Piamsomboon C, Laothavorn P, Saguanwong S, et al. Efficacy and safety of atorvastatin 10 mg every other day in hypercholesterolemia. J Med Assoc Thai. 2002;85:297-300.
37. Juszczyk MA, Seip RL, Thompson PD. Decreasing LDL cholesterol and medication cost with every-other-day statin therapy. Prev Cardiol. 2005;8:197-9.
38. Matalka MS, Ravnan MC, Deedwania PC. Is alternate daily dose of atorvastatin effective in treating patients with hyperlipidemia? The Alternate Day Versus Daily Dosing of Atorvastatin Study (ADDAS). Am Heart J. 2002;144:674-7.
39. Keleç T, Akar BN, Kayhan T, et al. The comparison of the effects of standard 20 mg atorvastatin daily and 20 mg atorvastatin every other day on serum LDL-cholesterol and high sensitive C-reactive protein levels. Anadolu Kardiyol Derg. 2008;8:407-12.
40. Mackie BD, Satija S, Nell C, et al. Monday, Wednesday, and Friday dosing of rosuvastatin in patients previously intolerant to statin therapy. Am J Cardiol. 2007;99:291.
41. Backes JM, Venero CV, Gibson CA, et al. Effectiveness and Tolerability of Every-Other-Day Rosuvastatin Dosing in Patients with Prior Statin Intolerance Ann Pharmacother. 2008;42:341-6.
42. Li J, Yang P, Liu J, et al. Impact of 10 mg rosuvastatin daily or alternate-day on lipid profile and inflammatory markers. Clin Chim Acta. 2012;413:139-42.
43. Gadaria M, Kearns AK, Thompson PD. Efficacy of rosuvastatin (5 mg and 10 mg) twice a week in patients intolerant to daily statins. Am J Cardiol. 2008;101:1747-8.
44. Backes JM, Moriarty PM, Ruisinger JF, Gibson CA. Effects of once weekly rosuvastatin among patients with a prior statin intolerance. Am J Cardiol. 2007;100:554-5.
45. Athyros VG, Tziomalos K, Kakafika AI, et al. Effectiveness of ezetimibe alone or in combination with twice a week Atorvastatin (10 mg) for statin intolerant high-risk patients. Am J Cardiol. 2008;101:483-5.
46. Keating AJ, Campbell KB, Guyton JR. Intermittent nondaily dosing strategies in patients with previous statin-induced myopathy. Ann Pharmacother. 2013;47:398-404.
47. Reindl EK, Wright BM, Wargo KA. Alternate-day statin therapy for the treatment of hyperlipidemia. Ann Pharmacother. 2010;44:1459-70.
48. Davidson MH, Donovan JM, Misir S, Jones MR. A 50-week extension study on the safety and efficacy of colesevelam in adults with primary hypercholesterolemia. Am J Cardiovasc Drugs. 2010;10:305-14.
49. Pandor A, Ara RM, Tumur I, et al. Ezetimibe monotherapy for cholesterol lowering in 2,722 people: systematic review and meta-analysis of randomized controlled trials. J Intern Med. 2009;265:568-80.
50. Gazi IF, Daskalopoulou SS, Nair DR, Mikhailidis DP. Effect of ezetimibe in patients who cannot tolerate statins or cannot get to the low density lipoprotein cholesterol target despite taking a statin. Curr Med Res Opin. 2007;23:2183-92.
51. Rivers SM, Kane MP, Busch RS, et al. Colesevelam hydrochloride-ezetimibe combination lipid-lowering therapy in patients with diabetes or metabolic syndrome and a history of statin intolerance. Endocr Pract. 2007;13:11-6.
52. Brooks EL, Kuvin JT, Karas RH. Niacin's role in the statin era. Expert Opin Pharmacother. 2010;11:2291-300.
53. Canner PL, Berge KG, Wenger NK, et al. Fifteen year mortality in Coronary Drug Project patients: long-term benefit with niacin. J Am Coll Cardiol. 1986;8:1245-55.
54. Blankenhorn DH, Nessim SA, Johnson RL, et al. Beneficial effects of combined colestipol-niacin therapy on coronary atherosclerosis and coronary venous bypass grafts. JAMA. 1987;257:3233-40.
55. Brown G, Albers JJ, Fisher LD, et al. Regression of coronary artery disease as a result of intensive lipid-lowering therapy in men with high levels of apolipoprotein B. N Engl J Med. 1990;323:1289-98.
56. Ma J, Li Y, Ye Q, et al. Constituents of Red Yeast Rice, a Traditional Chinese Food and Medicine. J Agri Food Chem. 2000;48:5220-5.
57. Becker DJ, Gordon RY, Halbert SC, et al. Red yeast rice for dyslipidemia in statin-intolerant patients: a randomized trial. Ann Intern Med. 2009;150:830-9.
58. Cicero AFG, Derosa G, Bove M, et al. Long-term effectiveness and safety of a nutraceutical based approach to reduce cholsterolemia in statin intolerant subjects with or without metabolic syndrome. Current Topicsin Nutraceutical Research. 2009;7:121-6.
59. Halbert SC, French B, Gordon RY, et al. Tolerability of red yeast rice (2,400 mg twice daily) versus pravastatin (20 mg twice daily) in patients with previous statin intolerance. Am J Cardiol. 2010;105:198-204.
60. Venero CV, Venero JV, Wortham DC, Thompson PD. Lipid-lowering efficacy of red yeast rice in a population intolerant to statins. Am J Cardiol. 2010;105:664-6.
61. Caso G, Kelly P, McNurlan MA, Lawson WE. Effect of coenzyme q10 on myopathic symptoms in patients treated with statins. Am J Cardiol. 2007;99:1409-12.
62. Fedacko J, Pella D, Fedackova P, et al. Coenzyme Q(10) and selenium in statin-associated myopathy treatment. Can J Physiol Pharmacol. 2013;91:165-70.
63. Zlatohlavek L, Vrablik M, Grauova B, Motykova E, Ceska R. The effect of coenzyme Q10 in statin myopathy. Neuro Endocrinol Lett. 2012;33(Suppl 2):98-101.
64. Marcoff L, Thompson PD. The role of coenzyme Q10 in statin-associated myopathy: a systematic review. J Am Coll Cardiol. 2007;49:2231-7.
65. Young JM, Florkowski CM, Molyneux SL, et al. Effect of coenzyme Q(10) supplementation on simvastatin-induced myalgia. Am J Cardiol. 2007;100:1400-3.
66. Bookstaver DA, Burkhalter NA, Hatzigeorgiou C. Effect of coenzyme Q10 supplementation on statin-induced myalgias. Am J Cardiol. 2012;110:526-9.
67. Bogsrud MP, Langslet G, Ose L, et al. No effect of combined coenzyme Q10 and selenium supplementation on atorvastatin-induced myopathy. Scand Cardiovasc J. 2013;47:80-7.

68. Parker BA, Gregory SM, Lorson L, et al. A randomized trial of coenzyme Q10 in patients with statin myopathy: rationale and study design. J Clin Lipidol. 2013;7:187-93.
69. Ahmed W, Khan N, Glueck CJ, et al. Low serum 25 (OH) vitamin D levels (<32 ng/mL) are associated with reversible myositis-myalgia in statin-treated patients. Transl Res. 2009;153:11-6.
70. Glueck CJ, Budhani SB, Masineni SS, et al. Vitamin D deficiency, myositis-myalgia, and reversible statin intolerance. Curr Med Res Opin. 2011;27:1683-90.
71. Riphagen IJ, van der Veer E, Muskiet FA, DeJongste MJ. Myopathy during statin therapy in the daily practice of an outpatient cardiology clinic: prevalence, predictors and relation with vitamin D. Curr Med Res Opin. 2012;28:1247-52
72. Kurnik D, Hochman I, Vesterman-Landes J, et al. Muscle pain and serum creatine kinase are not associated with low serum 25(OH) vitamin D levels in patients receiving statins. Clin Endocrinol (Oxf). 2012;77:36-41.
73. Gupta A, Thompson PD. The relationship of vitamin D deficiency to statin myopathy. Atherosclerosis. 2011;215:23-9.
74. Echaniz-Laguna A, Mohr M, Tranchant C, Neuromuscular Symptoms and Elevated Creatine Kinase after Statin Withdrawal N Eng J Med. 2010;362:564-5.
75. Sullivan D, Olsson AG, Scott R, et al. Effect of a Monoclonal Antibody to PCSK9 on Low-Density Lipoprotein Cholesterol Levels in Statin-Intolerant Patients The GAUSS Randomized Trial JAMA. 2012;308:2497-506.
76. Moriaty PM, Thompson PD, Cannon CP. Efficacy and safety of alirocumab vs ezetimibe in statin-intolerant patients, with a statin rechallenge arm: The ODYSSEY ALTERNATIVE randomized trial. J Clin Lipidology. 2015;9:758-69.
77. Nissen SE, Stroes E, Dent-Acosta RE, et al. Efficacy and Tolerability of Evolocumab vs Ezetimibe in Patients With Muscle-Related Statin Intolerance The GAUSS-3 Randomized Clinical Trial. JAMA. 2016;315(15):1580-90.

26. Sudden Cardiac Death: How to Predict and Prevent it?

Pankaj Manoria, PC Manoria, Piyush Manoria

INTRODUCTION

Sudden cardiac death (SCD) implies unexpected natural death from a cardiac cause within a short time period, generally within 1 hour from the onset of symptoms, in a person without any prior condition that would appear fatal.[1,2]

MAGNITUDE OF THE PROBLEM

Globally, every year 300,000 individuals die of SCD. Every 5th minute, one individual dies of SCD. Annual incidence is 0.36 to 1.28 per 1000 inhabitants.[3,4]

CAUSES OF SUDDEN CARDIAC DEATH

Coronary artery disease (CAD) is the most common cause in the developed world; while in younger patients, the major causes are hypertrophic cardiomyopathy, arrhythmogenic right ventricular cardiomyopathy (ARVC), anomalous coronary arteries, hereditary channelopathies like long QT syndrome (LQTS) **(Figs 1 and 2)**, etc. The prevalence of SCD is three-to-four folds higher in men. Approximately, 80% of victims of SCD do not survive to hospital discharge.[5]

MECHANISM OF SUDDEN CARDIAC DEATH

The most common sequence of events leading to SCD appears to be the degeneration of ventricular tachycardia (VT) into ventricular fibrillation (VF).

The first recorded rhythm in patients with a sudden cardiovascular collapse is VF in 75% to 80% of cases[6-7] **(Fig. 3)**.

The mechanism of SCD is complex and results from a complex interaction between abnormal myocardial substrate, transient triggering factors and arrythmogenic milieu. Successful identification of patients who are likely to benefit from implantable cardioverter defibrillator (ICD) prophylaxis will require the evaluation of all above three factors **(Fig. 4)**.

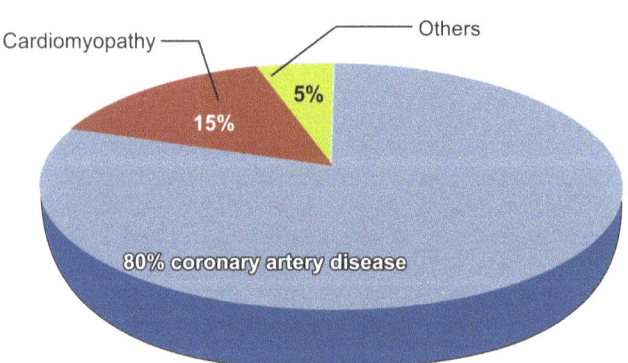

Fig. 1: Causes of sudden cardiac death in adults

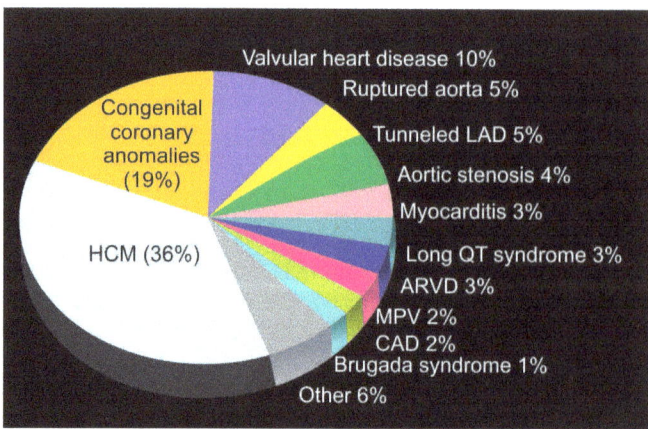

Fig. 2: Causes of SCD in young
Abbreviations: HCM, hypertrophic cardiomyopathy; LAD, left anterior descending artery; ARVD, arrhythmogenic right ventricular dysplasia; MPV, mitral valve prolapse; CAD, coronary artery disease

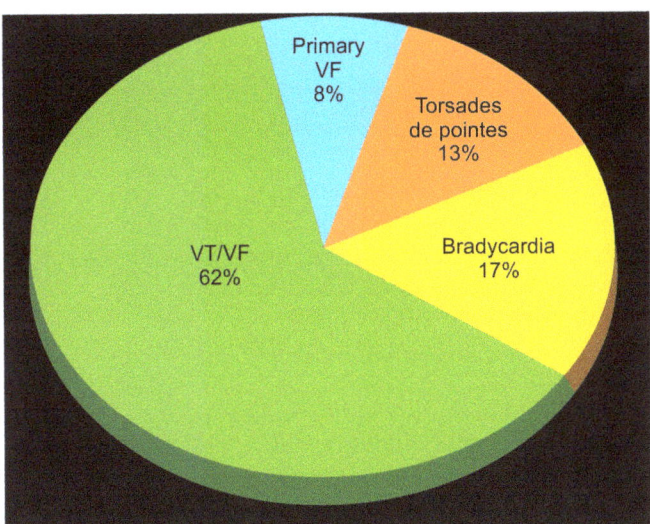

Fig. 3: Underlying arrhythmias in SCD
Abbreviations: VF, ventricular fibrillation; VT, ventricular tachycardia

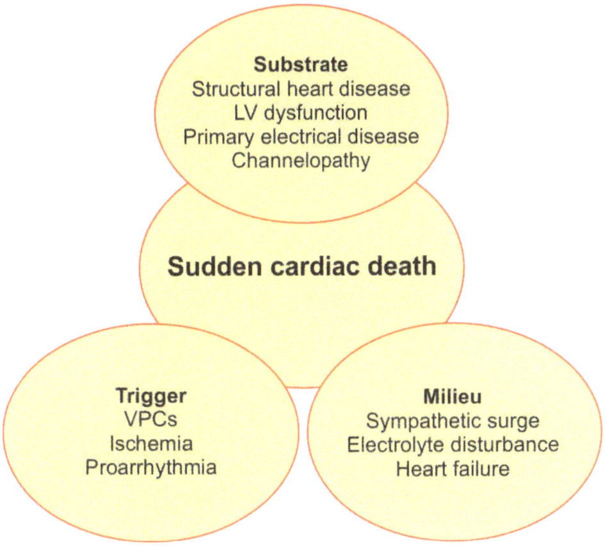

Fig. 4: Complex interplay of substrate, trigger and milieu leading to SCD
Abbreviation: VPC, ventricular premature complexes

RISK FACTORS FOR SUDDEN CARDIAC DEATH

Because up to 80% of individuals who suffer SCD have coronary heart disease (CHD), the epidemiology of SCD to a great extent parallels to that of coronary heart disease.[8] As such, the incidence of SCD increases with age in both men and women, whites and nonwhites, because the prevalence of CAD increases with age. However, among patients with CAD, the proportion of coronary deaths that are sudden decreases with age. SCD has a much higher incidence in men than women, reflecting sex differences in the incidence of CHD as well. Thus, 75% of SCD occur in men, with an annual incidence 3–4 times higher than in women.[9-10]

Risk Stratification of Sudden Cardiac Death

Evaluation of SCD survivors should always begin with a complete history and physical examination covering patient medications, family history, drug use and risk factors. Common cardiac risk factors, including smoking, hypertension and hyperlipidemia, are easily recognizable markers of increased risk for underlying ischemic cardiomyopathy. Other non-invasive useful tools for evaluation include holter monitor, echocardiogram, ECG, CT, MRI and coronary angiogram. The major non-invasive markers of SCD are shown in **Table 1**.

High-risk Factors for Sudden Cardiac Death

The high-risk factors for SCD are shown in **Table 2**.

TREATMENT

In view of the complexity of the mechanisms involved in SCD, there has been growing interest in the use of measures that may halt or delay progress of cardiac disease or prevent disturbances in the autonomic balance of the heart, such as the administration of anti-ischemic drugs, drugs to prevent plaque rupture or thrombus formation, and drugs that stabilize the autonomic balance or improve pump function (**Box 1**). Aggressive therapy using thrombolysis in acute ischemic syndromes or intracoronary interventions resulting in reduction of myocardial damage and scar formation and prevention of ventricular remodeling will diminish the occurrence of some of the mechanisms that play a role in a fatal arrhythmia.[17]

Role of ICD

Although the use of ICDs remains the mainstay of prevention of SCD, there remains challenges, especially in the identification of patients who are at high risk of SCD who will be benefited most from ICD implantation. This issue is of particular clinical importance in view of the fact that prophylactic ICD implantation is expensive in terms of device cost. In principle, ICD implantation will be more cost-effective when used for the patients at high risk of arrhythmic death.[18] Additional risk stratification of patients may improve patient selection for the ICD and thereby enhance its cost-effectiveness.

The indications of ICD are shown in **Table 3**.

The conditions in which ICD is not indicated are outlined in **Box 2**.

Table 1 Noninvasive markers of sudden cardiac death[11-16]

Noninvasive test	Markers of sudden death studies	Remarks
Abnormal myocardial substrate		
2DE	Reduced EF <35%	Predominant risk parameter in clinical trials involving ACDs
Cardiac MRI	Delayed gadolinium enhancement, perfusion defects	Useful prognostic value. Not a guide to treatment
ECG	Intraventricular conduction delay (QRS duration)	Useful prognostic value. Risk marker in ICD primary prevention trials. Also a criterion in cardiac resynchronization therapy
	Fragmented QRS complexes	Useful prognostic value. Not a guide to treatment
SAECG	Late potentials	Useful prognostic value. Not a guide to treatment
Autonomic nervous system		
I-MIBG scan	Uptake and washout of I-MIBG	Decreased uptake and increased washout associated with worse prognosis
ECG	Heart rate variability Heart rate turbulence Baroreflex sensitivity (BRS)	Useful prognostic value. Not a guide to treatment
Repolarization abnormalities		
Myocardial strain imaging	Mechanical dispersion	Useful prognostic value. Not guide to treatment
ECG	QT interval QT variability QT dispersion Microvolt electrical alternans	Short and long QT syndrome Useful prognostic value. Not a guide to treatment
	Early repolarization	Especially if localized to inferior leads
ECG	Disease specific conditions LVH Brugada Epsilon waves	HCM ST elevation pattern in V1-V2 ARVD

Abbreviations: 2DE, two-dimensional echocardiography; ECG, electrocardiogram; SAECG, single-averaged electrocardiography; I-MIBG, I-metaiodobenzylguanidine; LVH, left ventricular hypertrophy; ARVD, arrhythmogenic right ventricular dysplasia

Table 2 High-risk factors for SCD

Factor	Risk
Sudden death survivor	+++++
VT with syncope	++++
VT + EF < 40%	+++
VT with minimal symptoms	++
Previous MI, NSVT+ EF <35%	+

Table 3 Important Indications of ICD

Secondary prevention
1. Survivors of SCD
2. Structural heart disease and spontaneous sustained VT
Primary prevention
3. Post-MI NHYA II or III with LVEF <35%
4. DCMP NHYA II or III with LVEF <35%
5. Selected cases of HOCM, Brugada, ARVD, Long-QT syndrome

BOX 1 Clinical strategies to improve outcomes from sudden cardiac death

- Prevention of risk factor development for coronary artery disease
- Primary prevention and secondary prevention of SCD
  Appropriate use of β-blocker, ACE inhibitor, and statin therapy
  Implantable cardioverter-defibrillator in selected patients
- Community-based public access to defibrillation programs
- Regionalized systems of post-resuscitation hospital care

BOX 2 Contraindications for ICD

- VT due to a reversible cause
- Incessant VT
- Advance CHF and LV dysfunction NYHA-IV
- LVD with CAD amenable for revascularization
- VT resulting from arrhythmias amenable to surgical or catheter ablation

The treatment algorithm for patients resuscitated from SCD is shown in **Flow chart 1**.

Flow chart 1: Treatment algorithm for patient resuscitated from SCD

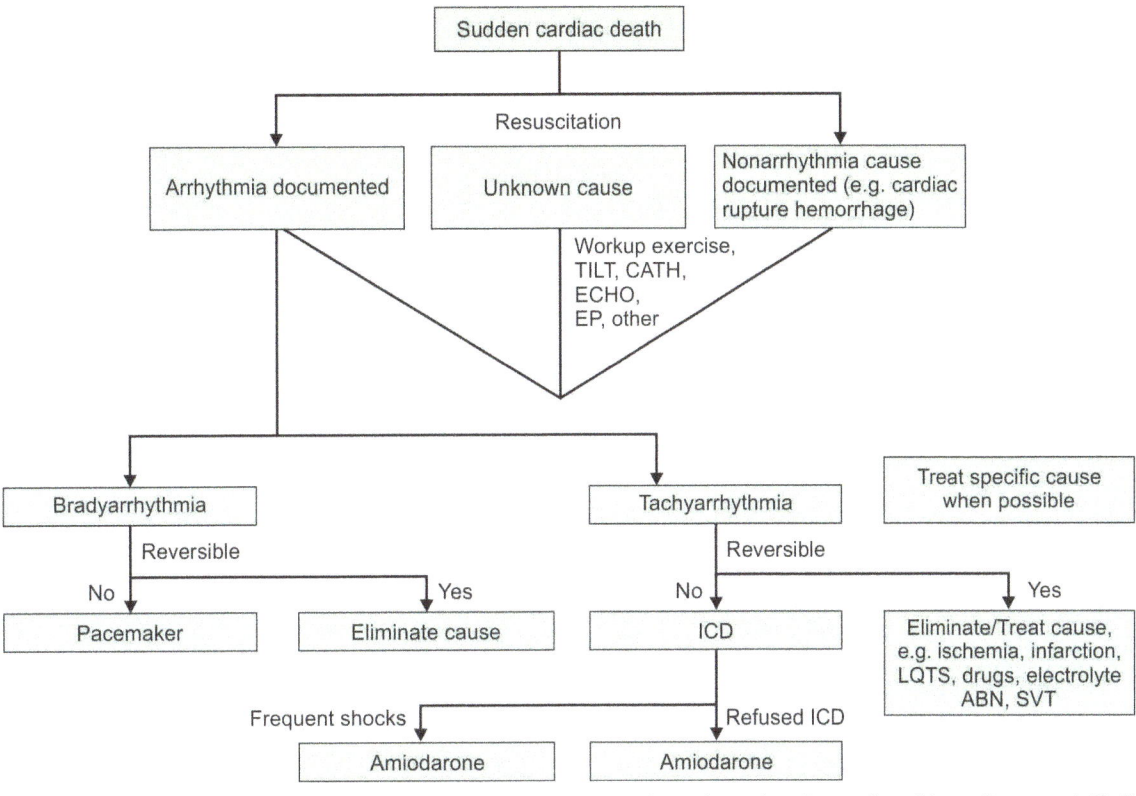

Abbreviations: EP, electrophysiology; ABN, abnormality; SVT, supraventricular tachycardia; ICD, implantable cardioverter defibrillator

Out-of-hospital Resuscitation

The majority of SCD victims have no symptoms and are not identified as being at high risk before the event. This stresses the enormous importance of improving the outcome of resuscitation attempts outside the hospital. The time frame after cardiac arrest during which circulation has to be restored to prevent death or irreversible cerebral damage is very short. In the so-called chain of survival, several steps are crucial[19-21] **(Fig. 5)**. The first step is to identify and locate the sudden cardiac arrest victim. Then the early CPR and early defibrillation is the key to survival. Much attention has recently been given to public access defibrillation, allowing nonphysicians to use widely distributed automated external defibrillators to defibrillate. In fact, it was suggested several years ago that external defibrillators be made "as common as fire extinguishers," and they should cover all public places. The last stage of chain of survival is to shift the patient for advanced care as soon as possible once the primary resuscitation is over.

Thus, SCD still remains a major health issue. Approximately, 80% of victims of SCD do not survive to hospital discharge. This high mortality underscores the importance of prevention of SCD. At the same time, more efforts are needed to improve out-of-hospital resuscitation by better warning systems and widespread availability of automated defibrillation devices. It is likely that these measures could increase the number of survivors of cardiac arrest. Following ICD implantation in certain instances, one also has to use concomitant drugs like amiodarone and beta blockers to minimize shocks.

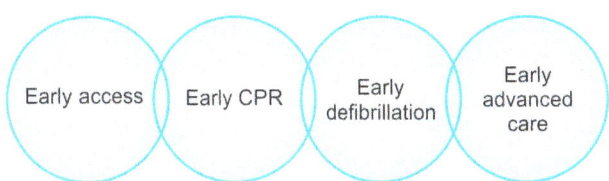

Fig. 5: Chain of survivals in sudden cardiac death

REFERENCES

1. Engelstein ED, Zipes DP. Sudden cardiac death. In: Alexander RW, Schlant RC, Fuster V (Eds). The Heart, Arteries and Veins. New York, NY: McGraw-Hill; 1998.pp.1081-112.
2. Myerburg RJ, Castellanos A. Cardiac arrest and sudden death. In: Braunwald E (Ed). Heart Disease: A Textbook of Cardiovascular Medicine. Philadelphia, Pa: WB Saunders; 1997.pp.742-79.
3. De Vreede Swagemakers JJM, Gorgels APM, Dubois-Arbouw WI, van Ree JW, Daemen MJAP, Houben LGE, Wellens HJJ. Out-of-

hospital cardiac arrest in the 1990s: a population-based study in the Maastricht area on incidence, characteristics and survival. J Am Coll Cardiol. 1997;30:1500-05.
4. Reddy KS, Yusuf S. Emerging epidemic of cardiovascular disease in developing countries. Circulation. 1998;97:596-601.
5. Camm AJ, Pakrashi T, Savelieva I. Sudden cardiac death: risk factors, treatment, and prevention. Dialogues in Cardiovascular Medicine. 2006;11(3).
6. Priori SG, Aliot E, Blomstrom-Lundqvist C, Bossaert L, Breithardt G, Brugada P, et al. Task Force on Sudden Cardiac Death, European Society of Cardiology. Summary of recommendations. Europace; 2002.
7. Zipes D, Wellens H. Sudden cardiac death. Circulation. 1998;98:2334-51.
8. Burke AP, Farb A, Malcom GT, Liang Y, Smialek J, Virmani R. Effect of risk factors on the mechanism of acute thrombosis and sudden coronary death in women. Circulation. 1998;97:2110-6.
9. James TN, St Martin E, Willis PW III, Lohr TO. Apoptosis as a possible cause of gradual development of complete heart block and fatal arrhythmias associated with absence of the AV node, sinus node, and intermodal pathways. Circulation. 1996;93:1424-38.
10. Burke AP, Farb BA, Malcom GT, Liang YH, Smialek J, Virmani R. Coronary risk factors and plaque morphology in men with coronary heart disease who died suddenly. N Engl J Med. 1997;336:1276-82.
11. Bello D, Fieno DS, Kim RJ, Pereles FS, Passman R, Song G, et al. Infarct morphology identifies patients with substrate for sustained ventricular tachycardia. J Am Coll Cardiol. 2005;45:1104-8.
12. Assomull RG, Prasad SK, Lyne J, Smith G, Burman ED, Khan M, et al. Cardiovascular magnetic resonance fibrosis, and prognosis in dilated cardiomyopathy. J Am Coll Cardiol. 2006;48:1977-85.
13. Iles L, Pfluger H, Lefkovits L, Butler MJ, Kistler PM, Kaye DM, et al.Taylor AJ Myocardial fibrosis predicts appropriate device therapy in patients with implantable cardioverter defibrillators for primary prevention of sudden cardiac death. J Am Coll Cardiol. 2011;57(7):821-8.
14. Bauer A, Watanabe MA, Barthel P, Schneider R, Ulm K, Schmidt G. QRS duration and late mortality in unselected postinfarction patients of the revascularization era. Eur Heart J. 2005;27:427-33.
15. Baldasseroni S, Opasich C, Gorini M, Lucci D, Marchionni N, Maurizio Marini, et al. (Italian Network on Congestive Heart Failure Investigators). Left bundle branch block is associated with increased 1-year sudden and total mortality rate in 5517 outpatients with congestive heart failure: A report from the Italian network on congestive heart failure. Am Heart J. 2002;143:398-405.
16. Bauer A, Watanabe MA, Barthel P, Schneider R, Ulm K, Schmidt G. QRS duration and late mortality in unselected post-infarction patients of the revascularization era. Eur Heart J. 2005;27:427-33.
17. Nichol G, Aufderheide TP, Eigel B, Neumar RW, Lurie KG, Bufalino VJ, Callaway CW, Menon V, Bass RR, Abella BS, Sayre M, Dougherty CM, Racht EM, Kleinman ME, O'Connor RE, Reilly JP, Ossmann EW, Peterson E. Regional systems of care for out-of-hospital cardiac arrest: a policy statement from the American Heart Association. Circulation. 2010;121:709-29.
18. Riegel, Tarkington LG, Yancy CW, et al. American College of Cardiology/American Heart Association Task Force on Practice Guidelines (Writing Committee to Revise the ACC/AHA/NASPE 2002 Guideline Update for Implantation of Cardiac Pacemakers and Antiarrhythmia Devices); American Association for Thoracic Surgery; Society of Thoracic Surgeons. ACC/ AHA/ HRS 2008 guidelines for device-based therapy of cardiac rhythm abnormalities: a report of the American College of Cardiology/American Heart. Association Task Force on Practice Guidelines (Writing Committee to Revise the ACC/AHA/NASPE 2002 Guideline Update for Implantation of Cardiac Pacemakers and Antiarrhythmia Devices): developed in collaboration with the American Association for Thoracic Surgery and Society of Thoracic Surgeons. Circulation. 2008;117:e350-e408.
19. Hallstrom AP, Ornato JP, Weisfeldt M, Travers A, Christenson J, McBurnie MA, Zalenski R, Becker LB, Schron EB, Proschan M; Public Access Defibrillation Trial Investigators. Public access defibrillation and survival after out-of-hospital cardiac arrest. N Engl J Med. 2004;351:637-46.
20. Nichol G, Huszti E, Birnbaum A, Mahoney B, Weisfeldt M, Travers A, Christenson J, Kuntz K. PAD Investigators. Cost-effectiveness of lay responder defibrillation for out-of-hospital cardiac arrest. Ann Emerg Med. 2009;54:226-35.
21. Rea T, Page RL. Community approaches to improve resuscitation after out-of-hospital cardiac arrest. Circulation. 2010;121:1134-40.

27

New Gadgets Knocking at the Door: Leadless Pacemakers, Subcutaneous Implantable Cardioverter Defibrillators, Wearable Defibrillators

Anitha G, Ulhas M Pandurangi

INTRODUCTION

The evolution of personalized electronic gadgets for cardiac care has been fascinating. Since the day of implantation of first permanent pacemaker in 1958 and the first implantable cardiac defibrillator (ICD) in 1980, millions of lives have been saved and the quality of life has been enhanced. Improved understanding of mechanism of benefit has resulted in smarter gadgets which are smaller, more efficient and devoid of fragile and error prone components.

Knocking at the door now are three such gadgets, viz. leadless pacemaker (LP), subcutaneous implantable cardioverter defibrillator (S-ICD) and wearable cardiac defibrillator (WCD). These smart gadgets seem to have overcome the common and potentially life-threatening complications of the existing devices without significant compromise on the lifesaving functions. Better understanding of the mechanisms and behavior of cardiac arrhythmia and also of the limitations of the gadgets, has led to several modifications over the last few years. The new gadgets have become compact, more intelligent, less invasive, longer lasting and most importantly are devoid of common vulnerabilities of present generation gadgets. The new gadgets may provide 'one-stop-solution' for not only cardiac but also other system disorders by donning multiple roles of poly-sensor, biochemical lab and drug house, etc. Three of the several advanced electronic implantable gadgets knocking at the door—leadless pacemakers, subcutaneous ICDs, wearable defibrillators have been described briefly below.

LEADLESS PACEMAKER

Most of the complications and malfunctions of the pacemaker can be attributed to the failing lead and hence the lead is considered as the Achilles heel of the pacemaker. A lead is a nidus for infection and can remain as a constant risk for infective endocarditis if not removed during the management of pacemaker pocket infection.[1] Inappropriate therapies and a premature battery drainage are almost always attributed to the malfunction of leads. A lead can potentially cause obstruction of the vessel and thromboembolism. A lead can make vessels inaccessible for future interventions. The removal of a malfunctioning or infected lead can be associated with significant morbidity and occasionally death. The overall incidence of complications related to the lead is about 8%.[2]

The attractive concept of leadless pacemaker (LP) was first reported as early as in 1970. However, it took more than four decades to miniaturize the device small enough to be implanted percutaneously and extracted or repositioned easily.[3] The development phase also saw improved battery technology, pacing and sensing abilities of the device. Currently there are two LPs which have been approved in Europe:

1. Nanostim™ Leadless Pacemaker (St Jude Medical Inc. Minnesota, USA—**Fig. 1A**).
2. Micra™ Tarascatheter pacing system (Medtronic Plc. Minnesota, USA—**Fig. 1B**).

The volume of the LP is about 1 cc and weighs approximately 2 g. The device is delivered percutaneously at the right ventricular (RV) apex via femoral vein through 18F introducer **(Fig. 1C)**. The lithiumcarbon monofluride battery (Li-CFX) has an equivalent longevity compared with conventional pacemaker. The first feasibility study to evaluate the safety and performance of the LP in the year 2009, paved way for further multicenter, randomized trials.[4] Currently, these gadgets are CE Mark approved. The present generation LPs are capable of only RV apical pacing. They can only be recommended in adults in whom VVIR mode of pacing is considered safe. Thin built adults, underlying ventricular dysfunction and in patients in whom long-term RV apical pacing is predicted to be detrimental are not the candidates for such devices.

WIRELESS CARDIAC STIMULATION SYSTEM

Wireless cardiac stimulation system for the left ventricle (WiCS-LV) is a 'hybrid leadless pacing system' **(Fig. 2)** that

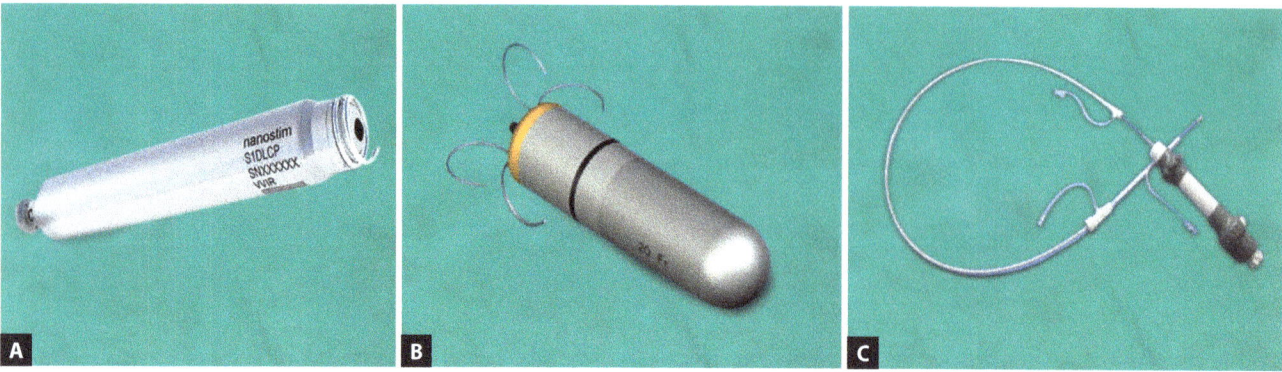

Figs 1A to C: (A) Nanostim LP (St Jude Medical Inc); (B) Micra LP (Medtronic Plc.); (C) 18F delivery system of LP

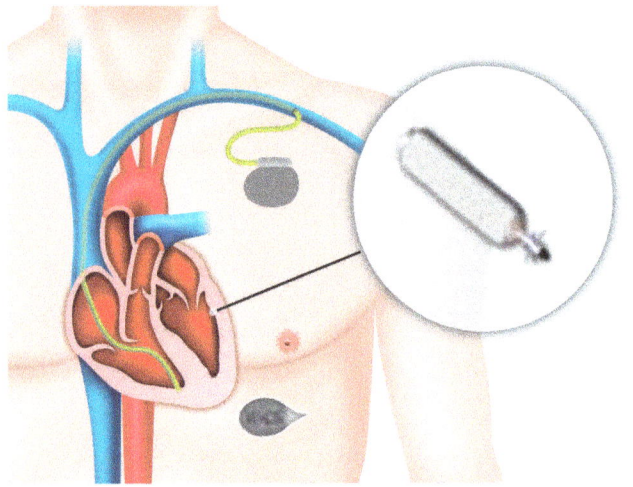

Fig. 2: The wireless cardiac stimulation for the left ventricle (WiCS-LV)

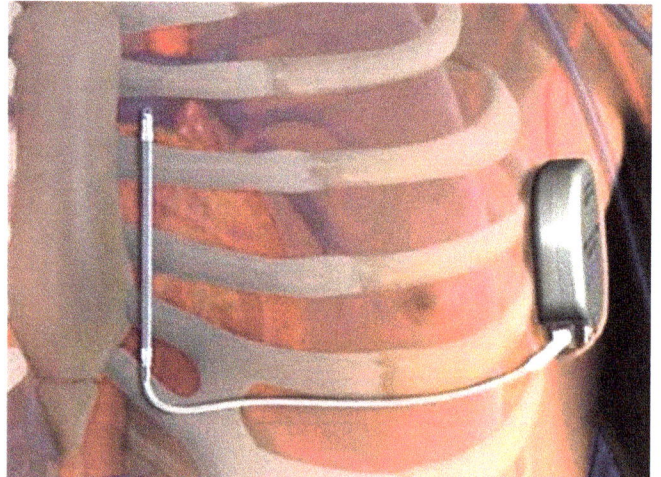

Fig. 3: The Subcutaneously implantable AICD

works with a conventional pacemaker and/or defibrillator to provide resynchronization therapy.[5] The WiCS-LV is a pulse generator implanted subcutaneously. It senses pacing pulse and transmits ultrasound energy to a receiver electrode implanted inside the LV. The receiver electrode then delivers electrical pulse in the LV at a time when RV is paced by the conventional system. Thus, it seems WiCS-LV system is set to obviate the need for endovenous LV lead responsible for procedure-related difficulties and complications.

SUBCUTANEOUS IMPLANTABLE CARDIOVERTER DEFIBRILLATOR

The automatic implantable cardioverter defibrillator (AICD) devices over the last three decades have proven to be the *only* effective therapy for sudden cardiac death due to ventricular arrhythmias. The AICD technology has gone through significant evolution from large patches covering heart requiring thoracotomy to a small box of the size of a match box implanted subcutaneously and thin electrodes mounted on wires which could be introduced endovenously. Over the years however, serious limitations mainly attributable to the leads have been recognized.[1,2,6] In addition to the fears of venous obstruction, thromboembolism, infection, etc. as described above in the section of LP, the bulkier AICD leads pose higher risk of fracture or insulation break, early battery depletion and higher morbidity and mortality during lead extractions. The leads are the reasons for serious complications during implant (hemopericardium, pneumothorax) and during follow-up (lead dislodgement, fracture, infection, etc.). The AICD lead malfunction is common and associated frequently with inappropriate therapies leading to adverse psychological and medical consequences. The need for more effective and safer therapies have become urgent. The need especially for an implantable defibrillator devoid of endovenous lead is acute. The earlier attempts to avoid endovenous leads in paediatric age group and in patients with inaccessible vascular system, adopted more invasive approach in the form of thoracotomy and epicardial placement of defibrillator patches with varying success. The S-ICD (Cameron Health, California—**Fig. 3**) is a

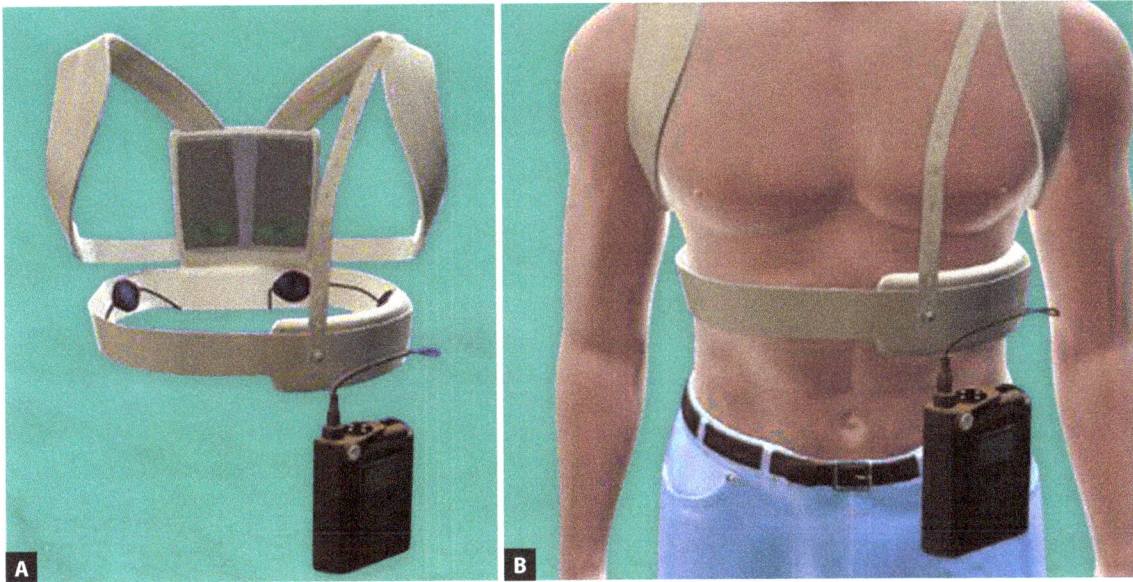

Figs 4A and B: Wearable cardiac defibrillator

novel defibrillator device which is devoid of endovenous leads. The device is tested over the past decade[7,8] and The European Union and Food and Drug Administration have approved the device for clinical use.

The pulse generator of S-ICD system is enclosed in a titanium case and the subcutaneous lead contains both sensing and defibrillating components. The generator is placed subcutaneously between the fourth and fifth intercostal space in the axillary region and the subcutaneous lead is placed parallel to the left border of the sternum. The device has the ability to deliver a biphasic DC shock of up to 80 J. The device also has the ability to pace ventricle up to 30 seconds during post-shock bradycardia. A recent study compared efficacy of S-ICD with conventional AICD. The S-ICD was found to be as effective to detect and terminate the ventricular arrhythmias.[9] The device, however, has still the limitations of inappropriate therapy, lead migration, infection and skin erosion either due to lead or generator.

WEARABLE CARDIOVERTER-DEFIBRILLATOR

Even though AICD is the *only* effective therapy for sudden cardiac death, there is an urgent need for more effective and safer therapy as discussed before. Its limitations had led to recommending AICD therapy only to those who have irreversible cause of sudden cardiac death and who are predicted to be at the highest level of risk stratification score. Such strategy of recommendation of AICD therapy may not protect many patients who are being observed for the reversibility of underlying pathology, patients waiting for cardiac transplantations and those patients who have temporary contraindication for AICD. The availability of wearable cardioverter-defibrillator (WCD) devices since the year 2000 has been shown to be useful in preventing SCD in such groups of patients. The commercially available WCD is the Life Vest (Zoll Medical, Pittsburgh, PA—**Figs 4A and B**) which has been approved by the Food and Drug Administration (FDA) in 2002.[10] The device weighing about 600 g is worn on a holster around the waist and the sensing and defibrillator electrodes are applied to the back and the front. The battery lasts for 24 hours and takes 2 hours to charge. Two batteries are provided for uninterrupted use. The device does not have pacing abilities. The biphasic shock energy may be programmed from 75 to 150 joules. Unlike the AICD device where the patient does not have control on therapies, the WCD device offers warning of an imminent shock and allows patient to lie down and receive the shock and avoid injuries. The device also allows the educated patient to even withhold the therapy in the context of hemodynamic stability or false diagnosis due to artefacts. At least three clinical trials have documented the efficacy of WCDs.[10]

CONCLUSION

The technology and understanding of the benefits of implantable electronic cardiac gadgets have increased significantly. At the same time the limitations of these gadgets have been exposed. The limitations may affect the outcomes more adversely than the natural course of the disease for which they were indicated. The newer gadgets knocking on the door hold promise to circumvent the limitations and increase the benefits.

REFERENCES

1. Klug D, Balde M, Pavin D, et al. Risk factors related to infections of implanted pacemakers and cardioverter-defibrillators: results of a large prospective study. Circulation. 2007;116:1349-55.
2. Lampert R. Managing with pacemakers and implantable cardioverter defibrillators. Circulation. 2013;128:1576.
3. Spickler JW, Rasor NS, Kezdi P, et al. Totally self-contained intracardiac pacemaker. J Electrocardiol. 1970;3:325-31.
4. Knops RE, Tjong FVY, Neuzil P, et al. Chronic Performance of a Leadless Cardiac Pacemaker - 1-Year Follow-Up of the LEADLESS Trial. JACC; 2015. pp. 1497-504.
5. Auricchio A, Delnoy PP, Regoli F, et al. First-in-man implantation of leadless ultrasound based cardiac stimulation pacing system: novel endocardial left ventricular resynchronization therapy in heart failure patients. Europace. 2013;15(8):1191-7.
6. Van Rees JB, de Bie MK, Thijssen J, et al. Implantation-related complications of implantable cardioverter-defibrillators and cardiac resynchronization therapy devices: a systemic review of randomized clinical trials. J Am Coll Cardiol. 2011;58:995-1000.
7. Hauser RG. The subcutaneous implantable cardioverter-defibrillator: should patients want one? J Am Cardiol. 2013;61:20-2.
8. Kobe J, Reinke F, Meyer C, et al. Implantation and follow-up of totally subcutaneous versus conventional implantable cardioverter-defibrillator: a multicentre case-control study. Heart Rhythm. 2013;10:29-36.
9. Aziz S, Leon AR, EL-Chami MF, et al. The subcutaneous defibrillator—A review of literature. JACC. 2014;63:1473-9.
10. Adler A, Halkin A, Viskin S, et al. New Drugs and Technologies: Wearable Cardioverter-Defibrillators. Circulation. 2013;127:854-860.

28. Echocardiographic Evaluation of Left Atrial Clot and its Utility in Clinical Practice

Asha Moorthy, Jain T Kallarakkal

The fundamentals of thrombogenesis were proposed 150 years ago by the report of Virchow's triad (blood stasis, endothelial injury, and hypercoagulability). However, the precise conditions under which thrombogenesis and thromboembolism occur in relation to the left atrium remain largely speculative. The tenets of Virchow hypothesis have been extrapolated to the left atrium and atrial fibrillation.

Thrombus formation occurs along a pathogenesis continuum that starts with spontaneous echo contrast (SEC) or "smoke" formation (erythrocyte rouleaux formation indicative of blood stasis), progresses to sludge formation (very dense smoke) and ends with complete thrombus formation.[1] Persistent SEC in the left atrium on transesophageal echocardiography (TEE) has been associated with later thrombus formation and systemic embolization. Sludge has an echocardiographic appearance that is more viscid than smoke but less dense than thrombus.

The anatomic structure of the left atrial appendage (LAA) and acquired enlargement and stretch of the left atrium or LAA in valvular and nonvalvular heart disease provide the milieu for blood stasis. Microscopic endocardial changes in the LAA have been reported in atrial fibrillation as compared with sinus rhythm and mitral stenosis as compared with mitral regurgitation. Edema, fibrinous transformation and endothelial denudation have been described in the LA tissue in patients with atrial fibrillation and thromboembolism.[2]

Impairment of extracellular matrix turnover has been implicated as a factor contributing to structural changes that occur in the left atrium. Patients with LA fibrillation have abnormal amounts of collagen and degradation products as well as concentrations of matrix metalloproteinases.[3]

Stasis of flow in the left atrium can also occur during sinus rhythm given the appropriate associated pathology (i.e. significant LA enlargement and/or mitral stenosis).[4]

The phenomenon of LAA "stunning" was demonstrated on TEE by an increase in the intensity of SEC and the decrease in LAA Doppler flow velocities immediately after cardioversion of atrial fibrillation to sinus rhythm.[5] Before this transesophageal echocardiographic observation, the prevailing theory was that stroke in the postcardioversion period resulted solely from dislodgement of a pre-existing thrombus (present before cardioversion and due to the underlying atrial fibrillation).[6] Further evidence for the role of postcardioversion stunning in the genesis of thromboembolism came from a series of patients who had postcardioversion strokes despite the absence of LA or LAA thrombus on precardioversion TEE.[7] These transesophageal echocardiographic studies formed the basis and rationale for the TEE-guided anticoagulation strategy used today when managing patients with atrial fibrillation undergoing electrical cardioversion.

The logic of echocardiographic imaging in atrial fibrillation is identifying one of the many underlying cardiac causes of atrial fibrillation, such as valvular heart disease, ventricular dysfunction and hypertension.

Once an associated etiology of atrial fibrillation has been identified or ruled out, attention turns to details of LA anatomy, specifically whether the left atrium is enlarged and, if so, how severely LA enlargement has significance relative to thromboembolic risk, maintenance of sinus rhythm, and prognosis.[8]

Although thrombus can be identified by TTE and the specificity is high, the sensitivity of TTE is unacceptably low, in part because most atrial thrombi are located in the LAA rather than the main LA cavity. The LAA is best viewed by TEE. LA size can be expressed as either the anterior-posterior LA diameter or LA area and measured according to the ASE guidelines on chamber quantification.[9] Investigation has demonstrated the superiority of LA volume measurements and more precisely LA volume indexed to body size as a more accurate measurement. In addition, atrial volumes have significant prognostic value relative to stroke risk, mortality, atrial fibrillation recurrence after electrical cardioversion, ablation and cardiac surgery.

It is believed that LA volumes obtained by 3D echocardiography may provide the ultimate quantification. However, this has not been routinely adopted in clinical practice at this time.

Because of its portability, relatively low cost, and non-invasive nature, TTE is recommended for evaluation of the left atrium, cardiac structure, and function in atrial fibrillation by the European Association of Echocardiography consensus guidelines, the American College of Cardiology, American Heart Association, and Heart Rhythm Society.

Because of its location immediately adjacent to the esophagus, the left atrium is the structure best suited to the strengths of TEE and its ability to visualize cardiac structures with high spatial resolution and good temporal resolution, all in real time. More specifically, TEE enables optimal visualization of LAA anatomy as well as interrogation of its function and physiology with Doppler interrogation. The introduction and addition of 3D imaging have added to our ability to interrogate Echocardiographic evaluation of the left atrium and LAA.

REFERENCES

1. Lowe BS, Kusunose K, Motoki H, Varr B, Shrestha K, Whitman C, et al. Prognostic significance of left atrial appendage "sludge" in patients with atrial fibrillation: a new transesophageal echocardiographic thromboembolic risk factor. J Am Soc Echocardiogr. 2014;27:1176-83.
2. Masawa N, Yoshida Y, Yamada T, Joshita T, Ooneda G. Diagnosis of cardiac thrombosis in patients with atrial fibrillation in the absence of macroscopically visible thrombi. Virchows Arch A Pathol Anat Histopathol. 1993;422:67-71.
3. Tziakas DN, Chalikias GK, Papanas N, Stakos DA, Chatzikyriakou SV, Maltezos E. Circulating levels of collagen type degradation marker depend on the type of atrial fibrillation. Europace. 2007;9:589-96.
4. Pollock C, Taylor D. Assessment of left atrial appendage function by transesophageal echocardiography. Implications for the development of thrombus. Circulation. 1991;84:223-31.
5. Grimm RA, Stewart WJ, Maloney JD, Cohen GI, Pearce GL, Salcedo EE, et al. Impact of electrical cardioversion for atrial fibrillation on left atrial appendage function and spontaneous echo contrast: characterization by simultaneous transesophageal echocardiography. J Am Coll Cardiol. 1993;22:1359-66.
6. Grimm RA, Stewart WJ, Black IW, Thomas JD, Klein AL. Should all patients undergo transesophageal echocardiography before electrical cardioversion of atrial fibrillation? J Am Coll Cardiol. 1994;23:533-41.
7. Black IW, Fatkin D, Sagar KB, Khandheria BK, Leung DY, Galloway JM, et al. Exclusion of atrial thrombus by transesophageal echocardiography does not preclude embolism after cardioversion of atrial fibrillation: A multicenter study. Circulation. 1994;89:2509-13.
8. Tsang TS, Abhayaratna WP, Barnes ME, Miyasaka Y, Gersh BJ, Bailey KR, et al. Prediction of cardiovascular outcomes with left atrial size: is volume superior to area or diameter? J Am Coll Cardiol. 2006;47:1018-23.
9. Lang RM, Badano LP, Mor-Avi V, Afilalo J, Armstrong A, Ernande L, et al. Recommendations for cardiac chamber quantification by echocardiography in adults: an update from the American Society of Echocardiography and the European Association of Cardiovascular Imaging. J Am Soc Echocardiogr. 2015;28:1-39.

29 Clinical Applications of Nuclear Cardiology Procedures and its Future Directions

GN Mahapatra

Over the past decade, advances in Nuclear Cardiology have provided a range of diagnostic tools for the practicing clinician. In the last few decades, numerous technological advances especially the development of new radionuclides, high resolution gamma scintillation cameras and sophisticated small computers have been responsible for improvement in the quality and scope of Nuclear Cardiology techniques for better identification and measurement of the extent of disease. A succession of new therapies for treating cardiac disease has impacted both cardiac morbidity and mortality which includes carvedilol, angiotensin converting enzyme inhibitors, statins and new generation of stents. In this text the value of nuclear imaging including new promising agents, improvement of gamma camera, improvement in software technology will also be discussed in addition to the existing routine technology to diagnose cardiac disease, to monitor the effects of therapy and to better stratify patients into different risk categories for cardiac death or MI ultimately the optimal integration of nuclear imaging with the other diagnostic modalities will allow the most accurate identification of patients who may benefit from more aggressive treatment such as myocardial revascularization or heart transplantation. In addition to these, Nuclear Cardiology procedures has distinct advantages over other diagnostic imaging modalities such as having a low radiation risk because low amount of radioactive are used. It is being relatively painless and noninvasive. It provides both structural and functional information of the organ of interest. It is definitely superior to other noninvasive tests like routine ECG, stress ECG and 2-D echocardiography with a sensitivity of 93% and specificity of 95%.

The various current concepts provide in a single noninvasive manner information about myocardial function (systolic, diastolic) perfusion, viability (ischemic, hibernating or stunned myocardium versus necrosed or scarred muscle), metabolism and neuroreceptor activity. In addition to these, with the introduction of newer radiopharmaceuticals and the improvement in software by Nuclear Cardiology scientists have further made Cardiovascular Nuclear Medicine a dynamic field. Every year new applications are introduced and the old ones are refined.

SCOPE OF RADIONUCLIDE IMAGING PROCEDURES

- Myocardial function, systolic and diastolic: global and regional
    - First pass radionuclide angiocardiography (FPRNA).
    - Stress multigated equilibrium blood pool imaging radionuclide ventriculography (RNV).
- Myocardial perfusion and measurement of coronary blood flow.
    - Stress-redistribution SPECT Tl-201 myocardial perfusion study with reinjection protocols.
    - Rest-redistribution Tl-201 myocardial perfusion scintigraphy/rest and IV NTG/ oral NTG study.
    - Stress gated SPECT Tc-99m sestamibi/tetrofosmin myocardial perfusion scintigraphy with rest IV/oral NTG gated SPECT study.
    - Pharmacological stress perfusion imaging.
    - Rubidium-82 PET myocardial perfusion study.
    - Stress N-13 ammonia/PET myocardial perfusion O-15 labelled water.
    - F-18 FDG PET myocardial ischemia imaging.
- Myocardial metabolism
    - F-18 FDG metabolic PET imaging
    - I-123 BMIPP Iodophenyl methyl pentadecanoic acid.
- Myocardial stunning and hibernation
- Myocardial infarct imaging
    - Tc-99m labelled pyrophosphate
    - Tc-99m labelled glucaric acid

- Tc-99m labelled annexin
- Indium-111 antimyosin antibody imaging
• Myocardial innervation: Parasympathetic and sympathetic
  - I-131 or I-123 MIBG planar/SPECT myocardial neuronal imaging
• Myocardial hypoxia imaging
• Myocardial apoptosis imaging
• Amyloidosis.

MYOCARDIAL PERFUSION

Before single photon emission computerized tomography (SPECT) technology became widely available, two dimensional planar was used for blood pool and myocardial perfusion imaging. Some of the early SPECT imaging tables would hold patient's up to 350 pounds but often obese patients found planar techniques more easy to tolerate. In certain situations, planar imaging will be the only option for obtaining a nuclear myocardial perfusion exam. Planar imaging may be acquired with gating, then summed to form composite images in three views. This is particularly useful for the morbidly obese patient, or a bed ridden individual who cannot tolerate a SPECT procedure. The morbidly obese patient will not always fit into the scan radians, even when a circular orbit is chosen especially when short stretcher unable to lie flat, or unable to hold arms out of the way. The body habitus of these morbidly obese men prevented diagnostic SPECT imaging with our dual head camera and in that case a gated planar exam may be completed successfully. Gating the images would enable our nuclear medicine physician to study the wall motion although we are unable to quantitate an ejection fraction.

Planar imaging techniques are important to master even today. Because of problem of overlapping structures of myocardium supplied by two independent coronary arteries and soft tissue artifact, nobody does this modality of imaging in the era of SPECT myocardial perfusion imaging unless and until the specific indications mentioned above.

Stress/Redistribution Stress Thallium Myocardial Perfusion Study (Fig. 1)

Thallium-201 was the only isotope available for the clinician to image the myocardium from 1970 through about 1990. It is a cyclotron produced radionuclide which decays by electron capture to mercury-201 with a half life of 73 hours, emitting mainly X-rays of 67/82 KeV (88% abundance) and gamma photons of 135 KeV and 167 KeV (12% abundance). It is supplied as thallous chloride and expires seven days after activity reference date and time. Due to excessive amount of impurities it should not be administered to patients after seven days.

Initially, used for planar imaging with a maximum dose 80 MBq (usually 1.5 mci), SPECT imaging needs higher dose (2.5 to 3 mci). The biological properties of thallium are similar to potassium. Because potassium is major intracellular cation in muscle and is essentially absent in scar tissue for which Thallium which is potassium analog is well suited for differentiating viable from nonviable scarred myocardium. Like potassium, thallium clashes the cell membrane via the active Na^+-K^+ ATPase transport system and by facilitative diffusion.

It remained popular even after Technetium 99m based tracers became available for single day imaging protocols. Viability studies or in conjunction with Tc-99m tracers in hybrid dual isotope protocols. It was common to do resting thallium perfusion imaging followed by Tc-99m Sestamibi Gated SPECT stress imaging, combining the best characteristics of both radiopharmaceuticals. Thallium imaging is historically significant as the epitome of myocardial perfusion imaging for decades, becoming a short of gold standard for its time.

Thallium-201 scintigraphy is most often performed either at rest or in conjunction with exercise stress in patients of suspected coronary artery disease to diagnose myocardial ischemia or known to have coronary artery disease for diagnosing the site and extent of myocardial infarction including impending ischemia leading to risk stratification and prognosis following myocardial infarction, assessment of thrombolytic therapy and assessment of myocardial viability.

For stress imaging 3–4 mci is administered at peak exercise and then 1.5–2 mci injection is given atleast 30 minutes prior to redistribution imaging. First pass myocardial extraction is 60–70% after stress injection and 80–90% after resting injection. The myocardium takes up around 5–15% of injected dose normally extracted by lungs before reaching systemic circulation and the remainder distribution into skeletal muscle, gastrointestinal tract and kidneys. In patients with left ventricular failure and raised left atrial pressure, pulmonary transit time is prolonged and greater quantity of tracer is deposited in lung a finding predictive of a poor prognosis.

In normally perfused myocardium, 80–90% of peak activity is reached within 1 minute following iv injection of thallium, peaking within 10–20 minutes. Thallium injection is usually given at peak exercise and exercise is continued for another minute longer to achieve maximum extraction in the myocardium. Imaging is initiated within 5 minutes of injection and procedure is completed within 30 minutes because in this period the redistribution of tracer in myocardium is relatively fixed, hence, this image reflects myocardial perfusion at peak exercise.

Over the subsequent hours there is a washout proportional to flow and slow equilibrium between thallium in the myocardial systole and systemic blood pool. This is independent of the flow rate but requires an intact myocyte cell membrane and is therefore a marker of myocardial viability.

Most redistribution occurs within 3–4 hours hence, an image at this time reflects resting perfusion. In resin supplied by

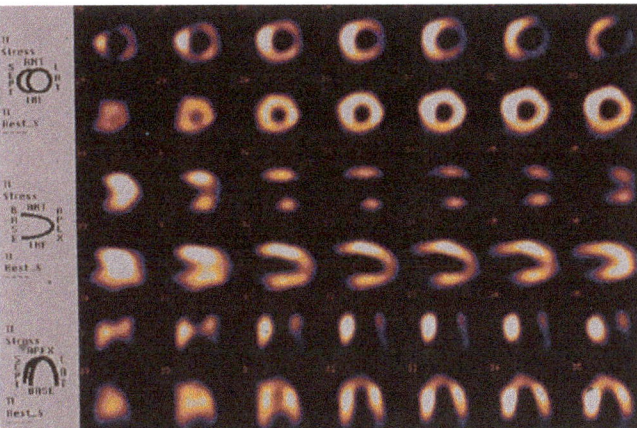

Fig. 1: Stress thallium myocardial perfusion scan showing a large area of stress perfusion defect involving anterolateral myocardial segments which shows fair amount of reperfusion in resting image suggestive of anterolateral myocardial ischemia

stenod's vessel, a stress perfusion defect is seen which improves in the distribution image. A stress defect which fails to improve on redistribution a fixed defect represents nonviable segment (infarct or old scar) most of time but hibernating myocardium may give the same appearance, hence importance of FDG PET imaging to differentiate viable hibernating myocardium from scar.

STRESS-GATED SPECT TC-99M MYOCARDIAL PERFUSION IMAGING AGENTS

The technetium labelled agents can be substituted for thallium in the rest and stress evaluation of myocardial perfusion. These agents are very different in behavior compared with thallous chloride. The technetium labelled agent is lost slowly from the myocardium with comparable clearance from normal and ischemic tissue. Since, Tc-99m labelled tracers are essentially fixed in the cells, separate injections are required for the rest and stress study. Same day studies or separate day studies are usually practiced. Usually, same day studies use as little as 8–10 mci for the stress study and up to 30 mci for the rest study. The second injection should contain 2.5–3 times the resting dose. The doses are adjusted as per the weight of the patient. There should be gap of at least three hours between the rest and stress study.

The advantage of using Technetium-99m labelled agents gives useful additional informations such as global ejection fraction, wall motion, wall thickening measurements in addition to pattern of myocardial tissue perfusion. If the particular segment of myocardial region appears to have a fixed perfusion defect and it demonstrates relatively preserved wall thickening and abnormal wall motion, it should be viable and may be a candidate for coronary revascularization. This method can also detect the stunned/hibernating myocardium which are labelled as viable myocardium. It can also differentiate a fixed defect in the stress and rest gated perfusion study in differentiating scar from an attenuation artifact as one observes breast attenuation commonly in females and diaphragmatic attenuation in males.

Sestamibi

Technetium-99m Sestamibi is a lipophilic monovalent cation which consists of six methoxy-isobutyl-isonitrile ligands surrounding a technetium central core. Sestamibi is cleared from blood very rapidly with T½ less than three minutes at stress and rest followed by a slow clearance phase. Less than 10% of injected dose remains in circulation at five minutes after injection. First pass myocardial extraction is about 40% after a stress injection and 60% after a rest injection. The myocardium takes up between 1.2–1.5% and retains it for hours. The myocardial distribution is proportional to blood flow up to about 2 mL/min/gram with a plateauing of extraction at higher flow rates which are achieved with vasodilatation (4 mL/min/gram) but this is not a constraint in detecting mild to moderate coronary stenose (50–70%). The most important clinical difference between Tl-201 and Sestamibi is that the latter undergoes minimal (10–15%) redistribution from initial pattern of uptake **(Figs 2 and 3)**.

Tetrofosmin

It is lipophilic diphosphine cation which can be labelled with Tc-99m. It has been developed to replace the Tl-201 in myocardial perfusion imaging. Preparation takes about 20 min of incubation at room temperature (but no boiling as required with Sestamibi). The radiation dose is slightly less than for Sestamibi and less than half that associated with Thallium.

The blood clearance of tetrofosmin is very rapid with less than 5% residual activity by 10 minutes. Its first pass extraction is 45%, total myocardial uptake is 1–1.2% of injected dose. Unlike thallium tetrofosmin is not potassium analog.

Tetrofosmin enters myocyte via passive transport driven by the negative membrane potential on the intact cell. The mitochondrial membrane potential plays a major role in the myocardial uptake and retention of tetrofosmin. Myocardial uptake is related to the metabolic status of the myocytes in particular the mitochondrial membrane and the plasma membrane potentials. Uptake is proportional to blood flow.

Hepatic clearance of tetrofosmin is more rapid than Sestamibi allowing to be started 15 minutes after stress injection.

Teboroxime

Technetium-99m teboroxime is a myocardial perfusion tracer, i.e. highly extracted and rapidly cleared by the myocardium. The first pass extraction fraction is 90% and the myocardial

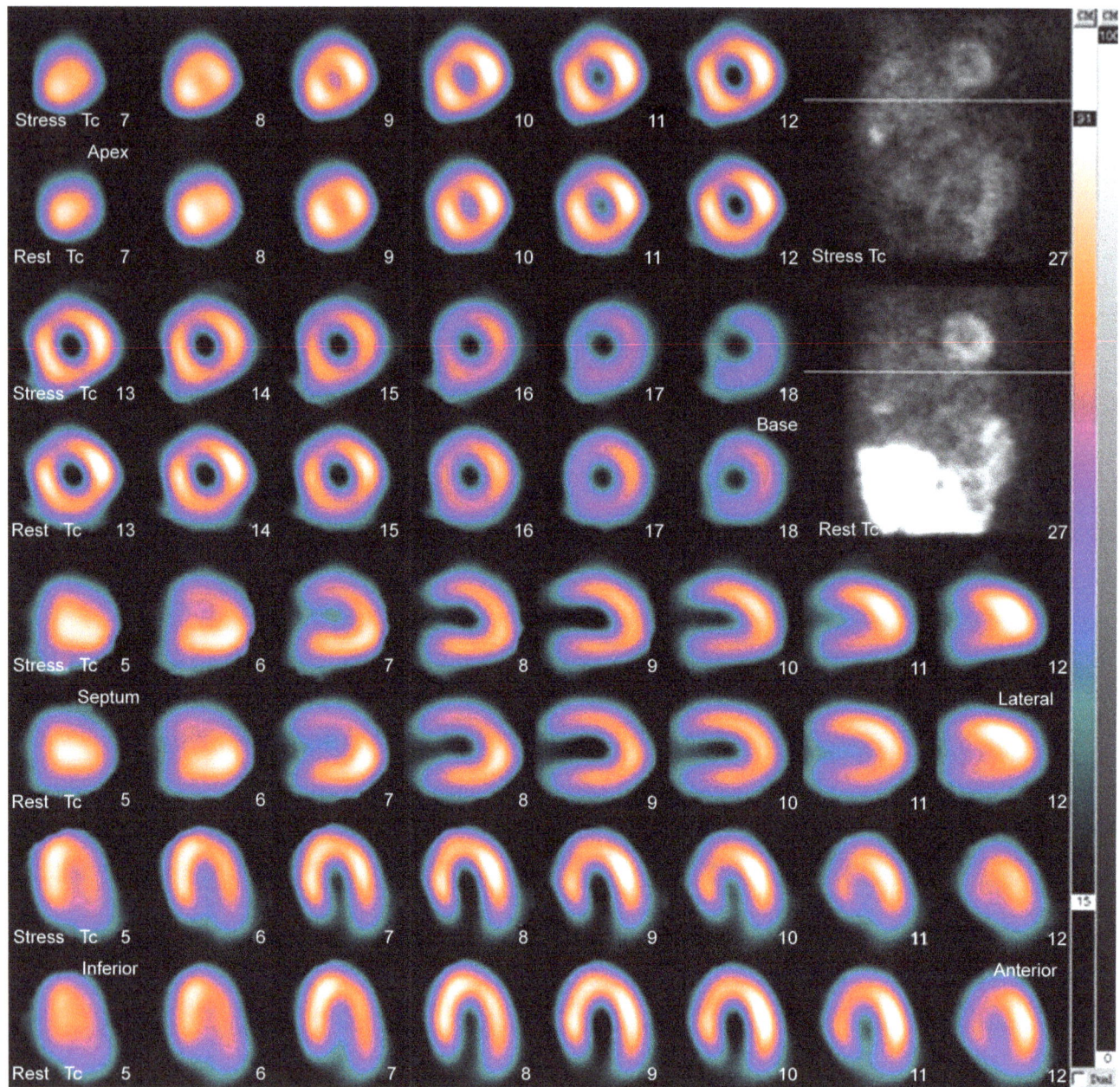

Fig. 2: Normal sestamibi myocardial perfusion scan

clearance T1/2 is equal to 10 minutes only which indicates the rapid clearance by the myocardium. The shorter duration protocol can be used for stress where we inject around 25 mci at peak exercise and around 60 minutes later resting perfusion can be evaluated. The advantage of Tc-99m teboroxime over other technetium-labeled perfusion agents are that the rapid biological half life amounting to around 5.3 minutes which allows studies to be completed in 60–90 minutes. It redistributes into ischemic myocardium like Tl-201. Technetium labelled teboroxime can detect coronary artery disease patients having two or three vessel disease. It can also detect one vessel disease to a great extent. The images can be compared with that of Tl-201 as an imaging. The injection to imaging time at stress is very short varies from 0.1 min to 2 min compared to tetrofosmin 10–15 minutes or Sestamibi from 30 min to 60 min. Because of the short duration of injection to imaging time as mentioned above, perfusion study should be completed within 10 minutes of administration due to rapid washout.

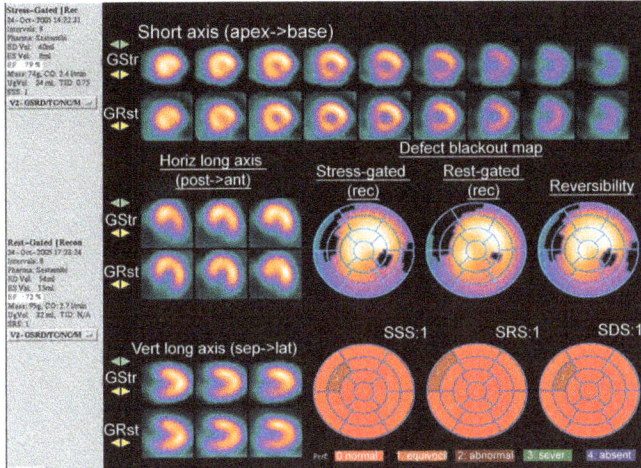

Fig. 3: Normal-gated SPECT

CLINICAL APPLICATIONS OF MYOCARDIAL PERFUSION IMAGING

The following are the important clinical subset of patients having suspected or proved coronary artery disease with or without history of heart attack in the past to diagnose and advocate further treatment planning including future risk stratification:

Suspected patients having strong family history of having one/ two risk factors (hypertension, diabetes, smoking, etc.): In this particular subset patients, if thallium stress test shows normal stress perfusion pattern with normal washout pattern in the 4 hours rest image (thallium has got a property to redistribute into the myocardium) it indicates that the suspected patient does not have any evidence of coronary artery disease (CAD) which would save him or her to go for further invasive test such as coronary angiography and the nuclear imaging is cost effective as the thallium stress test is approximately 1/3rd that of the cost of angiography.

Known case of coronary artery disease to evaluate ischemic/ infarction stratifying impending ischemia for future coronary events: Patient having a known history of previous myocardial infarction or recovering from acute myocardial infarction from the hospital, stress thallium myocardial scintigraphy delineates the area of ischemic/infarcted myocardium by revealing a stress perfusion defect in the part of the myocardium with evidence of redistribution (filling of the perfusion defect) in 4 hours image indicates viable myocardium, where revascularization procedure would convert completely the affected myocardium to its normal status/pattern. In an another group of patients fixed perfusion defect at stress and rest and even with the resting reinjection of Tl-201 is likely to have scarred myocardium (dead) where further angiography/ revascularization procedure would not help the patient as the dead myocardium cannot be recovered even if the circulation is re-established by angioplasty procedure. Tl-201 has got an unique property of not only evaluating the extent and viability of the affected segments resulting from myocardial infarction (MI), it can also detect the other impending ischemic zones in the myocardium for future coronary events (future myocardial infarct) which warns the patient for the future and also gives a clear cut guideline to the cardiologist to advocate his/her treatment planning.

To assess borderline lesions in coronary angiography: Most of the coronary artery lesions are eccentric unless and until it is viewed in multiple projections during angiography, one cannot assess the lesions correctly. In true sense, these lesions are originally borderline where cardiologists very commonly underestimates or overestimates the same lesions **(Figs 4A and B)**. The borderline lesions are 40% or 50% or 60% on coronary angiography, which needs the stress thallium myocardial scintigraphy to assess to have whether hemodynamic significant perfusion defect exists on the myocardial segments. In our experience we always routinely give this information whether the coronary intervention is necessary for these borderline lesions or nor by seeing a significant perfusion defect/normal on stress thallium test. This is considered to be an important subset of patients which cardiologists are aware of.

To assess myocardial blood flow in significant multi or single vessel lesion on coronary angiography: This is an important subset of patients where coronary angiography and stress thallium test do not match and it is called "mismatch pattern". In our experience of more than a decade on stress thallium studies, we have found normal stress thallium pattern in the myocardium, where multiple significant lesions are there in coronary angiography **(Figs 5A and B)**. This situation is due to the establishment of sufficient collaterals, which has been opened up as a result of significant lesion in coronary artery. The establishment of these collaterals is resulted due to the change in the life style of the patient pertaining to the regular exercise including *yoga* or *pranayama*, diet restriction and control of risk factors (diabetes, hypertension, etc.)

Equivocal or false positive treadmill stress test results: Suspected patients having false positive ST-T depression<3 mm or borderline ST-T changes or patients having LBBB or female patients not able to perform the treadmill quite effectively, all these types of patients can be subjected for a stress thallium test which clearly delineates, whether a stress perfusion defect is existing in any part of the myocardium or not **(Figs 6A and B)**. Depending on the stress thallium findings patient should be subjected for further invasive test or else, the normal stress thallium test does not indicate need for any further test such as angiography, etc **(Figs 7A and B)**.

Follow-up of patients of coronary artery bypass graft/balloon angioplasty/thrombolytic therapy

Cardiac patients who have undergone triple/four vessel bypass graft surgery or following post balloon angioplasty procedure complaints of shortness of breath, heaviness in the

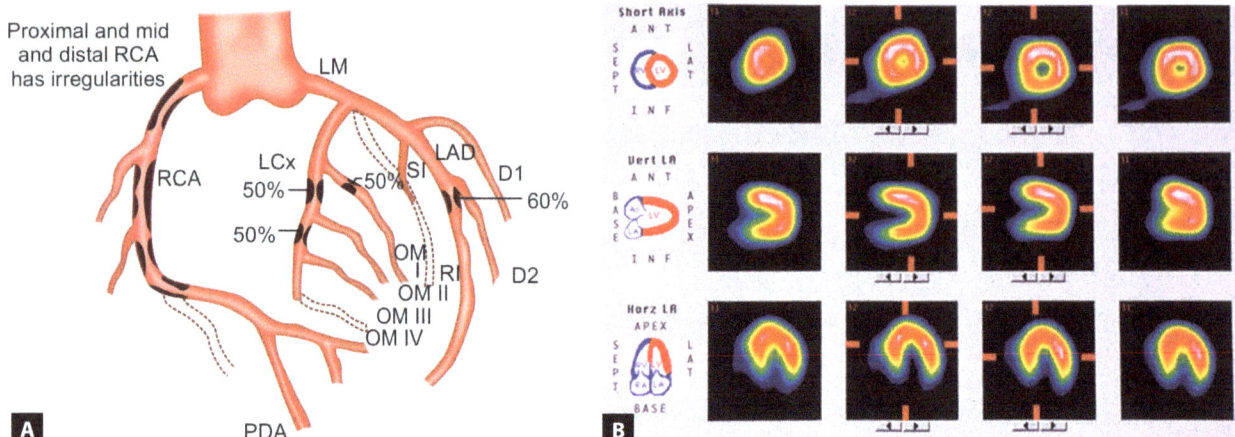

Figs 4A and B: (A) Coronary angiography showing borderline lesions in LAD, Cx and right coronary artery tree (B) Stress SPECT myocardial perfusion imaging showing almost uniform stress perfusion pattern in all the defined myocardial segments

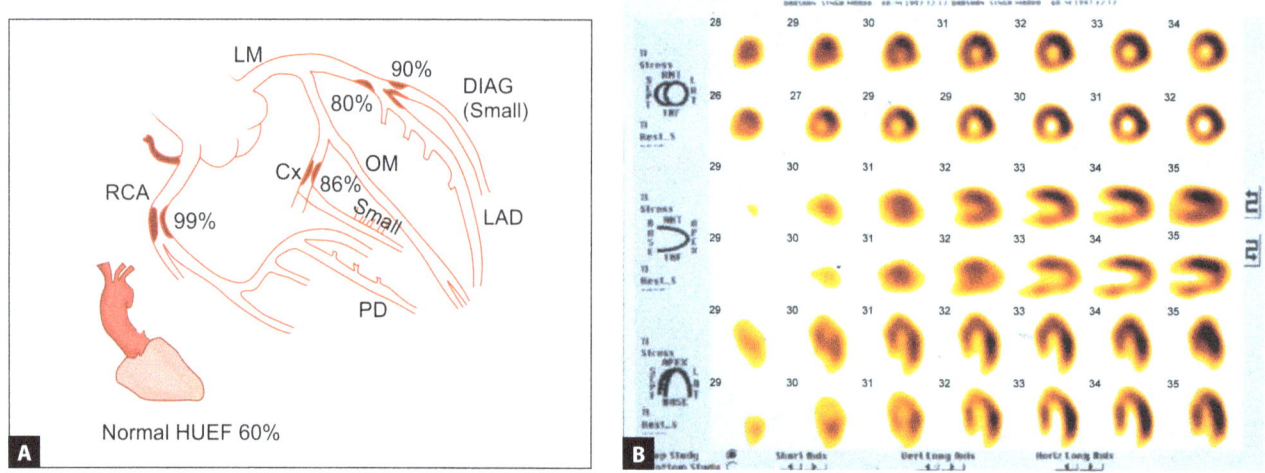

Figs 5A and B: (A) Coronary angiography showing significant lesions in LAD, Cx and right coronary artery tree; (B) Stress SPECT myocardial perfusion imaging showing almost uniform stress perfusion pattern

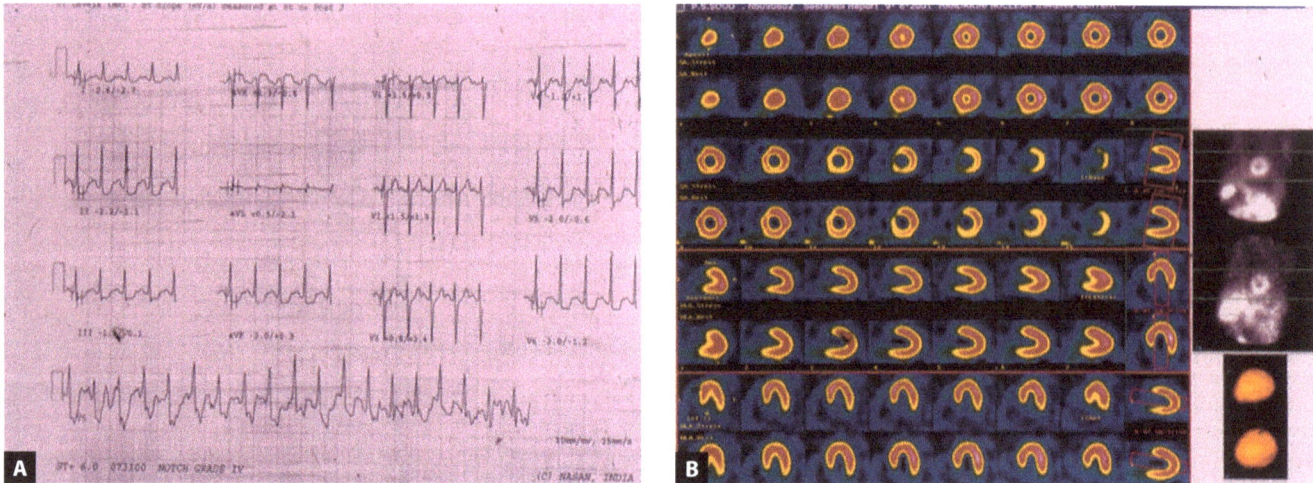

Figs 6A and B: (A) Treadmill stress test showing significant ST-T leads; (B) Stress sestamibi myocardial perfusion depression in all chest perfusion depression scan showing uniform stress

Chapter 29: Clinical Applications of Nuclear Cardiology Procedures and its Future Directions

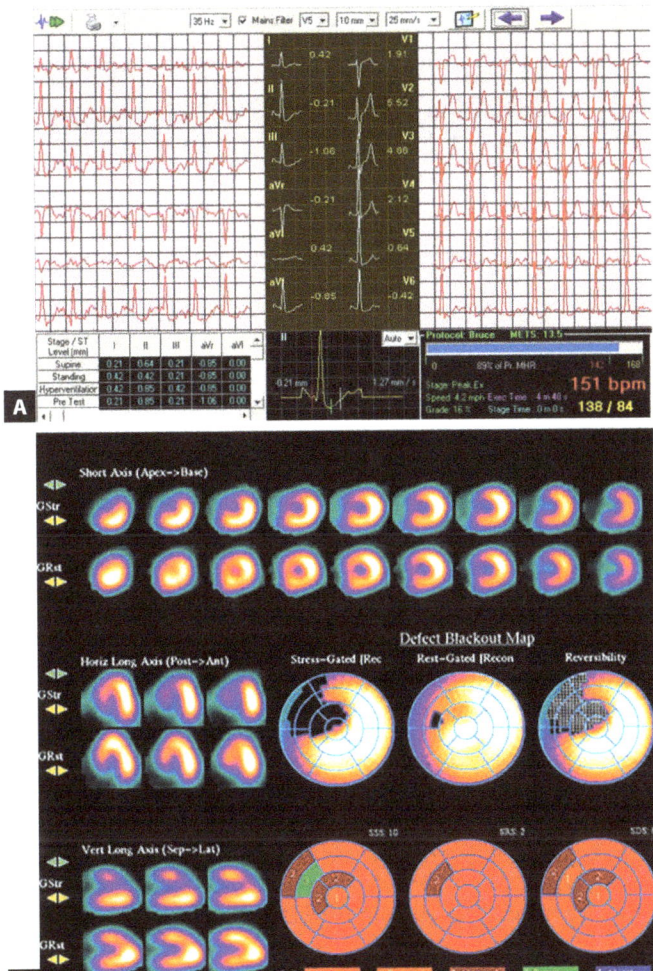

Figs 7A and B: (A) Treadmill stress test showing no significant ST-T depression in any of the chest leads; (B) Showing a definite area of stress perfusion defect in anteroseptal segment with evidence of adequate reversible ischemia

chest, transient short angina pain may be subjected to a stress thallium test to find out any significant perfusion defects at stress with evidence. Reversible ischemia that would definitely warrant redo-CABG/redo-angioplasty procedure as the restenosis of the arterial/venous graft has occurred. These types of patients even if they have undergone a routine treadmill stress test, literature review says if all the grafts are closed, stress test does not show any significant positive changes. Certainly stress thallium myocardium perfusion has an upper hand in this subset of patients.

PHARMACOLOGICAL STRESS PERFUSION IMAGING

The principle underlying myocardial perfusion imaging is to effect maximal exertion on the heart to attain maximum coronary blood flow. The purpose of stressing the heart is to create a disparity in blood flow between normal and stenosed arteries. This stress can result from increased oxygen demand in response to exercise or by vasodilatory effects on a pharmacological stress agent such as dipyridamole, adenosine, dobutamine, arbutamine, etc.

Pharmacological stress perfusion imaging is useful for patient who cannot exercise for various reasons including physical limitations, medications, lung diseases, peripheral vascular disease, severe osteoarthritis, elderly aged persons, aortic aneurysm, etc.

Pharmacological or physiologic stress is needed to detect coronary artery disease (CAD) when using myocardial perfusion imaging because even in the presence of high grade stenosis, resting blood flow is typically normal since distal arterial resistance is reduced to allow for a normal perfusion pattern. With dipyridamole/adenosine/dobutamine, myocardial regions supplied by normal or near normal arteries will experience increasing blood flow due to decrease coronary vascular resistance. In contrast, myocardium supplied by stenosed vessels may have only a minimum reserve capacity to dilate and will therefore be unable to increase blood flow at same rate seen in more normal territories.

There are three pharmacologic stress agents used today in cardiovascular nuclear medicine, viz. dipyridamole, adenosine, dobutamine/arbutamine.

DIPYRIDAMOLE MYOCARDIAL PERFUSION IMAGING

Protocol

Dipyridamole is administered in bolus, infusion with an optimal total dose of 0.56 mg/kg over a period of 4 min after stopping methylxanthine medication and caffeine consumption for 24 hours before the study is performed. During the cessation of dipyridamole infusion and the resultant stress on the heart interventions where patient can be encouraged to perform low level hand grip exercise and walking or sitting in place. These interventions stimulate catecholamine which reduces some splanchnic blood flow. This is an important consideration when using Tc-99m labelled compounds because they have more uptake in the splanchnic bed than Tl-201. The radiotracer either Tl-201/Tc-99m labelled agent is injected 7–9 min after dipyridamole infusion. The time for initiation or acquisition of image is started within 15 min following the injection of Tl-201 or 30–40 min following Tc-99m cardiolite/myoview injection.

Aminophylline is recommended as an antidote to any adverse reactions to dipyridamole infusion such as fall of blood pressure, etc. The routine use of this antidote is not recommended unless the side effect starts within 10–20 min after the infusion has been terminated. The patients should be supine and all the vital signs should be monitored during dipyridamole infusion.

MECHANISM OF ACTION OF DIPYRIDAMOLE

As dipyridamole is infused it blocks the reabsorption and metabolism of adenosine normally produced in the body. At basal condition normal adenosine level are relatively low. The biological half life of natural adenosine is normally 15–30 sec in the blood stream, increases with dipyridamole infusion, tripling or quadrupling the level of circulating adenosine. The increased level of natural adenosine actually produces the desired effect on the heart, i.e. coronary hyperemia with the increase of 20–40% of the heart rate. Blood pressure and diastolic blood pressure drops slightly.

Patients on effective antianginal therapy such as beta-blockers and calcium blocker will still have a positive myocardial perfusion image with dipyridamole despite adequate therapy.

Side Effects

- Systemic vasodilatation, i.e. headache, light headedness or symptoms like nausea, vomiting
- Myocardial ischemia
- Bronchospasm in case of asthmatic patients
- Patients with respiratory failure, severe chronic obstructive pulmonary disease (COPD).
- Major contraindication is allergy to dipyridamole or aminophylline.
- *Serious adverse reactions:*
  - Myocardial infarction (MI).
  - Bronchospasm.
  - Ventricular tachycardia.
  - Transient ischemic attack (TIA).

ADENOSINE MYOCARDIAL PERFUSION IMAGING

Adenosine myocardial perfusion image is useful in evaluating patients with CAD who cannot exercise. A review of clinical trials indicate that adenosine perfusion studies provide high sensitivity and specificity (80–90%) for identifying CAD.

Imaging Protocol

Intravenous infusion of adenosine at a dose of 140 ug/kg/min for 6 min procedure produces consistent hyperemia. The radiotracer is injected during adenosine infusion (at 3 min of 6 min infusion protocol) and then another 3 min infusion of adenosine is continued to have maximum vasodilatation in the myocardium followed by initiation of myocardial imaging under SPECT gamma camera **(Figs 8A and B)**. Adenosine has a very short half life of about 10 sec and so the hemodynamic changes disappear rapidly on completion of the injection. In the presence of coronary artery stenosis, regional flow differences are induced by adenosine which are revealed as perfusion defects in the scan. Adenosine protocol gives accurate result as exercise SPECT. Adenosine SPECT is a useful noninvasive test for the preoperative/intraoperative risk assessment of myocardial infusion in patients undergoing major surgery like joint replacement, kidney transplantation, peripheral vascular surgery, abdomino-pelvic surgery, etc.

Mechanism of Action

It directly act on A-1 receptor on vascular endothelial cells and A-2 receptor on vascular smooth muscles that result in vasodilatation.

Side Effect

The most common side effects are flushing, shortness of breath and chest pain. About 70–80% of patients experience one or more of these reactions. The vast majority of these reactions is transient and rarely requires a counter acting response. Interestingly older patients tolerate adenosine better than young patients.

Serious Adverse Effects

The adverse effect that has generated the most attention is a high degree AV block. This has been reported in < 1% of patients. In general, it always occurs during the first 2–3 min of adenosine infusion and is transient, first degree block (prolongation of PR interval) is more common occurring in 10% of patients. A second degree block occurs in 4–5% of patients. Adverse effects also occur in patients with bronchial asthma.

DOBUTAMINE MYOCARDIAL PERFUSION IMAGING

Since dipyridamole and adenosine work well to produce adequate hyperemia and causes maximal vasodilatation in the myocardium, one might ask why do we need a third pharmacologic stress agent. The patients selected for Dobutamine studies are those who cannot exercise and who are not good candidates for dipyridamole or adenosine because of history of chronic obstructive pulmonary disease or asthma. These patients are prime candidates for dobutamine stress perfusion imaging. Other candidates include patients who drink coffee or use medication containing theophylline (within 12 h) before a scheduled dipyridamole or adenosine myocardial perfusion study. Patients who use oral dipyridamole could attain dangerously high adenosine levels if adenosine is administered intravenously as pharmacologic stress. These patients are also candidates for dobutamine stress testing. In addition patients with heart failure who are already receiving low dose IV Dobutamine for ionotropic support are at times referred for stress perfusion imaging. In these patients it may be more reasonable to perform Dobutamine stress study by simply

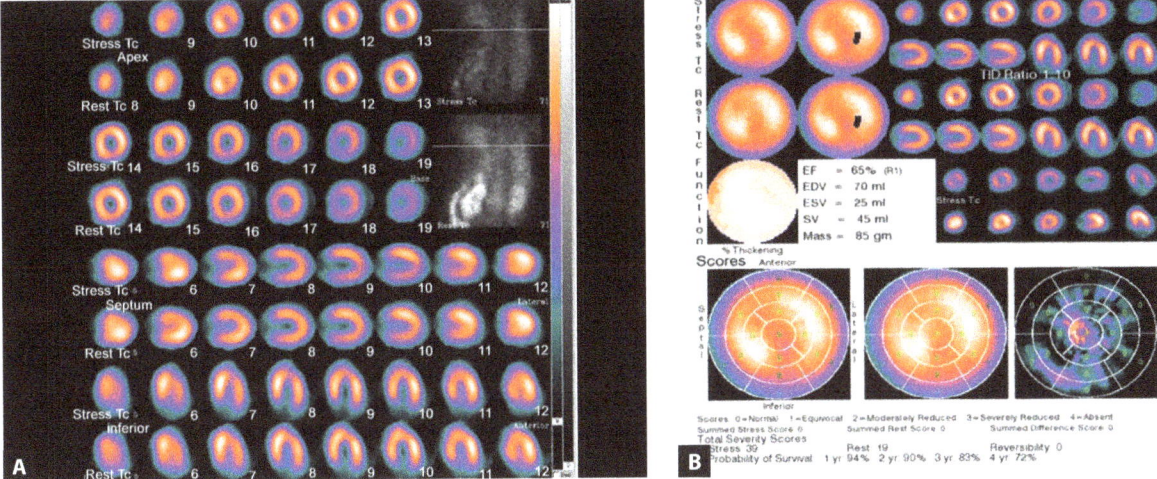

Figs 8A and B: IV adenosine infusion gated myocardial perfusion scan reveals uniform stress perfusion pattern with good systolic wall thickening is seen in all the defined myocardial segments

increasing its dose rather than a dipyridamole or adenosine perfusion scan.

Protocol

The protocol used begins with a low dose of dobutamine 10 ug/kg/min for 3 min and increases to maximum of 40 ug/kg/min every 3 min. Thallium-201/ Tc-99m Sestamibi is injected 5 min after starting the first dose of dobutamine with the infusion maintained for another 2 min. The infusion is stopped after 3 min and image acquired followed by delayed (or rest) image acquisition.

Mechanism of Action

Dobutamine is a predominant beta-1 agonist that increases heart rate and myocardial contractility at sufficiently high dose. Dobutamine also increases systolic blood pressure. The increases in three parameter results in increased myocardial oxygen demand. Normal coronary arteries dilate to increase perfusion in order to meet the demand, stenotic arteries may not be able to increase blood flow to the same degree as normal vessels creating a perfusion defect based on a similar physiologic response as that triggered by exercise stress.

Various data from series of patients who have undergone this dobutamine myocardial perfusion imaging indicated that an increase in heart rate is the most consistent effect of dobutamine. Systolic blood pressure increases, peaking around 20 ug/kg/min, diastolic blood pressure decreases due to the peripheral (beta-2) vasodilator effect of dobutamine.

Recent PET studies using 13N-ammonia show that changes in blood flow after administration of dobutamine myocardial blood flow with 40 ug/kg/min dose of dobutamine. The increase in blood flow is significantly related to heart rate a good correlation between increase in blood flow and oxygen demand.

This result is expected because the primary cause of increased coronary blood flow with dobutamine has increased oxygen demand; the direct effect of coronary vasodilatation produced by dobutamine is secondary. With dipyridamole and adenosine on the other hand, myocardial perfusion increases primarily because of the drug's vasodilatory effect on the coronary arteries.

Side Effects

- Palpitation due to patient's awareness of increased heart rate and force of contraction.
- Chest pain.
- Headache, flushing and dyspnea.
- Premature ventricular ectopic beats.
- Occasional ventricular tachycardia with atrial fibrillation.

Dobutamine has a longer biological half-life about 2 min than adenosine. Many of its adverse effects are similar to those reported with adenosine and usually last only a few mins. Rarely do patients require medication such as a rapidly acting beta blocker, i.e. esmolol to neutralize the side effects of dobutamine.

Sensitivity and Specificity in Detecting Coronary Artery Disease

Dobutamine perfusion imaging detects CAD with a greater accuracy in patients with multivessel disease (100%) than in patients with single vessel disease (84%). Another recent study using dobutamine–thallium SPECT in patient reported a sensitivity of 97% and specificity of 80% for detecting CAD. Another two studies using dobutamine Sestamibi imaging found sensitivities of 80% and 83% and specificities of 74% and 89% respectively. The same studies reported sensitivities of 85% and 75% respectively for echocardiography with dobutamine.

PHARMACOLOGICAL STRESS PERFUSION IMAGING WITH LOW LEVEL TREADMILL/BICYCLE EXERCISE

It has been seen that only pharmacological stress perfusion imaging interferes with image interpretation particularly of inferior wall/segment of myocardium because of frequent occurrence of side effects with pharmacological stress such as the splanchnic pooling of tracer. This can be overcome with clubbing the former with moderate or even low grade exercise. The risk of brady-arrhythmias is minimized with combination of exercise to adenosine infusion protocol. The exercise could be on bicycle ergometer (at a workload of 25 to 50 watts) or on the treadmill following modified Bruce or even a flat low-grade demonstration level exercise. Strict monitoring of ECG for any arrhythmia, close watch on the blood pressure and the patients symptoms is to be done **(Fig. 9)**.

NEW OPTIONS IN PHARMACOLOGICAL STRESS (FIG. 10)

Regadenoson is an effective new agent for pharmacological stress used for myocardial perfusion imaging. It has equal effectiveness for myocardial perfusion scan compared with adenosine. It has reduced side effects and better patient tolerability than adenosine. Unlike other pharmacological agent, there is no need to calculate the appropriate dose taking into consideration the weight and height of the patient. It is usually administered in single bolus injection, i.e. 400 ug in 5 mL normal saline for all patients. Immediately 5 mL normal saline is usually flushed following regadenoson administration. Immediately after, 10 second injection of either TC99m sestamibi or tetrofosmin is injected within a period of 10 second following which 5 mL of normal saline is flushed. Within 1 minute of the administration, the imaging can be started. It is usually indicated as an alternative to dobutamine or adenosine in asthma/COPD.

Mode of Action

It has low affinity A2A receptor agonist. It has highly selectivity at least 10-fold lower affinity for the A1 receptor and weak if any affinity for the A2B receptor and A3 receptors. Finally A2A activation produces coronary vasodilation and increases coronary flow.

REGADENOSON MYOCARDIAL PERFUSION SCINTIGRAPHY (FIG. 11)

Positron Emission Tomography Imaging

Positron emission tomography techniques are employed to map myocardial perfusion and detect ischemic response to stress in the presence of coronary artery disease, quantitate the regional coronary blood flow which can identify diffuse atherosclerosis often undetectable on an angiogram and in the assessment of myocardial tissue viability.

Positron emitting isotopes used in cardiac PET	
Category/compounds	Function (mechanism)
Tracers of blood flow	
13-N ammonia	Metabolic trapping
82Rb	Sodium-Potassium pump
15O-water	Diffusion
62 Copper PT SM	Lipophilicity
11C (gallium 68) albumin microsphere	Capillary blockage
Tracers of metabolism	
11C-palmitate	Fatty acid metabolism
18-F-FDG	Exogenous glucose metabolism
11C-acetate	Oxidative metabolism
15O-oxygen	Oxygen consumption
11C (13N) amino acid synthesis	Amino acid and protein metabolism
Other tracers	
18F-misonidazole	Hypoxic and ischemic tissue
11C-carbon monoxide	Blood pool

The most commonly used radiopharmaceutical for cardiac PET imaging are F-18 FDG, Rubidum-82 Chloride, N-13 ammonia, O-15 water.

Injury to the myocardium is typically caused by decreased blood flow, a consequence of arteriosclerosis. Such evaluations involve monitoring regional coronary blood flow and ongoing active metabolism. These procedures can help identify potential viability of injured myocardium, regions likely to benefit from revascularization to facilitate its return to its normal function, e.g. PET study showing increased glucose consumption (using

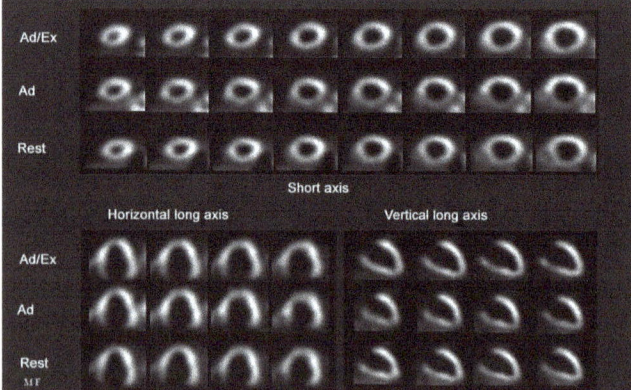

Fig. 9: IV adenosine infusion with low level treadmill exercise images showing improvement in the perfusion pattern particularly of the inferior myocardial segment which was showing a perfusion defect in the inferior segment in IV adenosine perfusion study without low level exercise

Chapter 29: Clinical Applications of Nuclear Cardiology Procedures and its Future Directions

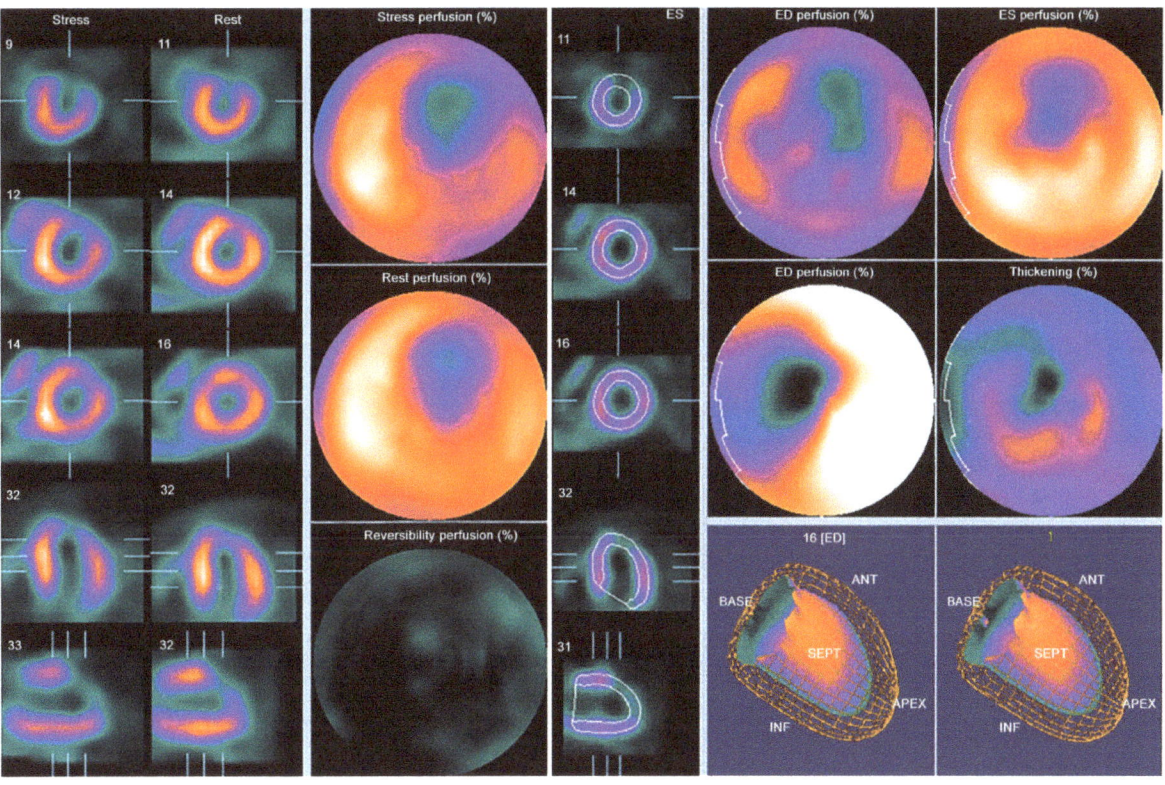

Fig. 10: IV regadenoson myocardial perfusion study showing fixed perfusion defect pertaining to anterior segment of the myocardium

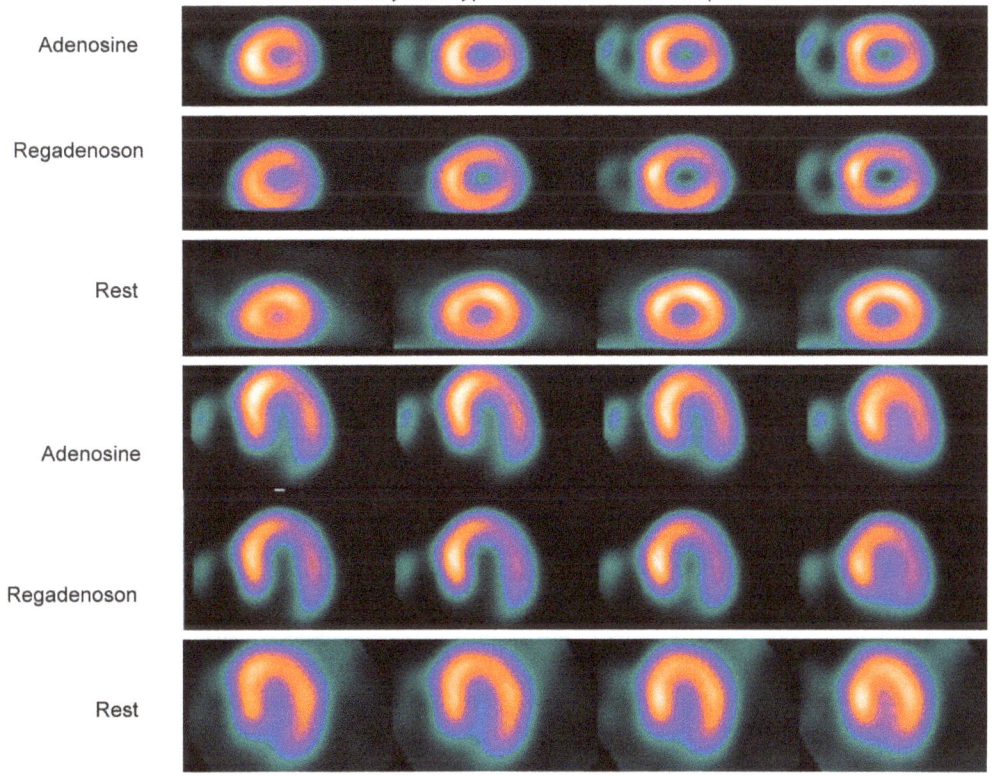

Fig. 11: Comparison MPI study showing the efficacy and superiority of IV regadenoson in defining the area of perfusion defect particularly anterolateral segment with respect to adenosine perfusion study

F-18 FDG) in myocardial areas of decreased blood flow (using N-13 ammonia or Rb-82) would indicate that restoration of cardiac function in those areas would be possible. Impaired contractile function in response to chronic reduction of resting blood flow may mask myocardial viability in some patients with severe CAD with the use of O-15 water, cardiologists obtain images of artery walls, where live tissue is designated by areas of illumination caused by high oxygen consumption.

Tracers of Myocardial Perfusion

Positron emitting radionuclides used for assessment of regional perfusion can be classified into two groups:
1. Tracers that are only partly extracted by the myocardium (Rb-82 chloride and N-13 ammonia).
2. Tracers that are freely diffusible (O-15 water).

Rubidium-82 PET Myocardial Perfusion Imaging (Fig. 12)

Myocardial perfusion imaging with positron emitter can be done without onsite cyclotron which is relatively complicated with an onsite source of generator produced tracer i.e. Rubidium-82.

Rb-82 is a monovalent cation and has ultra-short half-life 75 sec. Sr-82 decays to an elution column. Rb82 is eluted with 25 to 50 mL of normal saline by a computer controlled elution pump, connected by IV tubing to the patient. This generator has almost no breakthrough of strontium and has useful life of 4–6 weeks. Serial evaluations of regional myocardial perfusion can be made at intervals as short as 5 minutes. The short half-life of Rb82 taxes the performance limits of PET scanners; it facilitates the rapid completion of a series of resting and stress myocardial perfusion studies. Rb-82 is a very efficient imaging agent for routine clinical usage. Although the cost per patient at a low volume of studies per day is high, the cost with 6–10 studies per day is competitive with SPECT tracers.

The first pass extraction of Rb-82 at rest is approximately 50–60% and it is via Na^+/K^+ ATpase pump. Myocardial extraction of Rb-82 is similar to thallium–201 and slightly less than N-13 ammonia, decreasing during hyperemia. Rb-82 extraction can be altered by severe acidotic hypoxia and ischemia. Thus uptake of Rb-82 is a function of both blood flow and of myocardial cell integrity. Rb-82 perfusion imaging is usually performed before and after vasodilator stress rather than with exercise. Infarcted myocardium does not retain intravenously administered Rb-82. After administration, it washes out rapidly from damaged myocardial cells following the initial uptake phase. A mixture of reversible and irreversible myocardial tissue in the field of view results in an intermediate level of Rb-82 wash out that is proportional to the percentage of viable or infarcted tissue.

Imaging of Rb-82: Patient preparation for stress and rest myocardial PET perfusion imaging is identical to SPECT perfusion imaging. Despite the short half-life of Rb82, modern PET gamma cameras are able to obtain good quality images. The usual protocol takes approximately 15 minutes with a BGO crystal PET scanner and 35 minutes with LSO crystals PET scanner. The proper positioning is done with a low dose (20 mci) injection of Rb-82 and short 3 minutes scout acquisition and quick reconstruction. Subsequently, rest transmission imaging, rest perfusion 2D imaging and rest gated 3D imaging were done sequentially. Stress imaging is also done in similar manner. Transmission imaging is usually done with a germanium-68 pin or rod source, which takes about 8 minutes.

Tomographic data from Rb82 images can be displayed using polar maps utilizing the bulls eye approach with the apex located at the center and the base at the rim. Both relative and absolute flow reserve can be depicted on quantitative polar maps on Rb82 activity. In this manner, the rest and stress images are functionally interrelated. Three dimensional (3-D) topographic displays of Rb82 cardiac activity are more quantitative with respect to the polar maps. An automated quantitative analysis programmed may enhance accuracy and reproducibility of cardiac PET flow studies.

The sensitivity and specificity of PET MPI are superior to other noninvasive tests. Four studies involving a total of 342 patients have made direct comparisons of Tl-201 SPECT and PET MPI. In addition a survey of numerous studies of PET MPI in 1391 patients found excellent sensitivity (92%: CI = 90% to 94%) and specificity (90% CI = 88% to 92%). Churchwell et al. has also shown greater accuracy in a blinded analysis of the accuracy of 82 Rb PET in 194 patients with new quantitative software developed in their laboratory. Patterson et al. has also shown significantly better results with 82-Rb PET than their own SPECT Tl-201 results. These comparisons and Emory University's extensive clinical experiences are over 30,000 SPECT Tl-201 and over 2000 MPI. Though all patients with intermediate risk of coronary artery disease can undergo PET MPI, it is preferable to SPECT MPI in a subgroup of patients with attenuation problems i.e. large patients, women, breast implants or left mastectomy, chest wall deformity, left pleural or pericardial effusion. However, it must be emphasized that attenuation problems in SPECT cannot be predicted with confidence from examination of body habitus. There is an incremental benefit caused by greater specificity and sensitivity which gives rise to incremental economic benefit caused by more accurate tests like Rb82 PET MPI.

During the last 10 to 15 years, both SPECT and PET imaging have undergone significant improvements. A recent comparison between Tc-99m sestamibi SPECT and Rb82 PET MPI revealed a significant margin of improvement for CAD detection accuracy with Rb82 PET compared to SPECT. Given the proven value of PET myocardial perfusion imaging in the diagnosis of CAD, it is expected that the prognostic value of gated PET is also high, similar to SPECT imaging.

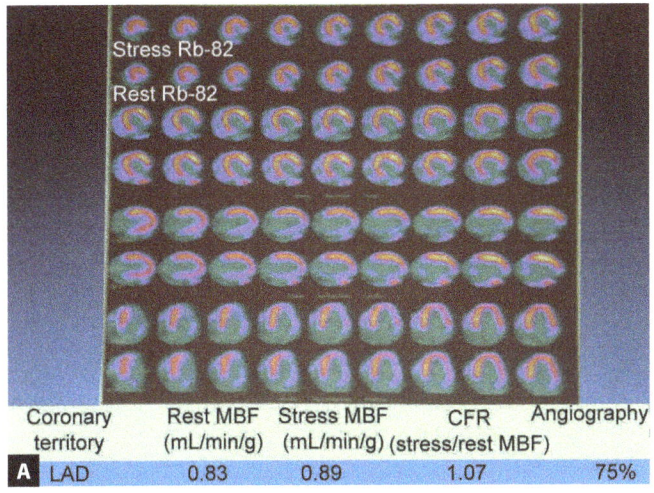
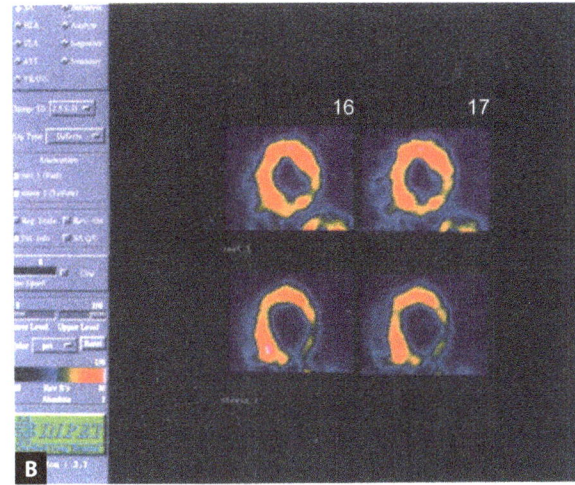

Figs 12A and B: (A) Rubidium-82 PET myocardial perfusion image showing defect involving inferolateral segments; (B) Rubidium-82 PET myocardial perfusion image a fixed showing a reversible perfusion defect involving small part of anterior and inferolateral myocardial segments

PET CT unit has become the preferred approach for PET imaging in oncology. The potential benefits of PET-CT in cardiac imaging are reduction in acquisition time by 10–12 minutes in comparison to a dedicated PET system. PET-CT imaging holds challenges and solution for the attenuation correction problem.

N-13 Ammonia/O-15 Labeled Water PET Perfusion Imaging (Fig. 14)

13N ammonia has been used for most of the scientific investigation in cardiac PET imaging for the past two decades. Its 10 minutes half-life requires an onsite cyclotron and radiochemistry synthesis capability. Imaging protocol from scout position to stress imaging takes 100–120 mins. Pharmacologic stress imaging usually follows resting injection and imaging, after the initial activity has been allowed to decay by staggering patients or using differential dose for rest and stress. Both rest and stress images can be gated. A dynamic acquisition is acquired for the quantification of blood flow. This can be accomplished by performing separate dynamic and gated acquisition with the same injection, or included list mode acquisitions. A third injection may be included for cold pressor testing. 13N ammonia imaging is time cumbersome, needs logistic and coordination.

In the blood stream, 13N ammonia consists of neutral ammonia (NH13) in equilibrium with its charged ammonium ion (NH4). The neutral NH3 molecule readily diffuses across plasma and cell membranes. Inside the cell, it re-equilibrates with its ammonium form which is trapped in glutamine via the enzyme glutamine synthase. Despite back diffusion, the first pass trapping of 13N ammonia at rest is high although decreasing with higher blood flow.

13N ammonia allows good quality gated and ungated images, taking full advantage of the superior resolution of PET imaging. Interestingly normal volunteers show mild heterogeneity or mild defect of 13N ammonia retention in the lateral wall of the left ventricle compared with other segments. The mechanism of this is not known. This must be taken in to account for both visual activity and increased lung activity in patient with lung congestion.

Myocardial Metabolism

A fundamental characteristic of the myocardium is its continuous requirement for oxygen and metabolic substrates to meet its energy demands. This process largely occurs by oxidizing fatty acids and glucose. Under normal conditions, fatty acids are the preferred energy source for overall oxidative metabolism. When blood flow is reduced to the heart muscle and ischemia ensues, fatty acids can no longer be oxidized and glucose becomes the preferred energy source. This metabolic phenomenon is useful for the identification of myocardium that is underperfused but still viable. Such tissue is often

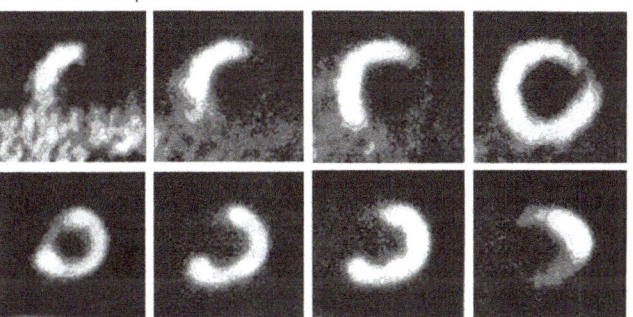

Fig. 13: Intense F-18 FDG uptake in inferior and lateral wall of the myocardium with a resting perfusion defect in the upper row of the image suggesting hybernating myocardium

hypokinetic or akinetic but returns to normal or near-normal function if blood flow is restored. Consequently, in patients with severely impaired ventricular function, combined with measurements of myocardial perfusion and glucose metabolism have been advocated. It may be noteworthy to mention that eating fat and protein shifts the heart away from using glucose as an energy source.

Metabolic Tracers

Fluorine-18 FDG, C-11 palmitate, and C-11 acetate are typical examples of PET radiopharmaceuticals used for metabolic cardiac studies. 'Deoxyglucose' is an analog of glucose that can be labeled with F-18, a cyclotron produced radionuclide, to form F18-FDG. Its myocardial uptake reflects overall myocardial utilization of glucose. Palmitate is a naturally occurring fatty acid that can be chemically synthesized and labeled with C-11, a cyclotron-produced radionuclide with a physical half-life of approximately 20.4 minutes. Its myocardial uptake and clearance reflect the myocardial utilization of fatty acids **(Fig. 13)**.

The utilization of fatty acids and glucose by the heart is exquisitely sensitive to the level of glucose, fatty acids, and insulin in the blood, as well as the level of blood flow to the myocardium. Consequently, the substrate environment must be standardized when these two tracers are used to study myocardial metabolism. FDG-6P is the trapped form of the compound. Injected after the patient has fasted, insulin forces FDG into muscle cells, including myocardium.

Acetate labeled with C-11 has emerged as a promising tracer of overall oxidative metabolism under diverse loading conditions levels of blood flow. Unlike C-11 palmitate and FDG, the myocardial kinetics of C-11 acetate are relatively insensitive to changes in the substrate environment.

Fluorine-18 FDG Metabolic Imaging (Fig. 14)

18F-FDG is a glucose analogue which crosses the capillary and sarcolemmal membrane at a rate proportional to that of glucose. Following myocardial uptake, FDG is phosphorylated to FDG phosphate and is then trapped in the myocardium unlike phosphorylated glucose. Regional myocardial uptake of FDG therefore reflects relative distribution of regional rates of exogenous glucose utilization, unlike the brain which mainly depends upon glucose metabolism. The myocardium is an omnivore. There are three major circulating substances which affect the myocardial metabolism: blood glucose, FFAs and insulin. Many other factors, such as the fasting period and age, also affect the FDG uptake. Even hospitalization status (in patient or outpatient) has an influence on the myocardial FDG uptake.

This complexity interferes with the interpretation of data obtained from FDG-PET imaging. To accommodate this complexity of metabolism, there are several different protocols for myocardial FDG PET imaging. These protocols can be divided into two major categories—One is imaging under low myocardial glucose metabolism which includes imaging under fasting conditions. The other protocol images the myocardium under high to maximum myocardial glucose metabolism which includes oral glucose loading and the euglycemic insulin clamp technique.

Under fasting conditions the normal myocardium primarily utilizes fatty acids, while glucose utilization and thus FDG uptake becomes minimal. Under this condition, ischemic myocardium with enhanced glucose metabolism markedly takes up FDG, which is displayed on PET images as hot spots. The problem of imaging under fasting conditions is the heterogeneous distribution of FDG in to normal myocardium. Usually the lateral wall of the left ventricle tends to show higher FDG uptake than the septum. High background activity with low tissue, FDG uptake also leads to poor image quality. For these reasons, FDG PET under fasting condition has recently not been recommended for clinical viability assessment.

The most commonly used protocol is oral glucose loading. Ingestion of about 50–70 g of glucose stimulates insulin secretion and increases the FDG uptake into normal myocardium to near maximum. This enhances the image quality with homogenous myocardial FDG uptake. Euglycemic insulin clamping is an alternative technique to oral glucose loading and is slightly more complex but guarantees more stable and controlled metabolic conditions. FDG uptake in to normal and ischemic but viable myocardium is enhanced and negative FDG uptake is considered to indicate scar tissue.

Thus hibernating myocardium therefore would demonstrate increased FDG uptake in the fasting state unlike the surrounding normal myocardium. But in the postprandial state (with oral glucose loading) hibernating myocardium would demonstrate FDG uptake. Therefore, either preserved or even enhanced FDG uptake in dysfunctional myocardial regions represent presence of myocardial viability by the help of most popular criterion of flow-metabolism mismatch methods. However, using this criterion requires a perfusion image preferably acquired either with PET or SPECT perfusion study.

Regional dysfunction due to stunned myocardium may be manifested by normal blood flow and normal, enhanced or reduced glucose utilization using FDG and flow images. Only criteria to diagnose this myocardium is the presence of regional myocardial wall motion abnormalities **(Fig. 15)**.

Myocardial Stunning and Hibernation

In 1975 Heyndrickx et al. demonstrated in a concuss dog model that a 15 min coronary occlusion (a period generally not associated with cell death) followed by reperfusion produced a marked depression in regional contractile function that persisted for atleast 6 hours after reperfusion. The term myocardial stunning was described this viability tissue that exhibits prolonged postischemic ventricular dysfunction even after the normal perfusion is restored. Stress-rest Tc-99m

Chapter 29: Clinical Applications of Nuclear Cardiology Procedures and its Future Directions

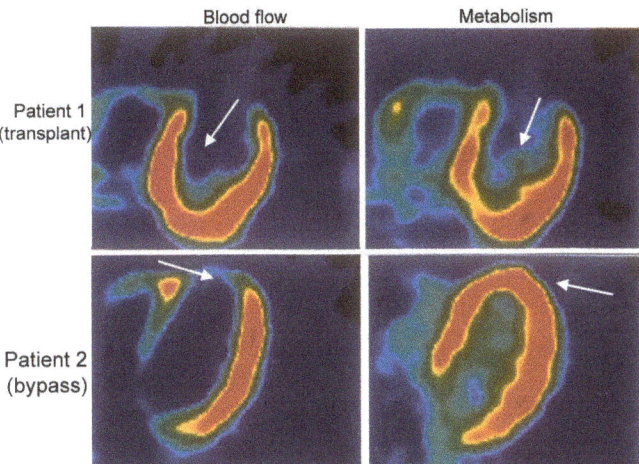

Fig. 14: Perfusion-metabolism mismatch using N-13 ammonia and F-18-FDG PET imaging tracer suggesting decreased perfusion with adequate metabolism in the involved myocardium

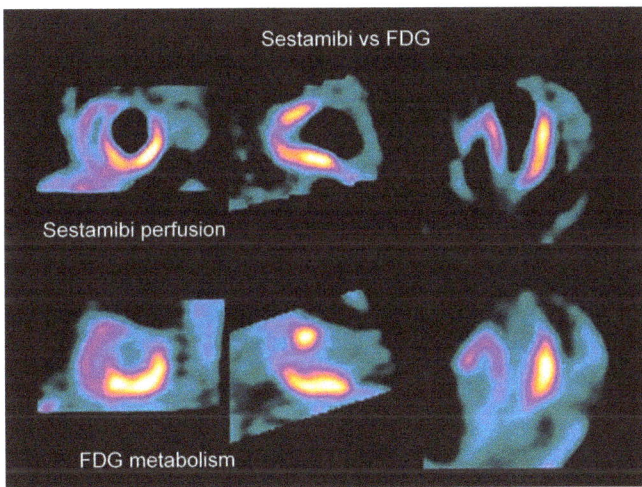

Fig. 15: Shows a significant area of resting perfusion defect involving anteroseptal segment of the myocardium without having significant FDG uptake suggesting scarred dead myocardium

SPECT MIBI/tetrofosmin myocardial function and perfusion study permits demonstration of stunning in patients with CAD after exercise and dobutamine induced ischemia contractile dysfunction despite restoration of normal function shown in the rest study.

The concept that stunning and hibernation may be casually related is supported by PET quantitative myocardial blood flow and flow reserved studies, which indicate that flow falls in chronically dysfunctional myocardium after a period of chronic stunning. Usually hibernating myocardium evident in FDG study has fair degree of FDG uptake is usually seen in resting fixed myocardial perfusion defects. Revascularization restores function in the functional hibernating state.

Myocardial Infarct Imaging

Myocardial infarct imaging agents are classified as:
- Hot-spot infarct-avid agents
- Cold spot markers of hypoperfused tissue.

Tc-99m Pyrophosphate

Tc-99m pyrophosphate planar imaging has been used for detection of myocardial infarction but used less commonly today with availability of better agents for imaging. During the ischemia there is increased flux of Ca^{++} ions across the cell membrane. So as the intracellular concentration of Ca^{++} ions increase it damages the cell irreversibility. So, this Ca^{++} ion provides the binding site for pyrophosphate. Pyrophospatase binds to the mitochondrial calcium complexes and proteins in region of necrotic myocardium.

The maximal uptake of pyrophosphate is by 24–48 hours after injection and scan may remain positive for six days. Some patients may show uptake by 12 hours. The scan to be positive in the uptake if the suspected lesion should be more than uptake in ribs. Sometimes a "doughnut pattern" of uptake is seen in large infarcts as less tracer reaches to central necrotic zone. Other than the infarct increased pyrophosphate uptake is also seen in cardiomyopathy, pericarditis, valvular calcification, amyloid heart, etc.

Tc-99m Labeled Glucarate

Glucaric acid, a six cycle dicarboxylic acid sugar is a small molecule which clears from the blood very rapidly and localizes in necrotic tissue by attachment to highly basic nuclear histones in the myocite. Acute MI can be visualized within 1–2 hours of onset of pain in patients with or without thrombolytic therapy. Technetium labeled glucaric acid will have an important role in the emergency room while evaluating the patient suffering from acute coronary syndrome.

Indium-111 Labeled Antimyosin Antibodies

Myosin is a larger intracellular protein present in abundance in myocardial cells. When the cell membrane is disrupted i.e. in acute myocardial infarction, these are exposed to outside. These antibodies are tagged with Indium-111 and used for imaging infarct. Nowadays fab fragments of these antibodies are used which is more specific thus pyrophosphate in infarct imaging.

Around 2 mci of injection of Indium-111-antimyosin antibodies immediately starts accumulating at the site of infarct. But its blood clearance is very slow (T1/2 =6–12 hours). So by 24 hours or later, images are acquired which will give a good diagnostic yield. Antimyosin antibodies have overall sensitivity of 92% in detection of acute MI. False positive findings are also seen in patients with myocarditis and idiopathic dilated cardiomyopathy.

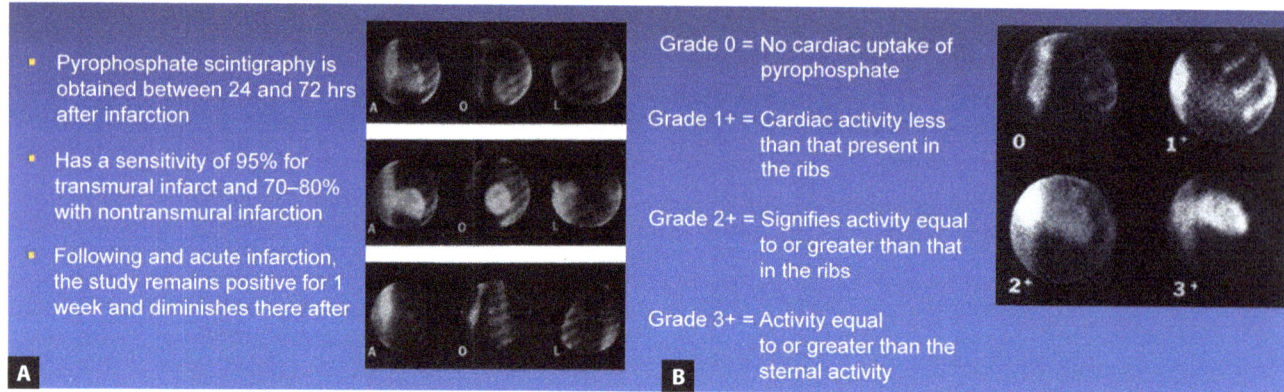

Figs 16A and B: (A) Technetium labeled pyrophosphate; (B) Various scoring grades in relation to myocardial lesions

Combined antimyosin and planar thallium imaging may provide prognostic information for risk stratification for future coronary events. A matched defect i.e. a fixed defect on thallium showing an area of antimyosin antibodies uptake confirm the irreversible damage to the area.

An unmatched defect i.e. absence of antimyosin uptake in thallium defect or patchy uptake of antimyosin antibodies in thallium defect confirms the presence of hibernating myocardium which warrants immediate intervention.

It has also been observed that antimyosin antibodies are picked by patients of unstable angina. So it can be used for prognostication in patients of unstable angina.

In patients receiving doxorubicin (a cardiotoxic drug), antimyosin antibodies can play a role in identifying cardiotoxicity in form of intense accumulation of this radiotracer.

Antimyosin antibodies can also be used in evaluation of heart transplant rejection and myocarditis or cardiomyopathy.

Technetium-99m Labeled Annexin V (Fig. 17)

Usually, cell death occurs through two very distinctive processes, necrosis or apoptosis. Apoptosis (programmed cell death/cell suicide) signal induced and result in progressive cell shrinkage and systemic cleavage of proteins and DNA. This is an energy dependent process. Hence, the cell membrane integrity is maintained unlike necrosis. Subsequently, cell breaks into finger like processes i.e. apoptotic bodies which are cleared by phagocytosis by neighboring cells or scavenger cells resulting in inflammation or scar. As compared to the cell necrosis where the damage occurs to the cell membrane integrity which results in denaturation of proteins and DNA damage. This results in release of intracellular contents and ultimately cell ruptures resulting in disintegration or scar. Annexin is a protein having similar structural and functional characteristics that have an affinity to bind phospholipids surfaces. It is a 34 kd protein binds to the phosphatidylserine expose in the cell surface. Tc-99m labeled Annexin V (22–30 mci with 0.5–1.0 mg Annexin) is injected and 4–6 hours following each injection imaging of myocardium can be initiated. Annexin accumulates in acute necrotic myocardium as a hot spot infarct-avid agent. The localization can be done by simultaneously doing a thallium-201 imaging **(Figs 18 and 19)**.

DUAL ISOTOPE IMAGING USING TL-201 AND F-18 FDG IMAGING

Assessment of metabolism by PET provides the sensitive detection of tissue viability based on the integrity of cardiac substrate metabolism. The increased FDG uptake in the hibernating myocardium appears to be an independent prognostic parameter identifying ischemically compromised myocardium and thus high risk clinical conditions. This metabolic signal of jeopardized myocardium is especially helpful in patients with advanced ischemic heart failure because revascularization is associated with higher risk. The most important functional recovery following revascularization of the failing heart is the amount of hibernating myocardium present.

Metabolic imaging with PET offers a sophisticated means of assessing regional tissue viability in patients with advanced coronary artery disease (CAD) and impaired left ventricular function. The assessment of relative and regional uptake covering the complete left ventricular volume represents an advantage over competing modalities. The classification of myocardial tissue into viable, hibernating or scarred can be performed with high sensitivity and specificity.

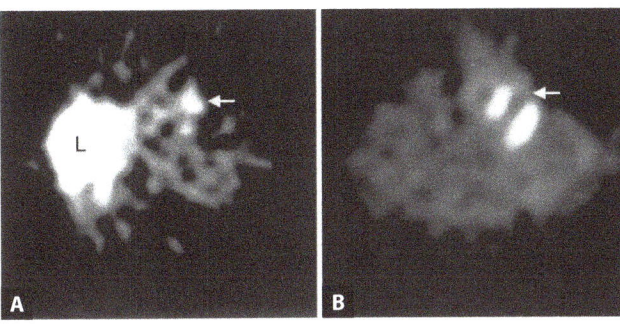

Figs 17A and B: Tc-99m labeled annexin myocardial infarct imaging showing a hot spot involving apical and lower septal segment of the myocardium which is showing a cold area in the regular thallium-201 myocardial perfusion imaging transaxial slices

Glucose Metabolism

^{18}F–fluorodeoxyglucose traces transmembranous transport as well as phosporylation of exogenous glucose. ^{18}F–fluorodeoxyglucose 6-phosphate does not enter any further metabolic pathways but accumulates in the myocardium, which is proportional to glucose transport and phosporylation.

Patient Preparation

Oral glucose loading is the most widely used approach for preparing patients for fluoro-2-deoxyglucose (FDG) imaging. FDG is administered 60–90 minutes after 50 g of oral glucose load. This switches the primary substrate for myocardial metabolism from free acids to glucose. This is facilitated by the release of insulin. Thus viable myocardium will preferentially take up glucose and hence FDG. In patients with diabetes, supplement insulin is necessary. Even with glucose loading protocols with bolus insulin, images are often sub-optimal in diabetics.

Most cardiac FDG studies are acquired 40–60 minutes after injection of tracer. This time period is required to reduce the FDG plasma concentration to ensure high contrast between the blood pool and the myocardium. In patients with diabetes mellitus, a longer waiting period is advised to enhance myocardium-to-blood contrast.

Data Interpretation

Matching of perfusion and FDG uptake of normal viable myocardium, which is not ischemic at rest whereas matched pattern of decreased perfusion and metabolism are indicative for irreversible tissue injury (scar). A mismatch pattern of reduced myocardial blood flow in presence of increased FDG uptake identifies viable but ischemically compromised myocardium. This helps to emphasize the clinician the true extent of viability and the potential for recoverable tissue.

Cardiac PET Scan Protocol

- Thallium perfusion scan at 8.30 am.
- FDG PET scan at 12 noon (blood sugar level should not be >130 mg/dL).

Where do we Ask for FDG PET Imaging in the Assessment of Myocardial Viability

One of the best-known disadvantages of PET is its low availability. PET scanners and on site cyclotron are too expensive for local hospitals. PET has only been available for a limited number of patients and researchers atleast in the last century. Because of this problem either stress-rest or rest-stress gated single photon emission computed tomography (SPECT) myocardial perfusion imaging with or without oral/IV augmented NG intervention with FDG SPECT imaging using ultra high energy collimator or dual isotope simultaneous acquisition (DISA) by injecting FDG at photo peak (511Kev) and Tc99m perfusion tracers such as IV tetrofosmin or MIBI allows simultaneous flow metabolism analysis with acceptable feasibility **(Figs 18 to 20)**.

The role of IV FDG PET with SPECT imaging should only be limited considering their higher cost to patients having fixed defects with stress-rest or rest-stress Tc99m tetrofosmin or rest-IV NTG intervention indicates a fixed defect which can be further confirmed by F-18 FDG imaging a gold standard myocardial viable method.

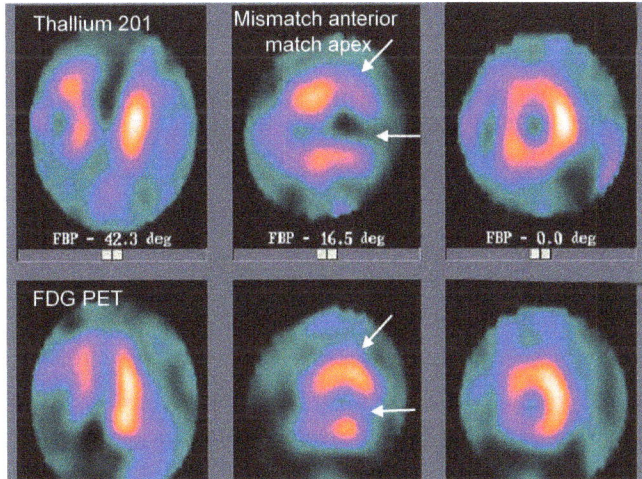

Fig. 18: Dual isotope myocardial imaging shows a stress defect involving part of anterior and apical myocardial segments which shows adequate metabolism involving anterior segments only. However, apical seems to have no metabolism suggesting scarred myocardium as evidenced from F-18 FDG metabolism study

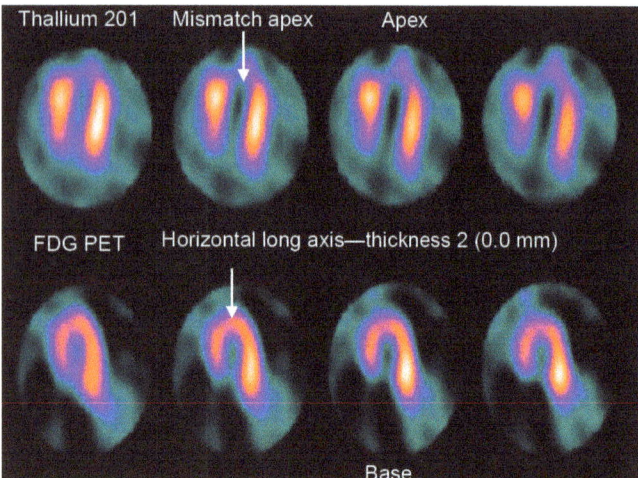

Fig. 19: Stress myocardial perfusion imaging with Thallium-201 perfusion showing an apical defect which shows adequate metabolism with F-18 FDG metabolism study as evidenced from the bottom row segments of images

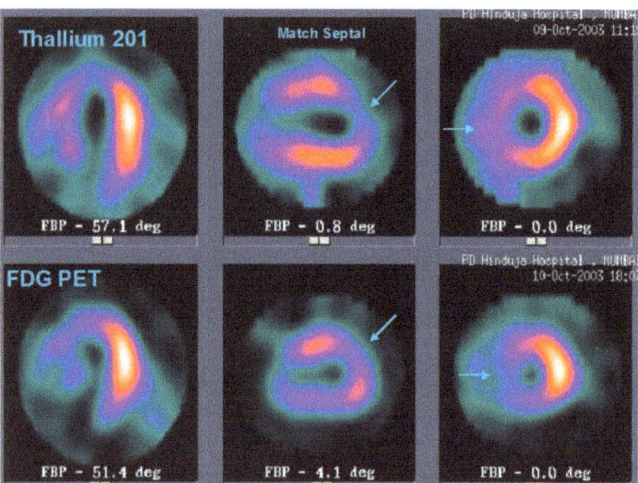

Fig. 20: Stress thallium myocardial perfusion study shows a perfusion defect involving anteroseptal segments which seems to have absent metabolism using F-18 FDG metabolic study

FLUORODEOXYGLUCOSE POSITRON EMISSION TOMOGRAPHY VERSUS FLUORODEOXYGLUCOSE SINGLE PHOTON EMISSION COMPUTED TOMOGRAPHY

A recent study by Sir Belink et al. compared the survival of patients randomized to PET-based or SPECT based management. The authors found only a very small and nonsignificant difference between these two management strategies. It seems from the result that it is not necessary to perform PET to make a Go/NoGo decision about coronary intervention in clinical practice. The PET cardiology community must make FDG PET imaging more accurate and sophisticated. There are several problems that need to be solved to make FDG PET more reliable and useful.

The one major problem in viability assessment using FDG PET is the absence of a standardized method. Both the imaging protocol (dynamic/static, loading/insulin clamp/ fasting) and data interpretation (mismatch/% uptake/metabolic rate) lacks standards. In 2003, American Society of Nuclear Cardiology (ASNC) issued a practice guideline for FDG/perfusion PET imaging. The requirement for standardization was partially solved by this guideline. However, more studies especially large scale multicentric trials are needed to establish the usefulness of FDG PET imaging in viability assessment.

One of the solutions for improving the accuracy of viability assessment with PET comes from the technology commonly used in SPECT. Applying the gated SPECT analysis techniques to FDG PET, evaluation becomes more precise. The big problem with this technique is the reliability of the analysis program, such as QGS, 4D-M SPECT or Emory cardiac tool box. These programs are all designed for clinical SPECT use. Thus parameters such as gamma fitting for wall detection are not optimized for PET. For several reasons, it is very hard for PET users to change and optimize such parameters. It is reported that ventricular volumes (EDV and ESV) measured by gated FDG PET are higher than those measured with MIBI SPECT, although there is a very good correlation between the former and latter. Even with this limited methodology, gated FDG PET shows significant incremental value over viability diagnosis as assessed by the perfusion- metabolism mismatch criterion.

Because of lower availability, increase cost and onsite cyclotron, FDG PET has limited utility in the present day clinical practice. FDG SPECT has taken a front seat for decades. Using an ultra high energy collimator, an FDG image could be obtained with routinely used relatively inexpensive gamma cameras, various studies has shown comparable results to conventional PET scanners. However, there are also results raising questions about the reliability of FDG SPECT particularly absence of photon attenuation correction in the imaging of SPECT camera. However, with the advent of CT containing (SPECT-CT) Hawk eye, Gamma camera system, the photon attenuation correction can be tackled efficiently especially while interpreting the inferior wall for viability assessment. Hence, FDG SPECT has one major benefit over PET namely that it allow dual isotope simultaneous acquisition (DISA). PET imaging uses only one photo peak (511 Kev) high energy photon and thus simultaneous dual-tracer acquisition is impossible. DISA using FDG and Tc99m perfusion tracer allows simultaneous flow and metabolism imaging in one sitting with acceptable feasibility.

EMERGING CONCEPTS IN NUCLEAR CARDIOLOGY (FIGS 21 AND 22)

- Cardiac software program
- Dedicated cardiac SPECT gamma camera
- New promising radiopharmaceuticals
- Useful combined nuclear cardiology techniques.

Cardiac Software Program

Several software packages available from a variety of vendors which are designed to process myocardial perfusion data and quantify various important parameters. We have been using quantitative gated SPECT (QGS) from Cedar-Sinai Medical center, 4D-M-SPECT. Emory cardiac tool box of Emory university where we calculate, end diastolic volume (EDV), end systolic volume (ESV), end systolic wall thickening and wall motion, ventricular global ejection fraction, perfusion scores i.e. defect size and reversibility, LV : RV count ratio, transient ischemic dilatation of LV (TID), heart lung ratio. Coronary flow reserve (CFR) = stress coronary flow reserve–rest coronary flow reserve.

Recently quatification of coronary blood flow through major artery, i.e. LAD, left circumplex and right coronary artery by the nuclear cardiology team of Brigham and Women hospital, Harvard Medical School, Boston.

Quantitation of Myocardial Blood Flow

This quantitation is particularly helpful in patient suffering from severe coronary artery disease having balanced ischemia. It is also helpful in patient having sub-clinical coronary artery disease where diagnosis is more important particularly in subset of patient having microvascular dysfunction. It is also helpful in monitoring the response to therapy, i.e. progression or regression of coronary artery disease. Here standard myocardial perfusion imaging may underestimate

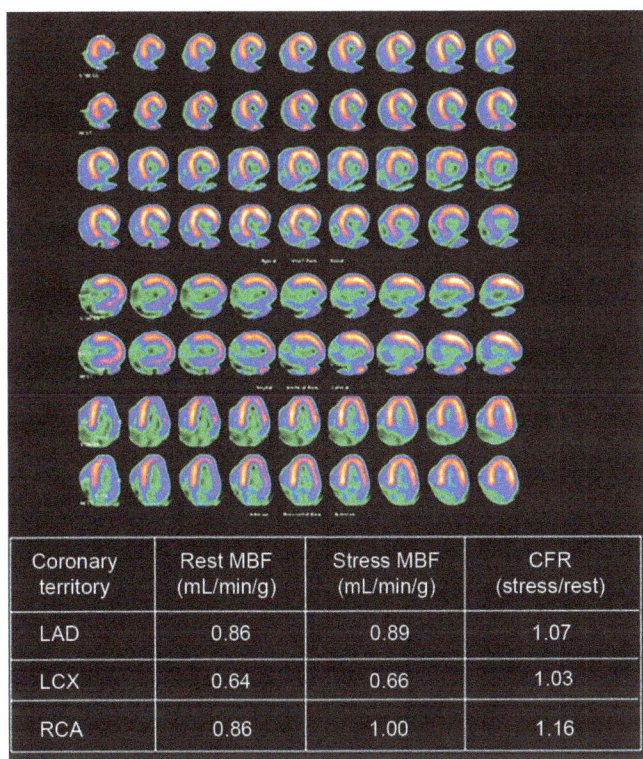

Coronary territory	Rest MBF (mL/min/g)	Stress MBF (mL/min/g)	CFR (stress/rest)
LAD	0.86	0.89	1.07
LCX	0.64	0.66	1.03
RCA	0.86	1.00	1.16

Fig. 22: Rubidium-82 myocardial perfusion study showing an area of fixed perfusion defect involving anteroseptal and inferior myocardial segments with the corresponding reduced coronary arterial blood flow in stress and rest study with coronary flow reserve (CFR) value

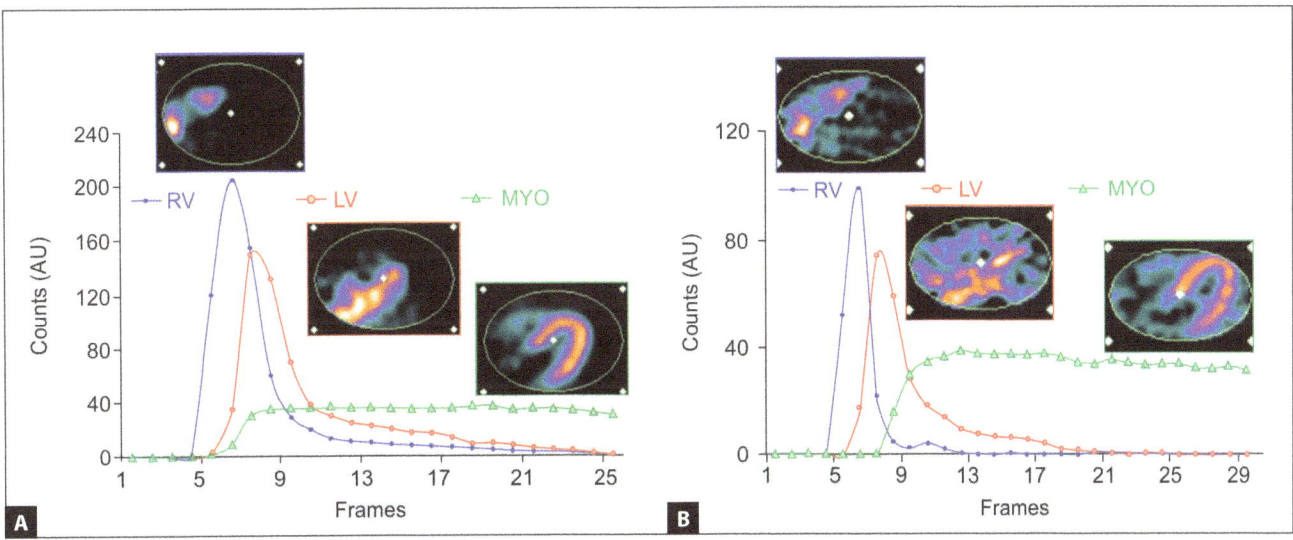

Figs 21A and B: Computation of myocardial blood flow with rubidium-82 and comparison to N13 ammonia

the extent of disease in 3 vessel coronary atherosclerosis here PET quantification of perfusion reserve (CFR) by use of Rb-82 net retention suggest a greater extent of the disease than the standard approach in patients with 3 vessel disease.

Protocol

Initially a scout scan is performed by administering a small dose of Rb-82 (10–20 mci). Next the attenuation correction image is acquired by using CT **(Fig. 23)**. List mode acquisition allowing for summed gated and dynamic image reconstruction from one injection. Most often rest scan is performed first followed by the stress scan. A single injection of Rb-82 40–60 mci in injected followed by emission scanning after permitting a pre-scan delay. This delay is important to allow for Rb-82 myocardial extraction from the blood pool and is usually 70–90 seconds. This will give highly accurate peak stress gated imaging the reflecting wall motion, E.F. at peak stress. IV dipyridamole is given as a weight based infusion over 4 minutes (0.56 mg/kg). Imaging is started as a list mode acquisition starting with the time of radiotracer injection (3 minutes after completion of dipyridamole infusion). Usually 40–60 mci of Rb-82 is given into the infusion.

COMPUTATION OF MYOCARDIAL BLOOD FLOW WITH RUBIDIUM-82 AND COMPARISON TO N13 AMMONIA (FIG. 21)

Reproducibility was evaluated in 22 subjects, accuracy was evaluated in 20 patients.

Myocardial Blood Flow Global Reduction in Flow, Coronary Steal (Fig. 24)

Dedicated Cardiac SPECT Gamma Camera

Dedicated cardiac SPECT gamma camera has come to the market. These are two types:
1. Dynamic SPECT cardiac gamma camera (DNM-530).
2. Solid state dedicated cardiac camera (D-SPECT).

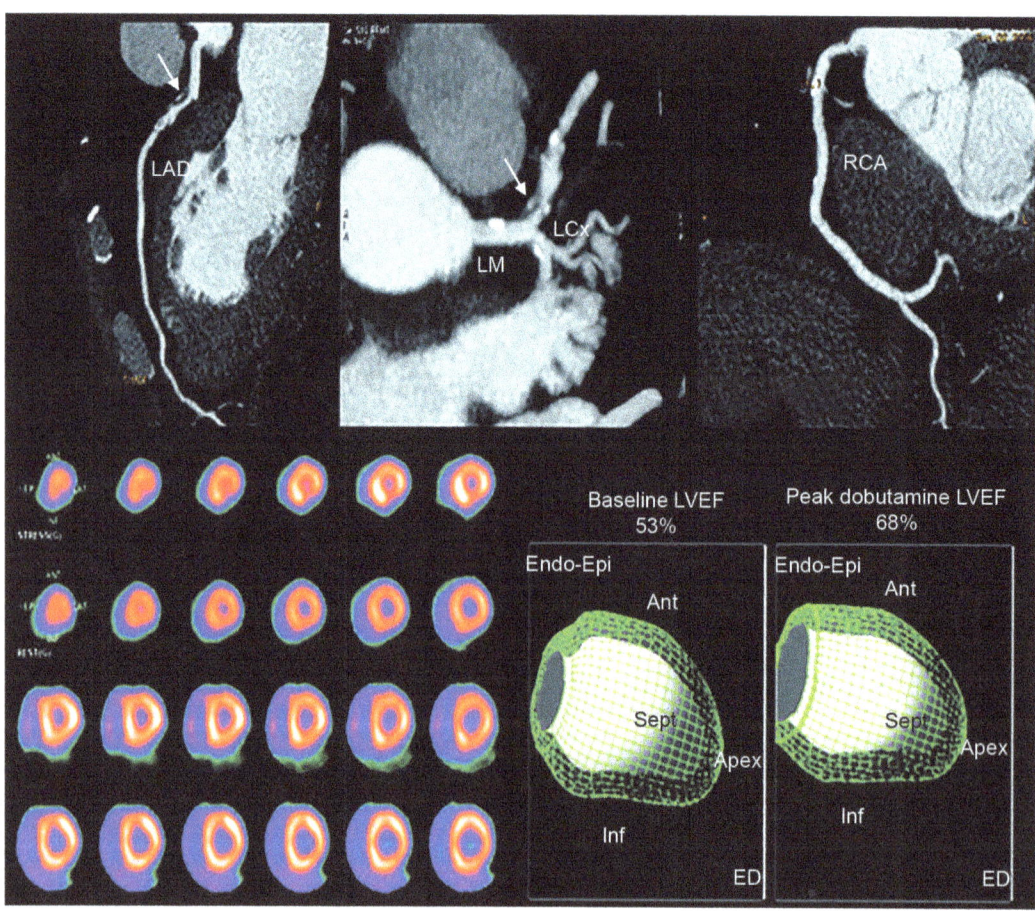

Fig. 23: Rubidium-82 myocardial perfusion study as well as CT of coronary arteries showing multiple plaques in LAD, LCx, RCA with having a small area of reduced perfusion pattern involving posterolateral segment with evidence of adequate reversible ischemia
Abbreviations: RCA, right coronary artery; LCx, left circumflex artery; LAD, left anterior descending; LVEF, left ventricular ejection fraction

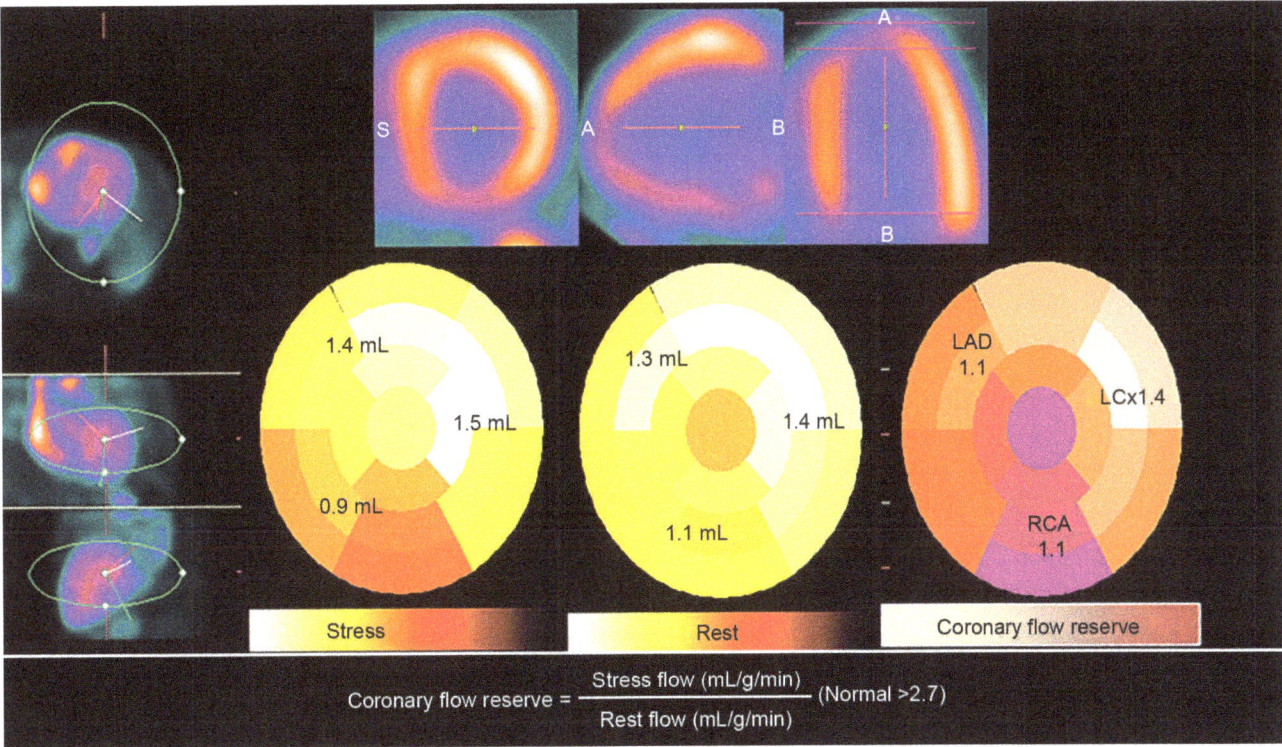

Fig. 24: Myocardial blood flow global reduction

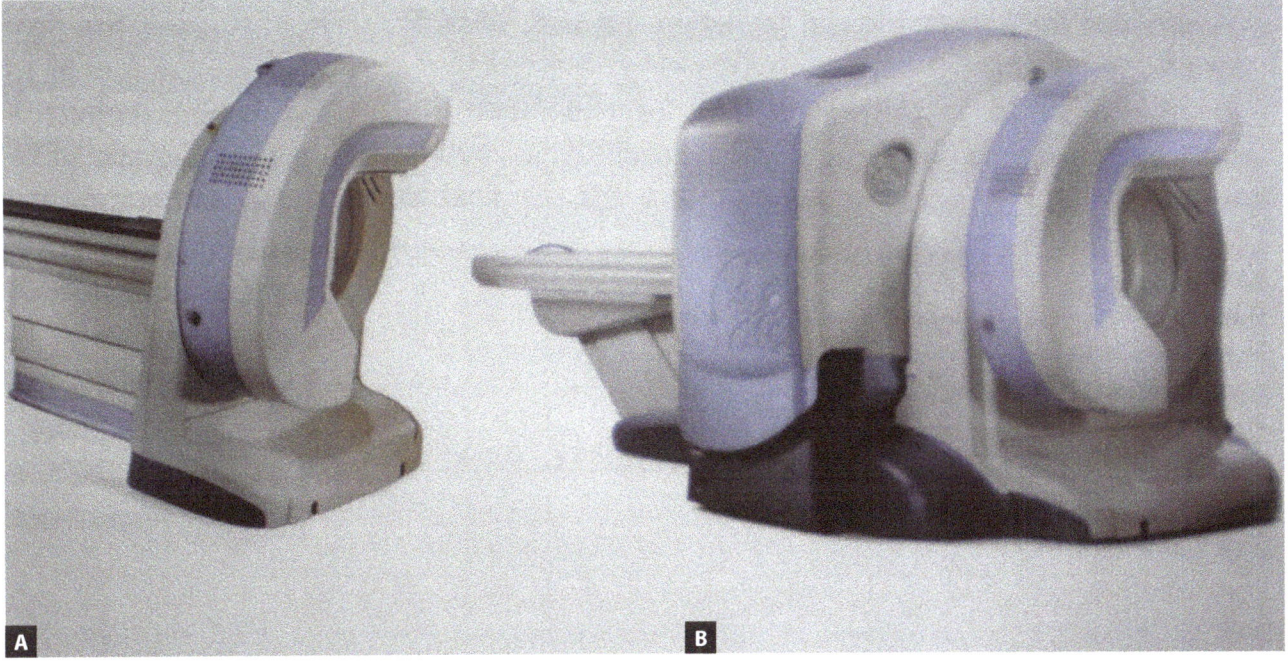

Figs 25A and B: (A) The discovery NM 530C (DNM) featuring a gantry, i.e. similar to a conventional cardiac SPECT camera with a different detector assembly. (B) Hybridization of the DNM camera with a multi detector CT camera

Dynamic SPECT Cardiac Gamma Camera (Figs 25A and B)

It is otherwise known as discovery NM 530 (DNM) SPECT marketed by GE it interfaces multi pinhole collimators with solid state modules aiming at slashing acquisition time without jeoparadizing quality.

DNM sensitivity, spatial resolution (SR), energy resolution (ER), counted response, cardiac uniformity and cardiac defect contrast as compared to conventional SPECT gamma camera which reveals sensitivity is higher spatial resolution is better and energy resolution is improved. The count rate is linear on DNM upto 612 KCPS as compared to severe dead time limitations as compared to conventional gamma camera **(Figs 26A and B)**. Additionally, it enables reduction of acquisition time thereby causing less radiation exposure to the patient with this fact acquisition protocol this may become a milestone in the evolution of nuclear cardiology as it assumes its key role in molecular imaging of the heart.

System Description

The DNM gantry is similar to that of an S-SPECT gamma camera. The detector assembly comprises a multi-pinhole collimator block, where each pinhole illuminates a solid state pixelated, gamma ray detector made of cadmium-zinc-telluride (CZT). Thus each pinhole and detector constitutes a complete miniature gamma camera. In CZT, an absorbed gamma camera ray is converted directly to an electric charge. In C-SPECT with scintillation crystals an absorbed gamma ray is first converted to ultraviolet light and only then to an. electrical change in an indirect process. The indirect process is inefficient and is then followed by a high amplification step in the photomultiplier tube resulting in limitation to the overall accuracy of the measured energy and position of the incident gamma rays. In CZT these limits are overcome by a direct signal of electron hole pairs that is 50 times bigger than the signal being amplified in the C-SPECT system.

Solid State Dedicated Cardiac Camera (D-Spect) (Figs 27 and 28)

Newly invented noninvasive methods for the assessment of ischemic heart disease. In clinical cardiac practice, MPI for evaluating regional myocardial blood flow and viability under rest or stress conditions has emerged with two clear roles:

1. Diagnosis of CAD and assessment of prognosis in patients with known CAD.
2. Long-term outcomes for making the most appropriate treatment decisions.

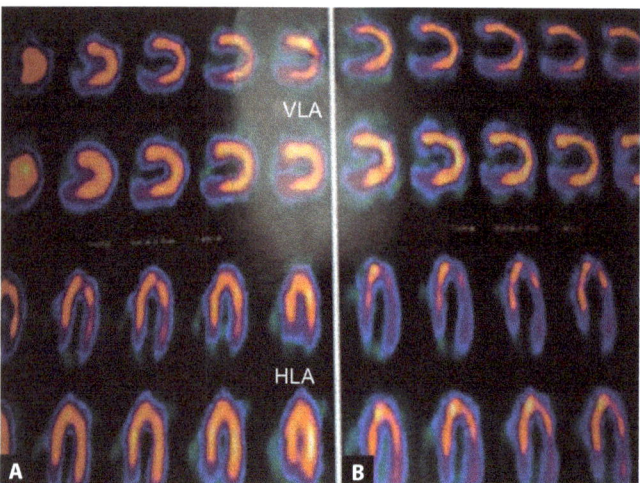

Figs 26A and B: Conventional SPECT images using 20 minutes acquisition for each stress or rest data DNM image using only 6 minutes acquisition for each data set

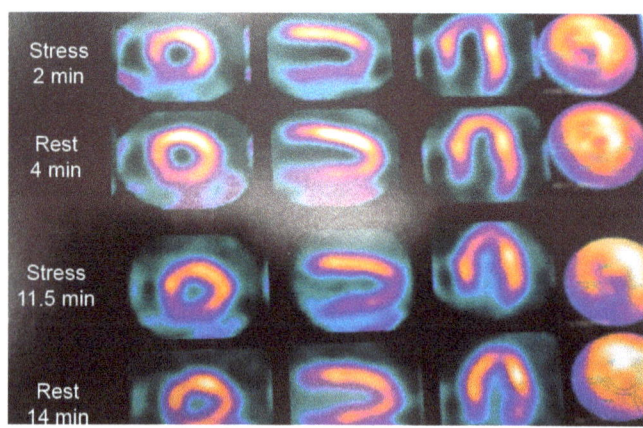

Fig. 27: Solid state dedicated cardiac camera (D-SPECT)

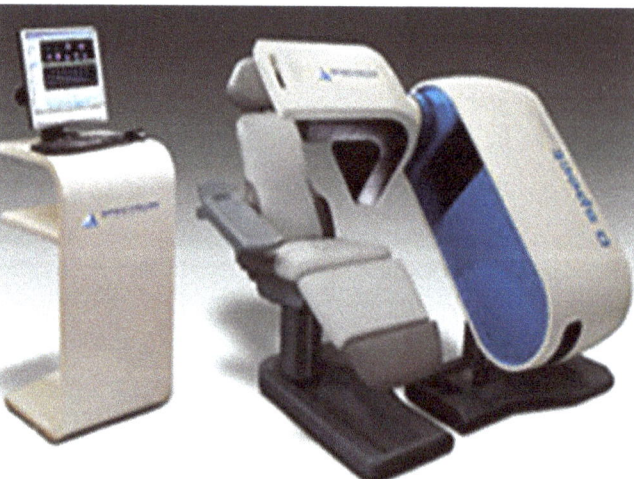

Fig. 28: D-SPECT cardiac scanner

DYNAMIC SINGLE PHOTON EMISSION COMPUTED TOMOGRAPHY (SPECT) (FIGS 29 TO 35)

Drawback of MPI

MPI is still affected by several drawbacks that are inherent to any nuclear techniques.
- Low photon flux
- Attenuation due to non-uniform tissues
- Motion artefacts due to time consuming scan
- Radiation exposure.

Suggestion

Shortening scan acquisition. Reducing radiation dose without decreasing imaging quality. Dedicated solid state cardiac camera (D-SPECT) represents an important answer for nuclear MPI.

Acquisition Protocol

All patients referred to MPI for suspected CAD, follow-up of a known CAD or preoperative risk assessment before major non cardiac surgery. 1-day Tc 99 tetrofosmin, adenosine or dobutamine stress/rest imaging protocol according to EANM guidelines. ECG gated images are first acquired on a conventional SPECT gamma camera with a 15 minute scan time each for stress and rest. They are immediately repeated on an ultra fast CZT D-SPECT camera with a 3 minutes acquisition time for stress and 2 minutes time for rest images. Reconstruction of image slices for both conventional SPECT

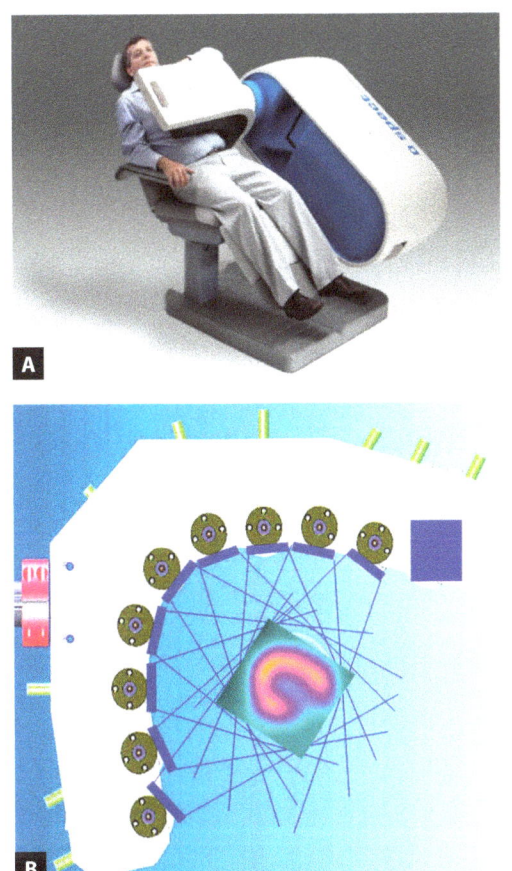

Figs 29A and B: (A) Positioning of D-SPECT camera on a sitting down posture of a cardiac patient; (B) Acquisition of MPI study in multi-detector system in D-SPECT cardiac camera

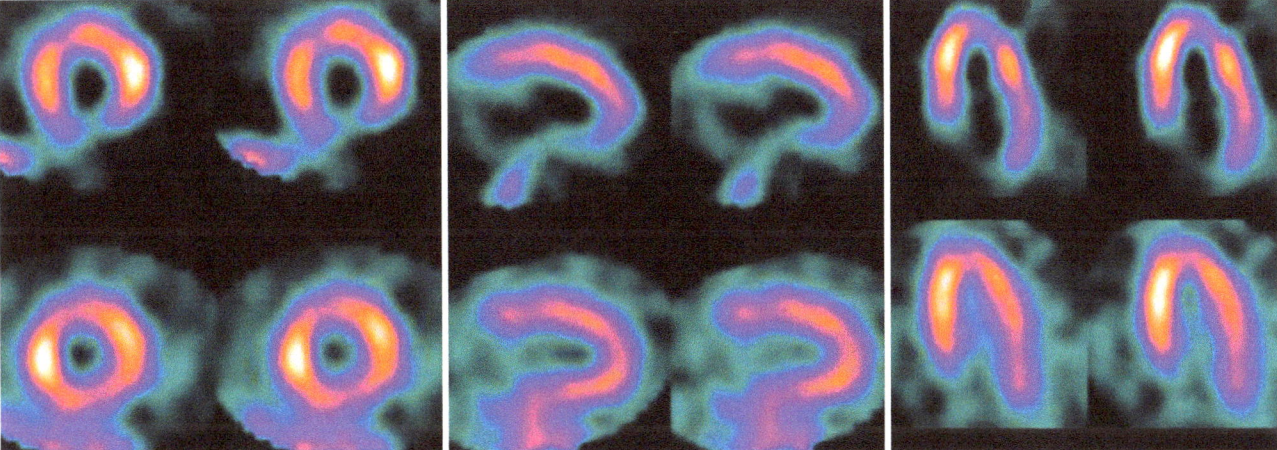

Fig. 30: Conventional SPECT

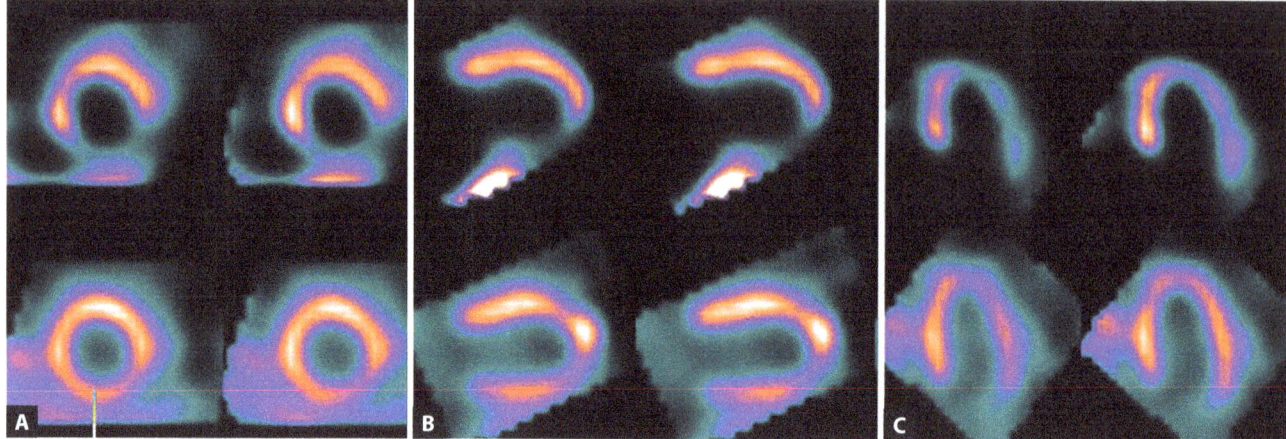

Figs 31A to C: DR-D SPECT

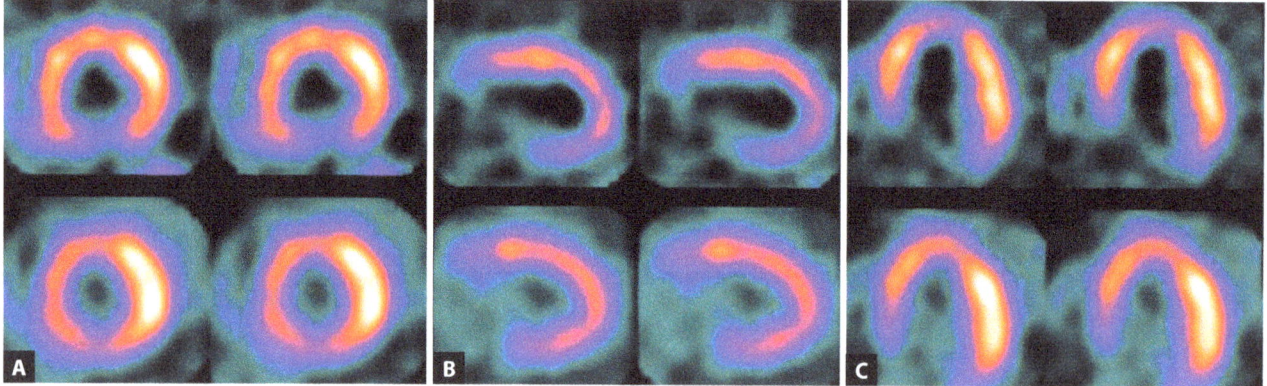

Figs 32A to C: Conventional SPECT (Stress and rest study)

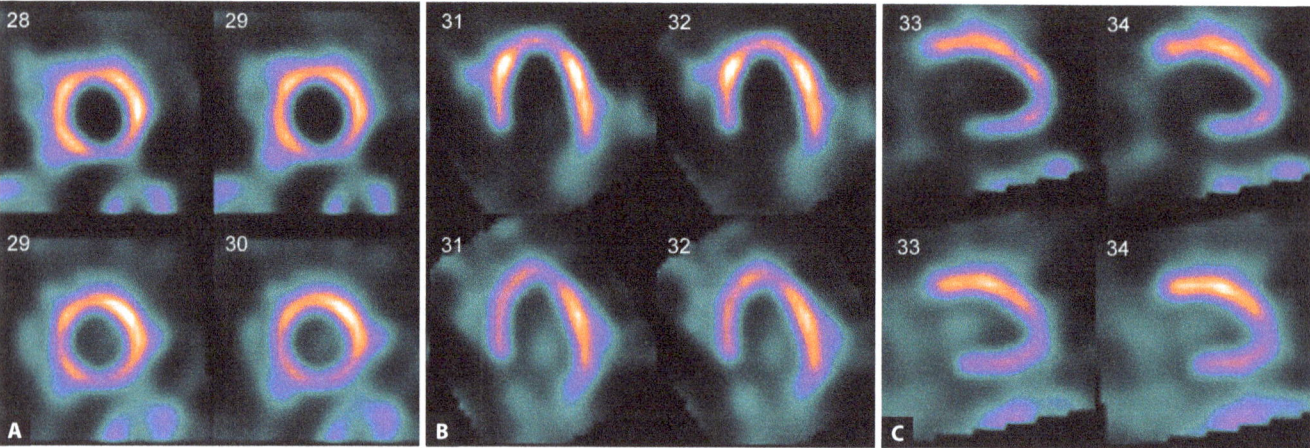

Figs 33A to C: DR-D SPECT (Stress and rest study)

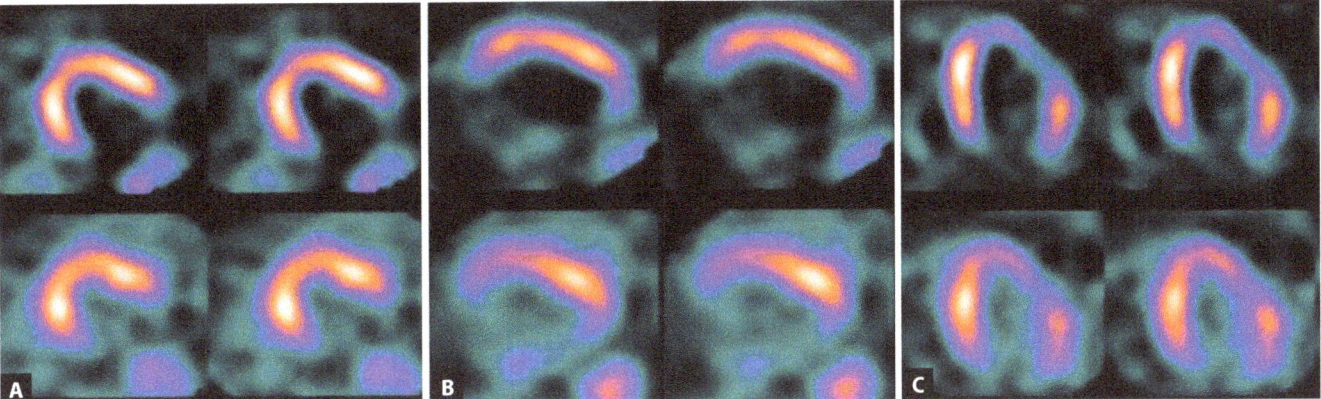

Figs 34A to C: Conventional SPECT (Stress and rest study)

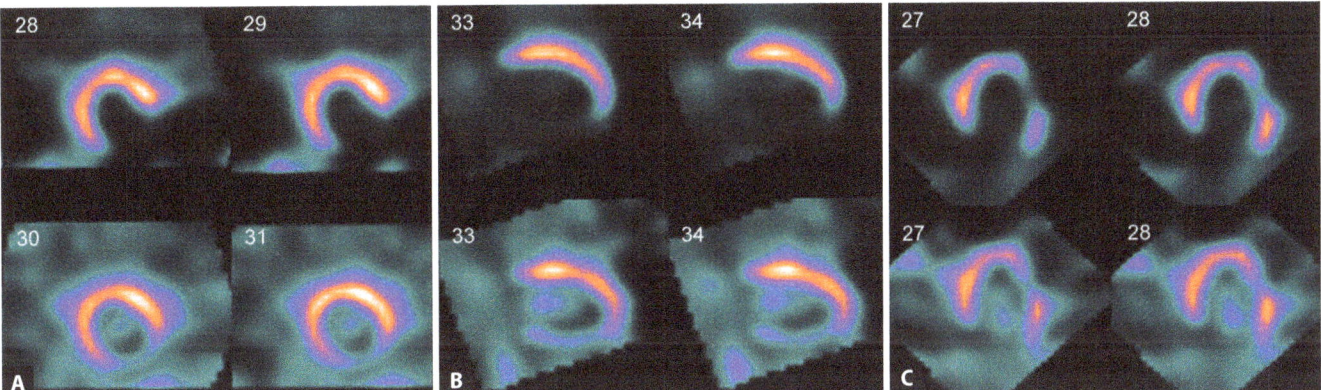

Figs 35A to C: DR-D SPECT (Stress and rest study)

and CZT D-SPECT images are made on a dedicated work station with quantitative segmental analysis using polar map for the left ventricle. Excellent clinical agreement (normal, ischemic scan) between CZT D-SPECT and conventional SPECT both on a per patient basis (96%) and on a per vessel territory basis (96.4%). Simultaneous acquisition of dual tracer with resting Tl-201 80 MBq and Tc 99m injection followed by D-SPECT for 6 minutes and stress with Tc 99 m Sestamibi injection of 250 MBq followed by 15 minutes acquisition time.

F-18 FLURPIRIDAZ POSITRON EMISSION TOMOGRAPHY MYOCARDIAL PERFUSION IMAGING TRACER

Flurpiridaz F-18 is a novel PET–MPI tracer also known as mitochondrial complex-1 (MC-1) of the electron transport chain. Flurpiridaz inhibits MC-1 by competing for binding with ubiquinone without affecting the viability of cardiomyocytes. It has been seen the uptake and washout kinetics of Flurpiridaz, which demonstrates a very rapid uptake, with a time to hold maximal uptake of 35 seconds and slow washout with a half time greater than 12 minutes.

The first uptake in isolated rabbit hearts, F18 flurpiridaz shows a significant myocardial uptake as compared to thallium-201 or TC 99m Sestamibi. Stress imaging is visible with both treadmill exercise and pharmacologic vasodilatation, Myocardium was clearly visualized for several hours after rest and stress with good myocardial to background ratio.

This radiotracer also permits evaluation of myocardial infarction (MI) size in rats. The advantage of this perfusion imaging in its unit dose availability from a regional cyclotron and can be delivered to the imaging centers in much the same way as F-18 FDG, thus obviating the need for onsite cyclotron.

Protocol

The longer half line also ensures that the radiotracer is presented long enough to allow a patient injected at peak treadmill to move to the camera and still we effectively image, using the relationship between rest-stress contamination

dosing. It is determined that for a same day rest exercise protocol a minimum dose ratio 3.0 is needed with 60 minutes waiting time between the two injection. The imaging can begin following adenosine stress protocol 2 minutes following injection of flurpiridaz F-18 during pharmacologic stress. With treadmill exercise protocol, imaging may begin as soon as patient is moved under the PET scanner following completion of exercise. Using flurpiridaz F-18, poststress imaging is therefore very closed to peak stress and has a higher chance of detecting stress-induced wall motion abnormalities. This is in contrast with the Tc99m SPECT MPI protocol in which poststress images are obtained 30–45 minutes following stress.

F-18 BMS MYOCARDIAL PET TRACER

New F-18 labeled pyridazinone analog (18-F-BMS) require on site tracer production. This has been successfully tried in a rat model of permanent and transient coronary occlusion using small animal PET scanner as well as recently been tried in human volunteers as well as patients. Both exercise and rest protocol can be performed as used in combination with exercise and rest perfusion SPECT. During a significant coronary occlusion this F-18 BMS produces a demonstrable perfusion defect which remains unchanged after resting tracer injection. In addition to this after transient ischemia the induced defect size decreases significantly after reperfusion suggesting potency of this new tracer as a new stress PET perfusion agent.

C-11 HYDROXYEPHEDRINE/C-11 EPINEPHRINE/I-123 MIBG AND Tc99M TETROFOSMIN/SESTAMIBI SPECT MPI

Cardiac sympathetic neuronal dysfunction has been shown to be abnormal in viable myocardium. The prediction of arrhythmic events with PET trail has shown that the extent of denervation determined by C-11 hydroxyephedrine PET in on independent predicator of cardiac arrest in patient with CAD and heart failure. These interesting findings suggest that the neurohormonal and viability hibernation.

Imaging may play complementary role in defining patients at risk needing an intervention.

There is some recent evidence suggesting that reverse mismatch seen in perfusion or FDG-PET with the extent of lateral scar and viability can be used to predict outcome response in patients undergoing cardiac resynchronization therapy **(Fig. 36)**.

TRACERS FOR DETECTING CHRONIC INFLAMMATORY DISORDERS SUCH AS CARDIAC SARCOIDOSIS/AMYLOIDOSIS

Inflammation is increasingly recognized as a key mechanism driving the progression or regression of variety of diseases, one approach of inflammation targeted molecular imaging that has entreated the clinical setting is imaging of cardiac sarcoidosis. Sarcoidosis is a systemic granulomatous disease, which may affect the heart in up to 40% of cases. Cardiac sarcoidosis may present as complete heart block, ventricular arrhythmias or congestive heart failure. Accordingly, cardiac involvement is a leading cause of death in patient with sarcoidosis emphasizing the need for accurate early detection and treatment.

Inflammation is generally detectable by F-18 FDG-PET owing to over expression of glucose transporters and over production of glycolytic enzymes in inflammatory cells but detection of myocardial inflammation is complicated by physiological uptake of FDG into myocytes owing to glucose sutras metabolism. Suppression strategies for myocardial glucose metabolism include prolonged fasting, dietary modifications and heparin loading. With these efficient patient preparation, FDG-PET is an accurate tool for diagnosis of

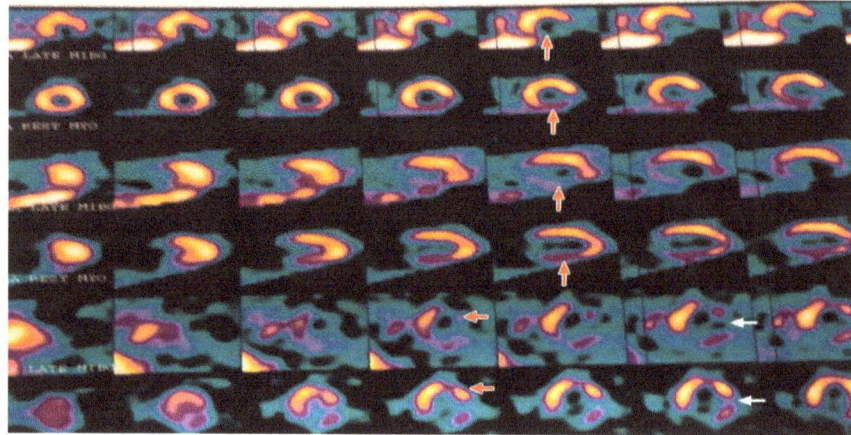

Fig. 36: I-131 MIBG (metaiodobenzylguanidine) and Tc-99m tetrofosmin SPECT images in a patient showing large MIBG defects involving inferior and lateral walls with almost preserved perfusion, which is an autonomic-perfusion mismatch

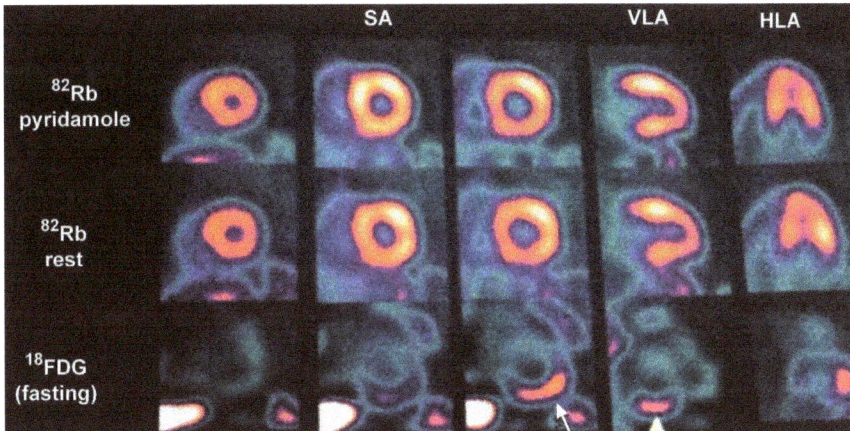

Fig. 37: PET imaging of cardiac sarcoidosis. Fasting F-18 FDG uptake is focally increased in basal inferior wall consistence with inflammatory foci and suppressed in others

cardiac sarcoidosis, therapy monitoring and biopsy guidance. A focal patchy myocardial uptake pattern typically suggests cardiac sarcoidosis. A meta-analysis of 7th studies with 164 patients showed a sensitivity of 89% and specificity of 78% **(Fig. 37)**.

TRACERS FOR DETECTING ATHEROMATOUS PLAQUE PARTICULARLY VULNERABLE PLAQUE IMAGING

Atherosclerosis, a leading cause of mortality, is characterized by fatty streak development, plaque (atheroma) formation and the potential of plaque rupture or erosion leading to myocardial infarction. SPECT imaging probes (tracers) are labeled with gamma-emitting radionuclides (e.g. Tc-99m, In-111, I-123, and I-131). PET tracers are labeled with positron-emitting radionuclides (O-15, C-11, F-18 FDG, F-18 NaF). Coregistration of SPECT/PET-CT images acquired sequentially allows anatomical localization **(Fig. 38)**.

TRACERS FOR STEM CELLS TRACKING

The newest targets for nuclear molecular imaging are stem cells. Clinical studies have demonstrated modest function benefits so far as stem cell tracking is concerned.

The molecular mechanism of stem cell engraftment and cardiac recovery in stem cell therapy need to be further elucidated. PET and SPECT imaging may help in this regard by noninvasively tracking the fate of cells.

Stem cells can be labeled directly and indirectly via reporter gene labeling. Direct labeling is adequate for short-term imaging, whereas reporting gene imaging is necessary for longitudinal studies.

In direct stem cell labeling, cells are incubated with radiopharmaceuticals *ex vivo* depending on the imaging modality. The radiopharmaceuticals that have been used are F-18 FDG for PET, In -111- oxine, Tc-99m HMPAO (hexamethylpropyleneamine oxime). The main advantage of direct cell labeling are that it can be translated directly into clinical studies owing to the use of approved radio-pharmaceuticals and that is provides high contrast owing to low background activity. Disadvantages are the limited observation period owing to decay, the loss of radiolabeled agent and possible radiotoxicity.

An alternative to direct labeling is the imaging of stem cells via a reporter gene. For this, a gene that encodes for an enzyme for a reporter that mediates accumulation of radiopharmaceutical is transfected into the cells before application. Because of accumulation of the reported probe requires expression of the transferred reporter gene, the imaging signal reflects cell viability. Another advantage is the possibility of repeated imaging over a longer period. Commonly used reporter genes include the HSV 1-tk and the sodium iodide symporter **(Fig. 39)**.

TRACERS FOR PATIENTS WITH INFECTIOUS ENDOCARDITIS AND AORTIC GRAFT PROSTHETIC INFECTION

18-F FDG PET-CT

Infectious endocarditis is a severe disease that is diagnosed using a combination of clinical, microbiologic and imaging modality such as CT, MR and USG. But, none of these modalities can identify metastatic complications, which may force the clinician to stop or early interruption of therapy, thus, triggering relapse and an unfavorable outcome. Infectious embolisms can be asymptomatic and difficult to recognize even in spite of multiple imaging techniques such as CT, MR and USG.

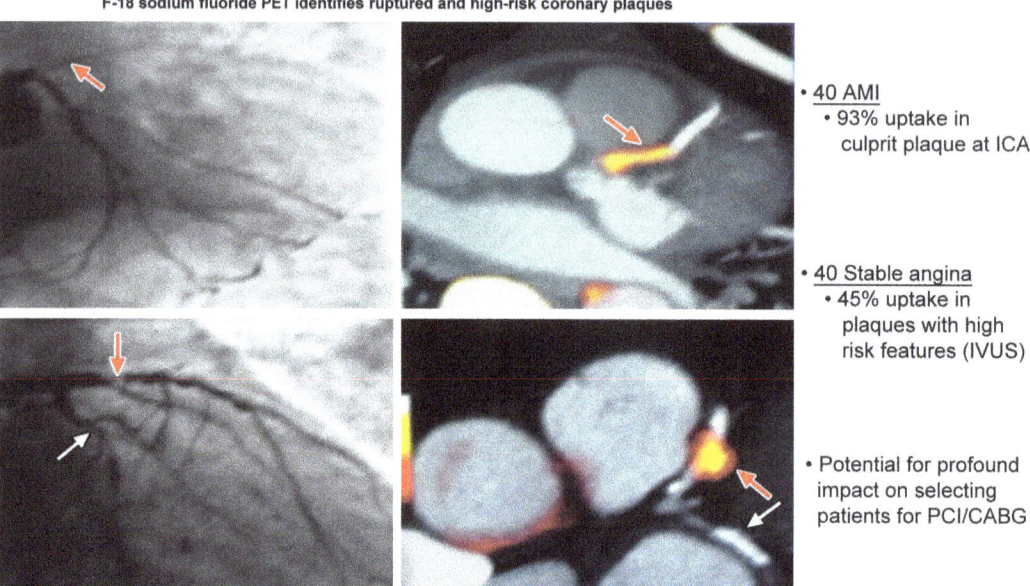

Fig. 38: F-18 NaF atheromatous plaque imaging showing adequate F-18 NaF uptake in the region of left anterior descending (LAD) and left circumflex artery suggesting unstable plaque imaging

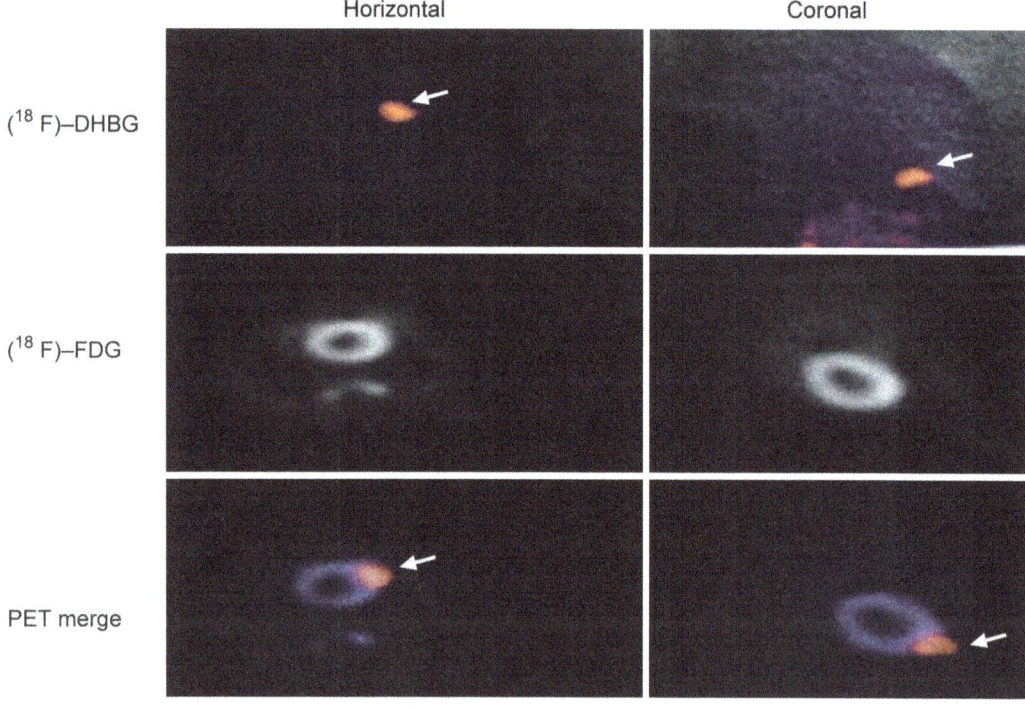

Fig. 39: Noninvasive tracking of embryonic stem cells (ESCs) showing the reporter gene labeled ESCs using F-18 FHBG reporter probe. The bottom row represents merged FHBG and FDG images showing the exact anatomical location of transplanted ESCs within the anterolateral wall of the heart

F-18 FDG PET-CT is wildly used on patient with oncohematologic conditions, since it can identify glucose uptake in areas with an increased metabolic rate.

It has a promising role in infectious endocarditic because of its high sensitivity, anatomic precision and lack of toxicity.

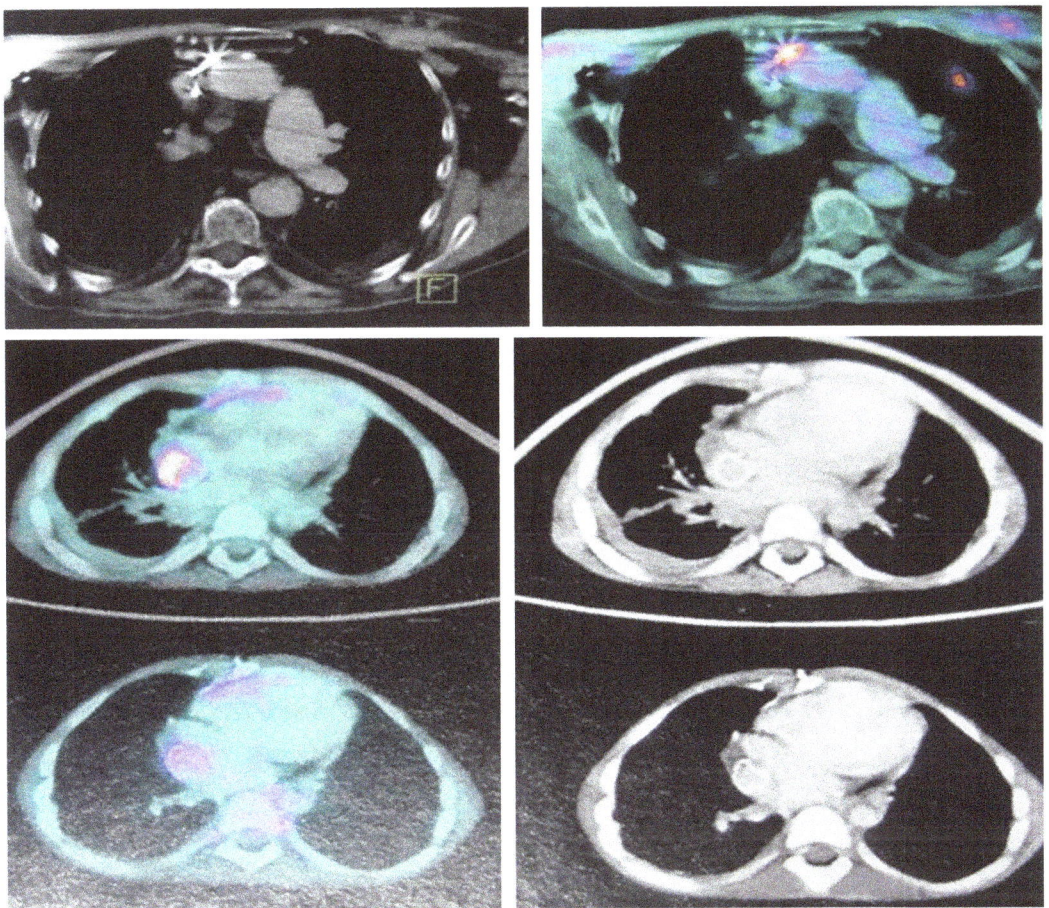

Fig. 40: PET-CT and CT (right) images of a patient with increased FDG uptake seen in the cardiac device and lower group of images showing almost complete recovery after 6 weeks of antibiotic treatment

The possibility of scanning, the whole body with a single test is particularly appealing for clinicians treating patient with, i.e. PET-CT. It reveals at least in one of the series showing pathologic uptake on the valves or cardiac devices. The validity values for the efficacy of PET-CT in the diagnosis of septic lesions are as follows, sensitivity 100%, specificity 80% positive predictive value 100%. It provides the clinician with whole body data, and it is quickly performed within less than an hour.

PET-CT images of case of pulmonary septic embolism is shown in **Figure 40**.

USEFUL COMBINED NUCLEAR CARDIOLOGY TECHNIQUES (FIGS 41 AND 42)

Dual Isotope Imaging using Tl-201 and F-18 FDG Imaging

Assessment of metabolism by PET provides the sensitive detection of tissue viability based on the integrity of cardiac substrate metabolism. The increased FDG uptake in the hibernating myocardium appears to be an independent prognostic parameter identifying ischemically compromised myocardium and thus high-risk clinical conditions. This metabolic signal of jeopardized myocardium is especially helpful in patients with advanced ischemic heart failure because revascularisation is associated with higher risk. The most important functional recovery following revascularization of the failing heart is the amount of hibernating myocardium present.

Metabolic imaging with PET offers a sophisticated means of assessing regional tissue viability in patients with advanced coronary artery disease (CAD) and impaired left ventricular function. The assessment of relative and regional uptake covering the complete left ventricular volume represents an advantage over competing modalities. The classification of myocardial tissue into viable, hibernating or scarred can be performed with high sensitivity and specificity.

Glucose Metabolism

18F-fluorodeoyglucose traces transmembranous transport as well as phosporylation of exogenous glucose. 18F-fluorodeoyglucose 6-phosphate does not enter any further

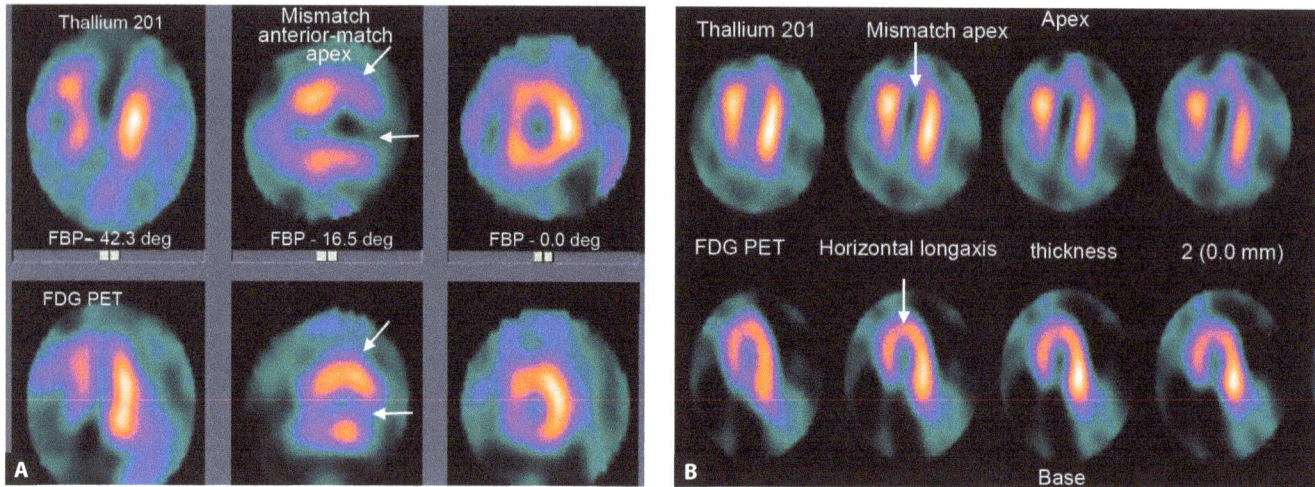

Figs 41A and B: (A) Dual isotope myocardial imaging shows a stress defect involving part of anterior and apical myocardial segments which shows adequate metabolism involving anterior segments only. However, apical segments seems to have no metabolism suggesting scarred myocardium as evidenced from F-18 FDG metabolism study; (B) Stress myocardial perfusion imaging with Thallium-201 perfusion showing an apical defect which shows adequate metabolism with F-18 FDG metabolism study as evidenced from the bottom row of images

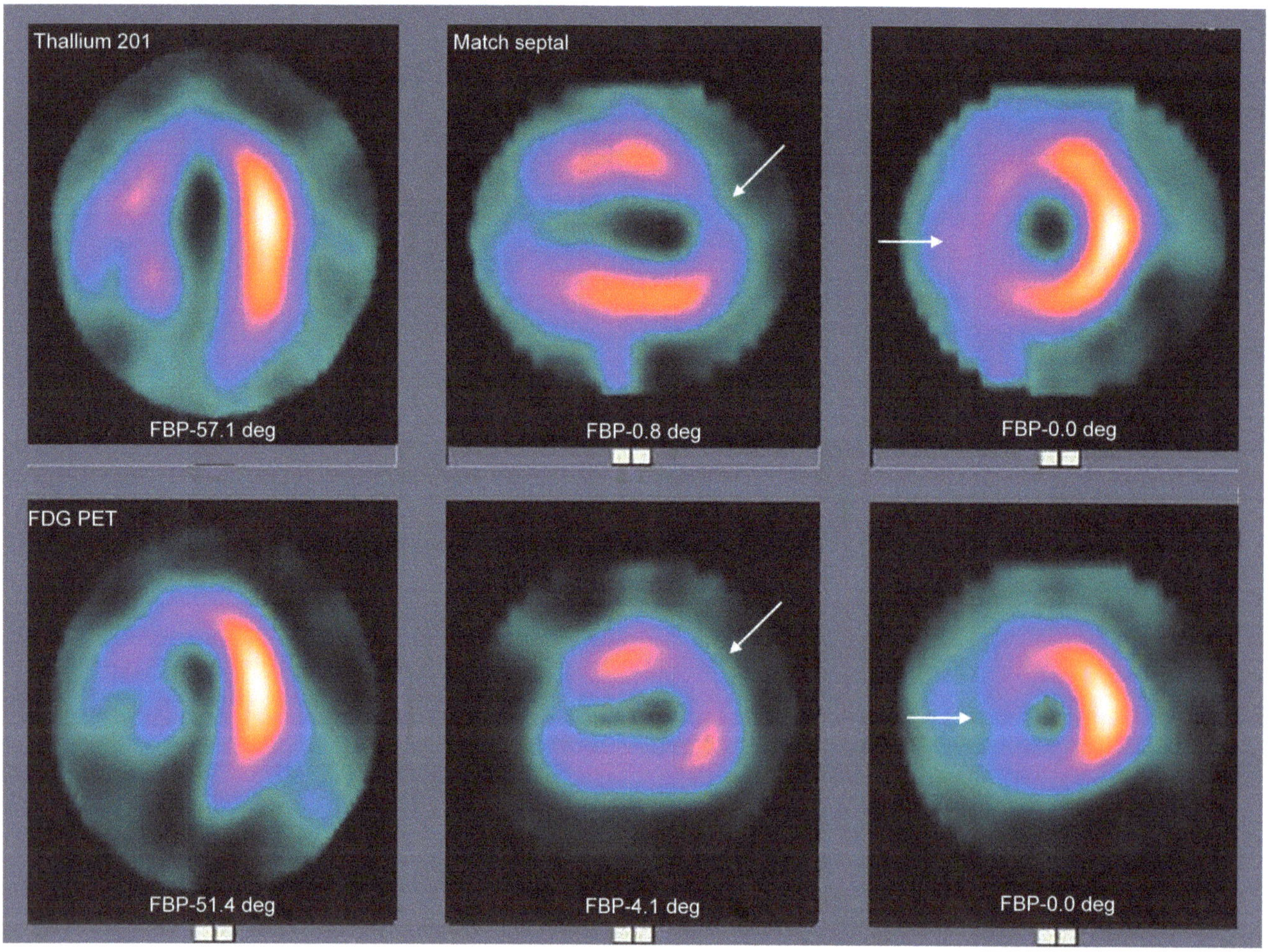

Fig. 42: Stress thallium myocardial perfusion study shows a perfusion defect involving anteroseptal segments, which seems to have absent metabolism using F-18 FDG metabolic study

metabolic pathways but accumulates in the myocardium, which is proportional to glucose transport and phosporylation.

Patient Preparation

Oral glucose loading is the most widely used approach for preparing patients for FDG imaging. FDG is administered 60 to 90 minutes after 50 gm of oral glucose load. This switches the primary substrate for myocardial metabolism from free acids to glucose. This is facilitated by the release of insulin. Thus viable myocardium will preferentially take up glucose, and hence FDG. In patients with diabetes, supplement insulin is necessary. Even with glucose loading protocols with bolus insulin, images are often suboptimal in diabetics.

Most cardiac FDG studies are acquired 40 to 60 minutes after injection of tracer. This time period is required to reduce the FDG plasma concentration to ensure high contrast between the blood pool and the myocardium. In patients with diabetes mellitus, a longer waiting period is advised to enhance myocardium-to-blood contrast.

Data Interpretation

Matching of perfusion and FDG uptake of normal viable myocardium, which is not ischemic at rest whereas matched pattern of decreased perfusion and metabolism are indicative for irreversible tissue injury (scar). A mismatch pattern of reduced myocardial blood flow in presence of increased FDG uptake identifies viable but ischemically compromised myocardium. This helps to emphasize the clinician the true extent of viability and the potential for recoverable tissue.

Cardiac PET Scan Protocol

- Thallium perfusion scan at 8.30 am.
- FDG-PET scan at 12 noon (blood sugar level should not be >130 mg/dL).

Combined or Dual Tracer Use of I-123-BMIPP and Perfusion Tracer (Tc-99m Tetrofosmin/ Sestamibi)

I-123-BMIPP Iodophenyl methyl-pentadecanoic acid is the most commonly used branched fatty acid tracer. It has a high myocardial extraction and retention with low background activity and low uptake in the liver and lungs after 60 minute injection. It maybe used for imaging of "Ischemia Memory" in patient's presenting with acquate chest pain. In subsequent face of MI suggesting myocardial stunning or delayed recovery of metabolism after recovery of perfusion can also be imaged. In patient with successful revascularization after acquate MI suggest discordant I-123 BMIPP uptake with resting normal n perfusion pattern reflects prior severe Ischemia after the recovery of perfusion or the so called "Ischemia Memory".

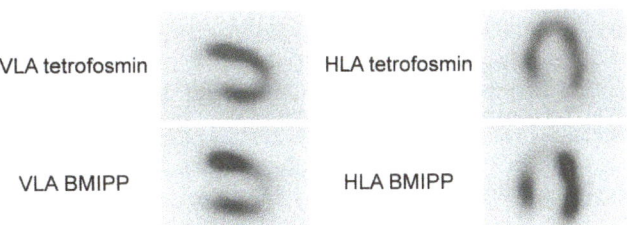

Fig. 43: Dual tracer

Follow-up studies shows delayed improvement in wall motion suggesting that they represent stunned myocardium.

Example (Fig. 43)

- A 65-year-old man presented with exertional chest pain.
- At the time of admission his chest pain was resolved a negative serologic and ECG evidence of acute MI.
- Resting myocardial perfusion SPECT images with Tc-99m tetrofosmin were obtained at the time of hospital admission without pain.
- 24-hours later following the chest pain I-123 BMIPP-SPECT imaging was performed with 32 images of 20 second/per stop.

CONCLUSION

Nuclear Cardiology specialty is no doubt a-state-of-art procedure in the present day clinical practice from its inception till date. Various nuclear techniques have proved their superiority in the form of sensitivity and specificity over other non-nuclear techniques such as CT angiography, dobutamine stress echocardiography (DSE), cardiovascular MRI and contrast echocardiography in the detection and further evaluation of patients suffering from coronary artery disease. In this context, Thallium-201 has been proved to be a potent radiotracer for the diagnosis and for the treatment planning of patients having CAD for more than three decades. The advent of various Technetium-99m labelled perfusion agents, particularly Tc-99m Sestamibi (Cardiolite) or Tc-99m Tetrofosmin (Myoview) have proved their increased specificity in detection of coronary artery disease. The advantage of using Technetium-labeled perfusion imaging agents has additional useful informations such as global ejection fraction, regional wall motion, and systolic wall thickening of left ventricle at rest/stress study. Pharmacological stress myocardial perfusion imaging which is an unique technique to evaluate myocardial perfusion during maximal coronary vasodilatation. In the early days of acute myocardial infarction, pharmacological intervention study can be substituted as submaximal predischarge exercise testing which is considered as a method for evaluating the extent of coronary artery disease and risk of future cardiac events. The role of Tl-201 reinjection and PET imaging, particularly, 18F-FDG, for myocardial viability have been used to correctly assess the amount of viable myocardium and would benefit patients undergoing revascularization procedures. The presence of reversible defects on rest/reinjection Tl-201 myocardial scintigraphy and PET pattern of perfusion metabolism mismatch are highly accurate fro identifying the presence of hibernating myocardium, and thus predicting the potential for recovery of left ventricular contractile dysfunction following revascularization. The evidence of three important parameters of myocardial perfusion imaging (presence of transient defects, the number of transient defects and increased lung uptake of either Tl-201 or Tc-99m agents) have emerged as strong predictors of future cardiac events in patients having post-myocardial infarction.

Cardiovascular MRI imaging uses ultrafast imaging sequence using Gadolinium-DTPA (Gd-DTPA) is a contrast agent itself and is expensive. Its rapid diffusion into interstitial space underestimates the assessment of degree of myocardial viability. Additionally, there is no quantitative assessment data is available till date and its absence availability of estimating simultaneous function and viability. The cost of CMR test is phenomenal in present day clinical practice, e.g. it is almost double the cost of the gated SPECT-myocardial perfusion scintigraphy. This specialty has grown tremendously for the last three decades with the introduction of new imaging agents, modification in techniques and innovation of new technology in the instruments as well as addition of various quantitative softwares, particularly, quantitation of coronary blood flow through the major coronary arteries has further widen its horizon in the era of multimodality imaging. The various procedures are cost effective and promising with an increased sensitivity and specificity. Every newer radiopharmaceutical are being invented along wth the improvement in the software and instrumentation as compared to other noninvasive modalities of investigation such as Cardiovascular MRI or MDCT or contrast echocardiography, etc. thereby keeping this modality as the leader of noninvasive diagnostic modality in patients suffering from coronary artery disease.

BIBLIOGRAPHY

1. Berman DS, Kiat H, Van Train K, et al. Tc99m Sestamibi in the assessment of chronic artery disease. Sem Nucl Med. 1991;XXT:190-212.
2. Bodenheimer MM, Banka VS, Fooshee C, et al. Relationship between myocardial perfusion and the presence of severity and reversibility of asynergy in patients with coronary heart disease. Circulation. 1976;53:792-800.
3. Brunken RC, Kottou S, Nienabar CA, et al. PET detection of viable tissue in myocardial segments with persistent defects at Tl201 SPECT. Radiology. 1989;172:65-73.
4. Chua T, Kiat H, Germano GF, et al. Rapid back adenosine stress/rest Technetium-99m teboroxime myocardial perfusion SPECT using a triple detector camera. J Nucl Med. 1993;34:1485-93.
5. Depuey EG, et al. Comparison to Tc-99m Sestamibi and Tl201 gated perfusion SPECT. J Nucl Cardiol. 1990;6:278-85.
6. Forster T, McNeilt Aj, Alustri A, et al. Simultaneously dobutamine stress echocardiography and Technetium-99m isonitrile single photon emission computed tomography in patients with suspected coronary artery disease. J Am Coll Cardiol. 1993;21:1591-6.
7. Gianrossi R, Detrane R, Mulvihill D, et al. Exercise induced ST depression in the diagnosis of coronary artery disease: a meta-analysis. Circulation. 1989;80:87-98.
8. Gracia E, Caake CD, Van Train KF, et al. Technetium 99m Sestamibi. Am J Cardiol. 1990;6G:80E-90E.
9. Gutman J, Berman DS, Freeman M, et al. Time to complete redistribution of Tl201 in exercise myocardial scintigraphy, relationship to the degree of coronary artery stenosis. Am Heart J. 1983;106:989-95.
10. Hays JT, Manmarian JJ, Cochran AJ, et al. Dobutamine Tl201 tomography for evaluating patients with suspected coronary artery disease unable to undergo exercise or vasodilatory pharmacologic testing. JA Coll Cardiol. 1993;21:1583-90.
11. Iskandrian AS, Heo J, Kong B, et al. Use of Tc99m isonitrile (RP 30A) in assessing left ventricular perfusion and function at rest during exercise in coronary artery disease and comparison with coronary arteriography and exercise Tl201 SPECT imaging. Am J Cardiol. 1989;64:270-5.
12. Kiat H, Maddahi J, Roy LT, et al. Comparison of Technetium-99m methoxy isobutyl isonitrile and Thallium-201 for evaluation of coronary heart disease by planar and tomographic methods. Am Heart J. 1989;117:1-11.
13. Mahapatra GN, et al. Nuclear techniques in assessing myocardial viability. J Cardiology Today. 1998;2:39-41.
14. Marwick T, Willemart B, D'Hondt AM, et al. Selection of the optimal non-exercise stress for the evaluation of ischemic regional myocardial dysfunction and Tc-99m MIBI single photon emission computed tomography. Circulation. 1993;87:345-54.
15. Ritchie JL, Albro PC, Caldwell JH, et al. Tl201 myocardial imaging: a comparison of the redistribution and rest images. J Nucl Med. 1979;20:477-83.
16. Rocco T, Dilsizian V, Maltais F, et al. Tl - 201 reinjection after delayed imaging demonstrates fill-in to region with "fixed "defect (abstract). J Nucl Med. 1988;29:76.
17. Taillefer R, Lamberi R, Dupras G, et al. Clinical comparison between Thallium-201 and Tc-99m methoxy-isobutyl isonitrile (Sestamibi) myocardial perfusion imaging for detection of coronary artery disease. Eur J Nucl Med. 1989;15:280-6.
18. Tamaki N, Yonekura Y, Mukai T, et al. Segmental analysis of stress Thallium of myocardial emission tomography for localisation of coronary artery disease. J Nucl med. 1984;9:99-105.
19. Tamaki N, Yonekura Y, Yamashita K, et al. SPECT Tl tomography and positron tomography using N13 Ammonia and F18 FDG in coronary artery disease. Am J Cardiac Imaging. 1989;3:3-9.
20. Verzjibergen FJ, Vermeersch PHM, et al. Inadequate exercise leads to suboptimal imaging 201-Thallium myocardial perfusion imaging after dipyridamole combined with low level exercise unmasks ischemia in symptomatic patients with nondiagnostic Tl-201 scan who exercise submaximally. J Nucl Med. 32;2071-8.

Cardiac Positron Emission Tomography Perfusion Tracers: Current Status and Future Directions

30

Jamshid Maddahi, René RS Packard

INTRODUCTION

In the past three decades, numerous studies have shown that positron emission tomography (PET) is superior to single photon emission tomography (SPECT) myocardial perfusion imaging (MPI) with respect to (1) shorter study acquisition time, (2) lower radiation dose to patients, (3) higher sensitivity and specificity for detection of coronary artery disease (CAD), and (4) assessment of coronary flow reserve (CFR). Nevertheless, several limitations of the currently available PET perfusion tracers have hampered their widespread use. The short half-life of these tracers necessitates either the availability of an on-site cyclotron or costly generators. This has also rendered exercise treadmill testing impractical in routine streamlined clinical practice. To address these limitations, ^{18}F-labeled PET radiotracers have been developed to take advantage of the much longer 109 minutes half-life of ^{18}F. This has led to a sharp growth in recent years in the development and experimental animal testing of ^{18}F-labeled PET MPI radiotracers.[1-3] In this article, we present an update to our earlier review[4] of currently available PET MPI tracers and ^{18}F flurpiridaz, the more thoroughly studied ^{18}F-labeled radiotracer.

CURRENT MYOCARDIAL PERFUSION POSITRON EMISSION TOMOGRAPHY TRACERS

The three currently available PET MPI tracers; ^{15}O water, ^{13}N ammonia, and ^{82}Rubidium, have different characteristics and use in the clinical setting as discussed below.

^{15}O Water

Physical and clinical features of the current PET MPI tracers and ^{18}F flurpiridaz are presented in **Table 1**. The physical half-life of this tracer is 2.06 minutes.[5] As such its production requires an on-site cyclotron. Image resolution of a PET MPI tracer depends on its positron energy; the higher the energy of the emitted positron, the longer the positron range and the lower the image resolution. ^{15}O has a 4.14 mm positron range[5] resulting in an intermediate image resolution **(Table 1)**. Perfusion defect contrast is influenced by the myocardial extraction fraction of the myocardial perfusion tracer that is used for imaging; the higher the extraction fraction, the higher the defect contrast.[4] The myocardial extraction fraction of ^{15}O water is 100%.[6] Theoretically, 100% myocardial extraction fraction of ^{15}O water should result in the highest perfusion defect contrast. However, poor myocardial-to-background ratio reduces defect contrast. Due to its very short half-life, stress imaging with ^{15}O water is only feasible in conjunction with pharmacologic stress, not treadmill exercise.

^{15}O water has been validated and extensively used for quantitation of myocardial blood flow (MBF) and coronary flow reserve (CFR).[4,6-9] However, ^{15}O water is not approved by the Food and Drug Administration (FDA) for clinical use and is not reimbursed by third party payers. The current clinical use of ^{15}O water is primarily for measuring MBF in research studies and in the academic setting.

^{13}N Ammonia

This tracer is taken up by the myocardium by passive free diffusion across cell membranes as ammonia (NH_3) where it equilibrates with its charged form ammonium (NH_4) and gets trapped inside the cell by conversion through glutamine synthase to ^{13}N-glutamine.[10-12] The physical half-life of ^{13}N ammonia is 9.96 minutes.[5] As such, its production has required an on-site cyclotron **(Table 1)**. Due to the 9.96 minutes half-life of ^{13}N ammonia, production and delivery of this tracer from a cyclotron a few miles away has been shown to be feasible. More recently, small, single site ^{13}N ammonia cyclotrons (*Ionetix*) have been developed that allow on-site production

Table 1 Characteristics of various cardiac positron emission tomography perfusion tracers. Reprinted with permission from Seminars in Nuclear Medicine

	^{15}O water	^{13}N ammonia	^{82}Rb	^{18}F flurpiridaz
Half-life (minutes)	2.06	9.96	1.25	109
Production	On-site cyclotron	On-site or nearby cyclotron	Generator	Regional cyclotron
Positron range (mm)	4.14	2.53	8.6	1.03
Image resolution	Intermediate	Intermediate-high	Lowest	Highest
Myocardial extraction fraction	100%	80%	65%	94%
Perfusion defect contrast	Intermediate*	Intermediate	Lowest	Highest
Pharmacological stress imaging protocol	Feasible	Feasible	Feasible	Feasible
Treadmill exercise Imaging protocol	Not feasible	Feasible but not practical	Not feasible	Feasible

* Theoretically 100% myocardial extraction fraction of ^{15}O water should result in the highest perfusion defect contrast. However, poor myocardial-to-background ratio reduces defect contrast.
Source: Maddahi J, Packard RR. Cardiac positron emission tomography perfusion tracers: current status and future directions. Semin Nucl Med. 2014;44(5):333-43.

and unit dose use of ^{13}N ammonia in the clinical setting. The positron range of ^{13}N ammonia is 2.53 mm[4,5] resulting in an intermediate-high image resolution as compared to other PET MPI tracers. The myocardial extraction fraction of ^{13}N ammonia is approximately 80% **(Table 1)**. Since the physical half-life of ^{13}N ammonia is longer than those of ^{15}O water and ^{82}Rb, it is feasible to use ^{13}N ammonia in conjunction with supine bicycle exercise[13,14] or treadmill exercise.[15] This approach, however, is not practical for routine clinical use. ^{13}N ammonia has been validated and extensively used for quantitation of MBF and coronary flow reserve in a variety of clinical conditions.[9,16-20] This tracer is approved by the FDA for clinical use and is reimbursed by third party payers.

^{82}Rb

This tracer is taken up by the myocardium as a potassium analog through active transport by the Na+/K+ ATPase-pump.[21-23] The physical half-life of ^{82}Rb is 1.25 minutes[4,5] and can be produced by a relatively small on-site generator **(Table 1)**. Availability of ^{82}Rb generators have been hampered by limited availability of ^{82}Sr and a single supplier for ^{82}Rb generators. Recently however, a new ^{82}Rb generator delivery system has been developed, comprised of $^{82}Sr/^{82}Rb$ generator and an elution system that may offer improvement in safety (Jubilant/DraxImage). This system has recently been approved by US FDA for clinical use. The positron range of ^{82}Rb is 8.6 mm[4,5] resulting in low image resolution as compared to other PET MPI tracers.[4] The myocardial extraction fraction of ^{82}Rb is lower than the other PET perfusion tracers, resulting in relatively lower defect resolution.[4]

The clinical imaging protocol for ^{82}Rb starts with initial scout and transmission CT scans obtained for orientation and attenuation correction. Beginning with the intravenous bolus administration of 50 mCi (1850 MBq) of ^{82}Rb, serial dynamic images are acquired for 6 minutes (14 × 5 sec, 6 × 10 sec, 3 × 20 sec, 3 × 30 sec and 1 × 90 sec). Rapidly after completion of the rest study, a standard intravenous vasodilator infusion is administered. At peak hyperemia, a second 50 mCi (1850 MBq) dose of ^{82}Rb is injected, and images recorded in the same manner.[24,25] Although the low myocardial extraction fraction of ^{82}Rb does not render it ideal for absolute quantitation of MBF and CFR, this tracer has been extensively validated for this purpose[23,26-28] and has provided useful information in the clinical setting.[29-32]

FUTURE DIRECTIONS

Among several ^{18}F labeled myocardial perfusion PET tracers, ^{18}F flurpiridaz, has undergone the most extensive clinical evaluation and has completed the first phase 3 multicenter clinical trial. As such, this review will focus on presentation of data on ^{18}F flurpiridaz. Further information on other promising F-18 labeled PET MPI tracers such as fluorodihydrorotenone (F18-FDHR), p-fluorobenzyl triphenyl phosphonium cation (F18-FBnTP) and 4-fluorophenyl triphenyl phosphonium ion (F18-FTPP) have been presented in our earlier review.[4]

^{18}F Flurpiridaz

^{18}F flurpiridaz is a novel PET MPI tracer which is a structural analog of pyridaben, a known inhibitor of mitochondrial complex-1 (MC-1) of the electron transport chain.[33] Experimental PET imaging in rats, rabbits and rhesus monkeys demonstrated a high and sustained cardiac uptake which was proportional to blood flow.[34] In a pig model, ^{18}F flurpiridaz exhibits significantly higher activity ratios of the myocardium versus the blood, liver and lungs compared to ^{13}N ammonia.[35] Finally, this radiotracer also permits evaluation of myocardial infarction (MI) size in rats.[36] Imaging characteristics and potential clinical advantages of ^{18}F flurpiridaz are described below.

Unit Dose Availability

^{18}F flurpiridaz has a half-life of 108 minutes and may be produced at regional cyclotrons and delivered to imaging centers in much the same way as ^{18}F-labeled fluorodeoxyglucose (FDG), thus obviating the need for an on-site cyclotron **(Table 1)**.

High Image Resolution

The positron range of ^{18}F is 1.03 mm and is shorter than those of ^{82}Rb (8.6 mm), H$_2$^{15}O (4.14 mm), and ^{13}NH$_3$ (2.53 mm) **(Table 1)**. Image resolution of ^{18}F flurpiridaz PET is also better than ^{99m}Tc SPECT. It is expected that improved image resolution leads to improved image quality and confidence of interpretation. In phase 2[37] and phase 3[38] clinical trials, a significantly higher percentage of images was rated as excellent/good by PET versus SPECT on stress and rest images. Diagnostic certainty of interpretation (define as percentage of cases with definitely abnormal/normal interpretation) was significantly higher for PET versus SPECT.

High Extraction Fraction and Perfusion Defect Resolution

The first-pass extraction fraction of ^{18}F flurpiridaz by the myocardium was determined in isolated rat hearts perfused with the Langendorff method.[39] The radiotracer demonstrated an elevated – 94% – and flow-independent extraction fraction of ^{18}F flurpiridaz, implying a linear relationship between uptake and MBF, an important attribute for stress MBF measurements. In comparison, ^{13}N ammonia has an extraction fraction of 82% at rest, and ^{82}Rb chloride one of 42% with a significant roll-off phenomenon, i.e. low extraction at high flows. The 94% extraction fraction of ^{18}F flurpiridaz did not change significantly at flows ranging from 5.0–16.6 mL/min, which were achieved using adenosine stress. This is a result of the high density of mitochondria in cardiac muscle (which comprise 20–30% of the myocardial intracellular volume) doubled by the lipophilicity of the compound and its high binding affinity to MC-1.[34] The primary route of excretion of the compound is renal, consistent with a rapid decrease in activity of the radiotracer in the kidneys. Higher myocardial extraction facilitates detection of milder perfusion defects.[40] In phase 2 clinical trials, the magnitude of reversible defects was greater with PET than SPECT in patients who had CAD on invasive coronary angiography.

Low Radiation Exposure

In the first phase 1 study,[41] the mean effective dose (ED) of ^{18}F flurpiridaz injected at rest was very similar to that of FDG, with a much lower exposure to the critical organ by a factor of 2.5. In the second phase 1 study,[42] dosimetry of ^{18}F flurpiridaz was evaluated in patients who were injected at rest and on a second day, at peak adenosine stress or at peak treadmill exercise. Excellent image quality was noted with both forms of stress imaging. Dosimetry results suggest that injection of up to 14 mCi (518 MBq) of ^{18}F flurpiridaz during a rest-stress protocol would provide a clinically acceptable ED at 6.4 mSv. This is significantly lower than EDs of stress-redistribution ^{201}Tl imaging (26 mSv) and rest-stress ^{99m}Tc SPECT imaging (11.5 mSv).[4]

Feasibility of Rest Treadmill Exercise Imaging

The longer half-life of ^{18}F also ensures that the radiotracer is present long enough to allow a patient injected at peak treadmill exercise to move to the camera and still be effectively imaged. Feasibility of rest-treadmill exercise ^{18}F flurpiridaz was initially shown in phase 1 clinical trials.[41,42] A very high target-to-background ratio was noted when ^{18}F flurpiridaz was injected at peak treadmill exercise. Using the relationship between rest-stress contamination and dosing, it was determined that for a same day rest-exercise protocol, a minimum dose ratio of 3.0 was needed, with a 60 minutes waiting time between the 2 injections. For an optimum same day rest-adenosine stress protocol, on the other hand, a dose ratio of 3 with a 30 minutes waiting time between the 2 injections was required.[41,42] These protocols were successfully implemented in the phase 2 and phase 3 clinical trials of ^{18}F flurpiridaz.

Peak Stress Function Imaging

Kinetic studies in phase 1 trials[42] have shown that imaging may begin 2 minutes following injection of ^{18}F flurpiridaz during pharmacological stress. With treadmill exercise protocol, imaging may begin as soon as the patient is moved under the PET imaging device following completion of exercise. Using ^{18}F flurpiridaz, poststress imaging is, therefore, very close to peak stress and has a higher chance of detecting stress-induced wall motion abnormalities. This is in contrast with ^{99m}Tc SPECT MPI protocol in which poststress images are obtained 30–45 minutes following stress.

Diagnostic Accuracy for Detection of CAD

In the phase 3 trial[38] of ^{18}F flurpiridaz, diagnostic performance of this tracer was compared to ^{99m}Tc SPECT-MPI for detection of CAD defined as ≥50% stenosis by invasive coronary angiography (ICA). Receiver-operating characteristic curve (ROC) area was 0.73 for PET and 0.66 for SPECT (p = 0.001).

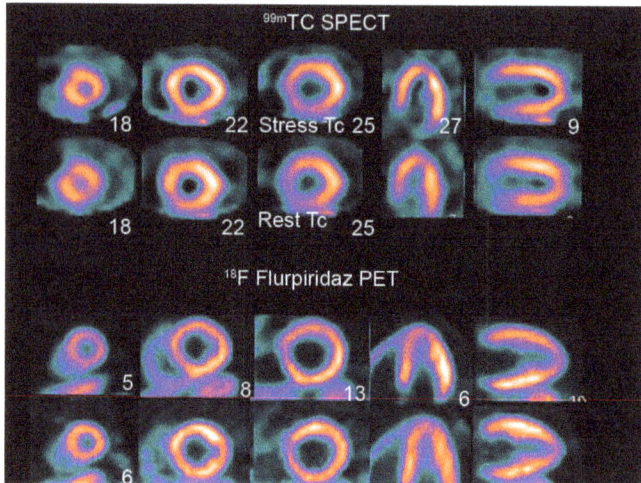

Fig. 1: Rest treadmill exercise ^{99m}Tc SPECT (upper rows) and flurpiridaz ^{18}F PET representative images (lower rows) from a patient with 70% stenosis in the proximal left anterior descending coronary artery. ^{99m}Tc SPECT images do not show a perfusion defect and were interpreted as normal. The flurpiridaz ^{18}F PET study, however, demonstrates superior image quality and reversible defects in the LAD territory

Of note, PET performance was superior to SPECT in subgroups of females and obese patients.[38] The patient shown in **Figure 1** had a normal SPECT-MPI. ^{18}F flurpiridaz MPI, however, showed reversible anterior, anteroseptal and apical defects that correlated with the presence of significant left anterior descending coronary disease on ICA.

Absolute Quantitation of Myocardial Blood Flow

The importance of absolute quantitation of myocardial flow, above and beyond relative perfusion imaging, has been well established and is progressively entering routine clinical practice.[9,43-45] ^{13}N ammonia CFR increases diagnostic sensitivity[44] and has a strong association with prognosis.[46,47] ^{82}Rb MBF and CFR correctly detects 3-vessel CAD[48] and predicts adverse cardiovascular events[29] beyond relative MPI.[30,31] Most importantly, absolute quantitation of MBF with ^{82}Rb is a strong and independent predictor of cardiac mortality in patients with known or suspected CAD, providing incremental risk stratification over established clinical variables and relative MPI.[32]

The elevated extraction fraction of ^{18}F flurpiridaz at different flow rates makes it an optimal candidate for absolute MBF quantitation. In an initial study, Nekolla and associates used a 3-compartmental modeling approach in a pig model for quantitation of MBF with ^{18}F flurpiridaz.[35] Another simplified method of absolute flow quantitation utilizing ^{18}F flurpiridaz and allowing radiotracer injection outside the PET scanner was proposed in a pig model.[49] Here, the authors posited that myocardial retention and standardized uptake values (SUV) based on late uptake could provide estimates of CFR.

Our group recently completed the first in human absolute quantitation of MBF with ^{18}F flurpiridaz.[50] We found that CFR in patients with a low likelihood of CAD and territories supplied by normal coronary arteries was 3.7 ± 0.39, while CFR was significantly lower in myocardial regions supplied by diseased coronary arteries (1.86 ± 0.59). Although the first-pass extraction fraction was taken directly from an animal study, its use in our approach gives human MBF values comparable to the commonly accepted values obtained by other methods. Indeed, our results are in a similar range as those measured with other radiotracers such as ^{82}Rb chloride, ^{13}N ammonia and ^{15}O water. Moreover, our results obtained with ^{18}F flurpiridaz do not necessitate a correction such as that often utilized in the case of ^{82}Rb for example.[51]

CONCLUSION

For decades, PET MPI was mostly limited to academic research centers and large hospital systems while SPECT MPI remained the default approach in routine clinical practice by which patients underwent cardiac risk stratification and evaluation of stress-inducible myocardial ischemia. The enhanced sensitivity and specificity of PET radiotracers compared to SPECT radiotracers, as well as their inherent attenuation correction and ability to quantitate flow in an absolute manner further increases the value of a PET-based approach. The major Achilles heel of routine PET MPI, however, has been the availability of radiotracers, with current requirement for either on-site or very nearby cyclotrons or costly generators. In this context ^{18}F-based PET radiotracers, taking advantage of the radioisotope's 108 minutes half-life, have garnered significant interest and have been developed by academic centers and biotechnology companies. Of the reported ^{18}F-based PET MPI radiotracers, only ^{18}F flurpiridaz is in advanced clinical evaluation with encouraging results.

FUNDING

^{18}F flurpiridaz clinical trials have been sponsored by Lantheus Medical Imaging. Lantheus Medical Imaging had no role writing of this manuscript. Dr Packard is supported by NIH grant T32 HL007895. Dr Maddahi is supported by a research grant from Lantheus Medical Imaging.

DISCLOSURE

Dr Maddahi is the lead Principal Investigator for ^{18}F flurpiridaz phase 1, 2, and 3 clinical trials, Chair of the Steering Committee and a Scientific Advisor to Lantheus Medical Imaging.

REFERENCES

1. Dilsizian V, Taillefer R. Journey in evolution of nuclear cardiology: will there be another quantum leap with the F-18-labeled myocardial perfusion tracers? JACC Cardiovasc Imaging. 2012;5:1269-84.
2. Rischpler C, Park MJ, Fung GS, Javadi M, Tsui BM, Higuchi T. Advances in PET myocardial perfusion imaging: F-18 labeled tracers. Ann Nucl Med. 2012;26:1-6.
3. Nekolla SG, Saraste A. Novel F-18-labeled PET myocardial perfusion tracers: bench to bedside. Curr Cardiol Rep. 2011;13:145-50.
4. Maddahi J, Packard RR. Cardiac PET perfusion tracers: current status and future directions. Semin Nucl Med. 2014;44(5):333-43.
5. Garcia EV, Galt JR, Faber TL, et al. Principles of nuclear cardiology imaging. In: Vasken Dilsizian, Jagat Narula (Eds). Atlas of Nuclear Cardiology, 4th edition. Chapter 1, pp 1-53, Springer Science, 2013.
6. Bol A, Melin JA, Vanoverschelde JL, et al. Direct comparison of [^{13}N] ammonia and [^{15}O]water estimates of perfusion with quantification of regional myocardial blood flow by microspheres. Circulation. 1993;87:512-25.
7. Kajander SA, Joutsiniemi E, Saraste M, et al. Clinical value of absolute quantification of myocardial perfusion with ^{15}O-water in coronary artery disease. Circ Cardiovasc Imaging. 2011;4:678-84.
8. Nitzsche EU, Choi Y, Czernin J, et al. Noninvasive quantification of myocardial blood flow in humans. A direct comparison of the [^{13}N] ammonia and the [^{15}O] water techniques. Circulation. 1996;93:2000-06.
9. Schindler TH, Schelbert HR, Quercioli A, et al. Cardiac PET imaging for the detection and monitoring of coronary artery disease and microvascular health. JACC Cardiovasc Imaging. 2010;3:623-40.
10. Bergmann SR, Hack S, Tewson T, et al. The dependence of accumulation of ^{13}NH$_3$ by myocardium on metabolic factors and its implications for quantitative assessment of perfusion. Circulation. 1980;61:34-43.
11. Schelbert HR, Phelps ME, Huang SC, et al. ^{13}N-ammonia as an indicator of myocardial blood flow. Circulation. 1981;63:1259-72.
12. Krivokapich J, Huang SC, Phelps ME, et al. Dependence of ^{13}NH$_3$ myocardial extraction and clearance on flow and metabolism. Am J Physiol. 1982;242:H536-542.
13. Tamaki N, Yonekura Y, Senda M, et al. Myocardial positron computed tomography with ^{13}N-ammonia at rest and during exercise. Eur J Nucl Med Mol Imaging. 1985;11:246-51.
14. Krivokapich J, Smith GT, Huang SC, et al. ^{13}N ammonia myocardial imaging at rest and with exercise in normal volunteers. Quantification of absolute myocardial perfusion with dynamic positron emission tomography. Circulation. 1989;80:1328-37.
15. Chow BJ, Beanlands RS, Lee A, et al. Treadmill exercise produces larger perfusion defects than dipyridamole stress N-13 ammonia positron emission tomography. J Am Coll Cardiol. 2006;47:411-6.
16. Czernin J, Muller P, Chan S, et al. Influence of age and hemodynamics on myocardial blood flow and flow reserve. Circulation. 1993;88:62-9.
17. Di Carli M, Czernin J, Hoh CK, et al. Relation among stenosis severity, myocardial blood flow, and flow reserve in patients with coronary artery disease. Circulation. 1995;91:1944-51.
18. Schindler TH, Nitzsche EU, Olschewski M, et al. Chronic inflammation and impaired coronary vasoreactivity in patients with coronary risk factors. Circulation. 2004;110:1069-75.
19. Prior JO, Quinones MJ, Hernandez-Pampaloni M, et al. Coronary circulatory dysfunction in insulin resistance, impaired glucose tolerance, and type 2 diabetes mellitus. Circulation. 2005;111:2291-8.
20. Schindler TH, Cardenas J, Prior JO, et al. Relationship between increasing body weight, insulin resistance, inflammation, adipocytokine leptin, and coronary circulatory function. J Am Coll Cardiol. 2006;47:1188-95.
21. Love WD, Burch GE. A comparison of potassium 42, rubidium 86, and cesium 134 as tracers of potassium in the study of cation metabolism of human erythrocytes in vitro. J Lab Clin Med. 1953;41:351-62.
22. Love WD, Romney RB, Burch GE. A comparison of the distribution of potassium and exchangeable rubidium in the organs of the dog, using rubidium. Circ Res. 1954;2:112-22.
23. Selwyn AP, Allan RM, L'Abbate A, et al. Relation between regional myocardial uptake of rubidium-82 and perfusion: absolute reduction of cation uptake in ischemia. Am J Cardiol. 1982;50:112-121.
24. El Fakhri G, Kardan A, Sitek A, et al. Reproducibility and accuracy of quantitative myocardial blood flow assessment with (82)Rb PET: comparison with (13)N-ammonia PET. J Nucl Med. 2009;50:1062-71.
25. Naya M, Murthy VL, Taqueti VR, et al. Preserved coronary flow reserve effectively excludes high-risk coronary artery disease on angiography. J Nucl Med. 2014;55:248-55.
26. Goldstein RA, Mullani NA, Marani SK, et al. Myocardial perfusion with rubidium-82. II. Effects of metabolic and pharmacologic interventions. J Nucl Med. 1983;24:907-15.
27. Huang SC, Williams BA, Krivokapich J, et al. Rabbit myocardial ^{82}Rb kinetics and a compartmental model for blood flow estimation. Am J Physiol. 1989;256:H1156-64.
28. Herrero P, Markham J, Shelton ME, et al. Noninvasive quantification of regional myocardial perfusion with rubidium-82 and positron emission tomography. Exploration of a mathematical model. Circulation. 1990;82:1377-86.
29. Fukushima K, Javadi MS, Higuchi T, et al. Prediction of short-term cardiovascular events using quantification of global myocardial flow reserve in patients referred for clinical ^{82}Rb PET perfusion imaging. J Nucl Med. 2011;52:726-32.
30. Ziadi MC, Dekemp RA, Williams KA, et al. Impaired myocardial flow reserve on rubidium-82 positron emission tomography imaging predicts adverse outcomes in patients assessed for myocardial ischemia. J Am Coll Cardiol. 2011;58:740-8.
31. Farhad H, Dunet V, Bachelard K, et al. Added prognostic value of myocardial blood flow quantitation in rubidium-82 positron emission tomography imaging. Eur Heart J Cardiovasc Imaging. 2013;14:1203-10.
32. Murthy VL, Naya M, Foster CR, et al. Improved cardiac risk assessment with noninvasive measures of coronary flow reserve. Circulation. 2011;124:2215-24.
33. Yalamanchili P, Wexler E, Hayes M, et al. Mechanism of uptake and retention of F-18 BMS-747158-02 in cardiomyocytes: a novel PET myocardial imaging agent. J Nucl Cardiol. 2007;14:782-8.
34. Yu M, Guaraldi MT, Mistry M, et al. BMS-747158-02: a novel PET myocardial perfusion imaging agent. J Nucl Cardiol. 2007;14:789-98.

35. Nekolla SG, Reder S, Saraste A, et al. Evaluation of the novel myocardial perfusion positron-emission tomography tracer 18F-BMS-747158-02: comparison to 13N-ammonia and validation with microspheres in a pig model. Circulation. 2009;119:2333-42.
36. Sherif HM, Saraste A, Weidl E, et al. Evaluation of a novel ^{18}F-labeled positron-emission tomography perfusion tracer for the assessment of myocardial infarct size in rats. Circ Cardiovasc Imaging. 2009;2:77-84.
37. Berman DS, Maddahi J, Tamarappoo BK, et al. Phase II safety and clinical comparison with single-photon emission computed tomography myocardial perfusion imaging for detection of coronary artery disease: flurpiridaz ^{18}F positron emission tomography. J Am Coll Cardiol. 2013;61:469-77.
38. Maddahi J, Udelson J, Heller GV, Lazewatsky JL, Orlandi C. The first phase 3 international multicenter clinical trial of flurpiridaz ^{18}F, a new radiopharmaceutical for PET myocardial perfusion imaging (abstract). J Nucl Cardiol. 2015;22:744.
39. Huisman MC, Higuchi T, Reder S, et al. Initial characterization of an ^{18}F-labeled myocardial perfusion tracer. J Nucl Med. 2008;49:630-6.
40. Maddahi J. Properties of an ideal PET perfusion tracer: new PET tracer cases and data. J Nucl Cardiol. 2012;19:S30-7.
41. Maddahi J, Czernin J, Lazewatsky J, et al. Phase I, first-in-human study of BMS747158, a novel ^{18}F-labeled tracer for myocardial perfusion PET: dosimetry, biodistribution, safety, and imaging characteristics after a single injection at rest. J Nucl Med. 2011;52:1490-8.
42. Maddahi J, Bengel FM, Czernin J, et al. Dosimetry, biodistribution, and safety of flurpiridaz ^{18}F in healthy subjects undergoing rest and exercise or pharmacological stress PET myocardial perfusion imaging. J Nucl Cardiol. 2017 in press.
43. Gould KL, Johnson NP, Bateman TM, et al. Anatomic versus physiologic assessment of coronary artery disease. Role of coronary flow reserve, fractional flow reserve, and positron emission tomography imaging in revascularization decision-making. J Am Coll Cardiol. 2013;62:1639-53.
44. Johnson NP, Gould KL. Integrating noninvasive absolute flow, coronary flow reserve, and ischemic thresholds into a comprehensive map of physiological severity. JACC Cardiovasc Imaging. 2012;5:430-40.
45. Fiechter M, Ghadri JR, Gebhard C, et al. Diagnostic value of ^{13}N-ammonia myocardial perfusion PET: added value of myocardial flow reserve. J Nucl Med. 2012;53:1230-4.
46. Tio RA, Dabeshlim A, Siebelink HM, et al. Comparison between the prognostic value of left ventricular function and myocardial perfusion reserve in patients with ischemic heart disease. J Nucl Med. 2009;50:214-9.
47. Herzog BA, Husmann L, Valenta I, et al. Long-term prognostic value of ^{13}N-ammonia myocardial perfusion positron emission tomography added value of coronary flow reserve. J Am Coll Cardiol. 2009;54:150-6.
48. Parkash R, deKemp RA, Ruddy TD, et al. Potential utility of ^{82}Rb PET quantification in patients with 3-vessel coronary artery disease. J Nucl Cardiol. 2004;11:440-9.
49. Sherif HM, Nekolla SG, Saraste A, et al. Simplified quantification of myocardial flow reserve with flurpiridaz ^{18}F: validation with microspheres in a pig model. J Nucl Med. 2011;52:617-24.
50. Packard RR, Huang SC, Dahlbom M, Czernin J, Maddahi J. Absolute quantitation of myocardial blood flow in human subjects with or without myocardial ischemia using dynamic flurpiridaz ^{18}F PET. J Nucl Med. 2014;55:1438-44.
51. Saraste A, Kajander S, Han C, et al. PET: Is myocardial flow quantification a clinical reality? J Nucl Cardiol. 2012;19:1044-59.

Index

Page numbers followed by *f* refer to figure and *t* refer to table

A

Abscess 5, 7, 7*t*
ACE inhibitors 145
Activated partial thromboplastin time 137
Acute coronary syndromes, treatment of 145
Adenosine
    infusion 201*f*
    myocardial perfusion imaging 200
    triphosphate transporter 70
Advanced coronary artery disease 208
Aggregatibacter 4
Alirocumab 129
Alteplase 155
Ambiguous angiographic lesions 113
Ambulance response interval 143
American College of Cardiology Foundation 24
American Heart Association 24, 109, 146, 156
Ammonia 225
Amyloidosis 218
Angioplasty 147
Anterior mitral leaflet, perforation in 9*f*
Anterolateral myocardial ischemia 195*f*
Antiarrhythmic therapy, prophylactic of 145
Antidote 136
Aortic
    abscess, multiple 8*f*
    dimensions 17
    disease 52
    graft prosthetic infection 219
    para-annular abscesses 8*f*
    pathology 17
    plaque 139
    regurgitation, severe 9*f*
    stenosis 17, 20
        diagnosis of 20
        evaluation of 17
        patients, echocardiographic information in 17*t*
        severe 19*f*
        true severe 21
    valve 6f
        abscess 9*f*
        area calculations 19
        large vegetation on 11*f*
Apixaban 135, 137*t*, 138
Arch of aorta 6*f*
Arrhythmia 55
Arrhythmogenic right ventricular
    cardiomyopathy 43, 46
    dysplasia 182, 184
Artery
    left circumflex 93, 94, 212, 220*f*
    posterior descending 59*f*, 93
    second diagonal 94
Artifacts 115
Aspirin administration 145
Assessing left ventricle contractile 20
Association of Coronary Stenosis 117
Association of Physicians of India 160
Atherosclerotic
    cardiovascular disease 179
    coronary artery disease 67
    plaques, imaging 76
Athlete's heart 39*t*
Atrial fibrillation 134, 135
Atrial septal defect 39
Atrial volume, left 27, 28*f*
Atrium, left 39
Automated external defibrillation 144
Automatic implantable cardioverter defibrillator 188

B

Balloon angioplasty 163, 197
Bare metal stent 163
Bicuspid 17
    aortic valve 6*f*, 8*f*
Bifurcation lesions 113, 166
Bioabsorbable vascular scaffold 112
    implantation of 114
Bioresorbable scaffold 169*t*
    advantages of 164*t*
Bioresorbable vascular scaffold 163, 164, 168
Bleeding 140
    risk assessment on anticoagulation 140*t*
    with newer agents, treatment of 137
Bococizumab 130
Body mass index 92
Bradycardia, treatment of 145
Breath, shortness of 52
Bronchospasm 200
Bull's eye 26*f*
Bypass surgery 59

C

Cadmium zinc telluride 104
Calcified coronary atherosclerosis 91
Calcium scoring 57
Cardiac
    amyloidosis 39, 45
        delayed enhancement in 46*f*
    camera 214
        solid state dedicated 214*f*
    computed tomography 57
    device 13, 55
    dyssynchrony 106
    emergencies, treatment for 143
    failure 139
    gamma camera 214
    imaging 1, 61
    implantable electronic devices 13
    magnetic resonance imaging 51, 57, 59, 61, 64, 85
    masses 52
    mechanical dyssynchrony 108
    muscle structure 31
    PET scan protocol 108, 209, 223
    resynchronization therapy 37-39, 108
    sarcoidosis 218, 219*f*
    sarcoidosis 39
    Software Program 211
    SPECT gamma camera 212
Cardiobacterium 4
Cardiological Society of India 160
Cardiomyopathy 43, 52
    dilated 43, 44*f*
    evaluation of 43
Chain of survival for cardiac arrest 144
Chemotherapy-induced cardiotoxicity, early detection of 38
Chest 198*f*
    pain 52
Chronic angina 95
Chronic chest pain 54
Chronic ischemic left ventricular dysfunction 88
Chronic kidney disease 69
Chronic pulmonary hypertension 38, 39
Chronic stable angina 72*f*
Coenzyme 178
Co-existent valvular disease 17
Cognitive adverse events 130
Comparable primary efficacy endpoints 140*f*
Complex interplay of substrate 183
Computed tomography coronary angiography 91
Concentric hypertrophy, increased 21
Congenital heart
    disease 38, 52, 55
    failure 27*f*, 139
Constrictive pericarditis 38
Conventional coronary angiography 57
Coronary angiography 57, 61, 118*f*, 197, 198*f*
Coronary arterial blood flow 211*f*
Coronary artery 59, 95
    bypass graft 165, 197
    calcium 95
    disease 54, 57, 67, 80, 90, 95, 100, 109, 182, 197, 199, 201, 221, 225
        diagnosis of 57, 100
    normal 58*f*
    right 212
Coronary computed tomographic angiography 95, 118

Coronary disease 90
Coronary flow reserve 67, 91, 101, 225
    in coronary artery disease, role of 100
Coronary heart disease 183
Coronary MR angiography 65
Coronary plaque, mixed density 61*f*
Coronary stenosis
    in heart transplant 38
    severity 121*f*
Coronary syndrome, acute 112, 113, 117
Coronary vascular tree 93*f*, 94*f*
Coronary vessels 52
Coxiella burnetii 4
Critical stenosis 8*f*
Cusp fenestration 10

D

Dabigatran 137*t*, 138
Descending artery, left anterior 58*f*, 92-95, 97*f*, 102
Diabetes mellitus 68, 139
Dimensionless velocity index 19
Dipyridamole, mechanism of action of 200
Dobutamine
    stress 65
    echocardiography 20
Dosimetry 71
Drug-eluting stent 163
Duke's criteria 3
Dyssynchronous left ventricular contraction 35*f*

E

Early advanced care 144
Early cardiopulmonary resuscitation 144
Early defibrillation 144
Early myocardial involvement 38
Early nausea, treatment of 145
Echocardiography 5, 17, 22
    during surgery 12
    in infective endocarditis, role of 4*t*
    two-dimensional 184
Echoes, abnormal 28
Edoxaban 138
Eikenella corrodens 4
Ejection fraction 24, 39, 53
Electrocardiogram 67, 100, 184
Electrocardiography 52
    single-averaged 184
Electron beam CT scanners 57
Electrophysiology 185
Embryonic stem cells, noninvasive tracking of 220*f*
Emergency medical service 144, 146
End-diastolic volume 39
Endocarditis 6
Energy metabolism 76
Epinephrine 218
Equilibrium radionuclide angiography 106
European Society of Cardiology 2015 4*t*
Evolocumab 129
Exercise, response to 17

F

Fatty acid 81
Fibrinolysis research, milestones of 154*t*
First diagonal artery 93-95
First obtuse marginal artery 93
Fistula 5
Flail mitral leaflet 10
Fluorine-18 FDG metabolic imaging 206
Fluorine-18-labeled deoxyglucose 85
Fluorodeoxyglucose 75
    positron-emission tomography 88
Flurpiridaz 226
Focal severe stenosis 59*f*
Fractional flow reserve 63, 117, 118, 118*f*, 121*f*
Fractional shortening 24

G

Gadolinium-based contrast media 55
Gain-of-function mutation 128
Gastrointestinal bleed 137
Gated myocardial perfusion 107
Gerbode ventricular septal defect 10*f*
Glucose metabolism 86*f*, 87*f*, 221

H

Haemophilus 4
Heart
    diastolic function of 25
    failure 4, 24
        echocardiography of 24
        symptoms, severe 52
        with normal LVEF 37
    Rhythm Society Guidelines 109
Hemodynamic consequences 18
Hibernating myocardium 55, 86*f*, 88
Hospital thrombolysis 147
Hybernating myocardium 205*f*
Hybrid cardiac imaging 98
    software, protocols of 90
Hybrid imaging 64
Hybrid myocardial imaging techniques 90
Hydroxyephedrine 218
Hypertension 39, 139, 140
Hypertrophic cardiomyopathy 39, 39*t*, 43, 44, 53, 182
Hypotension, treatment of 145

I

Idiopathic-dilated cardiomyopathy 43
Implantable cardiac defibrillator 187
Implantable cardioverter defibrillator 53, 185
Indian Medical Association 160
Infectious endocarditis 219
Infectious vegetations 7*t*
Infective endocarditis 3, 4
    diagnosis of 4*t*
    echocardiographic evaluation of 3
Inflammatory cardiomyopathy 43
In-hospital thrombolysis 147*f*
Integrated STEMI care systems 160
Intensive statin therapy 127*t*
Internal carotid artery 95
Interventricular dyssynchrony 106, 107*f*
Intracardiac pressure estimation 29
Intracoronary of streptokinase 154
Intraoperative echocardiography 4
Intra-right ventricular
    dyssynchrony 107*f*
    synchrony 107*f*
Intravascular ultrasonography 118
Intravascular ultrasound 112, 164, 167
    technique 101
Intravenous adenosine 51*f*
Intravenous drug abuser 13
Intravenous nitrate, prophylactic of 145
Intraventricular dyssynchrony, left 106
Invasive coronary angiography 67, 102
Iodine 81
Iron overload cardiomyopathy 46
Ischemia detected 118*f*
Ischemia using computer assisted tomography 62
Ischemia without significant stenosis 117
Ischemic heart disease 80
Ischemic left ventricular dysfunction 38

K

Kidney disease, chronic 175
Kingella 4

L

Lactic acid 164
Lambl's excrescences 7
Late gadolinium enhancement 53, 85
Later transesophageal echocardiography 3
Leadless pacemaker 187
Left anterior descending artery 182
Left main disease 113
Left ventricle 11, 17, 39, 106, 188
    systolic function, progression of 17
Left ventricular
    branch, posterior 93
    contractile reserve 17
    diastolic pressure, estimation of 29
    dysfunction 139
    dyssynchrony 38
    ejection fraction 17, 38, 106
    function after mitral clip implantation 38, 39
    geometry 28
    hypertrophy 184
        severity of 17
    myocardium, direction of movement of 33*f*
    noncompaction 38, 46
    noncompaction of 47*f*
    outflow tract calcification 7
    systolic dysfunction 20
    volume assessment 38
    wall-motion abnormalities 38
Lesion
    long 167
    severity 112
Lipoprotein cholesterol, high-density 127
Liver 87*f*
    function 140

Loss-of-function mutation 128
Low density lipoprotein cholesterol 174
Low photon flux 215
Low radiation exposure 227
Low reflection 168
Low-gradient aortic stenosis 20
Luminal stenosis
   degree of 118*f*
   severity of 117

M

Magnetic resonance spectroscopy 65
Main pulmonary artery 11
Major adverse cardiac events 164, 165
Male diabetic patient 103*f*
Maximum intensity projection 58*f*
Mean pulmonary wedge pressure 29
Mediastinal nodes 48*f*
Mediastinum 87*f*
Metabolic
   cardiomyopathy 43
   reserve 88
   tracers 206
Metabolism 81
   adequate 207*f*, 210*f*
Metaiodobenzylguanidine 218*f*
Minimal stent area 114
Mitral annular
   calcification 7
   velocity 27
Mitral regurgitation, severe 9*f*
Mitral valve 6*f*
   prolapse 182
   replacement 10*f*
Monitoring anticoagulant effect 136
Motion artefacts 215
Multidetector computed tomography 61
Muscular risk, prediction of 175
Myocardial blood flow 91, 102, 197, 212, 225
   absolute quantitation of 228
   computation of 212
   global reduction 213*f*
   quantitation of 211
Myocardial function 75
Myocardial imaging
   dual isotope 222*f*
   tracers for 82
Myocardial infarction 37, 117, 165, 200
   acute 38, 142, 142*f*, 143, 147, 153
   imaging 207
   increased 137
   rule out 62, 91
   thrombolysis in 156
Myocardial involvement in thalassemia 48*f*
Myocardial ischemia 37, 67
Myocardial metabolism 205
Myocardial perfusion 67, 75, 194, 197, 201*f*
   imaging 67, 75, 80, 90, 91, 92*f*, 94*f*, 95, 101, 117
      dipyridamole 199
      dobutamine 200
   marker 80, 81
   scan, normal sestamibi 196*f*
   tracers of 204

Myocardial PET tracer 218
Myocardial sarcoid, scar in 48*f*
Myocardial sarcoidosis 46
Myocardial segment, inferior 202*f*
Myocardial strain 25
Myocardial stunning and hibernation 206
Myocardial tumors 55
Myocardial viability 37, 52, 55, 65, 85, 209
   assessment 88
   marker of 82
Myocarditis 43, 52
Myocardium 87, 207*f*
   anterior segment of 203*f*
   inferior wall of 205*f*
   lateral wall of 205*f*
   normal 87*f*
Myopathy, persistence of 178

N

Native valve noninfectious vegetations 7
Necrotic core 115
Negative predictive value 91
Neointimal hyperplasia 114, 115
New oral anticoagulants 135
   pharmacokinetics of 136*t*
Newer agents, advantages of 156
Nonhomogeneous opacity 14*f*
Noninvasive cellular imaging 65
Nonischemic dilated cardiomyopathy 53
Nuclear cardiology 193, 211
   procedures 193
   techniques 221
Nuclear medicine techniques 106

O

Obstructive pulmonary disease, severe chronic 200
Odyssey alternative 129
Odyssey global programme 129*t*
Odyssey long-term study 130, 131*f*
Odyssey mono 129
Optical coherence tomography 114*f*, 115, 167
   depicting 113*f*
   role of 112
Oral nitrate, prophylactic of 145
Ortho/para iodo phenyl pentadecanoic acid 81
Out-of-hospital resuscitation 185

P

Pacemakers device 55
Papillary fibroelastoma 7
Particular positron-emission tomography 64
Patent ductus arteriosus 6*f*
Peak stress function imaging 227
Percutaneous coronary
   infarction 143
   intervention 95, 112, 115, 144, 147, 156, 163, 165
      evolution of 163
Perforation 5
Perfusion 58, 59
   imaging 62

Pericardial diseases 55
Pericardial effusion 53*f*
Peripheral artery disease 139
Perivalvular involvement 7
PET agents for imaging plaques 77*t*
PET tracers for cardiac imaging 76*t*
Pharmacoinvasive approach 157
Pharmacological stress 202
   perfusion imaging 199, 202
Plaque characterization 63
Plaque composition 112
Plaque erosion 113*f*
Plaque evaluation 58
Plaque morphology 117-119
Plaque rupture 113*f*
Post-cardiac surgery abnormal ventricular septal motion 39
Predisposing factors 175
Prehospital beta-blockade 145
Prehospital phase, management of 142
Prehospital thrombolysis 146, 147, 147*f*, 156, 157
   prerequisites for 146
Primary coronary angioplasty 147
Primary percutaneous coronary intervention 113
Prior myocardial infarction 139
Prosthetic valve 12
   dehiscence of 5
   endocarditis 3
   obstruction mechanism 12*t*
Prothrombin concentrate complex 137
Pseudoaneurysm 5
Pseudosevere aortic stenosis 21
Pulmonary artery, vegetation in 6*f*
Pulmonary hypertension 39
Pulmonary venous flow velocity 27
Pulmonary vessels 52
Pyrexia of unknown origin 3

R

Radial strain 34*f*
Radiation dosimetry 96, 97
Radiation exposure 215
Radionuclide 80
   for myocardial imaging agents 83*t*
   imaging procedures 193
Randomized controlled trials 147
Regadenoson myocardial perfusion 203*f*
   scintigraphy 202
Regadenoson stress 109*t*
Renal disease, advanced chronic 38
Renal dysfunction 136
Renal excretion 138*t*
Renal function, abnormal 140
Reperfusion therapy 146
Residual atherogenic risk poststatin therapy 127
Rest treadmill exercise imaging 227
Restrictive cardiomyopathy 38, 43, 45
Reteplase 156
Right atrial pressure, assessment of 29
Right coronary artery 88, 92-94

Right heart infective endocarditis 13
Right intraventricular dyssynchroy 106
Right ventricle 11, 106
Right ventricular
　fractional 28, 28*f*
　function 28
　　after mitral clip implantation 38, 39
　systolic pressure 29
Rivaroxaban 137*t*, 138
Rubidium 70
Rubidium-82 myocardial perfusion 204, 211*f*

S

Saphenous vein graft 59*f*
Septal subendocardial perfusion defect 54*f*
Sestamibi 195, 223
Shortened modified look-locker inversion-
　　recovery 65
Shoulder injury 6*f*
Sickle cell disease 39
Single-photon emission computed
　　tomography 64, 70, 215
　myocardial perfusion imaging 75
Specific cardiomyopathy 43
Speckle tracking echocardiography 31
Spectral computed tomography 63
Spire trials 130*t*
Staphylococcus aureus 4
　infection 7
Statin intolerance 174, 178
Statin myopathy
　incidence of 174
　mechanism of 175
　risk factors for 176*t*
ST-elevation anterior wall myocardial
　　infarction 159
ST-elevation myocardial infarction 153
　acute 142
　program, future directions for 160
　treatment of 158*t*
　trends in thrombolysis for 156
Stem cells tracking, tracers for 219
Stenosis without ischemia 117
Stent 57
　apposition, incomplete 114*f*
　coverage 115
　underexpansion 114*f*
Streptococcus bovis 4
Streptococcus equisimilis 153
Streptococcus gallolyticus 4
Streptokinase 154
　discovery of 153
　mechanism of action of 153
　source for 153
Stress
　cardiomyopathy 37
　cardiovascular 55*t*
　myocardial perfusion imaging 210*f*
　perfusion pattern 198*f*
　sestamibi myocardial perfusion depression
　　198*f*

single photon emission computed
　　tomography 101
　thallium myocardial perfusion 195, 210*f*,
　　222*f*
Stroke 134, 135, 139, 140
　and bleeding, risk of 135*f*
　in atrial fibrillation 134*f*
　　preventing 135*t*
　or systemic embolism 140*f*
　prevention of 138*t*
　risk assessment 139*t*
　risk, estimation of 139*t*
　volume 22, 24
　with atrial fibrillation 134*t*
Subclinical disease, detection of 38
Subcutaneous implantable cardioverter
　　defibrillator 187, 188
Subcutaneously implantable 188
Sudden cardiac death 53, 182, 184, 184*t*, 185
　causes of 182
　high-risk factors for 183
　in adults, causes of 182
　mechanism of 182
　risk factors for 183
　risk stratification of 183
Summed rest scores 67
Summed stress scores 67
Supraventricular tachycardia 185
Swedish registry 148
Synchrony parameters, values of 108*t*
Systemic embolism 10
Systolic arterial pressure 22
Systolic dysfunction, early left ventricular 38
Systolic function of heart 24
Systolic pulmonary arterial pressure,
　　estimation of 29
Systolic tricuspid annular velocity 29

T

Takotsubo cardiomyopathy 39
Target lesion revascularization 165
Target vessel revascularization 165
Tc-99m labeled glucarate 207
Tc-99m pyrophosphate 207
Teboroxime 195
Technetium-99m compounds 81
Tenecteplase 156
Tetralogy of Fallot 7*f*
Tetraphenylphosphonium 76
Tetrofosmin 195, 218, 223
Thallium-201 80
Thin cap fibroatheroma 115
Thromboembolic events 135
Thrombolysis 147
Thrombolytic agents for prehospital
　　thrombolysis 146
Thrombolytic therapy 197
　development of 153
Thrombus, large 10*f*
Tissue Doppler echocardiography 29

Tissue Doppler imaging 38
Tissue
　penetration 115
　type plasminogen activator 155
Transcatheter aortic valve replacement 39
Transesophageal echocardiography 4, 19
Transient ischemia
　attack 139, 200
　dilatation 67
Transmitral flow patterns, types of 27*f*
Transmitral flow velocity 26
Transthoracic echocardiography 3, 4
Treadmill stress test 197, 198*f*, 199*f*
Tricuspid 17
　annular plane systolic excursion 28

U

Unclassified cardiomyopathies 43
United States Food and Drug Administration
　　175
Urokinase 155

V

Valve
　anatomy 18
　aneurysm 5
　hemodynamics 18
　perforation 10
Valvular aortic stenosis, stages of 18*t*
Valvular disease 55
Valvular heart disease 38, 52
Valvular strands 7
Vascular disease 139
Vasomotion, restoration of 168
Vegetation 5
Vena cava, inferior 13
Ventricular dyssynchrony, intra-left 107*f*, 109
Ventricular ejection fraction, left 212
Ventricular fibrillation 182, 183
Ventricular premature complexes 183
Ventricular septal defect 13
Ventricular synchrony, intra-left 107*f*
Ventricular tachycardia 182, 183, 200
Ventricular thrombus 52
Ventriculoarterial impedance 22
Vienna STEMI registry 148, 148*f*
Viridans streptococci 4
Virtual computed tomography 63
Vitamin
　D 178
　K antagonist 134
Volume-rendered coronary CT angiogram 58*f*
Vomiting, treatment of 145

W

Wall motion abnormality 38
Warfarin 137*t*
Wearable cardiac defibrillator 189
Wireless cardiac stimulation 188
　system 187